Fourth Edition

Oncology Nursing Society

Manual for Radiation Oncology Nursing Practice and Education

Edited by
Ryan R. Iwamoto, ARNP, MN, AOCN®
Marilyn L. Haas, PhD, ANP-BC
Tracy K. Gosselin, RN, MSN, AOCN®

Oncology Nursing Society
Pittsburgh, PA

ONS Publishing Division
Executive Director, Professional Practice and Programs:
Elizabeth M. Wertz Evans, RN, MPM, CPHQ, CPHIMS, FACMPE
Publisher and Director of Publications: Barbara Sigler, RN, MNEd
Managing Editor: Lisa M. George, BA
Technical Content Editor: Angela D. Klimaszewski, RN, MSN
Staff Editor II: Amy Nicoletti, BA
Copy Editor: Laura Pinchot, BA
Graphic Designer: Dany Sjoen

First printing, December 2011
Second printing, April 2014
Third printing, March 2015

Library of Congress Cataloging-in-Publication Data

Manual for radiation oncology nursing practice and education. -- 4th ed. / edited by Ryan R. Iwamoto, Marilyn L. Haas, and Tracy K. Gosselin.
  p. ; cm.
Includes bibliographical references and index.
ISBN 978-1-935864-12-7 (alk. paper)
I. Iwamoto, Ryan R. II. Haas, Marilyn L. III. Gosselin, Tracy K. IV. Oncology Nursing Society.
[DNLM: 1. Oncologic Nursing--education--Outlines. 2. Radiation Oncology--education--Outlines. WY 18.2]
LC classification not assigned
616.99'40642--dc23
                                                                2011032186

Publisher's Note

This book is published by the Oncology Nursing Society (ONS). ONS neither represents nor guarantees that the practices described herein will, if followed, ensure safe and effective patient care. The recommendations contained in this book reflect ONS's judgment regarding the state of general knowledge and practice in the field as of the date of publication. The recommendations may not be appropriate for use in all circumstances. Those who use this book should make their own determinations regarding specific safe and appropriate patient-care practices, taking into account the personnel, equipment, and practices available at the hospital or other facility at which they are located. The editors and publisher cannot be held responsible for any liability incurred as a consequence from the use or application of any of the contents of this book. Figures and tables are used as examples only. They are not meant to be all-inclusive, nor do they represent endorsement of any particular institution by ONS. Mention of specific products and opinions related to those products do not indicate or imply endorsement by ONS. Web sites mentioned are provided for information only; the hosts are responsible for their own content and availability. Unless otherwise indicated, dollar amounts reflect U.S. dollars.

ONS publications are originally published in English. Publishers wishing to translate ONS publications must contact ONS about licensing arrangements. ONS publications cannot be translated without obtaining written permission from ONS. (Individual tables and figures that are reprinted or adapted require additional permission from the original source.) Because translations from English may not always be accurate or precise, ONS disclaims any responsibility for inaccuracies in words or meaning that may occur as a result of the translation. Readers relying on precise information should check the original English version.

Printed in the United States of America

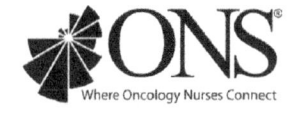

Oncology Nursing Society
Integrity • Innovation • Stewardship • Advocacy • Excellence • Inclusiveness

Contributors

Editors

Ryan R. Iwamoto, ARNP, MN, AOCN®
Oncology Nurse Educator
Cancer Information Service
National Cancer Institute
Seattle, Washington
Nurse Practitioner
Department of Radiation Oncology
Virginia Mason Medical Center
Seattle, Washington

Marilyn L. Haas, PhD, ANP-BC
Nurse Practitioner
CarePartners
Asheville, North Carolina
Evidence-Based Practice

Tracy K. Gosselin, RN, MSN, AOCN®
Associate Chief Nursing Officer
Duke Cancer Institute
Durham, North Carolina
IV.C. Skin Reactions; VIII.C. Intraoperative Radiation Therapy; VIII.H. Total Skin Irradiation; XII.B. American College of Radiology

Authors

Deborah Hutchinson Allen, MSN, RN, CNS, FNP-BS, AOCNP®
Oncology Clinical Nurse Specialist and Nurse Practitioner
Duke Cancer Institute
Durham, North Carolina
V.A. Brain and Central Nervous System

Karen J. Allen, MSN, RN, ANP-BC, OCN®
Nurse Practitioner, Department of Radiation Oncology
Duke Cancer Institute
Durham, North Carolina
V.A. Brain and Central Nervous System; VIII.D. Stereotactic Radiosurgery

Marylou S. Anton, MSN, RN, OCN®
Executive Director, Oncology Services
Holy Name Medical Center
Sister Patricia Lynch Regional Cancer Center
Teaneck, New Jersey
V.H. Female Pelvis

Andrea M. Barsevick, PhD, RN, AOCN®, FAAN
Associate Professor and Director of Nursing Research
Fox Chase Cancer Center
Philadelphia, Pennsylvania
IV.B. Fatigue

Susan Weiss Behrend, RN, MSN, AOCN®
Clinical Nurse Specialist
Department of Nursing
Fox Chase Cancer Center
Philadelphia, Pennsylvania
VI.C. Benign Conditions; XIII.D. National Comprehensive Cancer Network; XIII.E. National Cancer Institute

Janye Laird Blivin, RN, MSN
Oncology Clinical Nurse Specialist
Duke Cancer Institute
Durham, North Carolina
VIII.E. Hyperthermia

Rachel M. Bolton, RN, CPON®
Pediatric Radiation Oncology Nurse
Francis H. Burr Proton Therapy Center
Massachusetts General Hospital
Boston, Massachusetts
IX.A. Pediatric Radiation Oncology

Ingrid K. Bowser, MS, APRN-BC, AOCNP®, ADM-BC
Nurse Practitioner
Indiana University Health Goshen Center for Cancer Care
Goshen, Indiana
VIII.A. External Beam (Teletherapy)

Deborah Braccia, DNSc, MPA, RN, OCN®
Scientific Director, Oncology Scientific Operations, Managed Markets
Novartis Oncology
Hoboken, New Jersey
XIII.A.2. Oncology Nursing Society Web Site Resources; XIII.B. Additional Online Radiation Resources

Susan D. Bruce, RN, MSN, OCN®
Oncology Clinical Nurse Specialist
Duke Cancer Institute
Duke Raleigh Cancer Center
Raleigh, North Carolina
VIII.I. Photodynamic Therapy

Deborah Watkins Bruner, RN, PhD, FAAN
Independence Professor of Nursing Education
Director, Biobehavioral Research Center
University of Pennsylvania School of Nursing
Philadelphia, Pennsylvania
I. The Clinical Practicum; IV.E. Distress/Coping; IV.F. Sexual Dysfunction

Jennifer Dunn Bucholtz, RN, MS, GNP
Nurse Practitioner, Retired
The Sidney Kimmel Comprehensive Cancer Center at Johns Hopkins
Baltimore, Maryland
III. Radiation Protection and Safety

Denise Bundow, MN, ARNP
Advanced Registered Nurse Practitioner
Peninsula Cancer Center
Poulsbo, Washington
VII. Oncologic Emergencies

Jormain O. Cady, DNP, ARNP, AOCN®
Nurse Practitioner
Virginia Mason Medical Center
Seattle, Washington
V.E. Gastrointestinal/Abdomen; IX.B. Geriatric Radiation Oncology

Frances Cartwright-Alcarese, PhD, RN, AOCN®
Senior Director of Nursing Oncology Services
New York University Langone Medical Center
New York, New York
XI.D. Nursing Management in Radiation Oncology

Carrie F. Daly, RN, MSN, AOCN®
Oncology Nurse Manager
Radiation Oncology Department
Rush University Medical Center
Chicago, Illinois
X.A. Radioprotectors

Jennifer Deering, BScN, MN, NP
Head and Neck Radiation Oncology Nurse
Princess Margaret Hospital
Toronto, Ontario, Canada
IX.C. Radiation Therapy for People With Special Needs

Judith A. DePalma, PhD, RN
Professor
Rocky Mountain University of Health Professions
Provo, Utah
Consultant and Coach
Avanti Strategies
Pittsburgh, Pennsylvania
Evidence-Based Practice

Vanna M. Dest, MSN, APRN-BC, CBEC, AOCN®
Oncology Nurse Practitioner
Hospital of St. Raphael
Radiation Oncology Specialists of Southern Connecticut
New Haven, Connecticut
XIII.C. American Society for Radiation Oncology

Denice Economou, RN, MN, CNS, CHPN, AOCN®
Project Director, Survivorship Education for Quality Cancer Care
City of Hope
Duarte, California
XI.A. Survivorship

Barbara R. Fristoe, MN, ARNP
Nurse Practitioner
University of Washington Medical Center
Seattle, Washington
VIII.F. Total Body Irradiation and Hematopoietic Stem Cell Transplantation; VIII.G. Total Lymphoid Irradiation

Corsita Garraway, RN(EC), MScN, CON(C), CHPCN(C)
Nurse Practitioner–Adult
Palliative Radiation Oncology Program
University Health Network Princess Margaret Hospital
Adjunct Clinical Appointee, Lawrence S. Bloomberg Faculty of Nursing
University of Toronto
Toronto, Ontario, Canada
V.I. Bone Metastases; XI.B. Palliative Care

Maggie Leavitt Guerrero, MSN, RN, OCN®
Patient Care Supervisor
Radiation Oncology
Moffitt Cancer Center
Tampa, Florida
V.D. Thoracic

Laura J. Hanisch, PsyD
Clinical Psychologist
Patient Information Specialist
National Comprehensive Cancer Network
Fort Washington, Pennsylvania
IV.E. Distress/Coping; IV.F. Sexual Dysfunction

Debra J. Harris, BA, MSN, RN, OCN®
Nurse Manager, Inpatient Unit
Stem Cell Transplant–Hematological Malignancies
Oregon Health & Science University
Portland, Oregon
V.B. Head and Neck

Hilda Haynes-Lewis, MS, ANP-BC, AOCNP®
Nurse Practitioner
Department of Radiation Oncology
Montefiore Medical Center
Montefiore Einstein Center for Cancer Care
Bronx, New York
V.G. Male Pelvis/Prostate

Genevieve Hollis, MSN, CRNP, AOCN®, ANP-BC
Oncology Nurse Practitioner
Advanced Senior Lecturer B
Department of Radiation Oncology
Hospital of the University of Pennsylvania
Philadelphia, Pennsylvania
I. The Clinical Practicum

C.-M. Charlie Ma, PhD
Vice Chairman
Radiation Oncology Department
Fox Chase Cancer Center
Philadelphia, Pennsylvania
II. The Practice of Radiation Oncology

Catherine M. Mannix, RN, MSN, OCN®
Nursing Director, Radiation Oncology
Massachusetts General Hospital
Boston, Massachusetts
VIII.J. Proton Beam Radiation Therapy

Evie Matos, RN
Registered Nurse
Peninsula Cancer Center
Poulsbo, Washington
VII. Oncologic Emergencies

Beatrice Mautner, RN, MSN, OCN®
Vice President, Nursing and Clinical Services
Vantage Oncology
Manhattan Beach, California
XII.A. The Joint Commission

Susan Mazanec, PhD, RN, AOCN®
Nurse Scientist
Seidman Cancer Center
University Hospitals Case Medical Center
Instructor
Frances Payne Bolton School of Nursing
Case Western Reserve University
Cleveland, Ohio
IV.A. General Patient and Family Education

Maurene McQuestion, RN, BScN, MSc, CON(C)
Clinical Nurse Specialist, Advance Practice Nurse
Radiation Medicine Program and Head and Neck Site Group
Princess Margaret Hospital, University Health Network
Toronto, Ontario, Canada
*V.I. Bone Metastases; IX.C. Radiation Therapy for People With
    Special Needs; XIII.A.1. Radiation SIG*

Christine A. Miaskowski, RN, PhD, FAAN
Professor and Associate Dean
University of California
San Francisco, California
IV.D. Pain

Katherine Katen Moore, MSN, ANP-C, AOCN®
Associate Director, Health Services
Drew University
Madison, New Jersey
X.C. Radioimmunotherapy and Radiopharmaceuticals

Judith B. Nettleton, RN, BSN, OCN®
Radiation and Neuro-Oncology Nurse Coordinator
West Michigan Cancer Center
Kalamazoo, Michigan
V.F. Bladder

Tracey B. Newhall, RN, BS, OCN®
Nurse Navigator
Women's Cancer Center
Fox Chase Cancer Center
Philadelphia, Pennsylvania
IV.B. Fatigue

Natasha Hauptman Ng, RN, MSN, OCN®
Registered Nurse
Radiation Oncology, Hematology/Oncology
Virginia Mason Medical Center
Seattle, Washington
VI.A. Sarcomas

Maureen L. Oliveri, MSN, RN
Nurse Manager, Radiation Oncology
New York University
New York, New York
XI.D. Nursing Management in Radiation Oncology

Mary Ann Plambeck, RN, MSN, OCN®
Clinical Operations Director
Duke Cancer Institute
Durham, North Carolina
VI.B. Lymphoma; XII.A. The Joint Commission

Jessica Rearden, MS, RN
Predoctoral Student
University of Pennsylvania
Philadelphia, Pennsylvania
XI.C. Cancer Clinical Trials

Maria C. Romano, MS, RD, CDN
Adult Ambulatory Oncology Registered Dietitian
Montefiore Einstein Center for Cancer Care
Albert Einstein College of Medicine
Montefiore Medical Center
Bronx, New York
IV.G. Nutritional Issues

Beverly E. Smith, DNP, ANP-BC, NE-BC
Advanced Nurse Practitioner Radiation/Oncology
New York University Langone Medical Center
New York, New York
XI.D. Nursing Management in Radiation Oncology

Pamela Hallquist Viale, RN, MS, CS, ANP, AOCNP®
Oncology Nurse Practitioner
Editor-in-Chief, *Journal of the Advanced Practitioner in Oncology*
Goleta, California
*X.B. Radiosensitizers and Concurrent Chemotherapy and
    Biotherapy*

Jayne S. Waring, RN, BSN, OCN®
Clinical Nurse IV
Department of Radiation Oncology
Duke Cancer Institute
Durham, North Carolina
VIII.B. Low Dose Rate and High Dose Rate Brachytherapy

Stephanie A. Williams, RN, MSN, ACNP-BC, AOCNP®, CBCN®
Advanced Practice Nurse
Department of Surgical Oncology
Regional Care Center in Sugar Land
University of Texas MD Anderson Cancer Center
Sugar Land, Texas
V.C. Breast

Mary Ellyn Witt, MS, RN, AOCN®
Clinical Research Nurse
University of Chicago Medical Center
Chicago, Illinois
V.B. Head and Neck; XIII.A.1. Radiation SIG

Reviewers

Maria E. Bautista, MS, ANP-BC, CGRN
Adult Nurse Practitioner
Department of Radiation Oncology
Virginia G. Piper Cancer Center at Scottsdale Healthcare
Scottsdale, Arizona

Cynthia Briola, RN, OCN®, CBCN®
Penn CyberKnife Program Coordinator
Penn Medicne
Philadelphia, Pennsylvania

Jormain O. Cady, DNP, ARNP, AOCN®
Nurse Practitioner
Virginia Mason Medical Center
Seattle, Washington

Elise Carper, RN, MA, ANP-BC, AOCN®
Director of Nursing, Radiation Oncology
Adult Nurse Practitioner
Continuum Cancer Centers of New York
New York, New York

Vanna M. Dest, MSN, APRN-BC, CBEC, AOCN®
Oncology Nurse Practitioner
Hospital of St. Raphael
Radiation Oncology Specialists of Southern Connecticut
New Haven, Connecticut

Maurene McQuestion, RN, BScN, MSc, CON(C)
Clinical Nurse Specialist, Advance Practice Nurse
Radiation Medicine Program and Head and Neck Site Group
Princess Margaret Hospital, University Health Network
Toronto, Ontario, Canada

Disclosure

Editors and authors of books and guidelines provided by the Oncology Nursing Society are expected to disclose to the readers any significant financial interest or other relationships with the manufacturer(s) of any commercial products.

A vested interest may be considered to exist if a contributor is affiliated with or has a financial interest in commercial organizations that may have a direct or indirect interest in the subject matter. A "financial interest" may include, but is not limited to, being a shareholder in the organization; being an employee of the commercial organization; serving on an organization's speakers bureau; or receiving research from the organization. An "affiliation" may be holding a position on an advisory board or some other role of benefit to the commercial organization. Vested interest statements appear in the front matter for each publication.

Contributors are expected to disclose any unlabeled or investigational use of products discussed in their content. This information is acknowledged solely for the information of the readers.

The contributors provided the following disclosure and vested interest information:

Marilyn L. Haas, PhD, ANP-BC: Meniscus, Med Pharma, honoraria

Tracy K. Gosselin, RN, MSN, AOCN®: Clinical Care Options, Oncology Nursing Society, honoraria

Susan Weiss Behrend, RN, MSN, AOCN®: Jones and Bartlett, honoraria

Carrie F. Daly, RN, MSN, AOCN®: Roche, consultant; IMER, honoraria

Vanna M. Dest, MSN, APRN-BC, CBEC, AOCN®: EUSA Pharma, Myriad Laboratories, honoraria

Denice Economou, RN, MN, CNS, CHPN, AOCN®: Interactive Forums, honoraria

C.-M. Charlie Ma, PhD: Accuray Inc., honoraria and research funding; Varian Medical Systems, research funding

Pamela Hallquist Viale, RN, MS, CS, ANP, AOCNP®: Meniscus, Novartis, consultant; Amgen, Bristol-Myers Squibb, IMER, Meniscus, Merck, Novartis, honoraria

Table of Contents

List of Abbreviations

3DCRT: three-dimensional conformal radiation therapy

3DTPS: three-dimensional treatment planning system

5-FU: 5-fluorouracil

5-HT: 5-hydroxytryptamine (serotonin)

AASECT: American Association of Sexuality Educators, Counselors, and Therapists

ACR: American College of Radiology

ACS: American Cancer Society

ACTH: adrenocorticotropic hormone

ADL: activities of daily living

ADT: androgen deprivation therapy

AED: antiepileptic drug

AJCC: American Joint Committee on Cancer

ALARA: as low as reasonably achievable

ANA: American Nurses Association

APBI: accelerated partial breast irradiation

APN: advanced practice nurse

ARON: ASTRO Radiation Oncology Nurses

ASCO: American Society of Clinical Oncology

ASTRO: American Society for Radiation Oncology

ATP: adenosine triphosphate

AVM: arteriovenous malformations

BBB: blood-brain barrier

BCG: bacillus Calmette-Guérin

BMI: body mass index

CAM: complementary and alternative medicine

CBTRUS: Central Brain Tumor Registry of the United States

CDK: cyclin-dependent kinase

CFR: Code of Federal Regulations

CMS: Centers for Medicare and Medicaid Services

CMV: cytomegalovirus

CNS: central nervous system

CPR: cardiopulmonary resuscitation

CRF: cancer-related fatigue

CSF: cerebrospinal fluid

CT: computed tomography

CTCAE: Common Terminology Criteria for Adverse Events

CTV: clinical target volume

CTZ: chemoreceptor trigger zone

DPS: disintegration per second

DSB: double chromosomal strand break

DVH: dose-volume histogram

EBP: evidence-based practice

EBRT: external beam radiation therapy

EBV: Epstein-Barr virus

EGFR: epidermal growth factor receptor

ESA: erythropoietin-stimulating agent

ESCC: epidural spinal cord compression

ESTRO: European Society for Therapeutic Radiology and Oncology

FDA: U.S. Food and Drug Administration

FMEA: failure mode and effects analysis

GBM: glioblastoma multiforme

GFAP: glial fibrillary acidic protein

GI: gastrointestinal

GTV: gross tumor volume

GVHD: graft-versus-host disease

HAMA: human anti-mouse antibody

HDR: high dose rate

HIPAA: Health Insurance Portability and Accountability Act

HL: Hodgkin lymphoma

HPA: hypothalamic-pituitary-adrenal

HPV: human papillomavirus

HSCT: hematopoietic stem cell transplantation

HVL: half-value layer

IASLC: International Association for the Study of Lung Cancer

IBS: irritative bladder symptoms

ICRP: International Commission on Radiological Protection

ICRU: International Commission on Radiation Units and Measurements

IGRT: image-guided radiation therapy

IMRT: intensity-modulated radiation therapy

IORT: intraoperative radiation therapy

IPSS: international prostate symptom score

IRB: institutional review board

kVp: peak kilovolts

LDR: low dose rate

LET: linear energy transfer

LLLT: low-level laser therapy

MASCC: Multinational Association of Supportive Care in Cancer

MDM2: murine double minute 2

MeV: megaelectron volts

MLC: multileaf collimator

MRI: magnetic resonance imaging

MVAC: methotrexate, vinblastine, doxorubicin, and cisplatin

NCCN: National Comprehensive Cancer Network

NCI: National Cancer Institute

NCI CTEP: National Cancer Institute Cancer Therapy Evaluation Program

NCRP: National Council on Radiation Protection and Measurements

NHL: non-Hodgkin lymphoma

NK1: neurokinin-1

NLN: National Lymphedema Network

NPO: nothing by mouth

NRC: U.S. Nuclear Regulatory Commission

NSAID: nonsteroidal anti-inflammatory drug

NSCLC: non-small cell lung cancer

OAR: organ at risk

ONS: Oncology Nursing Society

PCNSL: primary central nervous system lymphoma

PDE5: phosphodiesterase type-5

PDT: photodynamic therapy

PET: positron-emission tomography

PG-SGA: Patient-Generated Subjective Global Assessment

PMB: photodynamic molecular beacons

PRIME-MD: Primary Care Evaluation of Mental Disorders

PSA: prostate-specific antigen

PTV: planning target volume

QA: quality assurance

RBE: relative biologic effectiveness

rhEGF: recombinant human epidermal growth factor

RION: radiation-induced optic neuropathy

RSO: radiation safety officer

RT: radiation therapy

RTOG: Radiation Therapy Oncology Group

SBRT: stereotactic body radiation therapy

SCC: spinal cord compression

SCLC: small cell lung cancer

SIG: special interest group

SNHL: sensorineural hearing loss

SNRI: serotonin norepinephrine reuptake inhibitor

SPF: sun protection factor

SRS: stereotactic radiosurgery

SSRI: selective serotonin reuptake inhibitor

SVC: superior vena cava

SVCS: superior vena cava syndrome

TBI: total body irradiation

TJC: The Joint Commission

TLI: total lymphoid irradiation

TMJ: temporomandibular joint

TNF: tumor necrosis factor

TNM: tumor, node, metastasis

TPN: total parenteral nutrition

TSH: thyroid-stimulating hormone

TURBT: transurethral resection of the bladder tumor

TURP: transurethral resection of the prostate

UTI: urinary tract infection

VHL: von Hippel-Lindau

WHO: World Health Organization

Introduction

Scientific and technologic advances in the field of radiation oncology and oncology have led to the introduction of new and updated treatment options, combined therapies across the cancer care continuum, and evidence-based symptom management. Radiation oncology nurses contribute and participate in the delivery of high-quality health care in multiple ways. They

1. Promote *practice* that is based upon the best available evidence to date. *Evidence-based practice* is defined as care that "integrates best scientific evidence with clinical expertise, knowledge of pathophysiology, knowledge of psychosocial issues, and decision-making preferences of patients" (Rutledge & Grant, 2002, p. 1)
2. Understand the physical, psychological, and social support needs of patients and their families to maintain a high level of the *art* of radiation oncology nursing practice
3. Communicate and advocate for patients and their families
4. Advocate for the role of oncology nurses in delivering quality cancer care to ensure that radiation oncology nursing services are available to patients.

In support of radiation oncology nurses' efforts nationally and internationally to provide quality care, the Oncology Nursing Society is providing the fourth edition of the *Manual for Radiation Oncology Nursing Practice and Education*. As with past editions, this manual covers the role of the radiation oncology nurse, the minimum qualifications for practice, and the revised and expanded scope of radiation oncology nursing practice. This edition includes seven new sections on bone cancer, benign conditions, oncologic emergencies, proton beam therapy, care of older adults, care of people with special needs, and survivorship.

This manual provides specific guidelines for the education of radiation oncology nurses, both new and experienced, and for the practice of quality nursing care. This manual can also assist with the articulation of the role of the radiation oncology nurse, justification of nursing positions in the department, and evaluation of radiation oncology nurses' performance.

This manual is not intended to serve as a comprehensive textbook but rather as an outline of the content necessary for the education and practice of radiation oncology nurses. Readers are encouraged to supplement this publication with the reference lists provided in the text and to continue to seek out new knowledge and skills that will provide the tools necessary for delivering high-quality, cost-effective patient care. Radiation oncology nurses also are encouraged to identify gaps in current knowledge and initiate or participate in quality improvement or research studies to fill those gaps in practice that will help to improve the quality of care and services delivered.

In preparing the update to these guidelines, the authors searched the PubMed database of the National Library of Medicine using the following key words: *radiation oncology, radiation therapy, symptom management for radiation therapy, radiation physics, radiation safety,* and *evidence-based practice*. Articles were limited to those published in the English language in peer-reviewed journals from 2000 forward. Older publications considered classic references were also included.

Further searches of the medical literature were conducted (based on initial findings, group feedback, and authors' experience) to identify additional relevant materials. In addition to searching peer-reviewed publications, the authors searched Web sites of known U.S. or international medical organizations or professional societies involved in producing relevant materials (e.g., reports, white papers, official announcements) pertinent to radiation-related topics. The authors sought to identify literature that would point to recommended evidence-based standards of practice or specific quality measures that had been developed by healthcare organizations or specialty societies. Web sites of the following organizations were searched:

- Oncology Nursing Society (www.ons.org)
- American Society for Radiation Oncology (www.astro.org)
- American College of Radiology (www.acr.org)
- National Comprehensive Cancer Network (www.nccn.org)
- National Cancer Institute (www.cancer.gov).

Findings derived from these searches were used to generate additional searches for guidelines published in the United States.

We hope that this manual will provide nurses with the knowledge to provide evidence-based practice to promote high-quality health care within the field of radiation oncology.

Ryan R. Iwamoto, ARNP, MN, AOCN®
Marilyn L. Haas, PhD, ANP-BC
Tracy K. Gosselin, RN, MSN, AOCN®

Reference

Rutledge, D.N., & Grant, M. (2002). Evidence-based practice in cancer nursing. Introduction. *Seminars in Oncology Nursing, 18,* 1–2.

Scope of Practice

The radiation oncology nurse is a registered professional nurse who functions independently and interdependently with the radiation oncology team in providing quality patient care. The radiation oncology nurse provides clinical care, education, psychosocial support, and consultation. The radiation oncology nurse may participate in the leadership roles of clinician, educator, administrative manager, consultant, or researcher. Using an evidence-based model of practice, the radiation oncology nurse provides nursing assessment, diagnosis, outcome identification, planning, implementation, and evaluation, focusing on the continuum of care to support patients receiving radiation therapy and their families and caregivers.

Radiation oncology nursing practice is based on the philosophic tenets identified in the Oncology Nursing Society's (ONS's) *Statement on the Scope and Standards of Oncology Nursing Practice* (Brant & Wickham, 2004). These standards and the ONS *Statement on the Scope and Standards of Advanced Practice Nursing in Oncology* (Jacobs, 2003) provide the framework from which these roles can be delineated. Critical components of professional practice are driven by the following core values: integrity, innovation, stewardship, advocacy, excellence, and inclusiveness (ONS, n.d.). ONS encourages radiation oncology nurses to assign personal meaning to each of these values.

Evidence-based practice (EBP) is the hallmark of 21st-century nursing. EBP "defines care that integrates best scientific evidence with clinical expertise, knowledge of pathophysiology, knowledge of psychosocial issues, and decision-making preferences of patients" (Rutledge & Grant, 2002, p. 1). Evidence specific to radiation oncology includes knowledge of the current and emerging technologies that are the foundation of radiation therapy, the symptoms associated with each therapy, and the growing number of biomarkers that help to predict patient outcomes. Oncology nurses recognize the levels of evidence, ranging from the highest level of well-designed and conducted meta-analyses and randomized controlled clinical trials to the lower, yet valuable, levels of evidence, including expert opinion. In practice, radiation oncology nurses evaluate the evidence based upon a hierarchy of sources including research. Radiation oncology nurses should incorporate and cite sources of current evidence in the topic area when developing policies, procedures, and guidelines for practice or publications.

It is *recommended* that the minimal education for the radiation oncology nurse is a baccalaureate degree in nursing. *Preferred* nursing experience should include two years of oncology nursing; alternatively, a 6–12-month didactic and clinically based preceptorship is highly *recommended*. Oncology nursing certification is also recommended.

The advanced practice nurse (APN) in radiation oncology has specialized knowledge and skills acquired through study and supervised practice. Educational preparation may include a master's degree, post-master's certificate, doctorate degree, administrative degree, or clinical research degree. The APN may function in the role of a clinical nurse specialist (CNS), nurse practitioner (NP), administrator, or researcher. The CNS is an expert clinician whose role includes components of patient care, leadership, education, consultation, and research. The NP is trained as a direct care provider and is qualified to diagnose and manage acute and chronic illness, either independently or collaboratively with a physician. The administrator role may include budgetary, human resource, program development, and strategic planning responsibilities. The clinical research role may incorporate participation in institutional review boards, cooperative group– and investigator-initiated studies, and quality assurance roles related to research. The role of the APN in radiation oncology is still evolving, and no practice standards are available (Shepard & Kelvin, 1999). Regardless of certification requirements, all oncology APNs must be licensed in their state as an RN and are subject to that state's legal restraints, regulations, and privileges for recognition and licensure of advanced practice nursing (Jacobs, 2003).

Standards of Care

Standards of Care pertain to professional nursing activities that the radiation oncology nurse demonstrates through the nursing process. The nursing process is the foundation of clinical decision making and encompasses all significant action taken by nurses in providing care to all patients and families (Brant & Wickham, 2004). The overall goal is to influence patients' and families' or caregivers' overall health, well-being, and quality of life across the care continuum.

Standard I. Assessment

The radiation oncology nurse assesses the needs of the patient and family throughout the continuum of care.

Standard II. Diagnosis

The radiation oncology nurse collaborates with other disciplines to analyze the assessment data and identify patient and family problems.

Standard III. Outcome Identification

The radiation oncology nurse identifies evidence-based nursing interventions that will guide expected patient and family outcomes.

Standard IV. Planning

The radiation oncology nurse, together with the patient, develops and communicates an individualized, comprehensive, measurable plan for interventions to attain expected patient outcomes.

Standard V. Implementation

The radiation oncology nurse implements a plan of care that incorporates evidence-based resources to achieve expected patient outcomes.

Standard VI. Evaluation

The radiation oncology nurse systematically evaluates patient and family responses to interventions and the process of care.

Standards of Professional Performance

Standards of Professional Performance describe a competent level of behavior in the professional nursing role. The radiation oncology nurse should be self-directed and purposeful in seeking the necessary knowledge and skills to enhance professional development and clinical outcomes (Moore-Higgs et al., 2003).

Standard I. Quality of Care

The radiation oncology nurse systematically evaluates and documents the effectiveness of clinical care.

Standard II. Accountability

The radiation oncology nurse evaluates his or her own nursing practice in relation to professional practice standards, relevant statutes, and regulations.

Standard III. Education

The radiation oncology nurse pursues ongoing professional development via educational activities that enhance critical thinking, knowledge, and skills related to the field of radiation oncology.

Standard IV. Leadership

The radiation oncology nurse serves as a leader, role model, and mentor for the professional development of peers and colleagues.

Standard V. Ethics

The radiation oncology nurse serves as a patient and family advocate, protecting personal health information and patient autonomy, dignity, and rights in a manner sensitive to spiritual, cultural, and ethnic practices based upon those put forth by the American Nurses Association (Fowler, 2008).

Standard VI. Collaboration

The radiation oncology nurse collaborates and consults with the patient and family, along with the multidisciplinary team, to enhance desired clinical outcomes for the patient.

Standard VII. Research

The radiation oncology nurse uses research as the scientific basis for nursing practice and participates in the conduct of research to improve patient outcomes.

Standard VIII. Resource Utilization

The radiation oncology nurse works with the multidisciplinary team to provide safe and effective patient care, securing appropriate services and financial resources as needed.

References

Brant, J.M., & Wickham, R.S. (Eds.). (2004). *Statement on the scope and standards of oncology nursing practice.* Pittsburgh, PA: Oncology Nursing Society.

Fowler, M.D.M. (2008). *Guide to the code of ethics for nurses: Interpretation and application.* Silver Spring, MD: American Nurses Association.

Jacobs, L.A. (Ed.). (2003). *Statement on the scope and standards of advanced practice nursing in oncology* (3rd ed.). Pittsburgh, PA: Oncology Nursing Society.

Moore-Higgs, G., Watkins-Bruner, D., Balmer, L., Johnson-Doneski, J., Komarny, P., Mautner, B., & Velji, K. (2003). The role of licensed nursing personnel in radiation oncology part A: Results of a descriptive study. *Oncology Nursing Forum, 30,* 51–58. doi:10.1188/03.ONF.51-58

Oncology Nursing Society. (n.d.). ONS's core values. Retrieved from http://www.ons.org/about/CoreValues

Rutledge, D.N., & Grant, M. (2002). Evidence-based practice in cancer nursing. Introduction. *Seminars in Oncology Nursing, 18,* 1–2.

Shepard, N., & Kelvin, J.F. (1999). The nursing role in radiation oncology. *Seminars in Oncology Nursing, 15,* 237–249.

Evidence-Based Practice

I. Definition and implications

A. Definition: *Evidence-based practice* (EBP) is the application of the most current evidence to clinical issues. The uniqueness of this process is that the application of the evidence is buffered through the clinician's expertise and the clients' (patients' and families') expectations. All three components must be in place to truly be EBP and to allow for the individualization of the evidence to the current clinical situation (DePalma, 2009; Melnyk & Fineout-Overholt, 2011; Sackett, Straus, Richardson, Rosenberg, & Haynes, 2000).

B. Implications for practice
 1. Regulatory and professional organizations support the importance of EBP.
  a) Regulatory and accrediting agencies have created new requirements, such as the Joint Commission's inclusion of evidence-based performance measures in its core measures phase of the ORYX initiative in healthcare settings (Joint Commission, 2010).
  b) The American Nurses Credentialing Center's Magnet Recognition Program® for excellence in nursing services: This program recognizes healthcare organizations that provide nursing excellence and provides dissemination of successful nursing practices and strategies (American Nurses Credentialing Center, n.d.). One of the 14 aspects of excellence includes research and EBP (Steinbinder & Scherer, 2010).
  c) Professional nursing organizations have included EBP in core competencies and standards of practice, especially related to the role of advanced practice nurses (APNs) (American Association of Colleges of Nursing, 2006, 2007, 2011; Jacobs, 2003; National Organization of Nurse Practitioner Faculties, 2011).
 2. The managed care environment, with its demands for quality care and cost-effectiveness, supports the adoption of an evidence-based approach to practice to avoid administering care that does not make a difference.
 3. APNs generally are ideal facilitators for EBP because they possess the clinical expertise, the awareness of patient, family, and healthcare providers' needs, and knowledge of the particular clinical system to be able to negotiate for both the basic process and the resultant practice changes (DePalma, 2009). APNs promote the value of evidence in clinical decision making by
  a) Being a role model by making clinical care decisions based on evidence
  b) Coordinating clinical interdisciplinary quality improvement groups that use evidence
  c) Effecting changes within the system to promote EBP, especially the removal of barriers in the environment (Hockenberry, Wilson, & Barrera, 2006; Marshall, 2006).
 4. Research-based evidence relevant to clinical practice can be accessed through an increasing variety of sources.
  a) Original individual research studies published in professional journals
  b) Professional conference proceedings or best practice consensus statements
  c) Evidence-based summaries
   (1) Published as integrated or systematic reviews (most credible)
   (2) Researched at sites such as the Cochrane Library (www.thecochrane library.com)
   (3) Located in the Oncology Nursing Society (ONS)-published Putting Evidence Into Practice (PEP) series in the *Clinical Journal of Oncology Nursing* and in *Putting Evidence Into Practice: Improving Oncology Patient Outcomes* (Eaton & Tipton, 2009; Eaton, Tipton, & Irwin, 2011)
   (4) EBP protocols or guidelines developed and available through sites such as
    (a) National Comprehensive Cancer Network (NCCN) at www.nccn.org/clinical.asp, catalogued by types of cancer, prevention, risk reduction, and supportive care
    (b) American Society of Clinical Oncology (ASCO) at www.asco.org, catalogued as types of cancer, supportive care, and survivorship
    (c) American College of Radiology (ACR) at www.acr.org, catalogued by modality, including radiation therapy (RT).
 5. EBP is extremely relevant in radiation oncology nursing, where an emphasis has always existed on two of the components of the EBP process:
  a) The clinical expertise of the radiation oncology nurse
  b) Appreciation of the patient's and family's values and expectations.

C. Advantages of evidence-based practice
 1. Advantages of adopting an evidence-based approach to practice exist from the adminis-

trative, clinical practice, regulatory, and legal perspectives.

2. Overall, EBP is
   a) Safe—Prevents errors caused by variation or lack of clarity in practice
   b) Therapeutic—Improves patient outcomes
   c) Ethical—Decreases variations in care based on patient populations or healthcare providers
   d) Cost-effective in the long term—Controls resource utilization and affects reimbursement
   e) Legally defensible—Limits liabilities because a rationale can be provided for "best" practice
   f) Satisfying—Promotes patient and caregiver satisfaction.

II. The process of evidence-based practice

A. EBP is considered a total process (see Figure 1) beginning with the statement of the clinical question and proceeding through the evaluation of the effectiveness of the practice change and continual improvement of the process with the caregiver and patient perspectives in mind (DePalma, 2009; Melnyk & Fineout-Overholt, 2011). EBP emphasizes research evidence but allows for the use of other levels of evidence, depending on the adopted hierarchy or levels of evidence (see Figure 2 for one example of a hierarchy of evidence listing both research and nonresearch evidence).

B. EBP is a natural process for the inquisitive radiation oncology nurse who wants to deliver the highest quality of care, but EBP also is a time-consuming and resource-intensive process. Practice settings that value an environment of inquiry and the use of new, credible knowledge are most likely to provide the resources for access and application of that new knowledge (Melnyk & Fineout-Overholt, 2011). The EBP process is similar to the nursing process because both involve similar steps.

Figure 1. Evidence-Based Practice Process

Evidence-based practice is a total process with the following steps:
1. Identify relevant clinical issues.
2. Format a searchable clinical question.
3. Find the best practice or most current evidence.
4. Appraise the evidence.
5. Synthesize the evidence to make a recommendation.
6. Implement the recommended practice change.
7. Evaluate the effectiveness of any practice change.
8. Continually improve practice based on new evidence.

Figure 2. Example of a Hierarchy or Levels of Evidence

Research
- Meta-analyses
- Systematic reviews of research articles
- Randomized controlled intervention studies
- Nonrandomized controlled intervention studies
- Qualitative studies

Nonresearch
- Evidence-based consensus statements
- Quality improvement data
- Risk or infection control data
- Program evaluation
- Expert opinion

---

1. Identify relevant clinical issues. The clinical problem should emerge from clinical situations where a knowledge gap or uncertainty exists regarding the "best" response or intervention. Therefore, the problem is a statement of a question that needs to be answered or a situation that needs a solution. Ideally, an interdisciplinary group of stakeholders coordinated by the physician and the APN decide upon the clinical issue.

2. Form a searchable problem. An ideal statement is succinct and uses searchable words. The PICO (population, intervention, comparison, and outcome) framework can be helpful in formulating the statement because it serves as a reminder of the key aspects to include (DePalma, 2009; Melnyk & Fineout-Overholt, 2011).

3. Find the best practice or most current evidence. Radiation oncology nurses should elicit help from reference librarians or professional colleagues in planning and initiating the search for evidence. The search should be based on the keywords in the statement of the problem.
   a) Prior to a search being done, several factors need to be decided to guarantee the best focused search.
      (1) Language: English or international publications
      (2) Time frame: Range of years to search; past five years preferred. In some instances, classic citations exist that need to be considered.
      (3) Sample: Age, sex, ethnicity, diagnosed with disease or not, in treatment or not
      (4) Setting: Home care, acute care, rehabilitation
      (5) Measurement: Specific variable measured; specific tool or diagnostic test used
      (6) Types of evidence: What types of articles will be acceptable, such as

research or systematic review articles, evidence-based clinical guidelines, or opinion articles

b) Initial searches often need to be refocused or expanded to locate a feasible amount of credible evidence to review. Ideal types of evidence are meta-analyses or systematic/integrative reviews (see Figure 2) that have already collected and synthesized relevant research studies and evidence-based clinical guidelines. Therefore, besides the general searching of bibliographic databases such as MEDLINE®, CINAHL®, and PsycINFO®, sites that offer systematic reviews, clinical guidelines, or specialty-specific standards are valuable resources and should be included in the search strategy (see Table 1 for key resources).

4. Appraise the evidence. Although initially difficult, this step determines the scientific merit, feasibility, and utility of the evidence. The radiation oncology nurse must critically appraise the evidence for its validity and usefulness within the specific clinical practice or setting.

a) Based on the hierarchy of evidence used, each study is assessed for the level of evidence.

b) Tools are available to help in the appraisal of the research and nonresearch evidence (Brown, 2009; Melnyk & Fineout-Overholt, 2011; Newhouse, Dearholt, Poe, Pugh, & White, 2007).

5. Synthesize the evidence to make a recommendation. This is combining the findings from all the sources of evidence (research and nonre-

Table 1. Evidence-Based Practice (EBP) Web Sites

Site/URL	Description
Academic Center for Evidence-Based Practice www.acestar.uthscsa.edu	Comprehensive list of EBP resources targeting nurses
ACP Journal Club www.acpjc.org	Searchable database with original studies and reviews from 130 clinical journals Palliative care content area
Agency for Healthcare Research and Quality www.ahrq.gov	Evidence report topics, evidence technical reviews, and clinical guidelines
American College of Radiology www.acr.org	Access to quality research and research links
American Society of Clinical Oncology (ASCO) www.asco.org	Cancer portals give access to disease-specific information, including research published in the *Journal of Clinical Oncology* and *Journal of Oncology Practice* and clinical practice guidelines developed by ASCO.
Centre for Health Evidence www.cche.net/che/home.asp	"User's Guides for EBP" series from *JAMA*; guidance on how to critique and use different types of evidence articles (Need to subscribe to be able to view and print articles)
Cochrane Library www.thecochranelibrary.com	Systematic reviews and guidelines; generally medically oriented *Cancer* is a search word in the database; at the time of this writing, 346 reviews were listed under that keyword. (Can browse titles and get abstracts for free but need to subscribe or pay a fee for documents)
Database of Abstracts of Reviews of Effects www.crd.york.ac.uk/crdweb	Systematic reviews produced and maintained by the National Health System's (United Kingdom) Centre for Reviews and Dissemination
National Comprehensive Cancer Network www.nccn.org	Practice guidelines for clinicians and patients, most based on cancer type; also outcomes and resource links
National Guideline Clearinghouse www.guideline.gov	A public resource for evidence-based clinical practice guidelines Guideline syntheses provide a comparison of guidelines on similar topics.
Oncology Nursing Society EBP Resource Area www.ons.org/Research/EBPRA	List of integrated reviews pertinent to cancer care Information on the EBP process and links to other resources
United Kingdom Database of Uncertainties about the Effects of Treatments (DUETs) www.library.nhs.uk/duets	Systematic reviews *Cancer* is one area that can be searched. (Use restricted to United Kingdom contributors)

search) and making a practice recommendation. This is the "so what" step. Whether a practice change recommendation can be made depends on the quality, amount, and currency of evidence. The recommendation must be faithful to the true state of the evidence, even when the evidence is contradictory or insufficient. The following decisions can be made based on the evidence.

a) Sufficient credible evidence exists to make a clear practice recommendation.

b) Contradictory evidence exists; therefore, the radiation nurse can make a decision about a practice change based on his or her clinical expertise, knowledge of the patient population, and what is feasible within the setting.

c) Insufficient evidence exists upon which to base a clear practice recommendation. This situation may lead to a research project at the clinical setting to determine whether a particular intervention can improve outcomes.

6. Implement the practice recommendation: Applying the results of the synthesis to actual practice often involves planning and making a change. Practice recommendations can be proposed as individual interventions or as protocols, guidelines, or pathways. It is important to adopt whatever format will be most readily accepted by the clinicians throughout the program or setting. The existing practice-change systems within the healthcare setting should be employed to facilitate the change and to keep all stakeholders informed and therefore invested. Two key points are to

a) Allow enough time for the education and reeducation of caregivers and patients.

b) Develop the evaluation plan simultaneously with the implementation plan so that no obvious points of evaluation are omitted.

7. Evaluate the effectiveness of any practice change. Evaluation provides essential data for decision making and assists the multidisciplinary team members in determining whether the intervention should be continued, rejected, or modified.

a) Data should include process issues, as well as the expected clinical outcomes and caregiver and organizational outcomes (Jennings, Staggers, & Brosch, 1999).

b) For example, after a change has been initiated to employ new patient education content regarding relaxation techniques aimed at improving breathlessness, evaluation points would include the following.

(1) The percentage of radiation oncology nurses who are including the content in their patient education

(2) The percentage of breathless patients who have appropriate patient education documented

(3) Improvement of patient outcomes (e.g., breathlessness, activity levels, quality of life)

8. Continually improve practice based on new evidence. Once the initial EBP change has been evaluated and deemed effective, that does not end the process. The interdisciplinary team needs to periodically revisit the issue based on the ongoing evaluation data and a search for new evidence. Either internal or external evidence can initiate further practice changes.

III. Evidence-based guideline implementation

A. As mentioned previously, one of the valuable bases for EBP is a clinical practice guideline. *Clinical practice guidelines* are classically defined as "systematically developed statements to assist practitioner and patient decisions about appropriate health care for specific clinical circumstances" (Institute of Medicine, 1990, p. 27). The increased adherence to clinical practice guidelines, the availability of guidelines via the Internet, and the expectation of improved quality and cost-effectiveness of health care based upon guidelines necessitate the evaluation of a guideline prior to adoption. Quality guidelines are those with a high degree of confidence in the method of development, the evidence base, and the applicability and feasibility for practice (AGREE Collaboration, 2001).

B. Evidence-based clinical practice guidelines serve as knowledge tools and decision aids for clinicians seeking to develop evidence-based decision making in a specific setting. The goals of using guidelines "are to provide an explicit, evidence-based description of the risks and benefits of an intervention and to outline areas where evidence is lacking" (Brouwers, Stacey, & O'Connor, 2010, p. E68).

C. Clinical practice guidelines are most valuable when they have been evaluated and adapted to local context. Acceptance and adherence to a clinical practice guideline are improved when it is customized to the particular organization (Brown, 2009; Harrison, Légaré, Graham, & Fervers, 2010).

D. Many tools and checklists exist to evaluate clinical practice guidelines. When these tools are compared, common points denote a quality guideline. A quality guideline should include
   1. Recommended interventions and the circumstances when these are most effective
   2. The extent, strength, and currency of evidence in support of the intervention (Griffiths & Feder, 1998)
   3. The role of patient preferences (AGREE Collaboration, 2001)
   4. How applicable and feasible the recommendations are (Brown, 2009; Melnyk & Fineout-Overholt, 2011).

E. A variety of implementation strategies also exist in the literature. Some examples include
   1. An audit and feedback intervention for nurse practitioners' implementation of cancer pain guidelines (Dulko, Hertz, Julien, Beck, & Mooney, 2010)
   2. The Educating Clinicians to Achieve Treatment Guideline Effectiveness (EDUCATE) intensive education intervention in community oncology practices nationally (Friedman et al., 2009).

References

AGREE Collaboration. (2001). Appraisal of Guidelines for Research and Evaluation (AGREE) instrument. Retrieved from http://www.agreecollaboration.org

American Association of Colleges of Nursing. (2006). Position statement on nursing research. Retrieved from http://www.aacn.nche.edu/Publications/positions/NsgRes.htm

American Association of Colleges of Nursing. (2007). White paper on the education and role of the clinical nurse leader. Retrieved from http://dms.dartmouth.edu/cms/resources/clinical_nurse_leader/cnl_white_paper.pdf

American Association of Colleges of Nursing. (2011). Essentials of master's education in nursing. Retrieved from http://www.aacn.nche.edu/education/pdf/Master'sEssentials11.pdf

American Nurses Credentialing Center. (n.d.). Program overview. Retrieved from http://www.nursecredentialing.org/Magnet/ProgramOverview.aspx

Brouwers, M., Stacey, D., & O'Connor, A. (2010). Knowledge creation: Synthesis, tools and products. *Canadian Medical Association Journal, 182,* E68–E72. doi:10.1503/cmaj.081230

Brown, S.J. (2009). *Evidence-based nursing: The research-practice connection.* Sudbury, MA: Jones and Bartlett.

DePalma, J.A. (2009). Research competencies. In A.B. Hamric, J.A. Spross, & C.M. Hanson (Eds.), *Advanced nursing practice: An integrative approach* (4th ed., pp. 217–248). Philadelphia, PA: Saunders.

Dulko, D., Hertz, E., Julien, J., Beck, S., & Mooney, K. (2010). Implementation of cancer pain guidelines by acute care nurse practitioners using an audit and feedback strategy. *Journal of the American Academy of Nurse Practitioners, 22,* 45–55. doi:10.1111/j.1745-7599.2009.00469.x

Eaton, L.H., & Tipton, J.M. (Eds.). (2009). *Putting evidence into practice: Improving oncology patient outcomes.* Pittsburgh, PA: Oncology Nursing Society.

Eaton, L.H., Tipton, J.M., & Irwin, M. (Eds.). (2011). *Putting evidence into practice: Improving oncology patient outcomes, volume 2.* Pittsburgh, PA: Oncology Nursing Society.

Friedman, L., Engelking, C., Wickham, R., Harvey, C., Read, M., & Whitlock, K.B. (2009). The EDUCATE study: A continuing education exemplar for clinical practice guideline implementation. *Clinical Journal of Oncology Nursing, 13,* 219–230. doi:10.1188/09.CJON.219-230

Griffiths, C., & Feder, G. (1998). Can we improve our management of acute asthma? An approach to using clinical guidelines. In L. Ridsdale (Ed.), *Evidence-based practice in primary care* (pp. 121–138). Edinburgh, Scotland: Churchill Livingstone.

Harrison, M.B., Légaré, F., Graham, I.D., & Fervers, B. (2010). Adapting clinical practice guidelines to local context and assessing barriers to their use. *Canadian Medical Association Journal, 182,* E78–E84. doi:10.1503/cmaj.081232

Hockenberry, M., Wilson, D., & Barrera, P. (2006). Implementing evidence-based nursing practice in a pediatric hospital. *Pediatric Nursing, 32,* 371–377.

Institute of Medicine. (1990). *Clinical practice guidelines: Directions for a new program.* Washington, DC: National Academies Press.

Jacobs, L.A. (Ed.). (2003). *Statement on the scope and standards of advanced practice nursing in oncology* (3rd ed.). Pittsburgh, PA: Oncology Nursing Society.

Jennings, B.M., Staggers, N., & Brosch, L.R. (1999). A classification scheme for outcome indicators. *Journal of Nursing Scholarship, 31,* 381–388. doi:10.1111/j.1547-5069.1999.tb00524.x

Joint Commission. (2010). 2010 ORYX performance measure reporting requirements for hospitals and guidelines for measure selections. Retrieved from http://www.jointcommission.org/assets/1/18/2010_ORYX_Performance_Measure_Reporting_Requirements.pdf

Marshall, M.L. (2006). Strategies for success: Bringing evidence-based practice to the bedside. *Clinical Nurse Specialist, 20,* 124–127.

Melnyk, B.M., & Fineout-Overholt, E. (2011). *Evidence-based practice in nursing and healthcare: A guide to best practice* (2nd ed.). Philadelphia, PA: Lippincott Williams & Wilkins.

National Organization of Nurse Practitioner Faculties. (2011). Nurse practitioner core competencies. Retrieved from http://www.nonpf.com/associations/10789/files/IntegratedNPCoreCompsFINALApril2011.pdf

Newhouse, R.P., Dearholt, S.L., Poe, S.S., Pugh, L.C., & White, K.M. (2007). *Johns Hopkins nursing evidence-based practice model and guidelines.* Indianapolis, IN: Sigma Theta Tau International.

Sackett, D.L., Straus, S.E., Richardson, W.S., Rosenberg, W., & Haynes, R.B. (2000). *Evidence-based medicine: How to practice and teach EBM* (2nd ed.). Philadelphia, PA: Churchill Livingstone.

Steinbinder, A., & Scherer, E. (2010). Creating nursing system excellence through the forces of magnetism. In K. Malloch & T. Porter-O'Grady (Eds.), *Introduction to evidence-based practice in nursing and health care* (2nd ed., pp. 235–274). Sudbury, MA: Jones and Bartlett.

Radiation Oncology Nursing Practice and Education

I. The clinical practicum

A. Course description: The didactic portion of this course is designed to prepare the RN to practice in a radiation oncology setting. Course topics include the following.
1. Brief overview of carcinogenesis
2. Properties and sources of ionizing radiation
3. Principles of radiobiology
4. Malignant and benign indications for RT
5. General principles of staging as a foundation for cancer treatment decisions
   a) Tumor, node, metastasis (TNM)
   b) Definitive
   c) Neoadjuvant
   d) Adjuvant
   e) Prophylactic
   f) Control
   g) Palliation
   h) Multimodality
6. Roles and responsibilities of radiation oncology team members (Bruner & Movsas, 2001; Oncology Nursing Certification Corporation, 2009)
   a) Physician
   b) APN and physician assistant
   c) RN
   d) Radiation physicist
   e) Dosimetrist
   f) Radiation therapist
   g) Social worker
   h) Nutritionist
   i) Counselors (psychiatric healthcare providers)
   j) Pastoral care provider
7. Radiation treatment planning
   a) Consultation
   b) Dose prescription (gross tumor volume, clinical target volume, planning target volume, organ at risk, dose-volume histogram, isodose, fractionation)
   c) Simulation (positioning, immobilization, tattoos, fiducial markers, image guidance)
   d) Creation and verification of plan (role of radiation physicists and dosimetrists, use of blocks and multileaf collimator)
   e) Setup
   f) Delivery and monitoring (role of radiation therapist, portal imaging, toxicity assessments)
8. Modalities of delivering RT
   a) External beam (three-dimensional conformal, intensity modulated, proton, stereotactic radiosurgery [SRS])
   b) Brachytherapy (low dose rate, high dose rate, interstitial, intracavitary)
   c) Miscellaneous (accelerated partial breast, total body irradiation [TBI], total nodal irradiation, intraoperative radiation, hyperthermia, photodynamic therapy)
   d) Chemical modifiers (radiosensitizers, radioprotectants, molecular targeted therapies)
   e) Radiopharmaceuticals
9. Comprehensive assessment and evidence-based management of general and site- and disease-specific radiation-related acute, delayed, and late toxicities
   a) General (e.g., fatigue, skin reactions)
   b) Site and disease specific (e.g., alopecia, mucositis, esophagitis, diarrhea)
10. Comprehensive assessment and evidence-based management of psychosocial issues experienced by patients receiving RT and their families and caregivers along the illness continuum
11. Post-treatment disease surveillance and survivorship issues associated with RT (Hewitt, Greenfield, & Stovall, 2006)
    a) Disease surveillance and follow-up
    b) Late effects
    c) Health promotion
    d) Legal protections regarding employment and health care
    e) Psychosocial services
    f) Transitioning to life after cancer
    g) Treatment summaries and survivorship care plans
12. Palliative RT and end-of-life care (Pituskin et al., 2010)
    a) Determining goals of care
    b) Pain and symptom management
    c) Supportive care referrals (e.g., physical therapy and occupational therapy for assistive devices, nutrition, hospice)
    d) Social work referrals (e.g., financial concerns, advance directives, wills, skilled care at home or in appropriate setting as needed)

e) Psychosocial needs (grief and bereavement process)

13. Education principles and theories relevant to addressing the needs of patients receiving RT and their family members

14. Implications of literacy level, ability to learn, and learning preference on patient and family education

15. Implications of cultural, ethnic, racial, socioeconomic, and gender variations in the RT experience

16. Documentation of patient care incorporating toxicity rating systems

17. Clinical trials and informed consent

18. Needs of special populations receiving RT
    a) Children (e.g., sedation, immobilization, support of parents)
    b) Older adults (e.g., comprehensive geriatric assessment) (Haas, 2004)

19. Radiation safety
    a) Standards and regulations
    b) Sources of radiation exposure (diagnostic, sealed, unsealed)
    c) Types of radionuclides
       (1) Cesium (^{137}Cs)
       (2) Cobalt (^{60}Co)
       (3) Gold (^{198}Au)
       (4) Iodine (^{125}I, ^{131}I)
       (5) Iridium (^{192}Ir)
       (6) Palladium (^{103}Pd)
       (7) Phosphorus (^{32}P)
       (8) Radium (^{226}Ra)
       (9) Radon (^{222}Rn)
       (10) Samarium (^{153}Sm)
       (11) Strontium (^{89}Sr, ^{90}Sr)
       (12) Tantalum (^{182}Ta)
       (13) Yttrium (^{90}Y)
    d) Potential health risks related to exposure
    e) Principles of radiation protection (as low as reasonably achievable [ALARA], radiation monitoring devices, restricted areas)

20. Quality improvement
    a) Standards
    b) Process

21. Current issues in RT
    a) Patient safety
    b) Reimbursement and healthcare reform
    c) Caregiver burden

22. Radiation oncology resources
    a) ONS
    b) ACR
    c) American Society for Radiation Oncology (ASTRO)
    d) ASCO
    e) NCCN
    f) National Cancer Institute (NCI)
    g) OncoLink (sponsored by the University of Pennsylvania)

B. Course objectives: At the completion of the didactic portion of this course, the nurse will be able to

1. Educate patients receiving RT and their families and caregivers about the
    a) Process of carcinogenesis
    b) Properties and sources of ionizing RT
    c) Principles of radiobiology.

2. Articulate benign and malignant indications for RT.

3. Apply principles of cancer staging in the determination of treatment purposes and goals for patients undergoing RT.

4. Describe the roles and responsibilities of the radiation oncology team members.

5. Describe the process of treatment planning and treatment delivery to patients undergoing RT and their families and caregivers, and anticipate their needs during this process.

6. Develop appropriate comprehensive nursing assessment and evidence-based management strategies in the care of a patient receiving various RT modalities.

7. Comprehensively assess the physical and psychosocial needs of patients undergoing RT and their family members, including actual or potential general and site- and disease-specific acute, delayed, and late toxicities related to RT.

8. Formulate an evidence-based and collaborative plan of care to address the physical and psychosocial needs of patients undergoing RT and their family members that includes measurable outcomes and an evaluation process.

9. Identify the post-RT survivorship needs of patients and their families and caregivers.

10. Describe evidence-based indications of palliative RT and the nursing management of patients receiving palliative RT.

11. Apply relevant education principles and theories to the plan of care across the illness

continuum, including appropriate self-care measures.

12. Tailor the plan of care according to cultural, ethnic, racial, socioeconomic, and gender variations.

13. Document key components of patient care, incorporating toxicity rating systems.

14. Describe the nurse's role in the informed consent process for clinical trials and the resources available to access clinical trials.

15. Describe the nursing assessment and management of special populations (e.g., children and older adults) across the illness continuum.

16. Describe radiation protection and safety precautions, procedures, and protocols.

17. Identify components of a comprehensive quality improvement program.

18. Articulate current technical, quality assurance, and reimbursement issues in RT.

19. Access radiation oncology resources.

C. Clinical activities

1. A qualified preceptor will supervise the nurse for a specified time period in a way that is individualized according to the nurse's ability and skill in meeting the specific objectives and institutional standards.

2. The preceptor and nurse will establish specific objectives at the beginning of the clinical practicum to meet previously defined course objectives. The nurse and preceptor may accomplish objectives by selecting a specific population of patients and providing the nurse with a period of supervised direct observation followed by independent responsibility for planning the care of these patients.

3. The nurse will observe the role of the radiation therapist, dosimetrist, and physicist and understand the interdisciplinary nature of therapeutic planning and treatment.

4. The nurse will observe multiple modalities for delivering RT for a variety of diagnoses, with various goals of care, and in patients from varied age and cultural groups.

5. The nurse will systematically assess the patient's physical, psychosocial, and educational needs specific to delivery of RT and its associated toxicities during consultation, treatment, and surveillance.

6. The nurse will use relevant educational principles and theories in the development of knowledgeable and effective patient and family teaching across the illness continuum, including appropriate self-care measures.

7. The nurse will develop a plan of care that is tailored according to the patient's cultural, ethnic, racial, socioeconomic, gender, and age variables and will communicate the plan of care to the patient, family, and multidisciplinary team.

8. The nurse will initiate appropriate evidence-based symptom management measures.

9. The nurse will make appropriate patient referrals.

10. The nurse will document, evaluate, and revise the plan of care as needed.

11. The nurse will be able to verbalize principles of radiation protection and will be observed using appropriate radiation safety procedures.

12. The nurse will assist in identifying appropriate clinical trial options and will assume an appropriate role in the informed consent process for patients interested in clinical trials.

13. The nurse will identify appropriate radiation oncology resources.

D. Evaluation

1. A competency-based evaluation tool developed from the practicum course objectives and individual objectives set with the preceptor can be used to determine competency during the consultation, treatment planning, treatment delivery, follow-up, and end-of-life phases of care. The evaluation documents the nurse's

   a) Understanding of the principles of carcinogenesis, disease staging, goals of care, radiobiology, and RT

   b) Knowledge of radiation toxicities, patient assessment, and evidence-based care management related to the treatment site and the radiotherapeutic modality used

   c) Ability to formulate, document, and evaluate individualized but comprehensive evidence-based care plans for patients during consultation and treatment planning, while receiving RT, and after completion of therapy

   d) Knowledge of patient education principles, including patient literacy, mental ability to learn, and age-specific and cultural variables

   e) Knowledge of radiation protection and safety principles

   f) Knowledge of radiation oncology resources.

2. The activities indicated in Figure 3 should be performed at a satisfactory level. If the nurse has not had an opportunity to carry out a particular activity, indicate "N/A" (not applicable). If the nurse has not achieved satisfactory competency for all activities, then a remediation and reevaluation plan should be developed.

Figure 3. Clinical Practicum Competency Evaluation Tool			
	Satisfactory		
	Yes **Date/Initials**	**No** **Date/Initials**	**N/A** **Date/Initials**
Basic Principles of Radiation Oncology			
Explains key principles of carcinogenesis, ionizing radiation therapy (RT), and radiobiology			
Articulates benign and malignant indications for RT			
Nursing Role Across Illness Continuum			
Identifies self and nursing role to patient			
Checks patient identification			
Assesses patient's literacy level, ability to learn, and learning preferences			
Educates patient and family members according to relevant education principles/theories and tailored to literacy			
Solicits questions to be sure patient and family understand teaching			
Determines cultural, ethnic, racial, socioeconomic, gender, and age variations and tailors plan of care accordingly			
Addresses the needs of special populations receiving RT a) Children (e.g., sedation, immobilization, support of parents) b) Older adults (e.g., comprehensive geriatric assessment)			
Documents assessment, intervention, and evaluation accurately and incorporates toxicity rating systems			
Accesses radiation oncology resources (e.g., Oncology Nursing Society, National Comprehensive Cancer Network, OncoLink, American Society for Radiation Oncology)			
Nursing Role During Consultation, Simulation, and Treatment Planning Phase			
Systematically assesses the patient's physical, psychosocial, and educational needs specific to delivery of RT and its associated toxicities			
Applies principles of cancer staging to identify treatment purposes/goals for a patient undergoing RT			
Describes process of radiation treatment planning a) Consultation b) Dose prescription (total dose, fractionation schedule) c) Simulation (positioning, immobilization, tattoos, fiducial markers, image guidance, gating) d) Creation and verification of plan (role of radiation physicists and dosimetrists) e) Setup			
Explains treatment modality appropriate to patient a) External beam (three-dimensional conformal, intensity-modulated, proton, stereotactic radiosurgery) b) Brachytherapy (low dose rate, high dose rate, interstitial, intracavitary) c) Miscellaneous (accelerated partial breast, total body irradiation, total nodal irradiation, intraoperative radiation, hyperthermia, photodynamic therapy) d) Chemical modifiers (radiosensitizers, radioprotectants, molecular targeted therapies) e) Radiopharmaceuticals			

(Continued on next page)

Figure 3. Clinical Practicum Competency Evaluation Tool *(Continued)*

	Satisfactory		
	Yes **Date/Initials**	**No** **Date/Initials**	**N/A** **Date/Initials**
Describes roles and responsibilities of members of radiation oncology team (physician, nurse, advanced practice nurse, physician assistant, radiation physicist, dosimetrist, therapist, social worker, nutritionist, counselor)			
Reinforces discussion of appropriate clinical trials and assists in informed consent process			
Verifies that informed consent has been obtained			
Explains and assists with simulation procedures			
Nursing Role During Treatment Phase			
Describes delivery of RT (role of radiation therapist, portal imaging)			
Assesses patient for acute general toxicities of RT (e.g., fatigue, altered nutrition, skin changes)			
Assesses patient for acute site-, disease-, and modality-specific toxicities of RT (e.g., alopecia, mucositis, esophagitis, diarrhea)			
Alerts patient to report potentially dangerous or uncomfortable symptoms immediately to nurse or physician			
Checks appropriate laboratory data and communicates results to other members of healthcare team as needed			
Monitors patient's psychological status and coping skills			
Teaches self-care measures to manage acute toxicities			
Initiates measures to manage acute general toxicities (e.g., energy conservation, nutritional supplements)			
Initiates measures to manage acute site-specific toxicities (e.g., mouth care, pain management)			
Collaborates with other members of the healthcare team in developing, evaluating, and modifying plan of care; demonstrates effective communication skills			
Refers patients and family members as needed to appropriate specialists (e.g., dietitian, counselor)			
Institutes appropriate radiation safety precautions			
Reviews follow-up schedule and discharge instructions with patient and family			
Nursing Role During Follow-Up Phase			
Assesses patient for delayed and late generalized toxicities of RT (e.g., fatigue)			
Assesses patient for delayed and late site-, disease-, and modality-specific toxicities of RT (e.g., lymphedema)			
Reinforces need for patient to continue to report potentially dangerous or uncomfortable symptoms			
Reinforces self-care measures to manage delayed and late toxicities of RT			
Initiates measures to manage delayed and late general RT toxicities (e.g., exercise)			

(Continued on next page)

Figure 3. Clinical Practicum Competency Evaluation Tool *(Continued)*	Satisfactory		
	Yes Date/Initials	No Date/Initials	N/A Date/Initials
Initiates measures to manage delayed and late site-, disease-, and modality-specific RT toxicities (e.g., lymphedema therapy)			
Reinforces disease surveillance and follow-up recommendations			
Assesses patient for symptoms of recurrent disease			
Checks appropriate laboratory and diagnostic data			
Evaluates and documents response to therapy			
Monitors patient's psychological status and coping skills			
Instructs patient in cancer-specific health promotion strategies, including cancer prevention and early detection measures			
Instructs patient in general health promotion strategies and those specific to increased risk for diseases associated with RT			
Provides resources regarding legal protections for employment and health care			
Offers formal treatment summaries and survivorship care plans			
Nursing Role During Palliative RT and End-of-Life Care			
Facilitates determination of goals of care			
Facilitates optimal pain and symptom management			
Initiates supportive care referrals to maximize function and quality of life and appropriate setting for skilled care as needed (e.g., physical therapy/occupational therapy for assistive devices, hospice)			
Initiates social work referral to address concrete services (e.g., financial concerns, advance directives, wills) and psychosocial support (grief and bereavement)			

References

Bruner, D.W., & Movsas, B. (2001). Role of the multidisciplinary team in radiation therapy. In D.W. Bruner, G. Moore-Higgs, & M. Haas (Eds.), *Outcomes in radiation therapy: Multidisciplinary management* (pp. 25–51). Sudbury, MA: Jones and Bartlett.

Haas, M.L. (2004). Utilizing geriatric skills in radiation oncology. *Geriatric Nursing, 25,* 355–360. doi:10.1016/j.gerinurse.2004.09.001

Hewitt, M., Greenfield, S., & Stovall, E. (Eds.). (2006). *From cancer patient to cancer survivor: Lost in transition* (Institute of Medicine report). Washington, DC: National Academies Press.

Oncology Nursing Certification Corporation. (2009). *A role delineation study of the radiation therapy nurse.* Pittsburgh, PA: Author.

Pituskin, E., Fairchild, A., Dutka, J., Gagnon, L., Driga, A., Tachynski, P., … Ghosh, S. (2010). Multidisciplinary team contributions within a dedicated outpatient palliative radiotherapy clinic: A prospective descriptive study. *International Journal of Radiation Oncology, Biology, Physics, 78,* 527–532. doi:10.1016/j.ijrobp.2009.07.1698

II. The practice of radiation oncology

A. Principles of radiation therapy
1. Definition of RT
   a) RT is the use of high-energy x-rays or other radiation particles to treat malignant and some benign diseases.
   b) Radiation with sufficient energy to disrupt atomic structures by ejecting orbital electrons is called *ionizing radiation* (Khan, 2003).
2. Types of ionizing radiation commonly used in treatment (see Figure 4)
   a) Electromagnetic radiation: X-rays and gamma rays have the same characteristics but differ in origin.
      (1) X-rays: Photons (i.e., "packets" of energy generated from an electrical machine, such as a linear accelerator)
      (2) Gamma rays: Photons emitted from the nucleus of a radioactive source (e.g., ^{60}Co, ^{137}Cs, ^{192}Ir)
   b) Particulate radiation: Consists of particles, including alpha particles, electrons, protons, and neutrons
      (1) Alpha particles: Large, positively charged particles with poor penetrating ability; emitted during disintegration (i.e., decay) of some radioactive sources (e.g., radium); have a mass approximately 8,000 times that of an electron
      (2) Electrons: Small, negatively charged particles accelerated to high energies by an electrical machine
      (3) Beta particles: Electrons emitted during disintegration of radioactive sources

      (4) Protons: Large, positively charged particles that may be generated by an electrical machine; have a mass approximately 2,000 times that of an electron
      (5) Neutrons: Large, uncharged particles that may be generated by a large machine (e.g., cyclotron)
3. Sources of radiation for treatment (see Figure 4) (Van Dyk, 1999)
   a) Megavoltage machines: Treatment machines used for external beam RT (EBRT) or teletherapy (treatment from a distance)
      (1) Linear accelerator: Machine that generates ionizing radiation from electricity. These machines are commissioned to treat with high-energy (1–50 MeV [megaelectron volts]) x-rays (intermediate to deep penetration and low to moderate skin dose) or (1–50 MeV) electrons (shallow penetration and high skin dose). The depth of treatment varies with energy and type of radiation. Linear accelerators may have multiple energies of both x-rays and electrons so that various depths of treatment may be selected.
      (2) ^{60}Co machine: Radioactive source (^{60}Co) emission of gamma rays; treatment depth is comparable to a 4 megavolt (MV) x-ray beam (intermediate penetration).
      (3) Cyclotron: Large, electrically powered machine that produces neutrons (large particles) or protons
   b) Radionuclides: Radioactive sources that emit radiation in the form of alpha particles, beta particles, gamma rays, or a combination; each radionuclide emits particles

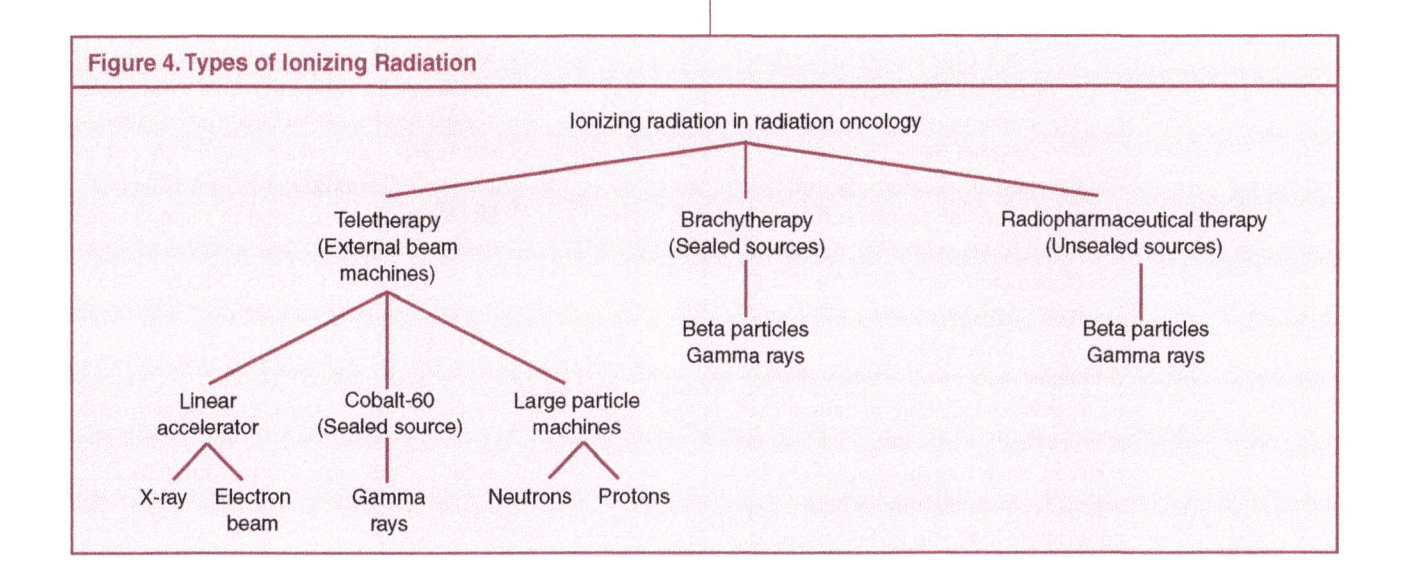

Figure 4. Types of Ionizing Radiation

Ionizing radiation in radiation oncology

- Teletherapy (External beam machines)
  - Linear accelerator
    - X-ray
    - Electron beam
  - Cobalt-60 (Sealed source)
    - Gamma rays
  - Large particle machines
    - Neutrons
    - Protons
- Brachytherapy (Sealed sources)
  - Beta particles
  - Gamma rays
- Radiopharmaceutical therapy (Unsealed sources)
  - Beta particles
  - Gamma rays

or rays with energies that are characteristic of that specific radionuclide.

(1) Brachytherapy (internal radiation): Therapy performed by placing radioactive material in or near the treatment volume. Sources are placed directly into (interstitial) or adjacent to (intracavitary, intraluminal, surface) tumors. Therapy may be administered with solid or liquid radioactive material. Brachytherapy is the therapeutic use of radionuclides that are sealed within metal containers; radioactive particles or rays penetrate the container to treat the disease. Small volumes of normal tissue and cancer can be irradiated to relatively high doses.

(a) Temporary: Sealed radioactive sources (e.g., ^{192}Ir, ^{137}Cs) are removed after the prescribed dose is reached in the calculated number of hours.

   i. High-dose-rate (HDR) treatment: One or several doses are administered and separated by at least six hours. Each dose is administered over a few minutes.

   ii. Low-dose-rate (LDR) treatment: Continuous LDR treatment is administered over several days in a protected lead-shielded room.

(b) Permanent: Sealed radioactive sources are left permanently in the tissue. Sources used for permanent placement (e.g., ^{125}I, ^{198}Au, ^{103}Pd) have relatively short half-lives and weak gamma emissions.

(2) Radiopharmaceutical therapy: Treatment with unsealed liquid radioactive sources that are ingested, injected, or instilled; each radionuclide has characteristics that determine where it can concentrate in the body. For example, oral ^{131}I is used to treat thyroid diseases, and IV ^{89}Sr and ^{153}Sm are used to treat multiple bone metastases.

4. Radioactivity

a) Isotope: The nucleus contains protons and neutrons. The number of protons and neutrons determines which "element." The number of neutrons determines which "isotope." An element may have both stable and radioactive isotopes (Khan, 2003).

b) Nuclei of radioactive elements have excess energy. Radioactive materials (also called radionuclides or radioactive sources/isotopes) decay and emit radiation in the form of alpha and beta particles and gamma rays until they become stable. *Radioactivity*, or *radioactive decay*, is the spontaneous emission (disintegration) of highly energetic particles or rays from the nucleus of an element. Radioactivity is measured in disintegration per second (DPS).

c) *Half-life* is the period of time required for a radioactive substance to lose one-half of its radioactivity through nuclear decay. The spontaneous decay or expulsion of particles and rays from a radionuclide occurs at a characteristic rate for each element.

d) A radioactive element radiates energy that is characteristic of that element. Some radioactive sources emit more penetrating radiation than others and therefore require more shielding to absorb the radiation. Fifty percent of the radioactivity from a source is absorbed by one half-value layer (HVL) of a substance, such as lead.

e) The characteristics of a radionuclide vary with the specific isotope. Table 2 shows the half-life, energy, and HVL of common elements.

5. Measurement of radiation (see Figure 5) (Khan, 2003)

a) Radiation-absorbed dose (rad) is the amount of energy absorbed per unit mass. Radiation previously had been prescribed in rad but is now prescribed in gray (Gy). 1 Gy = 100 centigray (cGy) = 100 rad.

b) Dose equivalent is used in radiation protection. Badge readings have been reported in millirem (mrem). Sievert (Sv) is the international unit for dose equivalent. 100 rem = 1 Sv.

c) Activity of radioactive sources has been measured in millicuries (mCi) and curies (Ci). Becquerel (Bq) is the international unit. Both units are measured as DPS. 1 Ci = 3.7×10^{10} dps. 1 Bq = 1 dps = 2.7×10^{-11} Ci.

Table 2. Characteristics of Radionuclides

Element	Half-Life	Energy	Half-Value Layer[a] (Lead)
Cesium-137 (^{137}Cs)	30 years	0.66 MeV (gamma)	0.65 cm
Cobalt-60 (^{60}Co)	5.2 years	1.25 MeV (gamma)	1.2 cm
Gold-198 ([198]Au)	2.7 days	0.41 MeV (gamma)	0.33 cm
Iodine-125 (^{125}I)	60.2 days	0.02 MeV (gamma)	0.02 cm
Iodine-131 (^{131}I)	8 days	0.36 MeV (gamma)	0.3 cm
Iridium-192 (^{192}Ir)	64.2 days	0.13–1.06 MeV (gamma)	0.6 cm
Radium-226 ([226]Ra)	1,620 years	1 MeV (gamma)	1.66 cm
Strontium-89 (^{89}Sr)	50.5 days	1.46 MeV (beta)	1 mm of lead blocks (100% of ^{89}Sr)

[a] One half-value layer blocks 50% of the radiation.

Note. Based on information from Cember, 1996; St. Germain, 1993a, 1993b.

Figure 5. Units of Measurement for Radiation

- Absorbed dose (gray [Gy], radiation-absorbed dose [rad]) (therapeutic doses)
  1 Gy = 100 rad; 100 centigray (cGy) = 100 rad
- Dose equivalent (sievert [Sv], rem) (radiation protection)
  1 Sv = 100 rem
- Activity (becquerel [Bq], curie [Ci]) (activity of radionuclides)
  1 Bq = 2.7 × 10^{-11} Ci = 1 dps; 1 Ci = 3.7 × 10^{10} dps

B. Radiobiology
1. *Radiobiology* is the study of events that occur after ionizing radiation is absorbed by a living organism. Ionizing radiation can result in breaking of chemical bonds and, eventually, in biologic change (see Figure 6). The nature and severity of effects and the time in which they appear depend on the amount and type of radiation adsorbed and the rate at which it is administered. Early- and late-responding tissues are affected differently by these factors. Interaction of radiation in cells is random and has no selectivity for any structure or site (Hall, 2000).
2. If critical sites are damaged by radiation, the probability of cell death is higher than if a noncritical site is damaged. DNA is considered to be the critical target for radiation damage. Cells can successfully repair much of the damage caused by ionizing radiation (Hall, 2000).
3. Response to ionizing radiation: Damage to DNA may lead to cell alteration or death. All living cells, whether normal or cancerous, are susceptible to the effects of radiation and may

be injured or destroyed by RT. Injury generally is expressed at the time of cell division (reproductive death).
a) Physical stage: Excitation and ionization of atoms or molecules
b) Radiochemical stage: Formation of free radicals, which are highly reactive
c) Biologic stage: Damage to critical target (DNA, which is composed of two strands that form a double helix)
   (1) Single chromosomal strand breaks: These generally are repaired readily and have little biologic consequence (Rossi, 1996). Misrepair (incorrect repair) may result in mutation.
   (2) Double chromosomal strand breaks (DSBs): DSBs are believed to be the most important damage produced in chromosomes by radiation and may result in cell death, mutation, or carcinogenesis. DSBs may activate an oncogene or inactivate a tumor suppressor gene (Hall & Cox, 1994).

Figure 6. Interaction of Ionizing Radiation in Tissue

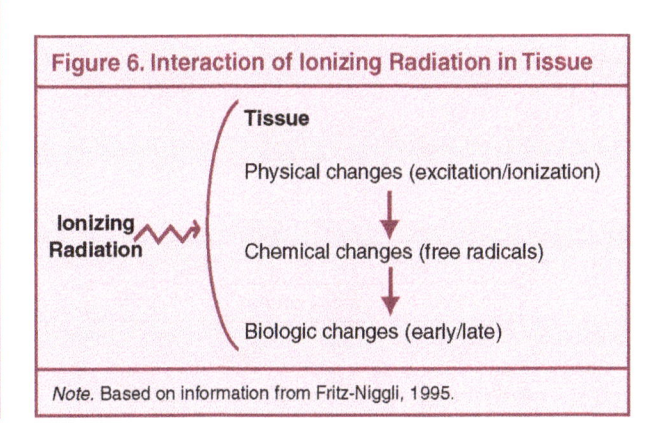

Note. Based on information from Fritz-Niggli, 1995.

4. Potential effects on a single cell in an irradiated volume of tissue (see Figure 7)
   a) No effect or no cell injury occurs in critical target.
   b) Radiation damage to critical target is repaired; cell continues to function and divide.
   c) Radiation damage to critical target is misrepaired, and mutation occurs.
   d) Cell death occurs.
5. Radiation-induced chromosome aberration effects (Bender, 1995; Hall, 1994, 2000; Hall & Cox, 1994)
   a) Cell death induced by radiation
      (1) Chromosome damage may cause reproductive failure (death at the time of cell division).
      (2) Apoptosis (programmed cell death), the process that occurs during normal development of organs and tissues, is enhanced by toxic treatments such as RT (Dewey, Ling, & Meyn, 1995).

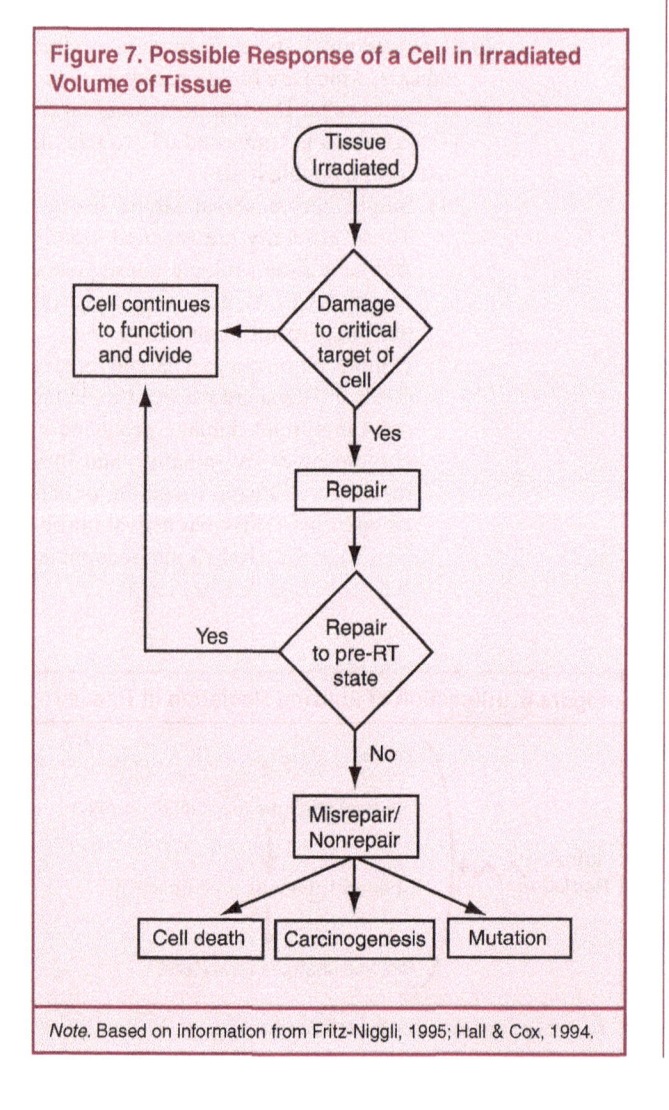

Figure 7. Possible Response of a Cell in Irradiated Volume of Tissue

Tissue Irradiated

Cell continues to function and divide

Damage to critical target of cell

Yes

Repair

Repair to pre-RT state — Yes

No

Misrepair/ Nonrepair

Cell death　Carcinogenesis　Mutation

Note. Based on information from Fritz-Niggli, 1995; Hall & Cox, 1994.

b) Mutation (germ cells): Heritable change in genes expressed in later generations; a large variation in mutation types exists.
c) Carcinogenesis (somatic cells): Chromosome aberration that may cause oncogene activation or suppressor gene loss (Hall, 1994)
6. *Radiosensitivity* is the innate sensitivity of cells, tissues, or tumors to radiation. Both normal and cancer cells are affected by radiation. Cells vary in their expressed sensitivity to radiation. Generally, rapidly dividing cells (e.g., mucosa) are most sensitive and are referred to as *radiosensitive*. Nondividing or slowly dividing cells (e.g., muscle cells, neurons) generally are less radiosensitive, or are *radioresistant*. Exceptions include small lymphocytes and salivary gland cells, which are nondividing but very radiosensitive. These may experience an interphase death (death prior to mitosis).
   a) Manifestations of radiation effects occur at different times for different tissues (Hall & Cox, 1994).
      (1) Acutely responding tissues demonstrate effects in hours to days and include the bone marrow, ovaries, testes, lymph nodes, salivary glands, small bowel, stomach, colon, oral mucosa, larynx, esophagus, arterioles, skin, bladder, capillaries, and vagina.
      (2) Subacutely responding tissues demonstrate effects in weeks to several months after RT and include the lungs, liver, kidneys, heart, spinal cord, and brain.
      (3) Late-responding tissues, including the lymph vessels, thyroid, pituitary gland, breasts, bones, cartilage, pancreas (endocrine), uterus, and bile ducts, rarely show acute effects and demonstrate effects months to years after RT.
   b) Factors that influence radiation sensitivity (Fritz-Niggli, 1995; Hall & Cox, 1994)
      (1) Cell cycle phase: Cells in the late G_2 and mitosis (M) phases are more sensitive. Cells in the late synthesis (S) phase are most resistant to radiation.
      (2) Oxygen: The presence of oxygen enhances radiation damage. When oxygen is not present, chemical damage in DNA may be repaired. Reoxygenation occurs as the tumor shrinks during RT, and previously hypoxic cells become better oxygenated. Hypoxia may contribute to radioresistance.
      (3) Differentiation: Poorly differentiated tumors generally are more sensitive. Far more radiation is required to destroy the function of a differentiat-

ed cell than to destroy a dividing cell (Hall, 2000). However, poor differentiation of a tumor is associated with a poor disease-free survival rate, perhaps because of a more aggressive natural history (Bentzen, 1993).

(4) Proliferative capacity: Rapidly dividing cells generally are more sensitive to the effects of radiation. Nondividing or slowly dividing cells usually are less sensitive, or are radioresistant.

(5) Repair of radiation damage: The greater the repair capability of the normal tissue, the greater the effectiveness of the treatment. DNA damage can be repaired to its original state or misrepaired with errors (mutation). Most repairs are believed to occur within six hours after a treatment.

(6) Tumor size: Tumor size is a major factor in dose-response outcomes of RT. Larger tumors generally are more difficult to control than small tumors of the same type. Control of large tumor masses may require a radiation dose that would result in unacceptable damage to normal tissue. Often, the tumor bulk indicates a poorly oxygenated mass that is less radiosensitive.

(7) Fractionation: This is the division of a total prescribed dose into smaller daily doses, or *fractions*. Daily fractions generally are 1.8–2 Gy. Fraction size is the dominant factor in determining late effects on tissue, with large fractions causing an increase in late effects (Hall, 2000). Fractionation varies depending on goal of therapy.

(a) Hyperfractionation: Multiple daily fractions (e.g., 1.2 Gy twice a day) are delivered, generally separated by at least six hours to allow for repair of damage to the normal tissues from the first dose before administration of the second dose. The intent is to decrease late effects while achieving equal or improved tumor control and equal or only slightly increased early effects. A higher total physical dose is administered.

(b) Hypofractionation: The total dose of radiation is divided into large doses, and treatments may be given less than once a day. Also called hypofractionated RT. A lower total physical dose is administered,

but a higher biologically equivalent dose is expected because of the larger fractional doses. Hypofractionation may have high potential for therapeutic gain as well as economic and logistic advantages for some tumors (e.g., RT for prostate cancer has been extensively investigated), but it may lead to increased late effects for surrounding normal tissues.

(8) Quality of radiation: Energy of various types of radiation is distributed differently in tissues. Heavy particles (e.g., neutrons, alpha particles) ionize densely and quickly; light particles (e.g., electrons) ionize sparsely in tissues.

(a) *Linear energy transfer* (LET) is the distribution of energy along the ionization track in irradiated material. High LET radiation is densely ionizing and is less influenced by the presence of oxygen (i.e., more effective on hypoxic cells than low LET radiation) and the cell cycle phase. Less repair occurs with high LET radiation. Low LET radiation is sparsely ionizing.

(b) Relative biologic effectiveness of a radiation type is dependent on LET. High LET radiation is more biologically damaging than low LET radiation.

7. Effect of radiation on normal cells versus cancer cells (Hall & Cox, 1994)

a) Although both normal cells and cancer cells are affected by radiation and respond similarly to RT, only cancer cells are believed to undergo reoxygenation.

b) Malignant tumors differ greatly in radiosensitivity because of innate sensitivity, mitotic activity, hypoxic component, and blood supply.

c) Dividing a dose into multiple daily fractions spares normal tissues because of damage repair between fractions and repopulation of cells if overall time is sufficient. Dose fractionation increases damage to cancer cells because of reoxygenation of the tumor and reassortment of cancer cells into more sensitive phases of the cell cycle.

d) Side effects are the result of radiation damage to normal cells.

8. Biomarkers for RT: A *biomarker*, or *biologic marker*, is a substance used as an indicator of a biologic state. It is a characteristic that is objectively measured and evaluated as an in-

dicator of normal biologic processes, pathogenic processes, or radiobiologic responses to RT treatments. Research is being conducted on biomarkers for tumor/tissue response and treatment assessment in predictive radiation oncology (Riesterer, Milas, & Ang, 2007).

C. Dose prescription, treatment planning, and simulation
1. Specification of dose and volume: The method of writing and interpreting a prescription is essential to the success of treatment.
   a) The International Commission on Radiation Units and Measurements (ICRU) Report 50 (ICRU, 1993) definition of the treatment volume is separated into three distinct boundaries: (a) visible tumor, (b) a region to account for uncertainties in microscopic tumor spread, and (c) a region to account for positional uncertainties. These boundaries create three volumes (see Figure 8).
      (1) Gross target volume, or GTV: This is the gross extent of the malignant growth as determined by palpation or an imaging study.
      (2) Clinical target volume, or CTV: This is the tissue volume that contains the GTV and/or subclinical microscopic malignant disease.
      (3) Planning target volume, or PTV: This volume is defined by specifying the mar-
      gins that must be added around the CTV to compensate for the effects of organ, tumor, and patient movements and inaccuracies in beam and patient setup.
   b) ICRU (1993) also defined two other dose volumes.
      (1) Treated volume: This is the volume enclosed by an isodose surface that is selected and specified by the radiation oncologist as being appropriate to achieve the purpose of treatment (e.g., 95% isodose surface).
      (2) Irradiated volume: This is the volume that receives a dose significant in relation to normal tissue tolerance (e.g., 50% isodose surface).
   c) *Organs at risk*, or OARs, are defined as normal tissues whose radiation sensitivity may significantly influence treatment planning or prescribed dose (e.g., rectum and bladder for prostate treatment).
   d) ICRU (1993) defined a series of doses including the minimum, maximum, and mean dose for dose reporting purposes. Additionally, an ICRU reference dose is defined at the ICRU reference point. The ICRU reference point is chosen based on the following criteria: it must be clinically relevant, be defined in an unambiguous way, and be located where the dose can be accurately determined (not in a region with steep dose gradients). In general, this point should be in the central part of the PTV.
   e) Dose-volume histograms (DVHs) play an essential role in evaluating and reporting three-dimensional RT dose distributions.
      (1) A cumulative DVH plots the fraction of a structure receiving at least a specified dose against the specified dose.
      (2) A differential DVH plots the fraction of a structure receiving a dose within a specified interval against the dose.
2. Treatment planning: RT is a complex procedure that requires comprehensive treatment planning and quality assurance (QA). Treatment planning entails interactions among the radiation physicists, dosimetrists, radiation oncologists, residents (if available on the team), and radiation therapists and the use of a large number of software programs and hardware devices for geometric and dosimetric planning and QA. The following are the steps in the treatment planning process (Fraass et al., 1998; Kutcher et al., 1994).
   a) Patient positioning and immobilization to ensure a consistent position during the course of imaging and treatment

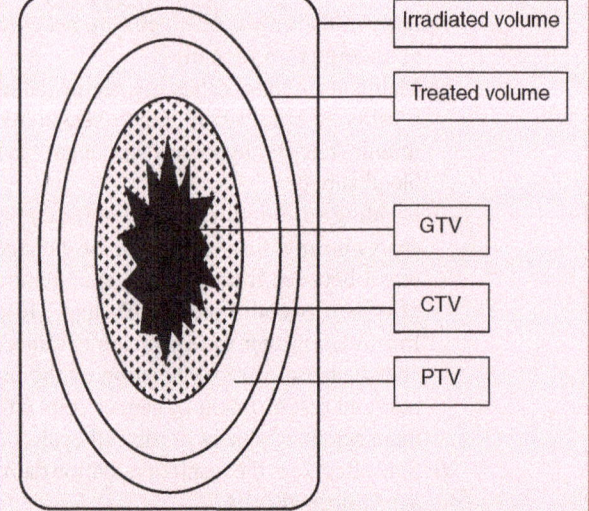

Figure 8. Schematic Illustration of the Boundaries of Tumor Volumes*

Irradiated volume

Treated volume

GTV

CTV

PTV

* As defined by International Commission on Radiation Units and Measurements (1993) Report 50

CTV—clinical target volume; GTV—gross tumor volume; PTV—planning target volume

b) Patient data acquisition (computed tomography [CT], magnetic resonance imaging [MRI], positron-emission tomography [PET], manual contouring)

c) Data transfer to treatment planning system

d) Definition of treatment volumes and OARs

e) Treatment design (modality, beam arrangements, modifiers)

f) Computation of dose distributions

g) Plan evaluation (review of isodose distributions, DVHs, or other physical or biologic dosimetric parameters)

h) Computation of monitor units or minutes based on the prescribed dose

i) Production of blocks and beam modifiers

j) Plan implementation (treatment simulation, data transfer to record and verify system)

k) Patient-specific treatment planning QA (review the plan, chart, monitor unit calculation, and port film, and perform additional calculations or measurements to verify the dose)

3. Simulation: This is the process of aiming and defining the radiation beams to meet the goals of the prescribed therapy. It is mainly concerned with geometric aspects of a treatment, such as the orientation of beams, their sizes, the placement of field-shaping blocks, and the placement of marks on the patient to allow for reliable reproduction of treatment geometry from day to day. Unforeseeable problems with a patient setup or treatment technique also can be solved during simulation.

a) A *treatment simulator* is an apparatus that uses a diagnostic x-ray tube but duplicates a radiation treatment unit in terms of its geometrical, mechanical, and optical properties.

b) By radiographic visualization of internal organs, correct positioning of fields and shielding blocks can be obtained in relation to external landmarks (Farmer, Fowler, & Haggith, 1963; Greene, Nelson, & Gibb, 1964; Van Dyk, 1999).

c) A *virtual simulator* is a piece of software that performs treatment simulation based on a digital representation of the patient derived from serial CT or other tomographic images (Sherouse, Mosher, Novins, Rosenma, & Chaney, 1987).

4. Three-dimensional conformal RT (3DCRT): The goal of 3DCRT is to conform the spatial distribution of the prescribed radiation dose to the precise three-dimensional configuration of the treatment volume while at the same time minimizing the dose to the surrounding normal tissues (Smith & Purdy, 1991).

a) A three-dimensional treatment planning system (3DTPS) is needed to plan a radiation treatment based on the three-dimensional treatment volume. A 3DTPS generally is characterized by acquisition of three-dimensional patient data, delineation of treatment portals based on a beam's eye view projection of the PTV, calculation of dose in three-dimensional patient geometry, and display of dosimetric information in volumes.

b) 3DCRT is commonly delivered with megavoltage photon and electron beams using multileaf collimators (MLCs) or custom-designed blocks (cutouts) to shape uniform open fields (to match the beam's eye view projection of the PTV) or using wedges or custom-designed compensators to account for the effect of surface irregularities and internal heterogeneities (to achieve uniform dose at a selected treatment depth, usually through the middle of the target volume).

5. Intensity-modulated RT (IMRT): IMRT is an advanced form of 3DCRT in which varying intensities (i.e., weights) of small subdivisions of beams (i.e., beamlets, field segments) are used to custom-design optimal radiation dose distributions (Webb, 2001). Because of the conformal dose distributions and steep dose gradients that can be achieved with IMRT, requirements for patient immobilization, target and structure delineation, treatment planning, beam delivery, and dose verification are more stringent (Boyer et al., 2000; Ma et al., 2000, 2003).

a) Special treatment planning software is needed to optimize the weights of individual beamlets (or field segments) via inverse planning (Bortfeld, Bürkelbach, Boesecke, & Schlegel, 1990; Brahme, 1988; Webb, 1992) or forward planning (Galvin, Croce, & Bednarz, 2000; Xiao, Galvin, Hossain, & Valicenti, 2000) to achieve superior target coverage and normal tissue sparing based on the specified dose requirements for the treatment volumes and dose constraints on the OARs.

b) IMRT fields are commonly delivered using a computer-controlled MLC (Convery & Rosenbloom, 1992; Ma, Boyer, Xing, & Ma, 1998; Spirou & Chui, 1994). However, beam intensity modulation also can be achieved using complex physical compensators.

c) IMRT is time- and resource-intensive. Adequate time to perform reviews and quality checks is essential. Therefore, as noted by Moran et al. (2011), "Team members need to acknowledge that initiation of [IMRT] treatment may need to be delayed to allow time for necessary quality assur-

ance checks and subsequent investigations of problems" (p. 195).

6. Image-guided radiation therapy (IGRT): IGRT is an advanced radiation treatment technique that uses imaging technology during treatment to ensure tumor location and beam delivery accuracy (Sharpe, Craig, & Moseley, 2007). The goal of IGRT is to decrease radiation dose to normal tissue and/or improve local control and quality of life by dose escalation or hypofractionation. Traditionally, diagnostic imaging technologies such as CT scans, x-rays, ultrasound, gamma cameras, PET scans, and MRI have been used to determine tumor location and size for treatment planning procedures. However, difficulty arises when trying to ensure accuracy of the beam delivery because many body parts may have moved from the time the original images were taken (e.g., bladder fullness, etc.). IGRT systems allow for frequent two- or three-dimensional imaging to correlate the actual tumor position with the radiation treatment plan to ensure accurate target dose delivery.

D. Purpose of radiation therapy
1. RT is used to treat local or regional disease and, rarely, systemic disease. The aim is to destroy malignant cells in the treated volume of tissue while minimizing damage to normal tissues.
2. RT can be selected for various purposes (Haas & Kuehn, 2001).
    a) Definitive treatment: RT is prescribed as the primary treatment modality, with or without chemotherapy, for the treatment of cancer. Examples can include cancers of the head and neck, lung, prostate, or bladder or Hodgkin lymphoma.
    b) Neoadjuvant treatment: RT is prescribed prior to definitive treatment, usually surgery, to improve the chance of successful resection. Examples include esophageal or colon cancers.
    c) Adjuvant treatment: RT is given after definitive treatment (either surgery or che-

motherapy) to improve local control. Examples may include breast, lung, or high-risk rectal cancers.
    d) Prophylaxis therapy: RT is delivered to asymptomatic, high-risk areas to prevent growth of cancer. Examples are prophylactic cranial irradiation in lung cancer or central nervous system (CNS) cancers to prevent relapse of certain forms of leukemia.
    e) Control: RT is given to limit the growth of cancer cells to extend the symptom-free interval for the patient. Examples may include pancreatic or lung cancers.
    f) Palliation: RT is given to manage symptoms of bleeding, pain, airway obstruction, or neurologic compromise to alleviate life-threatening problems in incurable illness or to improve the patient's quality of life. Examples may include relieving spinal cord compression, opening airways in patients with pneumonia, or relieving pain from bone metastases.

E. Tissue tolerance dose: The radiation dose to which a normal tissue can be irradiated and continue to function (see Table 3)
1. Organs vary in their ability to tolerate radiation injury. Normal tissue tolerance to radiation depends on the ability of the dividing cells to produce enough mature cells to maintain function of the organ. The tolerance dose is the dose of radiation that results in an acceptable probability of a treatment complication (Hall, 2000).
2. The dose prescribed to eradicate a cancer ultimately is dependent on the normal tissue tolerance of the dose.

F. Factors related to radiation-induced injury of normal tissue (Bentzen & Overgaard, 1994)
1. Patient-related factors
    a) Age
        (1) In children: Growth-related factors (e.g., growth retardation, endocrine changes)
        (2) In adults: Limited data available
    b) Hemoglobin level
        (1) Low hemoglobin has been found to decrease local control probability in cancers such as squamous cell carcinoma of the head and neck (Fein et al., 1995; Regueiro et al., 1995), carcinoma of the cervix (Werner-Wasik et al., 1995), and transitional carcinoma of the bladder (Cole et al., 1995).
        (2) Little information is available concerning hemoglobin level related to normal tissue reactions.

Table 3. Minimal and Maximal Tissue Tolerance to Radiation Therapy Dose

Tissue	Dose-Related Injury	Minimal Tolerance Dose TD 5/5[a] (Gy)	Maximal Tolerance Dose TD 50/5[b] (Gy)	Amount of Tissue Treated (Field Size or Length)
Bone marrow	Aplasia, pancytopenia	2.5	4.5	Whole
		30	40	Segmental
Brain	Infarction, necrosis	60	70	Whole
Eye	Blindness			
	Retina	55	70	Whole
	Cornea	50	> 60	Whole
	Lens	5	12	Whole
Fetus	Death	2	4	Whole
Heart	Pericarditis,	45	55	60%
	pancarditis	70	80	25%
Intestine	Perforation, ulcer,	45	55	400 cm²
	hemorrhage	50	65	100 cm²
Kidney	Acute and chronic	15	20	Whole (strip)
	nephrosclerosis	20	25	Whole
Liver	Acute and chronic	25	40	Whole
	hepatitis	15	20	Whole (strip)
Lung	Acute and chronic	30	35	100 cm²
	pneumonitis	15	25	Whole
Spinal cord	Infarction, necrosis	45	55	10 cm
Stomach	Perforation, ulcer, hemorrhage	45	55	100 cm²
Uterus	Necrosis, perforation	> 10	> 200	Whole
Vagina	Ulcer, fistula	90	> 100	Whole

[a] TD 5/5 = minimal tolerance dose; the dose, given to a population of patients under a standard set of treatment conditions, that will result in no more than a 5% rate of severe complications within five years after treatment.

[b] TD 50/5 = maximal tolerance dose; the dose, given to a population of patients under a standard set of treatment conditions, that will result in a 50% rate of severe complications within five years after treatment.

Note. Based on information from Bentel et al., 1989; Rubin et al., 1975.

c) Smoking: Can enhance some early and late side effects (Bentzen & Overgaard, 1994)

d) Tumor invasion: May interfere with normal tissue reactions

e) Infections: May increase normal tissue injury, especially when the immune system is compromised

2. Intrinsic radiosensitivity

a) Genetic syndromes: Some are associated with increased sensitivity to RT (e.g., ataxia telangiectasia).

b) Autoimmune diseases (e.g., systemic lupus erythematosus)

G. Considerations for radiation therapy

1. Diagnosis and staging: Tumor histology and extent of disease

2. General condition of the patient and comorbid conditions

3. Tumor site: Whether normal tissues are included in treatment fields

4. Combination therapy (e.g., chemotherapy, hyperthermia, immunotherapy, biotherapy): The goal is to improve the therapeutic ratio relative to the use of a single modality of treatment (Hall & Cox, 1994).

5. Available treatment facilities

H. Radioresponsiveness of normal tissue (see Figure 9)

1. Expression of normal tissue injury varies greatly from patient to patient.

2. Response of a tissue or organ primarily depends on the radiosensitivity of the cells and the

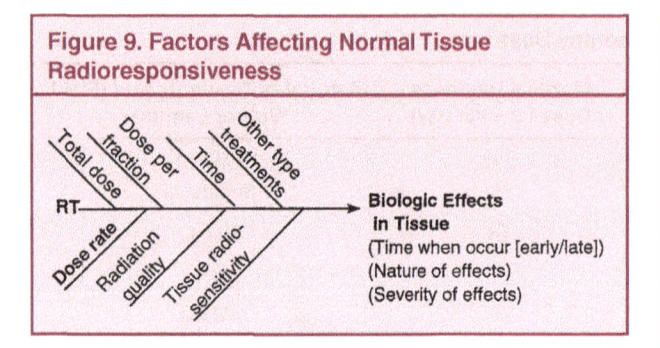

Figure 9. Factors Affecting Normal Tissue Radioresponsiveness

kinetics of the population in which the cells are functioning.

3. Treatment characteristics include total dose, dose per fraction or dose rate, and overall treatment time.
4. With combined-modality therapy (e.g., sequential or concomitant chemotherapy), interactions may substantially influence side effects of RT.

I. Side effects
1. Early side effects
   a) Occur during or immediately after RT
   b) Depend on total dose, dose per fraction, and overall treatment time (Bentzen, 1993)
   c) Do not predict for late side effects
2. Late side effects
   a) Occur months to years after RT and usually are the result of damage to the microcirculation
   b) Depend highly on dose per fraction. High dose per fraction results in more severe late effects.
   c) The time from RT to a specific late effect is the *latent period.*
   d) Late injury expression is time dependent. The severity and percentage of patients expressing the injury increase over time (Bentzen, 1993).

References

Bender, M.A. (1995). Cytogenetics research in radiation biology. *Stem Cells, 13*(Suppl. 1), 172–181.

Bentel, G.C., Nelson, C.E., & Noell, K.T. (1989). *Treatment planning and dose calculation in radiation oncology* (4th ed.). New York, NY: Pergamon Press.

Bentzen, S.M. (1993). Quantitative clinical radiobiology. *Acta Oncologica, 32,* 259–275.

Bentzen, S.M., & Overgaard, J. (1994). Patient-to-patient variability in the expression of radiation-induced normal tissue injury. *Seminars in Radiation Oncology, 4,* 68–80. doi:10.1053/SRAO00400068

Bortfeld, T., Bürkelbach, J., Boesecke, R., & Schlegel, W. (1990). Methods of image reconstruction from projections applied to conformation radiotherapy. *Physics in Medicine and Biology, 35,* 1423–1434. doi:10.1088/0031-9155/35/10/007

Boyer, A.L., Mok, E., Luxton, G., Findley, D., Chen, Y., Pawlicki, T., ... Xia, P. (2000). Quality assurance for treatment planning dose delivery by 3DCRT and IMRT. In A.S. Shiu & D.E. Mellenberg (Eds.), *General practice of radiation oncology physics in the 21st century* (pp. 187–230). Madison, WI: Medical Physics Publishing.

Brahme, A. (1988). Optimization of stationary and moving beam radiation therapy techniques. *Radiotherapy and Oncology, 12,* 129–140.

Cember, H. (1996). *Introduction to health physics* (3rd ed.). New York, NY: McGraw-Hill.

Cole, C.J., Pollack, A., Zagars, G.K., Dinney, C.P., Swanson, D.A., & von-Eschenbach, A.C. (1995). Local control of muscle-invasive bladder cancer: Preoperative radiotherapy and cystectomy versus cystectomy alone. *International Journal of Radiation Oncology, Biology, Physics, 32,* 331–340. doi:10.1016/0360-3016(95)00086-E

Convery, D.J., & Rosenbloom, M.E. (1992). The generation of intensity-modulated fields for conformal radiotherapy by dynamic collimation. *Physics in Medicine and Biology, 37,* 1359–1374. doi:10.1088/0031-9155/37/6/012

Dewey, W.C., Ling, C.C., & Meyn, R.E. (1995). Radiation-induced apoptosis: Relevance to radiotherapy. *International Journal of Radiation Oncology, Biology, Physics, 33,* 781–796. doi:10.1016/0360-3016(95)00214-8

Farmer, F.T., Fowler, J.F., & Haggith, J.W. (1963). Megavoltage treatment planning and the use of xeroradiography. *British Journal of Radiology, 36,* 426–435.

Fein, D.A., Lee, W.R., Hanlon, A.L., Ridge, J.A., Langer, C.J., Curran, W.J., Jr., & Coia, L.R. (1995). Pretreatment hemoglobin level influences local control and survival of T1–T2 squamous cell carcinomas of the glottic larynx. *Journal of Clinical Oncology, 13,* 2077–2083.

Fraass, B., Doppke, K., Hunt, M., Kutcher, G., Starkschall, G., Stern, R., & Van Dyke, J. (1998). American Association of Physicists in Medicine Radiation Therapy Committee Task Group 53: Quality assurance for clinical radiotherapy treatment planning. *Medical Physics, 25,* 1773–1829.

Fritz-Niggli, H. (1995). 100 years of radiobiology: Implications for biomedicine and future perspectives. *Cellular and Molecular Life Sciences, 51,* 652–664. doi:10.1007/BF01941263

Galvin, J.M., Croce, R., & Bednarz, G. (2000). Advanced forward planning techniques or forward planning is alive and well in the IMRT world. In A.S. Shiu & D.E. Mellenberg (Eds.), *General practice of radiation oncology physics in the 21st century* (pp. 73–100). Madison, WI: Medical Physics Publishing.

Greene, D., Nelson, K.A., & Gibb, R. (1964). The use of a linear accelerator "simulator" in radiotherapy. *British Journal of Radiology, 37,* 394–397.

Haas, M.L., & Kuehn, E.F. (2001). Teletherapy: External radiation therapy. In D.W. Bruner, G. Moore-Higgs, & M.L. Haas (Eds.), *Outcomes in radiation therapy: Multidisciplinary management* (pp. 55–66). Sudbury, MA: Jones and Bartlett.

Hall, E.J. (1994). Molecular biology in radiation therapy: The potential impact of recombinant technology on clinical practice. *International Journal of Radiation Oncology, Biology, Physics, 30,* 1019–1028. doi:10.1016/0360-3016(94)90305-0

Hall, E.J. (2000). *Radiobiology for the radiologist* (5th ed.). Philadelphia, PA: Lippincott Williams & Wilkins.

Hall, E.J., & Cox, J.D. (1994). Physical and biologic basis of radiation therapy. In J.D. Cox (Ed.), *Moss' radiation oncology: Rationale, technique, results* (7th ed., pp. 3–65). St. Louis, MO: Mosby.

International Commission on Radiation Units and Measurements. (1993). *Prescribing, recording, and reporting photon beam therapy* (Report No. 50). Bethesda, MD: Author.

Khan, F.M. (2003). *Physics of radiation therapy* (3rd ed.). Philadelphia, PA: Lippincott Williams & Wilkins.

Kutcher, G.J., Coia, L., Gillin, M., Hanson, W., Leibel, S., Morton, R.J., ... Svensson, G.K. (1994). Comprehensive QA for radiation oncology: Report of AAPM Radiation Therapy Committee Task Group 40. *Medical Physics, 21,* 581–618.

Ma, C.-M., Pawlicki, T., Jiang, S.B., Li, J.S., Deng, J., Mok, E., ... Boyer, A.L. (2000). Monte Carlo verification of IMRT dose distributions from a commercial treatment planning optimization system. *Physics in Medicine and Biology, 45,* 2483–2495. doi:10.1088/0031-9155/45/9/303

Ma, C.-M., Price, R., McNeeley, S., Chen, L., Li, J.S., Wang, L., ... Qin, L. (2003). Clinical implementation and quality assurance for intensity modulated radiation therapy (IAEA-CA-96/120). In *Standards and codes of practice in medical radiation dosimetry: Proceedings of an international symposium held in Vienna, Austria, 25–28 November 2002* (Vol. 2, pp. 369–380). Vienna, Austria: International Atomic Energy Agency.

Ma, L., Boyer, A.L., Xing, L., & Ma, C.-M. (1998). An optimized leaf-setting algorithm for beam intensity modulation using dynamic multileaf collimators. *Physics in Medicine and Biology, 43,* 1629–1643. doi:10.1088/0031-9155/43/6/019

Moran, J.M., Dempsey, M., Eisbruch, A., Fraass, B.A., Galvin, J.M., Ibbott, G.S., & Marks, L.B. (2011). Safety considerations for IMRT: Executive summary. *Practical Radiation Oncology, 1,* 190–195. doi:10.1016/j.prro.2011.04.008

Regueiro, C.A., Millán, I., de la Torre, A., Valcárcel, F.J., Magallón, R., Fernández, E., & Aragón, G. (1995). Influence of boost technique (external beam radiotherapy or brachytherapy) on the outcome of patients with carcinoma of the base of the tongue. *Acta Oncologica, 34,* 225–233.

Riesterer, O., Milas, L., & Ang, K.K. (2007). Use of molecular biomarkers for predicting the response to radiotherapy with or without chemotherapy. *Journal of Clinical Oncology, 25,* 4075–4083. doi:10.1200/JCO.2007.11.8497

Rossi, H.H. (1996). Radiation physics and radiobiology. *Health Physics, 70,* 828–831.

Rubin, P., Cooper, R., & Phillips, T.L. (1975). *Radiation biology and radiation pathology syllabus, set RT 1: Radiation oncology.* Chicago, IL: American College of Radiology.

Sharpe, M.B., Craig, T., & Moseley, D.J. (2007). Image guidance: Treatment target localization systems. *Frontiers of Radiation Therapy and Oncology, 40,* 72–93. doi:10.1159/000106029

Sherouse, G.W., Mosher, C.E., Novins, K.L., Rosenma, K.L., & Chaney, E.L. (1987). Virtual simulation: Concept and implementation. In I.A.D. Bruinvis, P.H. van der Giessen, H.J. van Kleffens, & F.W. Wittkamper (Eds.), *Ninth international conference on the use of computers in radiation therapy* (pp. 433–436). Scheveningen, Netherlands: NorthHollan Publishing.

Smith, A.R., & Purdy, J.A. (Eds.). (1991). *Three-dimensional photon treatment planning. Report of the Collaborative Working Group on the Evaluation of Treatment Planning for External Photon Beam Radiotherapy.* New York, NY: Pergamon Press.

Spirou, S.V., & Chui, C.S. (1994). Generation of arbitrary intensity profiles by dynamic jaws and multileaf collimators. *Medical Physics, 21,* 1031–1041.

St. Germain, J. (1993a). External monitoring within a medical environment. In G.G. Eichholz & J.J. Shonka (Eds.), *Hospital health physics: Proceedings of the 1993 Health Physics Society Summer School* (pp. 103–118). Richland, WA: Health Physics Society.

St. Germain, J. (1993b). Personnel protection in medicine. In G.G. Eichholz & J.J. Shonka (Eds.), *Hospital health physics: Proceedings of the 1993 Health Physics Society Summer School* (pp. 91–102). Richland, WA: Health Physics Society.

Van Dyk, J. (1999). *The modern technology of radiation oncology: A compendium for medical physicists and radiation oncologists.* Madison, WI: Medical Physics Publishing.

Webb, S. (1992). Optimization by simulated annealing of three-dimensional, conformal treatment planning for radiation fields defined by multileaf collimator: II. Inclusion of two-dimensional modulation of the x-ray intensity. *Physics in Medicine and Biology, 37,* 1689–1704. doi:10.1088/0031-9155/37/8/005

Webb, S. (2001). *Intensity-modulated radiation therapy.* Philadelphia, PA: Institute of Physics Publishing.

Werner-Wasik, M., Schmid, C.H., Bornstein, L., Ball, H.G., Smith, D.M., & Madoc-Jones, H. (1995). Prognostic factors for local and distant recurrences in stage I and II cervical carcinoma. *International Journal of Radiation Oncology, Biology, Physics, 32,* 1309–1317. doi:10.1016/0360-3016(94)00613-P

Xiao, Y., Galvin, J., Hossain, M., & Valicenti, R. (2000). An optimized forward planning technique for intensity modulated radiation therapy. *Medical Physics, 27,* 2093–2099.

III. Radiation protection and safety

A. Importance of knowing specific information regarding radiation protection regulations, principles, and practices
   1. Helps nurses avoid unnecessary radiation exposure
   2. Allows nurses to focus on the needs of patients receiving radionuclides versus possibly providing hasty care and minimal interaction (McQuestion, 2007)
   3. Allows nurses to adapt radiation safety practices to new therapeutic radionuclide procedures and treatments
   4. Assists nurses in teaching patients, families, and others in healthcare settings about radiation protection practices
   5. Allays possible fears and misconceptions regarding radiation exposure
   6. Helps put radiation exposure risks into perspective with other health risks

B. Purpose of radiation protection regulations (National Council on Radiation Protection and Measurements [NCRP], 1993, 2006).
   1. To prevent clinically significant radiation-induced deterministic effects by keeping exposed healthcare workers and the public at a certain threshold dose
      a) *Deterministic effects* are predictable detrimental health problems that occur in someone exposed to ionizing radiation.
      b) Effects usually are associated with a threshold dose.
      c) Severity of effects increases as dose increases.
      d) Effects are predictable and based on acute, large-dose exposures as seen in historical studies (e.g., atomic war survivors, Chernobyl nuclear power plant workers, individuals treated with RT decades ago for benign diseases) (Martin, Sutton, West, & Wright, 2009).
      e) A small group of deterministic effects appear beyond acute period (e.g., radiation-induced cataracts in occupational exposure and TBI).
      f) Acute, large-dose effects are rare in occupational exposure but can occur with major mishandling of radionuclide source, equipment problems, or nuclear power plant disasters.
   2. To limit the risk of stochastic effects to a reasonable level in relation to societal needs, values, and economic factors
      a) *Stochastic effects* are detrimental health effects that can occur in someone from low-level, long-term exposure to ionizing radiation.
      b) Effects occur regardless of total dose or threshold dose.
      c) Risk of effects is based on the linear no-threshold model, a statistical model that suggests that any increase in radiation exposure dose leads to an incremental increase in risk. Although the acceptance of this model has been heavily debated in the radiation protection scientific community, most recent reviews by NCRP and other scientific consensus panels hold this model to be true (Martin et al., 2009; NCRP, 2006).
      d) Main effect from exposure to low-dose radiation exposure is cancer (Martin et al., 2009).
      e) Leukemia and most solid cancers have been linked with radiation (Gilbert, 2009).
      f) Offspring of exposed individuals can have genetic effects as well.
      g) Several factors can influence cancer induction. These include age, genetic heritage, gender, and the individual's immune susceptibility.
   3. To keep radiation exposure to individuals or groups at a dose limit that is ALARA
      a) ALARA concept has been present for more than 30 years in radiation protection regulations.
      b) Regulations aim to keep the public and occupational workers safe from deleterious radiation exposure.
   4. To apply individual dose limits to ensure that radiation exposure does not result in individuals or groups of individuals exceeding levels of acceptable risk

C. Sources of radiation exposure (NCRP, 2009; Schauer, 2010): Recently, a dramatic shift and increase has occurred in the amounts of ionizing radiation the average person receives from various sources (NCRP, 2009). In the 1980s, natural background radiation represented 83% of an individual's exposure, and medical sources (mostly diagnostic) constituted 18%. By 2006, because of the increased use of diagnostic imaging, natural background radiation decreased to 50%, and medical source radiation increased to 48%.

1. Natural background radiation
    a) Radon, a naturally occurring gas from the soil and other places, is the leading source of natural radiation.
    b) Cosmic radiation exposure depends on the altitude of the geographic area in which the individual lives. Because air is thinner at higher altitudes, less cosmic air is filtered from outer space, and exposures are higher.
    c) Natural sources include very small amounts of radionuclides found in humans from ingesting food and water containing radionuclides, such as potassium-40.
2. Occupational exposure from the nuclear power industry and other industries using ionizing radiation represented 0.1% of public exposure in 2006 versus 0.3% in 1980 (NCRP, 2009).
3. Consumer products (televisions, microwave ovens) represented 4% of public radiation exposure in 2006 versus 2% in 1980.
4. Medical sources: The use of medical radiation sources has increased 600% in the United States since the early 1980s, mostly in the use of CT, interventional fluoroscopy, and nuclear medicine procedures (Schauer, 2010). Because of the dramatic increase in medical radiation exposure, radiation protection organizations and regulators are now focusing on reducing unnecessary radiation exposure. Steps taken to reduce excess medical imaging include advising consumers to keep track of medical imaging procedures and to question the need for these examinations (Amis et al., 2007; U.S. Food and Drug Administration [FDA], 2010).
    a) Diagnostic x-rays from external radiograph studies (general x-rays, including portable x-ray units, fluoroscopy, dental x-rays, CT scans, mammograms). In RT, this includes CT localization scans used in IGRT.
        (1) Fluoroscopy for diagnostic imaging represents the largest source of occupational exposure in medicine because the operator must be present in the examination room and the x-ray tube used may be energized for considerable periods of time.
        (2) General radiography poses little exposure if the operator is protected behind the shielded barrier.
        (3) Radionuclides used in nuclear medicine studies (bone scan, thyroid scan, heart scan, PET scan, radionuclide angiography, lymphoscintigraphy [sentinel lymph node localization])
        (4) Radionuclides used in laboratory departments (in vitro studies on blood, urine, or cells and radioimmunoassay and laboratory research studies that use radionuclides)
    b) Therapeutic sources of radiation
        (1) EBRT (teletherapy) sources (x-rays, gamma rays, electrons, protons, neutrons)
        (2) Because personnel are not permitted inside the treatment room for EBRT, this source represents little exposure risk unless lower-energy contact therapy orthovoltage sources are used and operated by personnel or if inadequate shielding is used for external beam equipment.
        (3) The patient receiving EBRT is not radioactive and poses no exposure risk to personnel, the public, or the family.
    c) Radionuclide sources used in internal RT
        (1) Sealed sources (brachytherapy) (e.g., ^{125}I, ^{192}Ir, ^{137}Cs): Seeds or ribbons placed directly into tissues (interstitial brachytherapy) or applicators in body cavities (intracavitary brachytherapy). Table 4 lists sealed radionuclides and their physical properties.
        (2) Remote afterloading brachytherapy: Radioactive sources (^{192}Ir) with highly specific activity that deliver HDR radiation in a short period of time. The radioactive source is housed in a shielded unit and poses no exposure risk to staff when inserted remotely into patients. It is crucial that proper safeguards and procedures are used to ensure that the radioactive source is returned to the machine. In the past 20 years, use of remote afterloading brachytherapy has increased, especially in the treatment of gynecologic malignancies, sarcomas, and other solid tumors, which has led to a dramatic decrease in radiation exposure to healthcare personnel.
        (3) Unsealed sources (oral, IV, colloidal radiopharmaceutical therapy) (e.g., ^{131}I, ^{89}Sr, ^{153}Sm, ^{90}Y, ^{32}P): Table 5 lists therapeutic radiopharmaceuticals and their physical properties.

Table 4. Physical Properties of Brachytherapy Radionuclides

Radionuclide	Half-Life	Photon Energy (MeV)	Half-Life Layer (mm Pb)	Exposure-Rate Constant[a] Γ_δ (R cm^2 mCi^1 h^1)	Physical Form
^{226}Ra[b]	1,600 y	0.83 (mean)	12	8.25[c]	Tubes, needles
^{222}Rn[b]	3.83 d	0.83 (mean)	12	8.25[c]	Seeds
^{60}Cs	5.25 y	1.25 (mean)	12	13	Plaques, needles
^{137}Cs	30 y	0.662	6.5	3.2	Tubes, needles
^{192}Ir	74.02 d	0.397(β max)	3	4.59	Seeds in ribbons, wires, source on cable
^{125}I	60.14 d	0.028	0.025	1.45	Seeds
^{103}Pd	17 d	0.020	0.008	0.86	Seeds
^{198}Au	2.7 d	0.412	3.3	2.35	Seeds
^{90}S/^{90}Y	28.2 y	2.24 (β max)	N/A[d]	N/A[d]	Plaques
^{241}Am	432 y	0.60	0.12	3.14	Tubes
^{169}Yb	32 d	0.093 (mean)	0.48	3.27	Seeds
^{131}Cs	9.69 d	0.030	0.030	1.24	Seeds
^{145}Sm	340 d	0.043	0.060	0.885	Seeds

[a] This subscript notation δ in Γ_δ is used to denote that the calculated value does not include the contributions of radiations removed (i.e., attenuated by the presence of encapsulating materials).

[b] Listed for historical significance only

[c] 0.5 mm platinum-iridium filtration

[d] N/A = not applicable

Note. From *Management of Radionuclide Therapy Patients* (NCRP Report No. 155, p. 43), by National Council on Radiation Protection and Measurements, 2006, Bethesda, MD: Author. Reprinted with permission of the National Council on Radiation Protection and Measurements, http://NCRPonline.org.

D. Major organizations involved in radiation protection guidelines and standards (although they lack regulatory authority)
1. NCRP (www.ncrp.org), a nongovernmental, nonprofit organization first chartered by the U.S. Congress in 1964
    a) Collects, analyzes, develops, and disseminates information to the public about protection against radiation and radiation measurements, quantities, and units, particularly those concerned with radiation protection
    b) Provides a means by which organizations concerned with the scientific and related aspects of radiation protection and radiation quantities, units, and measurements can cooperate for effective utilization of their combined resources and to stimulate the work of such organizations
    c) Develops basic concepts about radiation quantities, units, and measurements and the applications of these concepts and radiation protection
    d) Cooperates with ICRU and other national and international organizations, governmental and private, concerned with radiation quantities, units, and measurements and radiation protection
    e) Publishes guidelines concerning all aspects of radiation protection for both ionizing and nonionizing radiation exposure. Table 6 lists current NCRP limits of ionizing radiation exposure for radiation workers and the public.
    f) Regulatory agencies in the United States usually adhere to the NCRP guidelines.
2. International Commission on Radiological Protection (ICRP, www.icrp.org)
    a) An independent, registered nonprofit charity established in the United Kingdom to advance the science of radiation protection for the public benefit
    b) Involved with guidance on all aspects of radiation protection
    c) Offers recommendations to regulatory and advisory agencies intended to help manage-

Table 5. Physical Properties of Photon- and Beta-Emitting Radionuclides Commonly Used in Therapeutic Radiopharmaceuticals

Radionuclide	Physical Half-Life	Specific Gamma-Ray Constant[a,b] ($R\ cm^2\ mCi^1\ h^1$)	Maximum Beta-Ray Energy (MeV)	Specific Bremsstrahlung Constant[a,b] ($R\ cm^2\ mCi^1\ h^1$)	
				Soft Tissue $Z_{eff} = 7.9$	Bone (calcium) $Z_{eff} = 21$
Photon- and Beta-Emitters					
[131]I	8.04 d	2.23	0.81	0.000768	0.00204
[177]Lu	6.7 d	0.222		0.000385	0.00102
[153]Sm	47 h	0.712	0.497, 0.44	0.000597	0.0.00159
[186]Re	89 h	0.143	0.8	0.00121	0.00322
[188]Re	17 h	0.320	1.07	0.00154	0.00409
Beta-Emitters					
[32]P	14.3 d	-	1.71	0.00405	0.0108
[33]P	25.4 d	-	0.25	0.000658	0.00175
[89]Sr[c]	50.5 h	-	1.49	0.00314	0.00843
[90]Y	64.1 h	-	2.28	0.00564	0.015

[a] Values for constants from NUREG-1556, Vol. 9 (U.S. NRC, 2005), and for ^{177}Lu only (Unger & Trubey, 1982).

[b] The specific gamma-ray constant is a physical quantity that is expressed in conventional units of $R\ cm^2\ mCi^1\ h^1$. The specific gamma-ray constant and the analogous specific bremsstrahlung are therefore expressed in these conventional units.

[c] Although ^{89}Sr emits a gamma ray, it is grouped with the beta emitters because the frequency of its gamma-ray emissions, < 0.01% per decay, is negligibly low.

Note. From *Management of Radionuclide Therapy Patients* (NCRP Report No. 155, p. 75), by National Council on Radiation Protection and Measurements, 2006, Bethesda, MD: Author. Reprinted with permission of the National Council on Radiation Protection and Measurements, http://NCRPonline.org.

ment and professional staff with responsibilities for radiologic protection

   d) Radiation protection legislation in most countries adheres to ICRP recommendations.

E. Major agencies in the United States and Canada that have regulatory authority concerning medical uses of ionizing radiation

  1. U.S. Nuclear Regulatory Commission (NRC): All NRC regulations are now available online at www.nrc.gov.

   a) Provides direct regulatory authority over the medical use of reactor-produced radionuclides (therapeutic and diagnostic)

   b) Regulates use of by-product materials (materials made radioactive in a reactor)

   c) Regulates the use of radioactive materials used in medicine per the "Standards for Protection Against Radiation" in the *Code of Federal Regulations* (10 CFR Part 20), including requirements for

    (1) Dose limits for radiation workers and the public

    (2) Monitoring and labeling radioactive materials

    (3) Posting specific warning signs in places using radiation sources

    (4) Reporting theft or loss of radioactive materials

    (5) Penalties for noncompliance with NRC regulations

    (6) Tables of individual radionuclide exposure limits.

   d) Issues broad medical licenses to individuals using radionuclides for medical use in hospital and outpatient settings

   e) Specifies what instructions should be given to nursing staff who care for brachytherapy patients according to 10 CFR Part 35

    (1) Size and appearance of the brachytherapy sources

    (2) Safe handling and shielding instructions in case of dislodged sources

    (3) Procedures for visitor control

    (4) Procedures for patient or human research control

Table 6. Recommended Dose Limits

Population	Annual Effective Dose Limit (mSv)
Adult workers	50
Adult worker who declares her pregnancy	0.5 mSv month^{-1}
Members of the public	1
Family member of patient	5
Pregnant women and children	1
Trained and monitored family member of patient	50
Adult lifetime	Age × 10 mSv

Note. From *Management of Radionuclide Therapy Patients* (NCRP Report No. 155, p. 17), by National Council on Radiation Protection and Measurements, 2006, Bethesda, MD: Author. Reprinted with permission of the National Council on Radiation Protection and Measurements, http://NCRPonline.org.

 (5) Procedures for notifying the radiation safety officer (RSO) if the patient has a medical emergency or dies

2. FDA (www.fda.gov)
   a) Regulates the design and manufacture of radiation devices and equipment
   b) Regulates the development of radiopharmaceuticals

3. State radiation commission/agencies
   a) States can be licensed by the NRC or can be classified as agreement states. *Agreement states*, per state law, assign all responsibility for radiation protection to a state agency. Agreement states may require radiation protection practices in addition to the NRC guidelines. Figure 10 shows the current agreement and non-agreement states.
   b) Individual states have their own radiation protection agencies that are responsible for setting state guidelines and enforcing the national standards and guidelines. States also regulate radiation-producing equipment (e.g., linear accelerators). Nurses are encouraged to become familiar with their individual state's radiation regulation programs.

4. Canadian Nuclear Safety Commission (www.cnsc-ccsn.gc.ca)
   a) Regulates nuclear substances and radiation devices to protect the health and safety of Canadians and the environment
   b) Safeguards against loss of nuclear materials

c) Regulates and grants licenses to medical facilities that use radionuclides
d) Establishes exposure dose limits for the public and occupational workers

5. Canadian Radiation Protection Bureau (www.hc-sc.gc.ca)
   a) Manages the National Dose Registry, which contains the occupational radiation dose records of all radiation-monitored workers in Canada
   b) Conducts research on exposure trends for radiation workers and on the health outcomes of occupational exposures to radiation
   c) Provides advice to federal departments and agencies, other levels of government, industry, universities, hospitals, workers, and the public on health issues related to radiation exposure

6. Institutional committees/individuals responsible for radiation protection
   a) Institutional radiation safety program/radiation safety committee
      (1) Designated by hospital/institution administration and authorized by the state and/or NRC to oversee and monitor the radiation protection program of an institution
      (2) Must meet quarterly per year to review the hospital's/institution's radiation protection program and should have a nursing representative
   b) RSO or delegated trained personnel responsibilities (NCRP, 2009).
      (1) Implements and monitors the institution's radiation protection program
      (2) Trains personnel, including nurses, in radiation protection practices, as well as educates patients and families on discharge precautions with certain radionuclide procedures
      (3) Serves as the primary resource person regarding the institutional radiation protection practices/issues
      (4) Monitors radiation doses received by occupationally exposed individuals and the public in and around the medical facility
      (5) Monitors radiation exposure from patients who are receiving internal RT in both inpatient and outpatient settings
      (6) Determines when patients treated with radionuclides can be discharged from radiation isolation
      (7) Responsible for inventory and receipt of radioactive sources
      (8) Responsible for removal of radioactive waste/contamination

Figure 10. U.S. Nuclear Regulatory Commission Agreement States

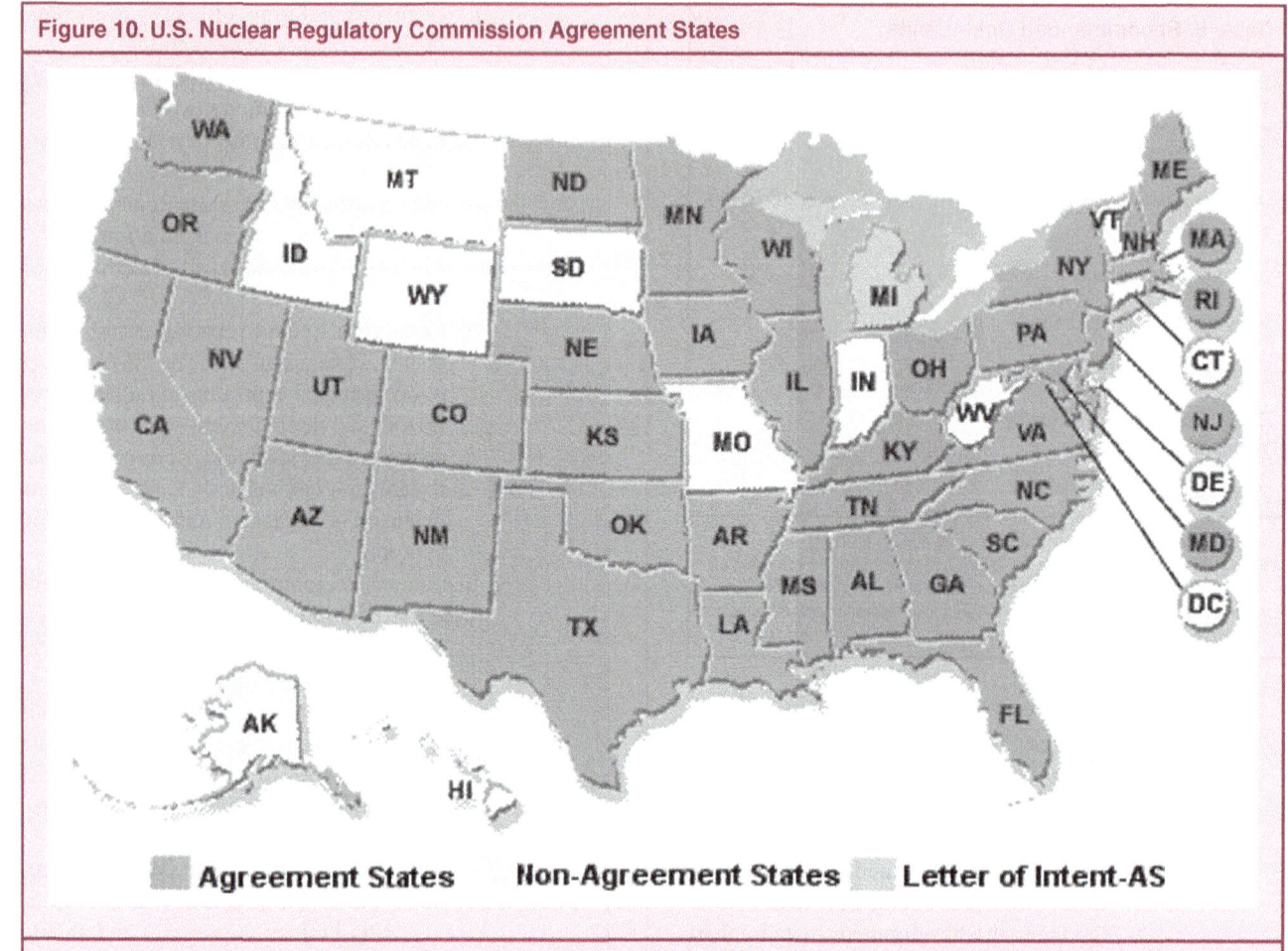

Agreement States   Non-Agreement States   Letter of Intent-AS

Note. From "Directory of Agreement State and Non-Agreement State Directors and State Liaison Officers: Agreement and Non-Agreement States," by the U.S. Nuclear Regulatory Commission, 2011. Retrieved from http://nrc-stp.ornl.gov/asdirectory.html.

F. Radionuclide factors that determine the type and amount of radiation protection practices
1. Type and energy of radiation emission from radionuclide (e.g., alpha, beta, gamma). Radionuclides can give off one or mixed emission spectra depending on the specific radionuclide (Kassis, 2008).
   a) Alpha: Particles of radiation composed of two protons and two neutrons that travel at great speed but have poor penetrating abilities because of their large size
      (1) Have energies ranging from 5 to 9 megaelectron volts (MeV) and travel in straight lines
      (2) Maximum distance is less than 5 cm in air.
      (3) A sheet of paper, clothes, or a distance of greater than 5 cm is adequate to shield a person from external alpha particle radiation.
      (4) Alpha particle sources inside the human body in high quantities when inhaled or swallowed (i.e., radon gas) can pose an internal hazard. They transfer relatively large amounts of ionizing energy to living cells (high LET and relative biologic effectiveness).
      (5) Alpha particles have a high dose equivalent. *Dose equivalent* is a quantity used in radiation protection to place all radiation on a common scale for calculating tissue damage. Dose equivalent is the absorbed dose times a quality factor. The quality factor accounts for the differences in radiation effects caused by different types of ionizing radiation. Alpha particles cause a greater amount of damage per unit of absorbed dose than other radiation, as the weighted quality factor is 20 times that of beta or gamma radiation (FDA, 2010).
      (6) Because of their poor penetrating range in tissues of only a few cell diameters, pure alpha emitters were not traditionally used in RT until the emer-

gence of radiolabeled antibodies. Experimental monoclonal antibodies labeled with pure alpha particles, such as bismuth-213, can be more cytotoxic than beta radiolabeled antibodies, as alpha emitters have a greater biologic effectiveness because of their high LET. Some evidence has also shown that alpha radiolabeled antibodies may kill tumor cells that are in hypoxic environments (NRC, Committee on State of the Science of Nuclear Medicine, 2007).

b) Beta: Particles are negatively charged electrons emitted from the nucleus of a decaying radioactive particle of radiation. They have deeper penetration than alpha particles and travel about one-half inch inside human tissue. They can be shielded by something as thin as a pad of paper.

 (1) Examples of pure beta particle radionuclides used in therapy are ^{32}P, ^{90}Y, ^{89}Sr, and ^{153}Sm.

 (2) Once a pure beta radionuclide is instilled or injected into the patient's body, the body will supply adequate shielding.

 (3) If a certain dose of some beta emitters is used systemically, the patient's body fluids may be temporarily radioactive.

 (4) Beta particles can pose an internal radiation hazard if inhaled or ingested.

c) Gamma: High-energy electromagnetic radiation given off by certain radionuclides when their nuclei transition from a higher to a lower energy state

 (1) Gamma rays have a wide range of energies and penetrating abilities. The higher the energy, the thicker the material needed to shield gamma radiation.

 (2) High-energy gamma-emitting radionuclides require both specified distances and shielding to reduce one's exposure.

 (3) Patients receiving high-energy gamma radionuclides (e.g., ^{137}Cs, ^{192}Ir) may be required to be in radiation isolation and behind lead shields.

 (4) Low-energy gamma emitters, such as ^{125}I and ^{103}Pd, do not require these same precautions (NCRP, 2006).

2. Half-life: The time required by a radioactive material to reduce to one-half of its radioactivity by radioactive decay. No chemical or physical operation can alter the decay rate of a radioactive substance.

a) Sealed radionuclides are chosen for either permanent implants (short half-life, low emissions) or temporary implants, which may have long half-lives.

b) Concern is given to the storage of the source if dislodged or if a spill or contamination occurs. Policies related to these incidents are based on the radionuclide's half-life.

c) Contaminated radioactive waste may require storage for decay for a time equal to 10 times the half-life. For example, if the half-life is 8 days, the storage requirement would be 80 days.

3. Amount of energy of the specific radionuclide used (NCRP, 2006).

a) In general, the greater the amount of the source used for high-energy radionuclides, the greater the amount of radiation safety protection measures needed.

b) The amount of energy that requires radiation isolation is determined by regulatory agencies, such as NRC, from guidelines established by the NCRP.

4. Radionuclide form: The two basic forms of radionuclides used are sealed (e.g., rods, ribbons, needles, seeds), which are surgically implanted into tumor tissues or in special applicators placed in body cavities, and unsealed (e.g., liquids, capsules, colloids), which can be ingested, injected, or instilled into the body.

a) Sealed sources

 (1) With sealed sources, the source, not the patient, is radioactive. The radioactive material is encapsulated, and safety measures are based on the source itself and the likelihood that it will become dislodged. The patient and his or her body fluids are not radioactive. For temporary implants, once the source has been removed and returned to safe storage and the area surveyed and checked for any dislodged sources, no further radiation protection measures are required.

(2) With permanent implants, dislodged source precautions may be in place for a specified time based on the energy of the source and the half-life. ^{125}I seeds with a half-life of 60 days may dictate longer time for dislodged source precautions than ^{103}Pd seeds with a half-life of 17 days (ICRP, 2005).

b) Unsealed sources

(1) With unsealed sources, the patient and his or her body fluids (blood, urine, feces, saliva, sweat) may be radioactive for a specified time, which is determined by the energy of the radionuclide, the amount used, and its half-life.

(2) Radiation safety measures are based on the specifics of the radionuclide used and the possibility of contamination from the patient's body fluids.

G. Principles of radiation protection (see Figure 11)

1. Time: The amount of exposure is directly related to the amount of time spent near the radioactive source. Nurses should continue to provide needed patient care while minimizing the time spent in close contact with a gamma radionuclide source inside a patient, which poses a radiation exposure risk. If there is a time limit for direct patient contact per nursing shift (determined by the RSO), this should be posted on the patient's hospital room door. The time limit for the patient's visitors also should be posted. Examples of strategies to minimize time include the following.

a) Provide necessary patient education before the procedure.

b) Teach, observe, and document the patient's ability to perform self-care measures before the procedure.

c) Evaluate the patient's understanding of the procedure. Discuss the reasoning for limiting staff and family exposure. This will help prevent the patient from feeling alienated.

d) Provide the maximum amount of direct nursing care before the radioactive source is placed or administered.

e) Assemble all necessary equipment and supplies in the patient's room before the procedure to avoid unnecessary trips, and ensure that equipment (e.g., telephone, television) in the patient's room works properly before the radioactive source is administered.

f) Check frequently on the patient via the intercom or telephone, anticipate the patient's needs, and encourage the patient to communicate any problems or concerns to the staff via the intercom or telephone.

g) Use time efficiently when in contact with the patient and organize care. Nurses caring for patients with specific radioactive procedures may want to practice routine care activities (e.g., logrolling the patient from side to side, visually checking the position of the gynecologic applicator, emptying a urine Foley bag).

h) Rotate the nursing and ancillary staff caring for the patient receiving radioactive implants, and reassure the family that care is a priority and the patient will not be neglected.

2. Distance: The amount of radiation exposure one receives is inversely related to the distance one is from the radioactive source/radioactive patient (inverse square law) (U.S. Environmental Protection Agency, 2010). By doubling the distance from the source, exposure is decreased by a factor of four (two squared). For example, an exposure rate of 40 mrem/hour at one meter would decrease to an exposure rate of 10 mrem/hour at a distance of two meters. The following are examples of nursing care measures that maximize distance from a radioactive source.

a) With direct patient contact, stand as far away from the sealed radioactive source as

---

Figure 11. Cardinal Principles of Time, Distance, and Shielding

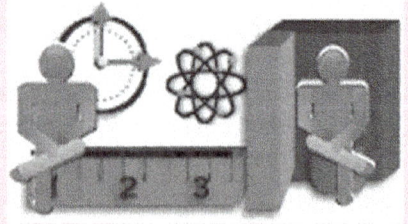

Time   Distance   Shielding

Time: To decrease exposure to penetrating beta and gamma ionizing radiation, decrease the time of exposure.

Distance: To decrease the amount of radiation exposure, increase the distance from the source. The intensity of the radiation is inversely proportional to the square of the distance from the source. For example, doubling the distance from the source will reduce the intensity of the radiation by a factor of 4.

Shielding: Shielding is useful for absorbing radiation exposure. Select the right shielding to stop the type of radiation being used (see Figure 12).

Note. From "Radiation Protection Basics," by the U.S. Environmental Protection Agency, 2010. Retrieved from http://www.epa.gov/radiation/understand/protection_basics.html.

possible. For example, stand at the head of the bed to take vital signs when in the room with a patient who has a gynecologic implant. Talk to the patient from the doorway rather than inside the room.

   b) Assist the patient with needed tasks (e.g., unwrapping food items) from a distance.

   c) Reinforce teaching of self-care activities while standing at a distance from the patient.

3. Shielding (U.S. Environmental Protection Agency, 2010): The amount of radiation exposure received from a specified radioactive source can be decreased by the use of an absorbing material (shield) placed between the source and the person receiving the exposure. Figure 12 shows the type of shielding that can stop different forms of ionizing radiation. The amount of exposure decreased by shielding will vary with the energy of the source and the thickness of the shielding material. *HVL* refers to the thickness of a material required to reduce radiation exposure to one-half of its original exposure amount. For example, the HVL of ^{137}Cs is 6 mm of lead or 10 cm of concrete. The following are common suggestions for using shielding to reduce exposure when shielding is appropriate.

   a) Keep the shielding between the source and the person exposed. Build shields into the walls and floors of designated treatment rooms that are used for radioactive procedures that use high-energy gamma sources.

   b) Continue to use principles of time and distance, even with shields, to further reduce radiation exposure.

   c) Consider that maneuvering the shield may require increased nursing time in the room, making some uses of shields unwarranted.

   d) Select the correct material for shielding based on the type of emitters (i.e., lead for high-energy gamma sources, plastic for pure beta sources).

   e) Use more shielding in institutions that perform large numbers of gamma-emitting radioactive procedures.

H. Radiation monitoring devices (see Figure 13)
  1. General information
    a) Even though ionizing radiation cannot be detected by the human senses, detection devices (personal monitoring device or survey monitor) can measure the amounts of radiation exposure received by an individual.
    b) Monitoring devices do not offer any radiation exposure protection. They only physically measure levels or amounts of exposure.
  2. Types of personal dosimetry monitors
    a) Personal monitoring devices are recommended for individuals who need constant radiation exposure monitoring in the occupational setting. Monitors are recommended for all occupationally exposed individuals who, in the judgment of the RSO, have the potential to receive greater than 10% of the annual effective dose limit during the normal course of their duties and individuals who enter radiation areas (NCRP, 2009).
      (1) Electronic personal dosimeters should be worn consistently at work during times of potential and actual exposure (and should not be worn outside of work).
      (2) The dosimeter is not to be shared or exchanged with other staff.
      (3) The dosimeter should not be exposed to excessive heat or moisture.
      (4) The dosimeter should not remain on lab coat or placed in a room with radiation sources when it is not being worn.
      (5) The dosimeter should be worn on the area of the body that the highest deep, shallow, and eye-dose equivalent is expected to be received. In general, this is on the front of the body between the waist and collar of the individual. For specialized work where the highest dose is at the head level, such as in fluoroscopy, the dosimeter should be worn at the collar.
      (6) The dosimeter should be read according to the institutional time schedule,

---

Figure 12. Type of Shielding That Can Stop Different Forms of Ionizing Radiation

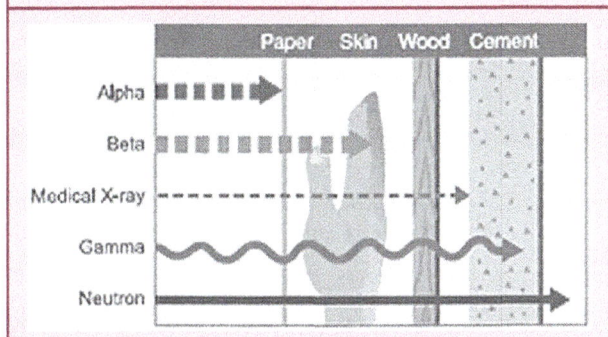

Note. From "Radiation Basics," by the U.S. Nuclear Regulatory Commission, 2010. Retrieved from http://www.nrc.gov/about-nrc/radiation/health-effects/radiation-basics.html#ionizing.

Figure 13. Examples of Radiation Monitoring Devices

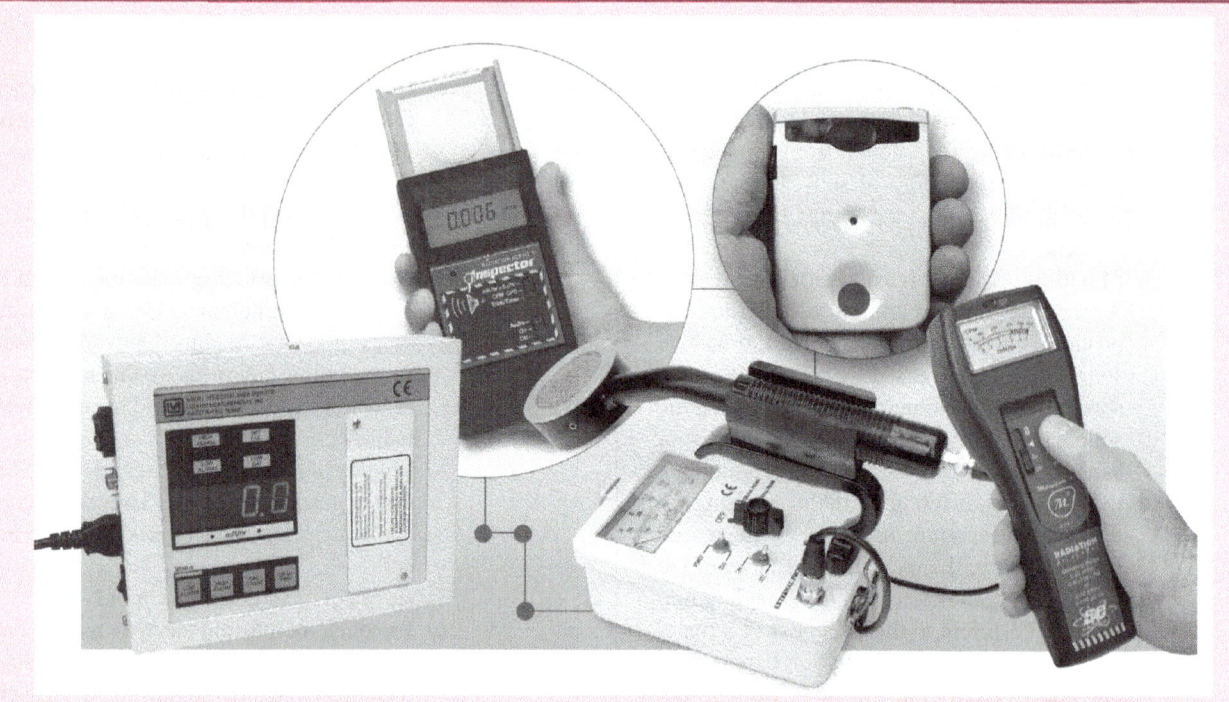

Clockwise from top left: inspector survey meter, electronic personal dosimeter, survey meter, survey meter with probe, and digital area monitor

Note. Photo courtesy of Biodex Medical Systems, Inc. Used with permission.

and the cumulative record of personal monitor readings should be kept on file at the institution.

b) Ring dosimeter: An individual monitoring device that is similar to a personal dosimeter but is worn on the finger and is used by personnel who are handling radioactive material. Guidelines are similar to those of a personal dosimeter.

c) Pocket ion chamber dosimeter: A lightweight radiation measurement instrument that gives similar readouts of radiation exposure as a personal dosimeter but is used by individuals who do not need continual radiation exposure monitoring but rather periodic monitoring for scheduled radioactive procedures. Unlike an individual monitor, different personnel can share pocket dosimeters. The amount of radiation exposure received is known immediately for each person who wears the monitoring device. Pocket dosimeters are especially useful for nursing/healthcare staff and family members who are in contact with people being cared for on inpatient or outpatient units that infrequently use diagnostic or therapeutic radioactive materials. Pocket ion dosimeters should

(1) Be left at the nurses' station or outside the patient's room with the exposure dose record sheet that keeps track of individual exposure amounts. These devices should not be kept near the radioactive source.

(2) Be worn the same place as a personal dosimeter, where the highest dose may be received.

(3) Be read before entering the patient's room and then again after leaving the patient's room. The readings should be recorded on the dose record sheet. Information to record includes the name of the person exposed, date, time, dosimeter readouts, time spent in the room, and the readings before entering and then after leaving the room.

(4) Be handled gently. If dropped, tapped, or knocked, pocket ion chamber dosimeters can show inaccurate readings and may need to be recalibrated by the radiation safety staff or radiation oncology dosimetry staff.

(5) Be read by holding them up toward the light in a horizontal position and reading the point at which the hairline crosses the numbered scale.

    (6) Have their records kept on file and monitored by the RSO/radiation safety staff.

I. Recognition of radiation-restricted areas: Federal and state laws require the posting of appropriate radiation protection warning signs in areas containing potential and real radiation exposure.
1. Radiation caution sign (see Figure 14)
   a) Has a yellow background with magenta lettering and should specify the specific radionuclide source and radiation precautions
   b) Should be placed on the door of the rooms, both inpatient and outpatient, that have any ionizing radiation present
   c) With rooms with patients containing radioactive sealed sources, the caution sign needs to specify any restrictions for staff and visitors and needs to remain in place until the source is removed and the room surveyed for possible source dislodgement, or until exposure risk is no longer present.
   d) With rooms with patients containing unsealed radioactive sources, the caution sign needs to specify restrictions for staff and visitors and remain in place until the room is surveyed and all contaminated articles removed.
2. Therapeutic radionuclide information sheets
   a) Should be placed in the patient's inpatient or outpatient chart
   b) Document radionuclide information (e.g., name of radionuclide, dose, specific activity, how administered, date of administration)

J. Special radiation protection considerations and issues involved in the discharge of patients treated with radiopharmaceuticals or permanent implants
1. Pure beta emitters (^{90}Y labeled antibody [anti-CD20 antibody], ^{89}Sr, ^{153}Sm)
   a) Because ^{90}Y is a pure beta emitter, administration is safely performed on an outpatient basis. Some patients need to be treated as inpatients for medical reasons, not because of radiation protection hazard. ^{153}Sm and ^{89}Sr, also pure beta emitters, can be given as an outpatient injection.
   b) There is no external radiation exposure risk to patients' family members and healthcare workers in contact with the patient.
   c) Because of possible internal exposure risk from ingesting urine or blood, healthcare staff need to follow universal precautions. Bags, vials, and tubes that are used and contain pure beta emitters absorb any radiation that may be present. In general, these supplies are handled, surveyed, and discarded by designated radiation safety personnel.
   d) Patients receiving pure beta emitters can be discharged immediately after treatment without any activity limits, and no dose rate limit measurements need to be taken.
   e) The person administering pure beta radiopharmaceuticals should wear gloves and use a plastic syringe cover over the medication and be careful to not spray or drip the medication.
   f) The patient should be encouraged to use regular toilet facilities, avoid urine leakage, and double flush the toilet. Anyone handling the patient's urine, especially in the first 24 hours after the injection, should wear gloves.
   g) Condoms are recommended for sexual relations for one week after injection.
   h) After discharge, patients should clean up any spilled urine and dispose of any urine- or blood-contaminated material (e.g., flush it down the toilet; place it in a plastic bag in household trash) to prevent it from being handled by others.
2. Radioactive ^{131}I for thyroid cancer/hyperthyroidism
   a) In 1997, the NRC revised its patient release regulations, allowing for larger activities of radioactive ^{131}I to be given as an outpatient administration. Previously, NRC required any individual receiving 30 mCi or greater of radioactive ^{131}I to be an inpatient in radiation isolation and discharged after an exposure rate of less than 5 mR (milliroentgen)/hour at one meter was obtained. The new regulation allows patients to be

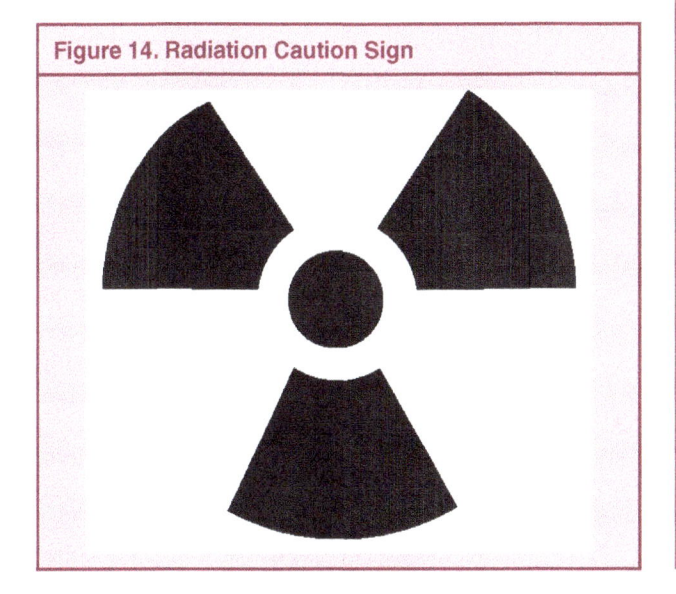

Figure 14. Radiation Caution Sign

released if the total effective dose equivalent to any other individual is not likely to exceed 5 mSv (NRC, 1997).

b) With systemic gamma-emitting radionuclides, such as ^{131}I, the patient's body fluids (blood, urine, saliva, feces, semen) pose a temporary radiation hazard, as well as the patient being an external hazard to individuals in close contact with the patient.

c) Studies have shown that the amounts of radiation exposure received by household members of patients discharged after receiving ^{131}I have been below the limit of 1 mSv/year (ICRP, 2005).

d) Discharge instructions are based on not only the amount of ^{131}I given but on several other factors such as where the patient will be discharged to, who will be in the home, including children, the sex and age of each household member, and sleeping partner information; workplace information and the presence of pregnant women or minors at work; transportation to and from the medical facility to the home; physical challenges; incontinence or ostomy care; and ability to comprehend instructions. Figure 15 provides an example of discharge instructions given to a patient who has received radioactive iodine therapy.

e) Discharge instructions for unsealed sources, such as radioactive iodine, can be determined by a computerized program specific to the particulars of outpatient radioiodine therapy. A copy of these should be given to the patient and family and placed in the patient's record (Reiman, 2005).

3. [125]I and [103]Pd prostate seed implants

a) Prostate implants can be inserted as an outpatient procedure. Once the seeds are in place, there is little radiation exposure risk to others.

b) NRC guidelines allow discharge of patients if the exposure rate at one meter is at or below 0.01 mSv/hour for ^{125}I and 0.03 mSv/hour for [103]Pd (NRC, 1997).

c) A study involving radiation exposure to family members of men who received ^{125}I seeds showed that spouses received an average of 14 mrem and other family members received less than 8 mrem over one year. With [103]Pd, spouses received 6 mrem and other family members received essentially 0 mrem (to put things into perspective, a person flying from New York to Tokyo receives 20 mrem, and someone flying from New York to Los Angeles receives 5 mrem) (Michalski, Mutic, Eichling, & Ahmed, 2003).

d) Discharge instructions to patients who received ^{125}I or [103]Pd vary per institution but should contain the following information (NRC, 2008).

(1) Name and description (for example, "small metallic seeds, about ⅓ to ½ inch long") of the radioactive source(s)

(2) Time schedule and activities to minimize exposure to others, including holding or cuddling children, closeness to pregnant women, sleeping restrictions with partner, and sexual intercourse

(3) Use of public transportation and being out in public

(4) Precautions regarding possible dislodged seeds (i.e., use of condom and how long, straining urine and how long, what to do if dislodged seed or pellet is found (Do not touch it with bare hands; pick it up with something like tweezers or a spoon. Place it in a container with a tight lid and keep in a location away from people, then notify contact person in treatment facility who placed sources.)

4. Patient information card/letter concerning radiopharmaceutical/radionuclide procedure

a) Patients discharged with radiopharmaceuticals/radionuclides in body should have a letter or wallet identification card from the physician or medical facility specifying radionuclide therapy

b) Patients may set off very sensitive alarms that detect radioactivity, such as those found in airports, train stations, government buildings, tunnels, and border crossings.

c) Patients treated with ^{131}I may set off alarms for up to 95 days after therapy for thyroid cancer (Reiman, 2005).

5. Special radiation protection considerations: In a freestanding facility not associated with a hospital, it is recommended that the local fire, emergency medical services, and police

Figure 15. Example Instruction Sheet

Radiation Safety Precautions for
Radiopharmaceutical Therapy Patients

<u>Note:</u> Please carefully read and follow the instructions in this document.

If you or your healthcare provider have any questions or concerns regarding the radionuclide therapy you have received, please contact:

<u>Dr. J. Smith</u>
Nuclear Medicine Attending Physician

at   <u>(111) 222-3333</u>
Telephone number

or   <u>0000</u>
Emergency or pager telephone number

Patient **John Q. Patient**, Medical Record Number **1111-11-111**, received a therapeutic dose of **6.475 MBq (175 mCi)** of **Iodine-131 Sodium Iodide** at **General Hospital** on **January 1, 2004**, at **9:00 am** and should observe the following radiation safety precautions at home as follows.

- Avoid close contact [less than 1 meter (3 feet) away from] with pregnant women and children until **1 day** after the administration of the radionuclide therapy.
- Do not hold or embrace children for more than 10 minutes a day until **21 days** after the day your radionuclide therapy was administered. *This requires that you avoid contact with these children altogether during your* **first day** *after the day your radionuclide therapy was administered.*
- Unless you work alone (for example, driving a truck), do not return to work until **1 day** after the day your radionuclide therapy was administered.
- Do not sleep in the same bed with your sleeping partner until **7 days** after the day your radionuclide therapy was administered.
- However, if your sleeping partner is pregnant, do not sleep in the same bed with your sleeping partner until **24 days** after the day your radionuclide therapy was administered. This requires that you avoid contact with your pregnant sleeping partner *altogether* during the **first day** after the day your radionuclide therapy was administered.

[Instruction Sheet Continued]

    Patient: **Patient, John Q.**

    MRN: **111-11-111**

In addition, the following precautions should be observed until 1 day after the administration of your radiopharmaceutical therapy.

- To the extent that is reasonable, generally try to remain as far away from individuals around you as possible.
- After using the toilet, flush twice and, as usual, wash your hands. If possible, use paper towels to dry your hands and dispose of the paper toweling in the trash.
- You should otherwise observe good personal hygiene and may shower, bathe, shave, etc., as you normally would, rinsing the shower stall, tub, or sink thoroughly after use.
- Wipe up any spills of urine, saliva, or mucus with tissues or a small amount of disposable (i.e., flushable) paper toweling, and dispose of the tissue or toweling down the toilet.
- Use nondisposable plates, bowls, spoons, knives, forks, and cups. If possible, you should use a separate sponge or washcloth from that used by the rest of your household to wash plates, bowls, spoons, knives, forks, and cups that you have used. Rinse the sink thoroughly after use, wipe the fixtures with paper towels, and dispose of the paper toweling in the trash.
- If you use a dishwasher, wash your plates, bowls, spoons, knives, forks and cups separately from those of the rest of your household.
- Use the same set of plates, bowls, spoons, knives and forks for **1 day** after your radionuclide therapy.
- Store and launder your soiled/used clothing and bed linens separately from those of the rest of your household, running the rinse cycle two times at the completion of the machine laundering.
- Do not share food or drinks with anyone.
- After using the telephone, wipe the receiver (especially the mouth piece) with paper towels, and dispose the paper towels in the trash.

Signature Section (example release form)
I have read this form and all of my questions have been answered.
By signing below, I acknowledge that I have read and accept all of the information above.

Signature of patient or patient representative   Print name of patient or representative   Date

_____   _____   _____

Relation of personal representative to patient _____

Note. From *Management of Radionuclide Therapy Patients* (NCRP Report No. 155, pp. 166–168), by National Council on Radiation Protection and Measurements, 2006, Bethesda, MD: Author. Reprinted with permission of the National Council on Radiation Protection and Measurements, http://NCRPonline.org.

are aware of radiation hazards. All freestanding facilities also are regulated by NRC and state radiation control organizations.

6. Special populations: Radiation exposure of pregnant employees (NCRP, 1994)

   a) Embryos/fetuses are the most radiosensitive living tissues.

   b) The most radiosensitive period of a fetus is in the first trimester.

   c) Because of the radiosensitivity of the embryo, a pregnant woman has a dose limit of 5 mSv (0.5 rem) during pregnancy per NCRP guidelines.

   d) Many institutions recommend that pregnant women do not provide care to patients who are receiving radionuclide therapy. However, by law, pregnant women cannot be restricted from providing this care, as long as NCRP guidelines for exposure limits are followed.

   e) The pregnant woman assumes all responsibility for the exposure of the fetus until the pregnancy is officially declared. Once a pregnancy is declared, the supervisors/RSO are responsible for ensuring that the woman's monitored radiation exposure does not exceed the 5 mSv (0.5 rem) dose limit. The RSO also is required to evaluate the work area and recommend further procedures to reduce exposure.

7. Emergency procedures: General guidelines for emergency procedures, including radioactive spills and loss or rupture of a sealed radioactive source, can be found in NCRP Report No. 155, 2006, pp. 130–131.

   a) Dislodged source guidelines

      (1) Notify the radiation oncologist and RSO regarding any dislodged source as soon as it is discovered.

      (2) Have a lead storage container available to store any dislodged source and have long-handled forceps available to pick up the source. Only individuals with training in handling radioactive sources should be permitted to handle dislodged sources. Bare hands should never be used to pick up a radioactive source.

      (3) The patient also should be instructed to never pick up a dislodged radioactive source and to immediately contact the staff if a dislodgment is suspected.

      (4) The time the source became dislodged should be recorded and communicated to the radiation oncology team to determine the therapeutic radiation dose that the patient received.

      (5) Radiation safety staff should survey all applicators, dressings, and linens that may contain a dislodged source before removing them from the room.

   b) Cardiopulmonary resuscitation (CPR) of patients who have received radionuclide therapy

      (1) CPR in patients with sealed radionuclides

         (a) Begin CPR immediately.

         (b) Immediately notify personnel who can properly remove the sealed source and place it in a lead/safe container.

         (c) Once the source is removed and properly stored and the area is surveyed, no additional risk of exposure is present.

      (2) CPR in patients with unsealed sources (^{131}I) (Health Physics Society, 2002)

         (a) Begin CPR immediately.

         (b) Notify radiation safety personnel/radiation oncologist.

         (c) Realize that the priority is the patient, and staff exposure is likely to be minimal. (Thirty minutes of resuscitation of a patient with 100 mCi of ^{131}I would result in approximately 100 mrem exposure at one foot, a 200 mrem/hour exposure rate.)

         (d) People performing CPR should wear gloves, a gown, and shoe covers.

         (e) All equipment used for CPR should be surveyed for radiation contamination before removal from the room.

         (f) All personnel involved in CPR should remain in the immediate location of the patient's room and be cleared to leave the area by radiation safety personnel.

8. Information on handling other situations involving patients with radionuclides, such as dialysis, emergency surgery, death, autopsy, cremation, and organ donation, can be found in NCRP Report No. 155, 2006, pp. 131–140.

K. Nursing education in radiation protection

   1. Nurses caring for patients receiving radionuclides should receive specific training in radiation protection and periodic review in radiation protection practices per institutional guidelines.

   2. Education has been shown to be effective in increasing nurses' knowledge about radiation

safety practices (Dauer, Kelvin, Horan, & St. Germain, 2006).

3. NRC regulations require that nurses caring for patients receiving radionuclides be instructed in radiation protection measures.

L. Related Web sites
1. ACR: www.acr.org
2. American Association of Physicists in Medicine: www.aapm.org
3. Canadian Nuclear Safety Committee: www.cnsc.gc.ca
4. FDA: www.fda.gov
5. Health Physics Society (Ask the Experts): www.hps.org
6. ICRP: www.icrp.org
7. NCRP: www.ncrponline.org
8. NRC: www.nrc.gov
9. Radiological Society of North America: www.rsna.org

References

Amis, E.S., Jr., Butler, P.F., Applegate, K.E., Birnbaum, S.B., Brateman, L.F., Hevezi, J.M., … Zeman, R.K. (2007). American College of Radiology white paper on radiation dose in medicine. *Journal of the American College of Radiology, 4,* 272–284. doi:10.1016/j.jacr.2007.03.002

Dauer, L.T., Kelvin, J.F., Horan, C.L., & St. Germain, J. (2006). Evaluating the effectiveness of a radiation safety training intervention for oncology nurses: A pretest-intervention-posttest study. *BMC Medical Education, 6,* 32. doi:10.1186/1472-6920-6-32

Gilbert, E.S. (2009). Ionising radiation and cancer risks: What have we learned from epidemiology? *International Journal of Radiation Biology, 85,* 467–482. doi:10.1080/09553000902883836

Health Physics Society. (2002). Answer to question #1753 submitted to "Ask the Experts": Where can I find a policy manual for a code situation in a ^{131}I high-dose therapy patient? Retrieved from http://hps.org/publicinformation/ate/q1753.html

International Commission on Radiological Protection. (2005). Radiation safety aspects of brachytherapy for prostate cancer using permanently implanted sources. A report of ICRP Publication 98. *Annals of the ICRP, 35*(3), iii–vi, 3–50.

Kassis, A.I. (2008). Therapeutic radionuclides: Biophysical and radiobiologic principles. *Seminars in Nuclear Medicine, 38,* 358–366. doi:10.1053/j.semnuclmed.2008.05.002

Martin, C.J., Sutton, D.G., West, C.M., & Wright, E.G. (2009). The radiobiology/radiation protection interface in healthcare. *Journal of Radiological Protection, 29*(2A), A1–A20. doi:10.1088/0952-4746/29/2A/S01

McQuestion, M. (2007). Radiation protection and safety. In M.L. Haas, W.P. Hogle, G.J. Moore-Higgs, & T.K. Gosselin-Acomb (Eds.), *Radiation therapy: A guide to patient care* (pp. 25–35). St. Louis, MO: Elsevier Mosby.

Michalski, J., Mutic, S., Eichling, J., & Ahmed, S.N. (2003). Radiation exposure to family and household members after prostate brachytherapy. *International Journal of Radiation Oncology, Biology, Physics, 56,* 764–768. doi:10.1016/S0360-3016(03)00002-6

National Council on Radiation Protection and Measurements. (1993). *Limitation of exposure to ionizing radiation* (NCRP Report No. 116). Bethesda, MD: Author.

National Council on Radiation Protection and Measurements. (1994). *Considerations regarding the unintended radiation exposure of the embryo, fetus, or nursing child* (NCRP Commentary No. 9). Bethesda, MD: Author.

National Council on Radiation Protection and Measurements. (2006). *Management of radionuclide therapy patients* (NCRP Report No. 155). Bethesda, MD: Author.

National Council on Radiation Protection and Measurements. (2009). *Ionizing radiation exposure of the population of the United States* (NCRP Report No. 160). Bethesda, MD: Author.

National Research Council, Committee on State of the Science of Nuclear Medicine. (2007). *Advancing nuclear medicine through innovation.* Washington, DC: National Academies Press. Retrieved from http://www.nap.edu/catalog/11985.html

Reiman, R.E. (2005, July). *Releasing nuclear medicine patients to the public: Dose computations and discharge instructions.* Lecture presented at the American Academy of Physicists in Medicine 47th Annual Meeting, Seattle, WA. Slides retrieved from http://www.aapm.org/meetings/05AM/pdf/18-2638-6734-583.pdf

Schauer, D.A. (2010, May). *NCRP activities related to radiation protection in medicine. Identifying the future: Exploring trends, changing direction.* Lecture presented at the 12th Annual Meeting of the Health Care Industry Advisory Council, Savannah, GA. Slides retrieved from www.ncrponline.org/PDFs/ASRT_HCIAC_May10_DAS.pdf

Unger, L.M., & Trubey, D.K. (1982). Specific gamma-ray dose constants for nuclides important to dosimetry and radiological assessment. Oak Ridge, TN: Oak Ridge National Laboratory.

U.S. Environmental Protection Agency. (2010). Radiation protection basics. Retrieved from http://www.epa.gov/radiation/understand/protection_basics.html

U.S. Food and Drug Administration. (2010, February 9). Initiative to reduce unnecessary radiation exposure from medical imaging [News release]. Retrieved from http://www.fda.gov/Radiation-Emitting-Products/RadiationSafety/RadiationDoseReduction/ucm199904.htm

U.S. Nuclear Regulatory Commission. (1997). Regulatory guide 8.39: Release of patients administered radioactive materials. Retrieved from http://www.nrc.gov/reading-rm/doc-collections/reg-guides/occupational-health/rg/

U.S. Nuclear Regulatory Commission. (2005). Consolidated guidance about materials licenses: Program-specific guidance about medical use licenses—Final report (NUREG-1556, Vol. 9). Retrieved from http://www.nrc.gov/reading-rm/doc-collections/nuregs/staff/sr1556/v9/nureg-1556-9.pdf

U.S. Nuclear Regulatory Commission. (2008). Consolidated guidance about materials licenses: Program-specific guidance about medical use licenses (NUREG-1556, Volume 9, Revision 2). Retrieved from http://www.nrc.gov/reading-rm/doc-collections/nuregs/staff/sr1556/v9/r2

IV. General symptom management

A. General patient and family education
   1. Definition: Patient education is a planned, systematic process that uses various techniques such as teaching, counseling, and behavior modification to assist people to learn health-related behaviors (e.g., knowledge, skills, attitudes, values) (Bartlett, 1985; Bastable, 2008b). Patient education is a dynamic and interactive process between the teacher and learner.
   2. Learning theories provide a framework for patient education (see Table 7) (Doak, Doak, & Root, 1996).
   3. Components of the patient education process include assessment, planning, implementation, and evaluation (Bastable, 2008b; Redman, 2001).
   4. Historically, patient education has been a core role component of the radiation oncology nurse (Bruner, 1993; Gosselin-Acomb, 2006; Hilderley, 1980; Moore-Higgs et al., 2003; Shepard & Kelvin, 1999; Strohl, 1988).
   5. Rationale for patient education
      a) The Patient Care Partnership establishes a patient's right to information about diagnosis, treatment, prognosis, procedures, medical consequences, personnel, and the hospital (American Hospital Association,

Table 7. A Summary of Key Education and Behavior Theories and Their Applications

Theory Name	Proponents/Reference	Description	Application
Health Belief Model	Becker, 1974; Harrison et al., 1992; Hochbaum et al., 1992; Rosenstock, 1974	Explains people's health behaviors: why they may accept preventive health services or adopt healthy behaviors.	This is a behavior research tool but can imply best content and topic sequence for educational materials.
Self-Efficacy	Bandura, 1977; Bandura & Adams, 1977; Bandura et al., 1977	People are more likely to adopt a health behavior if they think they can do it.	Intervention should give people confidence by building up to behavior step by step. Give them many little "successes" in the behavior change process.
Locus of Control Theory	Wallston et al., 1976	People who believe *they* are in control of their own health status are more likely to change behaviors in response to health education facts. The converse is also true.	For people who believe they are *not* in control, build more support into health education programs.
Cognitive Dissonance Theory	Festinger, 1957; Lewin, 1943	A high level of unhappiness (dissonance) is more likely to lead to behavior change. Theory points to readiness to change and how to cut probability of relapse.	Design intervention to foster unhappiness with present behavior status. To reduce relapse, reinforce to keep dissonance low.
Diffusion Theory	Rogers & Shoemaker, 1971	Some people will adopt new behaviors early, some late. Early adopters can influence others. Applies to a community or population.	Foster early adoption by making intervention consistent with beliefs, values, and social system of target population.
Stages of Readiness	Prochaska & DiClemente, 1983	A person goes through stages of readiness to adopt and to maintain a new health behavior. Education interventions work best if they match a person's stage of readiness.	Design intervention to fit the stages of readiness of your client population. If many stages are present, the intervention may need several different messages.
Adult Education Theories	Bruner, 1966; Coleman, 1988; Knowles, 1970	Main concern of adults is solving and managing their own problems. They care about self-fulfillment. Adults need active participation. Adults are less interested in facts about health as a subject.	1. Design education intervention to address the solution to their health problems. Give less information about other topics. 2. Build on adult's experience. 3. "Talk it out," teach via demonstrations, discussion, and examples.

Note. From *Teaching Patients With Low Literacy Skills* (2nd ed., p. 13), by C.C. Doak, L.G. Doak, and J.H. Root, 1996, Philadelphia, PA: Lippincott. Copyright 1996 by C.C. Doak and L.G. Doak. Adapted with permission.

_____

_____

_____

_____

_____

_____

_____

2003). The ONS (2009) position on quality cancer care outlines patients' rights to information throughout the cancer care continuum.

b) State nurse practice acts and the American Nurses Association's (ANA's) *Nursing: Scope and Standards of Practice* (ANA, 2010) define the scope of nursing practice and designate health or patient education as an independent function of the professional nurse.

c) Accreditation organizations, such as the Joint Commission, have delineated patient safety goals that include education components.

d) Interventional studies of preparatory education for patients receiving RT have measured various outcomes such as patient satisfaction, self-care behaviors, anxiety, and quality of life.

   (1) Studies testing various delivery methods for patient education have consistently reported increased patient satisfaction with preparatory information (D'Haese et al., 2000; Häggmark et al., 2001; Hoff & Haaga, 2006; Poroch, 1995). However, their findings did not concur regarding the effect of patient education on anxiety. Anxiety reduction was noted in a randomized study testing a stepwise information group approach (D'Haese et al., 2000) and in a study using a quasi-experimental design to evaluate a structured group education session (Poroch, 1995). Yet, a larger randomized trial of three information formats did not find any significant differences between the groups on outcomes of anxiety, depression distress, or quality of life (Häggmark et al., 2001). Similarly, in a randomized trial of an orientation program for both patients and their family members, no significant differences in anxiety or mood were

noted between the patient and family intervention group and the control group (Hoff & Haaga, 2006).

   (2) Other studies have explored a specific intervention's effect on self-care or the symptom experience. Hagopian (1996) found that patients who listened to informational audiotapes practiced more helpful self-care behaviors than those in the control group. Patients were noted to perform more self-care behaviors after receiving systematic information about side effect management techniques (Dodd, 1987). In another study, structured patient education in the form of a newsletter did not affect either the helpfulness or the number of self-care behaviors (Hagopian, 1991). The delivery of concrete objective information about treatment side effects via audiotape recordings was found to reduce symptom uncertainty and help patients maintain social activities during treatment (Christman & Cain, 2004).

   (3) Several randomized trials have described conflicting results regarding the impact of a preparatory videotape on reducing general anxiety. Although Thomas, Daly, Perryman, and Stockton (2000) reported that a video improved satisfaction and reduced treatment-related anxiety, Harrison et al. (2001) found that the additional provision of videotape did not significantly reduce pretreatment worry. Similarly, a study using a quasi-experimental longitudinal design found that a preparatory video increased patient satisfaction but had no effect on psychological distress, knowledge about RT, or self-efficacy for coping (Dunn, Steginga, Rose, Scott, & Allison, 2004).

6. Assessment

   a) *Learning needs* are gaps in knowledge, skills, or attitudes (Kitchie, 2008). Most patients want information primarily so they can be active participants in their therapy (Hinds, Streater, & Mood, 1995). Ongoing assessment is essential, as informational needs change over time (Hinds et al., 1995; Treacy & Mayer, 2000) and exist across the continuum of cancer care (Chelf et al., 2001).

   b) *Readiness to learn* is the time when the patient is both receptive and willing to learn and occurs in four realms of physical readiness, emotional readiness, experiential readiness, and knowledge readiness (Kitchie, 2008).

c) *Learning style* is defined as the way that the patient perceives and processes information (Moss, 1994). Many learning styles exist. One approach to describing learning styles uses the senses:

   (1) Visual learner
   (2) Auditory learner
   (3) Tactile learner
   (4) Vocal learner
   (5) Kinesthetic learner.

d) *Health literacy* is "the degree to which individuals have the capacity to obtain, process, and understand basic health information and services needed to make appropriate health decisions" (Selden, Zorn, Ratzan, & Parker, 2000, Health Literacy section, para. 7). Low literacy is a barrier to patient education and may adversely affect informed consent, self-management, treatment outcomes, and quality of life (Davis, Williams, Marin, Parker, & Glass, 2002; Kripalani et al., 2006; Merriman, Ades, & Seffrin, 2002).

   (1) Health literacy skills vary widely. The 2003 National Assessment of Adult Literacy assessed health literacy tasks related to clinical interactions and activities, prevention activities, and navigation of the health system (Kutner, Greenberg, Jin, & Paulsen, 2006). Most adults had *intermediate* (53%) or *proficient* (12%) health literacy, meaning they had the skills necessary to perform moderately challenging literacy tasks. The ability to perform simple literacy tasks, defined as *basic* health literacy, was noted in 22% of adults. The remaining 14% had *below basic* health literacy, indicating they were nonliterate in English or had simple, concrete literacy skills.

   (2) Screening tools for health literacy include the Rapid Estimate of Adult Literacy in Medicine, or REALM (Davis et al., 1991), and the Test of Functional Health Literacy in Adults, or TOFHLA (Parker, Baker, Williams, & Nurss, 1995). Descriptions of these tools, including benefits and limitations of their use, can be found in reviews by Mancuso (2009) and Quirk (2000).

   (3) The single screening questions, "How confident are you filling out medical forms by yourself?" and "How often do you have someone help you read hospital materials?" were found to be effective in identifying clinic patients with limited and marginal health literacy skills (Chew, Bradley, & Boyko, 2004; Wallace et al., 2007). Limitations in the studies, however, prevent generalization to other populations (Mancuso, 2009).

   (4) Informal, subtle cues that may indicate low literacy include lack of interest, expression of frustration, slow reading speed, desire to let someone else read first, claims to have forgotten glasses, and inability to complete forms completely (Davis et al., 2002).

   (5) Age older than 65 years is associated with lower health literacy than that of younger age groups (Kutner et al., 2006).

7. Planning: Formulate the patient teaching plan with objectives that are "SMART—specific, measurable, attainable, realistic, timed" (Agre, 2005, p. 894). Patients require sensory, procedural, and self-care information (Poroch, 1995) that is tailored to the individual (Chelf et al., 2001). The teaching plan may include the following topics.

   a) Goal of treatment (cure, control, palliation)

   b) Type of treatment (teletherapy [3DCRT, IMRT, IGRT, SRS, stereotactic body RT, proton therapy], brachytherapy, systemic RT [radiopharmaceuticals, radioimmunotherapy], intraoperative, hyperthermia, photodynamic therapy)

   c) Simulation

      (1) Purpose
      (2) Preparation (e.g., disrobing, use of contrast material, laxative, enema)
      (3) Description of procedure (e.g., duration, staff present, bowel preparation, indwelling catheter, oral/IV contrast, positioning, immobilization devices, x-rays, CT scan, tattoos)
      (4) Postsimulation care (e.g., care of markings, laxative)

   d) EBRT treatment schedule

      (1) Monday through Friday (e.g., once or twice daily)
      (2) Total number of fractions and days
      (3) Days to be seen for "status check" appointments with physician and nurse
      (4) Days to receive laboratory work, if necessary
      (5) Timing of concurrent chemotherapy, if necessary

e) EBRT treatment experience
  (1) Staff administering the treatment
  (2) Positioning
  (3) Video and audio monitoring system
  (4) Sensory aspects (e.g., size of machine, sounds of machine, temperature of the room)
  (5) Duration
  (6) Port films

f) Possible side effects
  (1) General and site-specific side effects that may occur
  (2) Causes of symptoms
  (3) Expected onset and duration
  (4) Use of medications
  (5) Reassurance that patient is not radioactive with EBRT

g) Self-care activities
  (1) Preventive measures to initiate at start of treatment
  (2) Interventions to initiate as symptoms develop
  (3) Use of complementary therapies
  (4) Activity and nutrition recommendations

h) Physician and nurse contact information
  (1) Indications for calling
  (2) Telephone numbers to call during business hours, evenings, and weekends

i) Resources for assistance (e.g., support groups, dietitian, social worker, spiritual care counselor, community agencies)

j) Instructions at the completion of treatment
  (1) Treatment side effects, including patterns of recovery and self-care
  (2) Possible emotional effects (i.e., anxiety, worry, distress) during the post-treatment transition related to resumption of social responsibilities, desire to regain a sense of "normalcy," loss of continued contact with oncology team, persistent physical symptoms, and fears of cancer recurrence (Allen, Savadatti, & Levy, 2009; Costanzo et al., 2007; Deshields et al., 2005; Lethborg, Kissane, Burns, & Snyder, 2000; Rose & Yates, 2001; Wells, 1998).
  (3) Resources for psychosocial support/counseling; survivorship programs
  (4) Indications for calling the oncology team prior to a scheduled follow-up visit

k) Instructions during the post-treatment or follow-up phase to enhance self-management of living with cancer as a chronic illness. These instructions should be incorporated into the patient's comprehensive sur-

vivorship care plan (Institute of Medicine, 2006).
  (1) Cancer type and treatment received
  (2) Potential late effects of treatment and self-care practices to mitigate late effects
  (3) Recommended follow-up schedule and practices, including cancer screening guidelines
  (4) Cancer prevention measures; health promotion activities related to diet, exercise, and smoking cessation; and other behaviors to enhance well-being
  (5) Community psychosocial resources
  (6) Legal protections regarding employment and access to health insurance

8. Implementation
  a) Include significant others in teaching.
  b) Build a trusting relationship.
  c) Use teaching strategies appropriate for the developmental stage of the learner (Bastable & Dart, 2008) (see Table 8). Teaching techniques to optimize learning in older adults include rest periods, pacing, rehearsing, positive reinforcement, cueing, and setting personalized goals (Rendon, Davis, Gioiella, & Tranzillo, 1986).
  d) Schedule time for patient education to occur.
  e) Create an effective learning environment that is private, quiet, and free from distractions.
  f) Attend to patient's comfort needs before initiating teaching session.
  g) Provide verbal instructions.
    (1) Avoid using medical or technical terminology.
    (2) Divide complex information or tasks into smaller subunits of instruction.
    (3) Use advanced organizers or simple category names that are meaningful to the patient (Redman, 2001).
    (4) Tailor or personalize the instruction.
    (5) Allow time for questions and answers.
    (6) Provide contact information for staff.
  h) Use tools to reinforce verbal instructions.
    (1) Print materials matched to the reading skills of the patient
    (2) Videotapes
    (3) Audiotapes
    (4) Computer-assisted instruction
    (5) Internet
    (6) Flip charts
    (7) Models
    (8) Calendars or journals
  i) Use various methods of teaching.
    (1) Personal session

Table 8. Stage-Appropriate Teaching Strategies

Learner	General Characteristics	Teaching Strategies	Nursing Interventions
Infancy–toddlerhood Approximate age: Birth–2 years Cognitive stage: Sensorimotor Psychosocial stage: Trust versus mistrust (birth–12 months) Autonomy versus shame and doubt (1–2 years)	Dependent on environment Needs security Explores self and environment Natural curiosity	Orient teaching to caregiver. Use repetition and imitation of information. Stimulate all senses. Provide physical safety and emotional security. Allow play and manipulation of objects.	Welcome active involvement. Forge alliances. Encourage physical closeness. Provide detailed information. Answer questions and concerns. Ask for information on child's strengths/limitations and likes/dislikes.
Early childhood Approximate age: 3–5 years Cognitive stage: Preoperational Psychosocial stage: Initiative versus guilt	Egocentric Thinking is precausal, concrete, literal Believes illness is self-caused and punitive Limited sense of time Fears bodily injury Cannot generalize Animistic thinking (objects possess life or human characteristics) Centration (focus is on one characteristic of an object) Separation anxiety Motivated by curiosity Active imagination, prone to fears Play is his/her work	Use warm, calm approach. Build trust. Use repetition of information. Allow manipulation of objects and equipment. Give care with explanation. Reassure not to blame self. Explain procedures simply and briefly. Provide safe, secure environment. Use positive reinforcement. Encourage questions to reveal perceptions/feelings. Use simple drawings and stories. Use play therapy, with dolls and puppets. Stimulate senses: visual, auditory, tactile, and motor.	Welcome active involvement. Forge alliances. Encourage physical closeness. Provide detailed information. Answer questions and concerns. Ask for information on child's strengths/limitations and likes/dislikes.
Middle and late childhood Approximate age: 6–11 years Cognitive stage: Concrete operations Psychosocial stage: Industry versus inferiority	More realistic and objective Understands cause and effect Deductive/inductive reasoning Wants concrete information Able to compare objects and events Variable rates of physical growth Reasons syllogistically Understands seriousness and consequences of actions Subject-centered focus Immediate orientation	Encourage independence and active participation. Be honest; allay fears. Use logical explanation. Allow time to ask questions. Use analogies to make invisible processes real. Establish role models. Relate care to other children's experiences; compare procedures. Use subject-centered focus. Use play therapy. Provide group activities. Use drawings, models, dolls, painting, and audio- and videotapes.	Welcome active involvement. Forge alliances. Encourage physical closeness. Provide detailed information. Answer questions and concerns. Ask for information on child's strengths/limitations and likes/dislikes.
Adolescence Approximate age: 12–19 years Cognitive stage: Formal operations Psychosocial stage: Identity versus role confusion	Abstract, hypothetical thinking Can build on past learning Reasons by logic and understands scientific principles Future orientation Motivated by a desire for social acceptance Peer group is important Intense personal preoccupation; appearance is extremely important (imaginary audience) Feels invulnerable, invincible/immune to natural laws (personal fable)	Establish trust and authenticity. Know their agenda. Address fears/concerns about outcomes of illness. Identify control focus. Include in plan of care. Use peers for support and influence. Negotiate changes. Focus on details. Make information meaningful to life. Ensure confidentiality and privacy. Arrange group sessions. Use audiovisuals, role-play, contracts, and reading materials. Provide for experimentation and flexibility.	Explore emotional and financial support. Determine goals and expectations. Assess stress levels. Respect values and norms. Determine role responsibilities and relationships. Allow for 1:1 teaching without parents present, but with adolescent's permission, inform family of content covered.

(Continued on next page)

Table 8. Stage-Appropriate Teaching Strategies *(Continued)*

Learner	General Characteristics	Teaching Strategies	Nursing Interventions
Young adulthood Approximate age: 20–40 years Cognitive stage: Formal operations Psychosocial stage: Intimacy versus isolation	Autonomous Self-directed Uses personal experiences to enhance or interfere with learning Intrinsic motivation Able to analyze critically Makes decisions about personal, occupational, and social roles Competency-based learner	Use problem-centered focus. Draw on meaningful experiences. Focus on immediacy of application. Encourage active participation. Allow to set own pace and be self-directed. Organize material. Recognize social role. Apply new knowledge through role-playing and hands-on practice.	Explore emotional, financial, and physical support system. Assess motivational level for involvement. Identify potential obstacles and stressors.
Middle-aged adulthood Approximate age: 41–64 years Cognitive stage: Formal operations Psychosocial stage: Generativity versus self-absorption and stagnation	Sense of self well-developed Concerned with physical changes At peak in career Explores alternative lifestyles Reflects on contributions to family and society Reexamines goals and values Questions achievements and successes Has confidence in abilities Desires to modify unsatisfactory aspects of life	Focus on maintaining independence and reestablishing normal life patterns. Assess positive and negative past experiences with learning. Assess potential sources of stress due to midlife crisis issues. Provide information to coincide with life concerns and problems.	Explore emotional, financial, and physical support system. Assess motivational level for involvement. Identify potential obstacles and stressors.
Older adulthood Approximate age: 65 years and older Cognitive stage: Formal operations Psychosocial stage: Ego integrity versus despair	**Cognitive changes** Decreased ability to think abstractly and process information Decreased short-term memory Increased reaction time Increased test anxiety Stimulus persistence (afterimage) Focuses on past life experiences	Use concrete examples. Build on past life experiences. Make information relevant and meaningful. Present one concept at a time. Allow time for processing/response (slow pace). Use repetition and reinforcement of information. Avoid written exams. Use verbal exchange and coaching. Establish retrieval plan (use one or several clues). Encourage active involvement. Keep explanations brief. Use analogies to illustrate abstract information.	Involve principal caregivers. Encourage participation. Provide resources for support (respite care). Assess coping mechanisms. Provide written instructions for reinforcement. Provide anticipatory problem solving (what happens if . . .).
	Sensory/motor deficits Auditory changes Hearing loss, especially high-pitched tones, consonants (*S, Z, T, F*, and *G*), and rapid speech Visual changes Farsighted (needs glasses to read) Lenses become opaque (glare problem) Smaller pupil size (decreased visual adaptation to darkness) Decreased peripheral perception Yellowing of lenses (distorts low-tone colors: blue, green, violet)	Speak slowly, distinctly. Use low-pitched tones. Face client when speaking. Minimize distractions. Avoid shouting. Use visual aids to supplement verbal instruction. Avoid glares, use soft white light. Provide sufficient light. Use white backgrounds and black print. Use large letters and well-spaced print. Avoid color coding with blues, greens, purples, and yellows. Increase safety precautions/provide safe environment. Ensure accessibility and fit of prostheses (i.e., glasses, hearing aid). Keep sessions short. Provide for frequent rest periods.	

(Continued on next page)

Table 8. Stage-Appropriate Teaching Strategies *(Continued)*

Learner	General Characteristics	Teaching Strategies	Nursing Interventions
Older adulthood *(cont.)*	Distorted depth perception Fatigue/decreased energy levels Pathophysiology (chronic illness)	Allow for extra time to perform. Establish realistic short-term goals.	
	Psychosocial changes Decreased risk taking Selective learning Intimidated by formal learning	Give time to reminisce. Identify and present pertinent material. Use informal teaching sessions. Demonstrate relevance of information to daily life. Assess resources. Make learning positive. Identify past positive experiences. Integrate new behaviors with formerly established ones.	

Note. From *Nurse as Educator: Principles of Teaching and Learning for Nursing Practice* (3rd ed., pp. 152–156), by S.B. Bastable and M.A. Dart, 2008, Sudbury, MA: Jones and Bartlett. Copyright 2008 by Jones and Bartlett Learning, www.jblearning.com. Reprinted with permission.

(2) Group instruction or class

(3) Family conference

(4) Role-play

(5) Demonstration

j) Provide immediate feedback to the learner to increase motivation or the desire to learn (Moss, 1994). Feedback consists of positive reinforcement or suggestions for improvement (Smeltzer, Bare, Hinkle, & Cheever, 2010).

k) Strategies for teaching patients with low literacy skills include using multiple teaching methods and tools, partitioning information into small pieces, using vivid visuals, encouraging interaction during the educational session, offering examples or testimonials, and using videotapes (Bastable, 2008a; Doak, Doak, Friedell, & Meade, 1998; Meade, 1996).

9. Evaluation

a) Obtain verbal feedback from patient.

b) Observe return demonstration.

c) Modify the teaching plan to enhance learning (Smeltzer et al., 2010).

d) Reinforce learning at subsequent patient visits.

10. Documentation: Use the ONS *Radiation Therapy Patient Care Record* (Catlin-Huth, Haas, & Pollock, 2002) or similar documentation tool

a) Assessment: Document identified learning needs and any factors that may influence the patient's learning in the medical record.

b) Planning: Document learning objectives.

c) Implementation: Document the person(s) taught, topics, and methods used.

d) Evaluation: Document the patient's response to teaching, and plan for reinforcement and further evaluation.

11. Selected online resources

a) American Cancer Society (ACS): www.cancer.org

b) ASTRO RT Answers: www.rtanswers.org

c) National Center for Complementary and Alternative Medicine: http://nccam.nih.gov

d) National Coalition for Cancer Survivorship: www.canceradvocacy.org

e) National Institute for Literacy LINCS (Literacy Information and Communication System): http://lincs.ed.gov

f) National Library of Medicine MedlinePlus®: www.nlm.nih.gov/medlineplus

g) NCI: www.cancer.gov

h) NCI Office of Cancer Survivorship: http://cancercontrol.cancer.gov/ocs

i) ONS: www.ons.org

References

Agre, P. (2005). The education process. In J.K. Itano & K.N. Taoka (Eds.), *Core curriculum for oncology nursing* (4th ed., pp. 893–898). St. Louis, MO: Elsevier Saunders.

Allen, J.D., Savadatti, S., & Levy, A.G. (2009). The transition from breast cancer "patient" to survivor." *Psycho-Oncology, 18,* 71–78. doi:10.1002/pon.1380

American Hospital Association. (2003). The patient care partnership: Understanding expectations, rights and responsibilities. Retrieved from http://www.aha.org/aha/content/2003/pdf/pcp_english_030730.pdf

American Nurses Association. (2010). *Nursing: Scope and standards of practice* (2nd ed.). Washington, DC: Author.

Bandura, A. (1977). Self-efficacy: Toward a unifying theory of behavioral change. *Psychological Review, 84,* 191–215.

Bandura, A., & Adams, N.E. (1977). An analysis of self-efficacy theory of behavior change. *Cognitive Therapy and Research, 1,* 125–139.

Bandura, A., Adams, N.E., & Beyer, J. (1977). Cognitive processes mediating behavior change. *Journal of Personality and Social Psychology, 35,* 125–139.

Bartlett, E.E. (1985). At last, a definition. *Patient Education and Counseling, 7,* 323–324. doi:10.1016/0738-3991(85)90041-2

Bastable, S.B. (2008a). Literacy in the adult client population. In S.B. Bastable (Ed.), *Nurse as educator: Principles of teaching and learning for nursing practice* (3rd ed., pp. 229–283). Sudbury, MA: Jones and Bartlett.

Bastable, S.B. (2008b). Overview of education in health care. In S.B. Bastable (Ed.), *Nurse as educator: Principles of teaching and learning for nursing practice* (3rd ed., pp. 3–23). Sudbury, MA: Jones and Bartlett.

Bastable, S.B., & Dart, M.A. (2008). Developmental stages of the learner. In S.B. Bastable (Ed.), *Nurse as educator: Principles of teaching and learning for nursing practice* (3rd ed., pp. 147–198). Sudbury, MA: Jones and Bartlett.

Becker, M.H. (1974). The Health Belief Model and personal health behavior. *Health Education Monographs, 2,* 324–473.

Bruner, D.W. (1993). Radiation oncology nurses: Staffing patterns and role development. *Oncology Nursing Forum, 20,* 651–655.

Bruner, J.S. (1966). *Toward a theory of instruction.* Cambridge, MA: Belknap Press of Harvard University.

Catlin-Huth, C., Haas, M., & Pollock, V. (Eds.). (2002). *Radiation therapy patient care record: A tool for documenting nursing care.* Pittsburgh, PA: Oncology Nursing Society.

Chelf, J.H., Agre, P., Axelrod, A., Cheney, L., Cole, D.D., Conrad, K., ... Weaver, C. (2001). Cancer-related patient education: An overview of the last decade of evaluation and research. *Oncology Nursing Forum, 28,* 1139–1147.

Chew, L.D., Bradley, K.A., & Boyko, E.J. (2004). Brief questions to identify patients with inadequate health literacy. *Family Medicine, 36,* 588–594.

Christman, N.J., & Cain, L.B. (2004). The effects of concrete objective information and relaxation on maintaining usual activity during radiation therapy [Online exclusive]. *Oncology Nursing Forum, 31,* E39–E45. doi:10.1188/04.ONF.E39-E45

Coleman, J.S. (1988). Social capital in the creation of human capital. *American Journal of Sociology, 94,* S95–S121.

Costanzo, E.S., Lutgendorf, S.K., Mattes, M.L., Trehan, S., Robinson, C.B., Tewfik, F., & Roman, S.L. (2007). Adjusting to life after treatment: distress and quality of life following treatment for breast cancer. *British Journal of Cancer, 97,* 1625–1631. doi:10.1038/sj.bjc.6604091

D'Haese, S., Vinh-Hung, V., Bijdekerke, P., Spinnoy, M., De Beukeleer, M., Lochie, N., ... Storme, G. (2000). The effect of timing of the provision of information on anxiety and satisfaction of cancer patients receiving radiotherapy. *Journal of Cancer Education, 15,* 223–227.

Davis, T.C., Crouch, M.A., Long, S.W., Jackson, R.H., Bates, P., George, R.B., & Bairnsfather, L.E. (1991). Rapid assessment of literacy levels of adult primary care patients. *Family Medicine, 23,* 433–435.

Davis, T.C., Williams, M.V., Marin, E., Parker, R.M., & Glass, J. (2002). Health literacy and cancer communication. *CA: A Cancer Journal for Clinicians, 52,* 134–149. doi:10.3322/canjclin.52.3.134

Deshields, T., Tibbs, T., Fan, M.-Y., Bayer, L., Taylor, M., & Fisher, E. (2005). Ending treatment: The course of emotional adjustment and quality of life among breast cancer survivors immediately following radiation therapy. *Supportive Care in Cancer, 13,* 1018–1026. doi:10.1007/s00520-005-0801-z

Doak, C.C., Doak, L.G., Friedell, G.H., & Meade, C.D. (1998). Improving comprehension for cancer patients with low literacy skills: Strategies for clinicians. *CA: A Cancer Journal for Clinicians, 48,* 151–162. doi:10.3322/canjclin.48.3.151

Doak, C.C., Doak, L.G., & Root, J.H. (1996). *Teaching patients with low literacy skills* (2nd ed.). Philadelphia, PA: Lippincott.

Dodd, M.J. (1987). Efficacy of proactive information on self-care in radiation therapy patients. *Heart and Lung, 16,* 538–544.

Dunn, J., Steginga, S.K., Rose, P., Scott, J., & Allison, R. (2004). Evaluating patient education materials about radiation therapy. *Patient Education and Counseling, 52,* 325–332. doi:10.1016/S0738-3991(03)00108-3

Festinger, L. (1957). *A theory of cognitive dissonance.* Stanford, CA: Stanford University Press.

Gosselin-Acomb, T.K. (2006). Role of the radiation oncology nurse. *Seminars in Oncology Nursing, 22,* 198–202. doi:10.1016/j.soncn.2006.07.001

Häggmark, C., Bohman, L., Ilmoni-Brandt, K., Näslund, I., Sjödén, P.O., & Nilsson, B. (2001). Effects of information supply on satisfaction with information and quality of life in cancer patients receiving curative radiation therapy. *Patient Education and Counseling, 45,* 173–179. doi:10.1016/S0738-3991(01)00116-1

Hagopian, G.A. (1991). The effects of a weekly radiation therapy newsletter on patients. *Oncology Nursing Forum, 18,* 1199–1203.

Hagopian, G.A. (1996). The effects of informational audiotapes on knowledge and self-care behaviors of patients undergoing radiation therapy. *Oncology Nursing Forum, 23,* 697–700.

Harrison, J.A., Mullen, P.D., & Green, L.W. (1992). A meta-analysis of studies of the Health Belief Model with adults. *Health Education Research, 7,* 107–116. doi:10.1093/her/7.1.107

Harrison, R., Dey, P., Slevin, N.J., Eardley, A., Gibbs, A., Cowan, R., ... Hopwood, P. (2001). Randomized controlled trial to assess the effectiveness of a videotape about radiotherapy. *British Journal of Cancer, 84,* 8–10. doi:10.1054/bjoc.2000.1536

Hilderley, L.J. (1980). The role of the nurse in radiation oncology. *Seminars in Oncology, 7,* 39–47.

Hinds, C., Streater, A., & Mood, D. (1995). Functions and preferred methods of receiving information related to radiotherapy. Perceptions of patients with cancer. *Cancer Nursing, 18,* 374–384.

Hochbaum, G.M., Sorenson, J.R., & Lorig, K. (1992). Theory in health education practice. *Health Education Quarterly, 19,* 295–313. doi:10.1177/109019819201900303

Hoff, A.C., & Haaga, D.A.F. (2006). Effects of an education program on radiation oncology patients and families. *Journal of Psychosocial Oncology, 23*(4), 61–79. doi:10.1300/J077v23n04_04

Institute of Medicine. (2006). *From cancer patient to cancer survivor: Lost in transition.* Washington, DC: National Academies Press.

Kitchie, S. (2008). Determinants of learning. In S.B. Bastable (Ed.), *Nurse as educator: Principles of teaching and learning for nursing practice* (3rd ed., pp. 93–146). Sudbury, MA: Jones and Bartlett.

Knowles, M.S. (1970). *The modern practice of adult education.* New York, NY: Association Press.

Kripalani, S., Henderson, L.E., Chiu, E.Y., Robertson, R., Kolm, P., & Jacobson, T.A. (2006). Predictors of medication self-management skill in a low-literacy population. *Journal of General Internal Medicine, 21,* 852–856. doi:10.1111/j.1525-1497.2006.00536.x

Kutner, M., Greenberg, E., Jin, Y., & Paulsen, C. (2006). *The health literacy of America's adults: Results from the 2003 National Assess-*

ment of Adult Literacy (Report No. NCES 2006-483). Washington, DC: National Center for Education Statistics.

Lethborg, C.E., Kissane, D., Burns, W.I., & Snyder, R. (2000). "Cast adrift": The experience of completing treatment among women with early stage breast cancer. *Journal of Psychosocial Oncology, 18*(4), 73–90. doi:10.1300/J077v18n04_05

Lewin, K. (1943). Defining the "field at a given time." *Psychological Review, 50,* 292–310. doi:10.1037/h0062738

Mancuso, J.M. (2009). Assessment and measurement of health literacy: An integrative review of the literature. *Nursing and Health Sciences, 11,* 77–89. doi:10.1111/j.1442-2018.2008.00408.x

Meade, C.D. (1996). Producing videotapes for cancer education: Methods and examples. *Oncology Nursing Forum, 23,* 837–846.

Merriman, B., Ades, T., & Seffrin, J.R. (2002). Health literacy in the information age: Communicating cancer information to patients and families. *CA: A Cancer Journal for Clinicians, 52,* 130–133. doi:10.3322/canjclin.52.3.130

Moore-Higgs, G.J., Watkins-Bruner, D., Balmer, L., Johnson-Doneski, J., Komarny, P., Mautner, B., & Velji, K. (2003). The role of licensed nursing personnel in radiation oncology. Part B: Integrating the ambulatory care nursing conceptual framework. *Oncology Nursing Forum, 30,* 59–64. doi:10.1188/03.ONF.59-64

Moss, V.A. (1994). Assessing learning abilities, readiness for education. *Seminars in Perioperative Nursing, 3,* 113–120.

Oncology Nursing Society. (2009). Quality cancer care [Position statement]. Retrieved from http://www.ons.org/Publications/Positions/Quality

Parker, R.M., Baker, D.W., Williams, M.V., & Nurss, J.R. (1995). The test of functional health literacy in adults: A new instrument for measuring patients' literacy skills. *Journal of General Internal Medicine, 10,* 537–541.

Poroch, D. (1995). The effect of preparatory patient education on the anxiety and satisfaction of cancer patients receiving radiation therapy. *Cancer Nursing, 18,* 206–214.

Prochaska, J.O., & DiClemente, C.C. (1983). Stages and processes of self-change of smoking: Toward an integrative model of change. *Journal of Consulting and Clinical Psychology, 51,* 390–395.

Quirk, P.A. (2000). Screening for literacy and readability: Implications for the advanced practice nurse. *Clinical Nurse Specialist, 14,* 26–32.

Redman, B.K. (2001). *The practice of patient education* (9th ed.). St. Louis, MO: Mosby.

Rendon, D.C., Davis, D.K., Gioiella, E.C., & Tranzillo, M.J. (1986). The right to know, the right to be taught. *Journal of Gerontological Nursing, 12*(12), 33–38.

Rogers, E.M., & Shoemaker, F.F. (1971). *Communication of innovations* (2nd ed.). New York, NY: Free Press.

Rose, P., & Yates, P. (2001). Quality of life experienced by patients receiving radiation treatment for cancers of the head and neck. *Cancer Nursing, 24,* 255–263.

Rosenstock, I.M. (1974). The Health Belief Model and preventive health behavior. *Health Education Monographs, 2,* 354–386.

Selden, C.R., Zorn, M., Ratzan, S.C., & Parker, R.M. (2000). Current bibliographies in medicine 2000-1: Health literacy. Retrieved from http://www.nlm.nih.gov/archive//20061214/pubs/cbm/hliteracy.html

Shepard, N., & Kelvin, J.F. (1999). The nursing role in radiation oncology. *Seminars in Oncology Nursing, 15,* 237–249.

Smeltzer, S.C., Bare, B.G., Hinkle, J.L., & Cheever, K.H. (2010). *Brunner & Suddarth's textbook of medical-surgical nursing* (12th ed., Vol. 1). Philadelphia, PA: Wolters Kluwer/Lippincott Williams & Wilkins.

Strohl, R.A. (1988). The nursing role in radiation oncology: Symptom management of acute and chronic reactions. *Oncology Nursing Forum, 15,* 429–434.

Thomas, R., Daly, M., Perryman, B., & Stockton, D. (2000). Forewarned is forearmed—Benefits of preparatory information on video cassette for patients receiving chemotherapy or radiotherapy—A randomised controlled trial. *European Journal of Cancer, 36,* 1536–1543. doi:10.1016/S0959-8049(00)00136-2

Treacy, J.T., & Mayer, D.K. (2000). Perspectives on cancer patient education. *Seminars in Oncology Nursing, 16,* 47–56. doi:10.1016/S0749-2081(00)80007-8

Wallace, L.S., Cassada, D.C., Rogers, E.S., Freeman, M.B., Grandas, O.H., Stevens, S.L., & Goldman, M.H. (2007). Can screening items identify surgery patients at risk of limited health literacy? *Journal of Surgical Research, 140,* 208–213. doi:10.1016/j.jss.2007.01.029

Wallston, B.S., Wallston, K.A., Kaplan, G.D., & Maides, S.A. (1976). Development and validation of the health locus of control (HLC) scale. *Journal of Consulting and Clinical Psychology, 44,* 580–585. doi:10.1037/0022-006X.44.4.580

Wells, M. (1998). The hidden experience of radiotherapy to the head and neck: A qualitative study of patients after completion of treatment. *Journal of Advanced Nursing, 28,* 840–848. doi:10.1111/j.1365-2648.1998x.00714.x

B. Fatigue
  1. Pathophysiology
      a) The underlying etiology of fatigue in patients receiving RT is multifactorial; several theories have been proposed (Ryan et al., 2007).
          (1) Serotonin dysregulation: Cancer or its treatment may cause an increase in serotonin (5-hydroxytryptamine, or 5-HT) levels and/or upregulation of 5-HT receptors (Andrews, Morrow, & Hickok, 2004). The influence of 5-HT on appetite, sleep, memory, learning, temperature regulation, mood, behavior, cardiovascular function, muscle contraction, endocrine regulation, and depression suggests that 5-HT may have an effect on central fatigue. Proinflammatory cytokines such as tumor necrosis factor (TNF)-alpha may dysregulate the feedback loop, causing an increase of 5-HT release.
          (2) Hypothalamic-pituitary-adrenal (HPA) axis dysfunction: Cancer or its treatment may change the pattern of cortisol release by the HPA axis (the central regulatory system of cortisol). Serum cortisol varies, with the most concentration observed after waking and then tapering during the day (Posener, Schildkraut, Samson, & Schatzberg, 1996). Patients receiving RT may have fatigue associated with decreased serum cortisol levels, although the cor-

relation of cancer, fatigue, and HPA axis dysregulation is ambiguous.

(3) Circadian rhythm disruption: Changes in cortisol secretion rhythm and rest-activity pattern have been associated with increased fatigue in patients with cancer (Rich, 2007). A flatter diurnal cortisol slope was observed in those with greater fatigue. Fluctuating or depressed circadian rhythms may increase fatigue levels. Circadian dysregulation caused by cancer is complex: it may be related to genetic factors or psychosocial, environmental, and behavioral components, as well as host response to the tumor. Changes in immune functioning of patients with breast cancer have been linked with a flattened cortisol rhythm (Ryan et al., 2007).

(4) Muscle metabolism/adenosine triphosphate (ATP) dysregulation: ATP is the basis for energy needed for skeletal muscle functioning. Cancer-related fatigue (CRF) causes weakness or lack of energy, leading to peripheral fatigue. Regeneration of ATP in skeletal muscle may be compromised by the cancer or its treatment, resulting in decreased functional capacity. As a result of decreased intake of food and fluid because of changes in appetite and treatment side effects, replacement of ATP may be minimized. Patients with cancer, especially those with anorexia and cachexia, may have a greater likelihood of developing changes in metabolism of muscle protein (Giordano et al., 2003).

(5) Vagal afferent nerve activation: Signals transmitted from the viscera to the brain stem are dependent upon the vagal nerve. The vagal afferent nerve hypothesis suggests that somatic muscle activity inhibition and occurrence of "sickness behavior" is due to cancer or treatment stimulating vagal afferent nerves (Seruga, Zhang, Bernstein, & Tannock, 2008). This may contribute to a decrease in skeletal muscle tone, general weakness, fatigue, and a decreased ability to concentrate.

(6) Cytokine dysregulation: Increases in plasma levels of proinflammatory cytokines resulting from cancer tumor by-products or treatment are associated with increased fatigue (Ryan et al., 2007). In a pooled analysis of 18 studies, some of which included patients treated with RT, positive associations were found between fatigue and circulating levels of inflammatory markers (Schubert, Hong, Natarajan, Mills, & Dimsdale, 2007). Cytokines including TNF and interferon-alpha have been specifically linked with increased lethargy, anorexia, and fatigue.

b) Risk factors

(1) Anemia: Defined as a hemoglobin level of 11 g/dl or lower, anemia may be the result of cancer or its treatment (NCCN, 2011). Cancer-related anemia is attributable to a number of factors, including bleeding, hemolysis, bone marrow infiltration, and suboptimal nutrition. Decreased oxygenation of vital organs is a likely cause of fatigue.

(2) Nutritional disturbances: Cancer cachexia includes decreases in adipose tissue and skeletal muscle mass, leading to anorexia, weight loss, and fatigue.

(3) Emotional distress: Patients with cancer frequently experience depression. Studies have observed interruption in rest-activity rhythms (Berger, 1998), 5-HT dysfunction (Ryan et al., 2007), and changes in HPA axis activity (Bower, Ganz, & Aziz, 2005; Bower, Ganz, Dickerson, et al., 2005). The relationship between depression and fatigue is unclear; current research shows mixed results of the origin of these two symptoms. Greater mental fatigue has been correlated with anxiety for individuals with brain tumors (Purcell et al., 2010).

(4) Sleep disorders: Sleep disorders are strong predictors of fatigue in patients with cancer (Berger, 1998; Roscoe et al., 2007). Symptoms including light

sleep, increased wakefulness, early awakening, and difficulty falling asleep contribute to fatigue.

(5) Nutritional deficits occur because of alterations in taste, leading to food aversions, decreased food intake, and weight loss (Ravasco, 2005). Gastrointestinal (GI) tissue within the RT field may develop inflammatory changes, resulting in nausea, diarrhea, constipation, pain, and weight loss (McGough, Baldwin, Frost, & Andreyev, 2004).

(6) Therapies received prior to RT may influence the level of fatigue at the initiation of treatment (Purcell et al., 2010). Treatment with chemotherapy followed by RT may result in greater fatigue than RT alone (Bower et al., 2006; Dhruva et al., 2010; Donovan et al., 2004). RT to the head and neck correlates with a more severe increase in fatigue during treatment compared to those receiving pelvic radiation (Purcell et al., 2010). Fatigue was found to be worse on treatment days, with decrease in severity of symptoms on days off of treatment. Concomitant treatment is a potential contributing factor to radiation-related fatigue (Jereczek-Fossa, Marsiglia, & Orecchia, 2001).

(7) Comorbidities that may contribute to increased fatigue include diabetes, hypertension, heart disease, arthritis, hypothyroidism, malnutrition, and emotional distress (Bower et al., 2006; Morrow, 2007). Poirier's (2007) investigation showed that comorbidities in addition to a lack of social support may contribute to decreased functioning in patients with cancer.

2. Incidence and prevalence

a) No population-based studies exist on the incidence (identification of new cases) of fatigue related to RT for cancer. An incidence study conducted in two institutions evaluated women undergoing treatment for breast cancer (N = 288) who completed a diagnostic interview to identify cases of CRF prior to initiating chemotherapy or RT and after completing treatment (Andrykowski, Schmidt, Salsman, Beacham, & Jacobsen, 2005). Sixty women (21% of the entire sample) who did not meet the criteria for CRF before therapy were identified as "incident" or new cases of CRF after treatment completion; about one-third

(35%) of these new CRF cases had been treated with RT.

b) Two prevalence studies relevant to RT for cancer that were population based showed that the prevalence of fatigue varied depending on the patients studied, the timing of measurement, and the definition/measure of fatigue. Based on these studies and one systematic review, strong evidence supports that fatigue is a significant problem during and after cancer treatment.

(1) Vogelzang et al. (1997) conducted a telephone survey of 419 patients treated with RT or chemotherapy who were recruited from 100,000 randomly selected households in the United States. Fatigue during the course of treatment was reported by 78%; 32% reported having it on a daily basis and said it interfered with work, physical and emotional well-being, and enjoyment of life.

(2) Forlenza, Hall, Lichtenstein, Evengard, and Sullivan (2005) studied 30,525 individuals in the Swedish Twin Registry who had previously answered questions about fatigue in their daily lives; 1,103 of these individuals were also listed in the Swedish Cancer Registry, indicating they had been treated for cancer at some time in the past. Using various definitions of fatigue, 11.2%–23.2% of the cancer survivor group reported feeling "abnormally tired" during the most recent six months, which was higher than the prevalence of fatigue in the group without cancer (7.9%–19.7%). The association between fatigue in the survivor group and type of treatment was not investigated.

(3) Prue, Rankin, Allen, Gracey, and Cramp (2006) conducted a systematic review of the prevalence of fatigue related to cancer (including 11 studies of RT). Fatigue was apparent during and after RT, although the prevalence varied. In one study that was reviewed, prevalence differed by cancer diagnosis, with 65%–93% reporting fatigue during RT and 14%–46% reporting it three months later (King, Nail, Kreamer, Strohl, & Johnson, 1985). In a study of women receiving RT for breast cancer, 43% reported significant fatigue (Wratten et al., 2004). In a sample of men studied two or more years after

RT for prostate cancer, 19% reported severe fatigue (Vordermark, Schwab, Flentje, Sailer, & Kölbl, 2002).

3. Assessment: NCCN (2010) recommends that patients with cancer be screened for fatigue at regular intervals and that those who screen positive should have a comprehensive evaluation.

a) Screening: The first step is to screen for the presence or absence of fatigue using a question such as, "Are you experiencing fatigue?" If fatigue is present, a 0–10 numeric rating scale can be used to rate the severity of fatigue. A score of 0–3 indicates mild fatigue, 4–6 indicates moderate fatigue, and 7–10 indicates severe fatigue. NCCN recommends that a score of 4 or greater should trigger a more comprehensive evaluation of fatigue (NCCN, 2010).

b) Comprehensive evaluation

(1) Focused history

(a) Disease and treatment status (rule out recurrence or progression; obtain information on current medications, nonprescription drugs, or supplements, chemotherapy, RT, last date of treatment)

(b) Review of systems

(c) In-depth fatigue history (onset, pattern, duration, change over time, associated or alleviating factors, interference with function)

(2) Assessment of treatable contributing factors

(a) Pain

(b) Emotional distress (anxiety, depression)

(c) Anemia

(d) Sleep disturbance

(e) Nutritional status (weight, intake, fluid/electrolyte balance)

(f) Activity level (decreased activity or fitness)

(g) Medication side effects

(h) Alcohol or substance abuse

(i) Comorbid conditions (infection; cardiac, pulmonary, renal, hepatic, neurologic, or endocrine dysfunction)

c) Fatigue assessment tools: Few valid and reliable measures of fatigue are available that are appropriate for use in clinical practice. Desirable characteristics of a clinical practice tool include brevity, ease of completion and scoring, and information to guide interpretation of scores.

(1) The NCCN fatigue screening tool is a 0–10 scale (0 = no fatigue and 10 = extreme fatigue) (NCCN, 2010). Based on consensus within the NCCN fatigue guidelines panel, a score of 4 or greater (defined as moderate fatigue) is the threshold for further evaluation. Research to define groups with mild, moderate, or severe fatigue has shown inconsistent results, leaving the NCCN consensus-based recommendation as the most logical choice (Butt et al., 2008; Chang et al., 2007; Given et al., 2008).

(2) The ONS fatigue scale is a 1–5 scale (1 = no fatigue, 2 = mild fatigue, 3 = moderate fatigue, 4 = extreme fatigue, and 5 = worst fatigue (Catlin-Huth, Haas, & Pollock, 2002). No empirically based cut score is available.

(3) The "fatigue" criterion of the *Common Terminology Criteria for Adverse Events* (CTCAE) is a 1–3 scale (1 = fatigue relieved by rest; 2 = fatigue not relieved by rest, limiting instrumental activities of daily living [ADL]; and 3 = fatigue not relieved by rest, limiting self-care ADL) (NCI Cancer Therapy Evaluation Program [CTEP], 2010). No empirically based cut score is available.

(4) Numerous multi-item questionnaires have been evaluated as valid and reliable measures of fatigue. Several recent reviews of published CRF instruments highlight the validity and reliability, as well as the strengths and weaknesses, of each measure (Barsevick et al., 2010; Minton & Stone, 2009; Mota & Pimenta, 2006; Whitehead, 2009).

(5) A set of diagnostic criteria for CRF syndrome was proposed to standardize fatigue assessment and identify cases of fatigue (Alexander, Minton, Andrews, & Stone, 2009; Alexander, Minton, & Stone, 2009; Cella, Davis, Breitbart, & Curt, 2001; Sadler et al., 2002; Servaes, Prins, Verhagen, & Bleijenberg, 2002). To fulfill the diagnostic criteria, an individual must report 6 of 11 symptoms on most days for two weeks, and at least one symptom must be "significant fatigue, lack of energy, or increased need to rest" (Cella et al., 2001, p. 3386). Also, fatigue must be severe enough to affect daily functioning, must be a consequence of cancer

or cancer therapy, and must not be primarily related to a psychiatric disorder (see Figure 16). This set of criteria was submitted and accepted for inclusion in the *International Classification of Diseases* (ICD-10) (Portenoy & Itri, 1999).

d) Follow-up assessment is used to track fatigue over time and evaluate the effectiveness of fatigue management strategies. Fatigue assessment should be conducted at regular intervals during treatment and after treatment completion (NCCN, 2010). Although fatigue may resolve after treatment, some patients experience chronic fatigue that is negatively associated with quality of life (Bower, 2005; Bower et al., 2006; Jereczek-Fossa et al., 2001; Visser & Smets, 1998; Vordermark et al., 2002).

4. Management of treatable causes
   a) Pharmacologic management
      (1) Anemia
         (a) NCCN (2010) recommended using the cancer- and chemotherapy-induced anemia guidelines in evaluating and managing anemia as a treatable cause of fatigue.
         (b) Treatments for anemia may include iron replacement for iron-deficiency anemia and/or transfusion of packed red blood cells.
         (c) Although good evidence supports erythropoietin-stimulating agents (ESAs) as effective treatment for anemic patients receiving chemotherapy (Minton, Richardson, Sharpe, Hotopf, & Stone, 2008), the use of these agents is restricted by FDA-labeled indications. Revisions and a "black box" warning in 2010 do not include the use of ESAs in RT.
      (2) Pain: A summary of a Cochrane review (Potter, 2005) investigating the best strategy to manage cancer pain cited the World Health Organization's three-step analgesic ladder (Kumar, 2007) as the established guide.
         (a) Use acetaminophen or nonsteroidal anti-inflammatory drugs (NSAIDs) for mild cancer pain.
         (b) For moderate, weak, or episodic pain, add short-acting opioids.
         (c) Pain that is severe or intractable requires stronger, long-acting opioid medication.

         (d) Pain control should target the root cause of pain, with additional analgesics or other therapies, including antidepressants, anticonvulsants, and corticosteroids. Bisphosphonates have been shown to delay the median time to skeletal events in breast cancer, as well as providing better control of bone pain (Pavlakis, Schmidt, & Stockler, 2005).
      (3) Depression: Literature supporting pharmacologic management of depression indicates that depression affects 10%–14% of patients seen by general practitioners (Adams, Miller, & Zylstra, 2008). Studies in patients with cancer point to a prevalence rate of 25% with rates decreasing to that of the general population once patients have been in remission for a year (Navari, Brenner, & Wilson, 2008). Medi-

---

Figure 16. Proposed Criteria for Diagnosis of Cancer-Related Fatigue

The following symptoms have been present every day or nearly every day during the same 2-week period in the past month:
- Significant fatigue, diminished energy, or increased need to rest, disproportionate to any recent change in activity level

Plus five (or more) of the following:
- Complaints of generalized weakness or limb heaviness
- Diminished concentration or attention
- Decreased motivation or interest in engaging in usual activities
- Insomnia or hypersomnia
- Experience of sleep as unrefreshing or nonrestorative
- Perceived need to struggle to overcome inactivity
- Marked emotional reactivity (e.g., sadness, frustration, or irritability) to feeling fatigued
- Difficulty completing daily tasks attributed to feeling fatigued
- Perceived problems with short-term memory
- Post-exertional malaise lasting several hours

The symptoms cause clinically significant distress or impairment in social, occupational, or other important areas of functioning.

There is evidence from the history, physical examination, or laboratory findings that the symptoms are a consequence of cancer or cancer-related therapy.

The symptoms are not primarily a consequence of comorbid psychiatric disorders such as major depression, somatization disorder, somatoform disorder, or delirium.

Note. Based on information from Cella et al., 1998.

From "Cancer-Related Fatigue: Guidelines for Evaluation and Management," by R.K. Portenoy and L.M. Itri, 1999, *Oncologist, 4,* p. 2. Copyright 1999 by AlphaMed Press. Reprinted with permission.

cation use has increased as the number of available agents has grown. Several well-known classes of drugs commonly prescribed include the following.

(a) Selective serotonin reuptake inhibitors (SSRIs) and serotonin norepinephrine reuptake inhibitors (SNRIs) are used most often with good safety and tolerability (Adams et al., 2008). SSRIs, such as fluoxetine, sertraline, paroxetine, citalopram, and escitalopram, inhibit presynaptic serotonin reuptake (To, Zepf, & Woods, 2005). SNRIs slow down the reuptake of serotonin and norepinephrine at higher doses; these include venlafaxine and duloxetine (Adams et al., 2008).

(b) Tricyclic antidepressants enhance the availability of norepinephrine and serotonin neurotransmitters. This class includes nortriptyline, desipramine, and imipramine (Adams et al., 2008).

(c) Monoamine oxidase inhibitors prevent monoamine oxidase from breaking down neurotransmitters. These include phenelzine, isocarboxazid, and tranylcypromine (To et al., 2005).

(d) Additional therapies include bupropion, which prevents presynaptic reuptake of norepinephrine and dopamine, and mirtazapine, which blocks serotonin receptors (To et al., 2005).

(4) Sleep disturbance: The prevalence of insomnia in patients with cancer is greater than in the general population, ranging from 23% to 61% (Fiorentino & Ancoli-Israel, 2006). Two classes of drugs have shown effectiveness in alleviating insomnia in this group.

(a) Benzodiazepines, including lorazepam, temazepam, diazepam, and clonazepam, are a widely used class of drugs to treat insomnia. A meta-analysis showed they were superior to placebo for insomnia in healthy people (Holbrook, Crowther, Lotter, Cheng, & King, 2000). However, these drugs may be slow to bring on sleep and may cause daytime sedation and depressive symptoms following use (Lader, 2009).

(b) Nonbenzodiazepine hypnotics, such as eszopiclone, zolpidem and zolpidem extended-release, and zaleplon, are useful in decreasing sleep latency, increasing total sleep time, and providing greater continuity of sleep (Calamaro, 2008; Fiorentino & Ancoli-Israel, 2006; Joffe et al., 2010). A National Institutes of Health state-of-the-science conference on insomnia concluded that nonbenzodiazepines are as efficacious as benzodiazepines but have fewer side effects ("National Institutes of Health State of the Science Conference Statement," 2005).

(c) Antidepressants, such as mirtazapine, have shown effectiveness for the improvement of insomnia due to antihistaminergic effects (Cankurtaran et al., 2008).

(5) Nutrition: A meta-analysis of the use of progestational steroids to decrease CRF did not demonstrate any advantage when compared to placebo (Minton et al., 2008).

(6) Comorbid conditions: NCCN recommends evaluation and optimal management of noncancer comorbidities throughout the course of treatment (NCCN, 2010). This may necessitate new medications, adjustment of current medications, or both.

b) Nonpharmacologic management: Strong evidence supports that a variety of nonpharmacologic interventions reduce fatigue.

(1) Exercise has the strongest evidence to support its benefits in managing CRF during and after treatment (Mitchell, Beck, Hood, Moore, & Tanner, 2009). Fourteen meta-analyses support the efficacy of exercising several times per week. Walking, cycling, swimming,

resistance exercise, or a combination of aerobic and resistance exercise was effective in reducing fatigue.

(a) The exercise prescription should include the type of exercise; initial intensity, duration, and frequency; and rate of progression to higher levels (NCCN, 2010). Consensus-based recommendations suggest that an exercise program should be tailored to the person's age, sex, and fitness level.

(b) Safety precautions: A professional with appropriate expertise should prescribe exercise. For deconditioned individuals and those with bone metastases, referral to a rehabilitation program may be appropriate. Patients should avoid exercising one to two days after receiving chemotherapy or during periods of neutropenia, low platelets, anemia, or fever. Exercise should be discontinued and medical attention sought if dyspnea, chest pain, dizziness, pain, or nausea and vomiting occur during activity (NCCN, 2010).

(2) Psychosocial interventions: A variety of psychosocial interventions are likely to be effective in managing fatigue (Jacobsen, Donovan, Vadaparampil, & Small, 2007; Kangas, Bovbjerg, & Montgomery, 2008; Mitchell et al., 2009). Combination interventions have been more successful, whereas single interventions, such as education alone or relaxation techniques alone, have been less effective (Kangas et al., 2008).

(a) Education about fatigue: Providing concrete objective information to prepare individuals for healthcare experiences that are likely to cause fatigue has been shown to be beneficial (Mitchell et al., 2009). Concrete objective information includes a description of physical sensations, causes, patterns, and consequences of a problem such as fatigue. This enables the individual and family to plan for it and maintain a sense of control over their experiences (Barsevick et al., 2004).

(b) Energy conservation: Teaching energy conservation strategies has been shown to reduce CRF during cancer treatment (Barsevick et al., 2004; Yates et al., 2005). The goal of energy conservation is to maintain valued activities through a balance of rest and activity. Strategies include delegation of less important activities, priority setting, pacing oneself, use of short rest periods, and performing demanding activities when energy is high.

(c) Behavioral interventions to optimize sleep: Beneficial interventions include stimulus control (go to bed when sleepy; maintain regular arising time; get out of bed when unable to sleep; avoid daytime napping), sleep restriction (limit amount of time in bed to closely approximate time asleep), and cognitive therapy (reduce or eliminate unrealistic sleep expectations and misconceptions about the cause of insomnia; emphasize the consequences of sleeplessness and anxiety resulting from failed attempts to control sleep) (Berger, 2009).

(d) Relaxation training: Behavioral techniques used to achieve a relaxed state have shown some benefit in combination with other approaches to reduce fatigue (Cohen & Fried, 2007; Decker, Cline-Elsen, & Gallagher, 1992; Jacobsen et al., 2002; Kim & Kim, 2005; Kim, Roscoe, & Morrow, 2002). These include progressive muscle relaxation (flexing and relaxing each body part in succession), guided imagery (imagining a restful scene with all the senses), diaphragmatic breathing (taking slow deep breaths that expand the whole diaphragm and push out the abdomen), body scan (focusing attention on each body part while in a relaxing position), and meditation (focusing on a word, sound, or object while clearing other thoughts from one's mind). Related interventions that have some evidence of effectiveness include massage and healing touch (Mitchell et al., 2009).

5. Documentation of fatigue at regular intervals (NCCN, 2010)

a) NCCN fatigue assessment: 0–10 scale (NCCN, 2010)

b) ONS fatigue scale 1–5 (Catlin-Huth et al., 2002)

c) CTCAE 1–3 scale (NCI CTEP, 2010)

d) Additional documentation should include

 (1) Treatable factors that contribute to fatigue

 (2) Impact of fatigue on daily activities

 (3) Recommended interventions for fatigue

 (4) Outcomes of intervention.

e) Desirable patient and family education outcomes

 (1) Adequate knowledge of fatigue and strategies for managing fatigue

 (2) Demonstration of fatigue management skills (e.g., energy conservation, relaxation strategies)

 (3) Self-report of decreased fatigue

 (4) Ability to maintain important activities despite fatigue

 (5) Family support for modification of patient activities

f) Teaching tools

 (1) Symptom diary (Nail, 2004): In this diary, fatigue and 14 other symptoms are rated each day on a 0–10 scale. The diary documents patterns of fatigue and other symptoms.

 (2) "Facts About Fatigue" self-care guide (Nail, 2004): This guide provides factual information about fatigue and self-care instructions.

 (3) Web sites: Many health-related sites contain accurate updated information about fatigue.

 (a) The Cancer Journey: www.thecancerjourney.org

 (b) "Seven Ways to Manage Cancer-Related Fatigue" from ACS (see ACS, 2010)

 (c) NCCN's "Living with Cancer" information: www.nccn.com/living-with-cancer.html

 (d) Cancer.Net information for patients on coping with cancer and managing side effects, including fatigue: www.cancer.net

 (e) NCI information on fatigue: www.cancer.gov/cancertopics/coping/physicaleffects#fatigue

References

Adams, S.M., Miller, K.E., & Zylstra, R.G. (2008). Pharmacologic management of adult depression. *American Family Physician, 77,* 785–792.

Alexander, S., Minton, O., Andrews, P., & Stone, P. (2009). A comparison of the characteristics of disease-free breast cancer survivors with or without cancer-related fatigue syndrome. *European Journal of Cancer, 45,* 384–392. doi:10.1016/j.ejca.2008.09.010

Alexander, S., Minton, O., & Stone, P.C. (2009). Evaluation of screening instruments for cancer-related fatigue syndrome in breast cancer survivors. *Journal of Clinical Oncology, 27,* 1197–1201. doi:10.1200/JCO.2008.19.1668

American Cancer Society. (2010). Seven ways to manage cancer-related fatigue. Retrieved from http://www.cancer.org/Treatment/TreatmentsandSideEffects/PhysicalSideEffects/Fatigue/seven-ways-to-manage-cancer-related-fatigue

Andrews, P.L.R., Morrow, G.R., & Hickok, J.T. (2004). Mechanisms and models of fatigue associated with cancer and its treatment. Evidence of pre-clinical and clinical studies. In J. Armes, M. Krishnasamy, & I.J. Higginson (Eds.), *Fatigue in cancer* (pp. 51–87). New York, NY: Oxford University Press.

Andrykowski, M.A., Schmidt, J.E., Salsman, J.M., Beacham, A.O., & Jacobsen, P.B. (2005). Use of a case definition approach to identify cancer-related fatigue in women undergoing adjuvant therapy for breast cancer. *Journal of Clinical Oncology, 23,* 6613–6622. doi:10.1200/JCO.2005.07.024

Barsevick, A., Beck, S.L., Dudley, W.N., Wong, B., Berger, A.M., Whitmer, K., … Stewart, K. (2010). Efficacy of an intervention for fatigue and sleep disturbance during cancer chemotherapy. *Journal of Pain and Symptom Management, 40,* 200–216. doi:10.1016/j.jpainsymman.2009.12.020

Barsevick, A.M., Dudley, W., Beck, S., Sweeney, C., Whitmer, K., & Nail, L.M. (2004). A randomized clinical trial of energy conservation for cancer-related fatigue. *Cancer, 100,* 1302–1310. doi:10.1002/cncr.20111

Berger, A.M. (1998). Patterns of fatigue and activity and rest during adjuvant breast cancer chemotherapy. *Oncology Nursing Forum, 25,* 51–62.

Berger, A.M. (2009). Update on the state of the science: Sleep-wake disturbances in adult patients with cancer [Online exclusive]. *Oncology Nursing Forum, 36,* E165–E177. doi:10.1188/09.ONF.E165-E177

Bower, J.E. (2005). Prevalence and causes of fatigue after cancer treatment: The next generation of research [Editorial]. *Journal of Clinical Oncology, 23,* 8280–8282. doi:10.1200/JCO.2005.08.008

Bower, J.E., Ganz, P.A., & Aziz, N. (2005). Altered cortisol response to psychologic stress in breast cancer survivors with persistent fatigue. *Psychosomatic Medicine, 67,* 277–280. doi:10.1097/01.psy.0000155666.55034.c6

Bower, J.E., Ganz, P.A., Desmond, K.A., Bernaards, C., Rowland, J.H., Meyerowitz, B.E., & Belin, T.R. (2006). Fatigue in long-term breast carcinoma survivors: A longitudinal investigation. *Cancer, 106,* 751–758. doi:10.1002/cncr.21671

Bower, J.E., Ganz, P.A., Dickerson, S.S., Petersen, L., Aziz, N., & Fahey, J.L. (2005). Diurnal cortisol rhythm and fatigue in breast cancer survivors. *Psychoneuroendocrinology, 30,* 92–100. doi:10.1016/j.psyneuen.2004.06.003

Butt, Z., Wagner, L.I., Beaumont, J.L., Paice, J.A., Peterman, A.H., Shevrin, D., … Cella, D. (2008). Use of a single-item screening tool to detect clinically significant fatigue, pain, distress, and anorexia in ambulatory cancer practice. *Journal of Pain and Symptom Management, 35,* 20–30. doi:10.1016/j.jpainsymman.2007.02.040

Calamaro, C. (2008). Sleeping through the night: Are extended-release formulations the answer? *Journal of the American Academy of Nurse Practitioners, 20,* 69–75. doi:10.1111/j.1745-7599.2007.00279.x

Cankurtaran, E.S., Ozalp, E., Soygur, H., Akbiyik, D.I., Turhan, L., & Alkis, N. (2008). Mirtazapine improves sleep and lowers anxiety and depression in cancer patients: Superiority over imipramine. *Supportive Care in Cancer, 16*, 1291–1298. doi:10.1007/s00520-008-0425-1

Catlin-Huth, C., Haas, M., & Pollock, V. (Eds.). (2002). *Radiation therapy patient record: A tool for documenting nursing care.* Pittsburgh, PA: Oncology Nursing Society.

Cella, D., Davis, K., Breitbart, W., & Curt, G. (2001). Cancer-related fatigue: Prevalence of proposed diagnostic criteria in a United States sample of cancer survivors. *Journal of Clinical Oncology, 19*, 3385–3391.

Cella, D., Peterman, A., Passik, S., Jacobsen, P., & Breitbart, W. (1998). Progress toward guidelines for the management of fatigue. *Oncology, 12*(11A), 369–377.

Chang, Y.J., Lee, J.S., Lee, C.G., Lee, W.S., Lee, K.S., Bang, S.-M., … Yun, Y.H. (2007). Assessment of clinical relevant fatigue level in cancer. *Supportive Care in Cancer, 15*, 891–896. doi:10.1007/s00520-007-0219-x

Cohen, M., & Fried, G. (2007). Comparing relaxation training and cognitive-behavioral group therapy for women with breast cancer. *Research on Social Work Practice, 17*, 313–323. doi:10.1177/1049731506293741

Decker, T.W., Cline-Elsen, J., & Gallagher, M. (1992). Relaxation therapy as an adjunct in radiation oncology. *Journal of Clinical Psychology, 48*, 388–393.

Dhruva, A., Dodd, M., Paul, S.M., Cooper, B.A., Lee, K., West, C., … Miaskowski, C. (2010). Trajectories of fatigue in patients with breast cancer before, during, and after radiation therapy. *Cancer Nursing, 33*, 201–212. doi:10.1097/NCC.0b013e3181c75f2a

Donovan, K.A., Jacobsen, P.B., Andrykowski, M.A., Winters, E.M., Balducci, L., Malik, U., … McGrath, P. (2004). Course of fatigue in women receiving chemotherapy and/or radiotherapy for early stage breast cancer. *Journal of Pain and Symptom Management, 28*, 373–380. doi:10.1016/j.jpainsymman.2004.01.012

Fiorentino, L., & Ancoli-Israel, S. (2006). Insomnia and its treatment in women with breast cancer. *Sleep Medicine Reviews, 10*, 419–429. doi:10.1016/j.smrv.2006.03.005

Forlenza, M.J., Hall, P., Lichtenstein, P., Evengard, B., & Sullivan, P.F. (2005). Epidemiology of cancer-related fatigue in the Swedish twin registry. *Cancer, 104*, 2022–2031. doi:10.1002/cncr.21373

Giordano, A., Calvani, M., Petillo, O., Carteni, M., Melone, M.R., & Peluso, G. (2003). Skeletal muscle metabolism in physiology and in cancer disease. *Journal of Cellular Biochemistry, 90*, 170–186. doi:10.1002/jcb.10601

Given, B., Given, C.W., Sikorskii, A., Jeon, S., McCorkle, R., Champion, V., & Decker, D. (2008). Establishing mild, moderate, and severe scores for cancer-related symptoms: How consistent and clinically meaningful are interference-based severity cut-points? *Journal of Pain and Symptom Management, 35*, 126–135. doi:10.1016/j.jpainsymman.2007.03.012

Holbrook, A.M., Crowther, R., Lotter, A., Cheng, C., & King, D. (2000). Meta-analysis of benzodiazepine use in the treatment of insomnia. *Canadian Medical Association Journal, 162*, 225–233.

Jacobsen, P.B., Donovan, K.A., Vadaparampil, S.T., & Small, B.J. (2007). Systematic review and meta-analysis of psychological and activity-based interventions for cancer-related fatigue. *Health Psychology, 26*, 660–667. doi:10.1037/0278-6133.26.6.660

Jacobsen, P.B., Meade, C.D., Stein, K.D., Chirikos, T.N., Small, B.J., & Ruckdeschel, J.C. (2002). Efficacy and costs of two forms of stress management training for cancer patients undergoing chemotherapy. *Journal of Clinical Oncology, 20*, 2851–2862. doi:10.1200/JCO.2002.08.301

Jereczek-Fossa, B.A., Marsiglia, H.R., & Orecchia, R. (2001). Radiotherapy-related fatigue: How to assess and how to treat the symptom. A commentary. *Tumori, 87*, 147–151.

Joffe, H., Petrillo, L., Viguera, A., Koukopoulos, A., Silver-Heilman, K., Farrell, A., … Cohen, L.S. (2010). Eszopiclone improves insomnia and depressive and anxious symptoms in perimenopausal and postmenopausal women with hot flashes: A randomized, double-blinded, placebo-controlled crossover trial. *American Journal of Obstetrics and Gynecology, 202*, 171.e1–171.e11. doi:10.1016/j.ajog.2009.10.868

Kangas, M., Bovbjerg, D.H., & Montgomery, G.H. (2008). Cancer-related fatigue: A systematic and meta-analytic review of non-pharmacological therapies for cancer patients. *Psychological Bulletin, 134*, 700–741. doi:10.1037/a0012825

Kim, S.-D., & Kim, H.-S. (2005). Effects of a relaxation breathing exercise on anxiety, depression, and leukocyte in hemopoietic stem cell transplantation patients. *Cancer Nursing, 28*, 79–83.

Kim, Y., Roscoe, J.A., & Morrow, G.R. (2002). The effects of information and negative affect on severity of side effects from radiation therapy for prostate cancer. *Supportive Care in Cancer, 10*, 416–421. doi:10.1007/s00520-002-0359-y

King, K.B., Nail, L.M., Kreamer, K., Strohl, R.A., & Johnson, J.E. (1985). Patients' descriptions of the experience of receiving radiation therapy. *Oncology Nursing Forum, 12*(4), 55–61.

Kumar, N. (2007). *WHO normative guidelines on pain management: Report of a Delphi Study to determine the need for guidelines and to identify the number and topics of guidelines that should be developed by WHO.* Geneva, Switzerland: World Health Organization.

Lader, M.H. (2009). Hypnotics: How effective are they for insomnia? *Psychiatric Times, 26*(5), 23–25.

McGough, C., Baldwin, C., Frost, G., & Andreyev, H.J. (2004). Role of nutritional intervention in patients treated with radiotherapy for pelvic malignancy. *British Journal of Cancer, 90*, 2278–2287. doi:10.1038/sj.bjc.6601868

Minton, O., Richardson, A., Sharpe, M., Hotopf, M., & Stone, P. (2008). A systematic review and meta-analysis of the pharmacological treatment of cancer-related fatigue. *Journal of the National Cancer Institute, 100*, 1155–1166. doi:10.1093/jnci/djn250

Minton, O., & Stone, P. (2009). A systematic review of the scales used for the measurement of cancer-related fatigue (CRF). *Annals of Oncology, 20*, 17–25. doi:10.1093/annonc/mdn537

Mitchell, S.A., Beck, S.L., Hood, L.E., Moore, K., & Tanner, E.R. (2009). ONS PEP resource: Fatigue. In L.H. Eaton & J.M. Tipton (Eds.), *Putting evidence into practice: Improving oncology patient outcomes* (pp. 155–174). Pittsburgh, PA: Oncology Nursing Society.

Morrow, G.R. (2007). Cancer-related fatigue: Causes, consequences, and management. *Oncologist, 12*(Suppl. 1), 1–3. doi:10.1634/theoncologist.12-S1-1

Mota, D.D., & Pimenta, C.A. (2006). Self-report instruments for fatigue assessment: A systematic review. *Research and Theory for Nursing Practice, 20*, 49–78.

Nail, L.M. (2004). Fatigue. In C.H. Yarbro, M.H. Frogge, & M. Goodman (Eds.), *Cancer symptom management* (3rd ed., pp. 47–60). Sudbury, MA: Jones and Bartlett.

National Cancer Institute Cancer Therapy Evaluation Program. (2010). *Common terminology criteria for adverse events* [v.4.03]. Retrieved from http://evs.nci.nih.gov/ftp1/CTCAE/About.html

National Comprehensive Cancer Network. (2010). *NCCN Clinical Practice Guidelines in Oncology: Cancer-related fatigue* [v.1.2011]. Retrieved from http://www.nccn.org/professionals/physician_gls/pdf/fatigue.pdf

National Comprehensive Cancer Network. (2011). *NCCN Clinical Practice Guidelines in Oncology: Cancer- and chemotherapy-induced anemia* [v.2.2011]. Retrieved from http://www.nccn.org/professionals/physician_gls/pdf/anemia.pdf

National Institutes of Health State of the Science Conference statement on Manifestations and Management of Chronic Insomnia in Adults, June 13–15, 2005. (2005). *Sleep, 28,* 1049–1057.

Navari, R.M., Brenner, M.C., & Wilson, M.N. (2008). Treatment of depressive symptoms in patients with early stage breast cancer undergoing adjuvant therapy. *Breast Cancer Research and Treatment, 112,* 197–201. doi:10.1007/s10549-007-9841-z

Pavlakis, N., Schmidt, R.L., & Stockler, M.R. (2005). Bisphosphonates for breast cancer. *Cochrane Database of Systematic Reviews* 2005, Issue 3. Art. No.: CD003474. doi:10.1002/14651858.CD003474.pub2

Poirier, P. (2007). Factors affecting performance of usual activities during radiation therapy. *Oncology Nursing Forum, 34,* 827–834. doi:10.1188/07.ONF.827-834

Portenoy, R.K., & Itri, L.M. (1999). Cancer-related fatigue: Guidelines for evaluation and management. *Oncologist, 4,* 1–10.

Posener, J.A., Schildkraut, J.J., Samson, J.A., & Schatzberg, A.F. (1996). Diurnal variation of plasma cortisol and homovanillic acid in healthy subjects. *Psychoneuroendocrinology, 21,* 33–38. doi:10.1016/0306-4530(95)00033-X

Potter, M.B. (2005). NSAIDs alone or with opioids as therapy for cancer pain. *American Family Physician, 72,* 436–437.

Prue, G., Rankin, J., Allen, J., Gracey, J., & Cramp, F. (2006). Cancer-related fatigue: A critical appraisal. *European Journal of Cancer, 42,* 846–863. doi:10.1016/j.ejca.2005.11.026

Purcell, A., Fleming, J., Bennett, S., McGuane, K., Burmeister, B., & Haines, T. (2010). A multidimensional examination of correlates of fatigue during radiotherapy. *Cancer, 116,* 529–537. doi:10.1002/cncr.24731

Ravasco, P. (2005). Aspects of taste and compliance in patients with cancer. *European Journal of Oncology Nursing, 9*(Suppl. 2), S84–S91. doi:10.1016/j.ejon.2005.09.003

Rich, T.A. (2007). Symptom clusters in cancer patients and their relation to EGFR ligand modulation of the circadian axis. *Journal of Supportive Oncology, 5,* 167–174.

Roscoe, J.A., Kaufman, M.E., Matteson-Rusby, S.E., Palesh, O.G., Ryan, J.L., Kohli, S., … Morrow, G.R. (2007). Cancer-related fatigue and sleep disorders. *Oncologist, 12*(Suppl. 1), 35–42. doi:10.1634/theoncologist.12-S1-35

Ryan, J.L., Carroll, J.K., Ryan, E.P., Mustian, K.M., Fiscella, K., & Morrow, G.R. (2007). Mechanisms of cancer-related fatigue. *Oncologist, 12*(Suppl. 1), 22–34. doi:10.1634/theoncologist.12-S1-22

Sadler, I.J., Jacobsen, P.B., Booth-Jones, M., Belanger, H., Weitzner, M.A., & Fields, K.K. (2002). Preliminary evaluation of a clinical syndrome approach to assessing cancer-related fatigue. *Journal of Pain and Symptom Management, 23,* 406–416. doi:10.1016/S0885-3924(02)00388-3

Schubert, C., Hong, S., Natarajan, L., Mills, P.J., & Dimsdale, J.E. (2007). The association between fatigue and inflammatory marker levels in cancer patients: A quantitative review. *Brain, Behavior, and Immunity, 21,* 413–427. doi:10.1016/j.bbi.2006.11.004

Seruga, B., Zhang, H., Bernstein, L.J., & Tannock, I.F. (2008). Cytokines and their relationship to the symptoms and outcome of cancer. *Nature Reviews Cancer, 8,* 887–899. doi:10.1038/nrc2507

Servaes, P., Prins, J., Verhagen, S., & Bleijenberg, G. (2002). Fatigue after breast cancer and in chronic fatigue syndrome: Similarities and differences. *Journal of Psychosomatic Research, 52,* 453–459. doi:10.1016/S0022-3999(02)00300-8

To, S.E., Zepf, R.A., & Woods, A.G. (2005). The symptoms, neurobiology, and current pharmacological treatment of depression. *Journal of Neuroscience Nursing, 37,* 102–107.

Visser, M.R., & Smets, E.M. (1998). Fatigue, depression and quality of life in cancer patients: How are they related? *Supportive Care in Cancer, 6,* 101–108. doi:10.1007/s005200050142

Vogelzang, N.J., Breitbart, W., Cella, D., Curt, G.A., Groopman, J.E., Horning, S.J., … Portenoy, R.K. (1997). Patient, caregiver, and oncologist perceptions of cancer-related fatigue: Results of a tripart assessment survey. Fatigue Coalition. *Seminars in Hematology, 34*(3, Suppl. 2), 4–12.

Vordermark, D., Schwab, M., Flentje, M., Sailer, M., & Kölbl, O. (2002). Chronic fatigue after radiotherapy for carcinoma of the prostate: Correlation with anorectal and genitourinary function. *Radiotherapy and Oncology, 62,* 293–297. doi:10.1016/S0167-8140(01)00492-3

Whitehead, L. (2009). The measurement of fatigue in chronic illness: A systematic review of unidimensional and multidimensional fatigue measures. *Journal of Pain and Symptom Management, 37,* 107–128. doi:10.1016/j.jpainsymman.2007.08.019

Wratten, C., Kilmurray, J., Nash, S., Seldon, M., Hamilton, C.S., O'Brien, P.C., & Denham, J.W. (2004). Fatigue during breast radiotherapy and its relationship to biological factors. *International Journal of Radiation Oncology, Biology, Physics, 59,* 160–167. doi:10.1016/j.ijrobp.2003.10.008

Yates, P., Aranda, S., Hargraves, M., Mirolo, B., Clavarino, A., McLachlan, S., & Skerman, H. (2005). Randomized controlled trial of an educational intervention for managing fatigue in women receiving adjuvant chemotherapy for early-stage breast cancer. *Journal of Clinical Oncology, 23,* 6027–6036. doi:10.1200/JCO.2005.01.271

C. Skin reactions
    1. Pathophysiology
        a) Skin is composed of two main layers and serves as a protective barrier.
            (1) Epidermis (superficial layer): During normal skin regeneration, superficial cells are shed through normal desquamation, and new cells are formed in the basal layer of the epidermis, migrate to the superficial layer, and continuously replace those that are lost. The basal layer of the epidermis proliferates rapidly; therefore, it is particularly sensitive to RT.
            (2) Dermis (deep layer containing blood vessels, glands, nerves, and hair follicles): This layer provides the supportive structure required for the epidermis to renew.
        b) Ionizing radiation damages the mitotic ability of stem cells within the basal layer, thus preventing the process of repopulation and weakening the integrity of the skin. Repeated radiation impairs the cell division within the basal layer, and skin reaction develops (Archambeau, Pezner, & Wasserman, 1995).

c) The skin is very sensitive to RT. Basal cell loss begins at 20–25 Gy (visible at two to three weeks), and maximum depletion occurs at 50 Gy (usually peaking at the end of treatment) (Chao, Perez, & Brady, 2002).

d) Temporary and partial hair loss occurs at 30 Gy, and permanent hair loss can occur at 55 Gy (Chao et al., 2002).

e) Types of skin reactions and approximate dosage at which they occur
   (1) Epilation—20 Gy
   (2) Erythema—20–40 Gy
   (3) Dry desquamation/pruritus—45 Gy
   (4) Moist desquamation—45–50 Gy
   (5) Hypopigmentation—45 Gy
   (6) Hyperpigmentation—45 Gy (Archambeau et al., 1995)

f) The healing process is considered to be a continuous process of three to four overlapping phases (Broughton, Janis, & Attinger, 2006).
   (1) Hemostasis (may or may not be considered one of the steps)
   (2) Clotting and inflammation
   (3) Cell migration and proliferation
   (4) Skin remodeling

g) A variety of cellular mediators are involved in the healing process (Cohen, Jorizzo, & Kircik, 2007).

2. Incidence
   a) Increasing use of concomitant chemotherapy and high-dose RT means that skin reactions are still a major problem for patients. The use of epidermal growth factor receptor (EGFR) inhibitor agents may also act as a radiosensitizer.
   b) Incidence rate is difficult to predict and monitor, as the severity and occurrence are not well documented.
      (1) Breast cancer: 87%–95% of women experience a skin reaction (Gosselin, Schneider, Plambeck, & Rowe, 2010; Williams et al., 1996).
      (2) Head and neck cancer: 94.3% of patients with head and neck cancer experience a skin reaction, and 98.1% who are also taking an EGFR inhibitor experience a skin reaction (Bonner et al., 2010).
   c) Impacting factors
      (1) Treatment related: Type of energy (electrons versus photons), use of tangential fields (higher doses received within thinner areas), use of parallel opposed fields (two skin surfaces are proximal), skin bolus (gel-like sheets build up skin to ensure higher dose),

skin types (the scalp has a higher tolerance than the trunk or groin), more oxygenated cells than hypoxic cells, size of treatment field, RT dose, and use of a radiosensitizer or previous radiation exposure (Chao et al., 2002; Porock, Kristjanson, Nikoletti, Cameron, & Pedler, 1998)
      (2) Non–treatment related: General skin condition, moist areas of the body causing friction (axilla, inframammary areas, groin, or perineum), skin folds and bony prominences, age, nutritional status (hydration), prior exposure to chemotherapy agents that cause a reaction known as *radiation recall* (e.g., doxorubicin), and underlying medical conditions (scleroderma, lupus, diabetes). Healing also may be affected in those with elevated blood pressure and in those who smoke (Chao et al., 2002; Porock et al., 1998).

3. Staging/assessment of symptoms
   a) Radiation-induced skin reactions are dependent on time-dose factors (amount of radiation that is prescribed over a set amount of time) rather than on the total dose delivered (Archambeau, 1987).
   b) Radiation-induced skin reactions range from erythema, where different shapes of redness occur from the release of histamine-like substances from damaged germinal cells, to dry desquamation (dry, flaky, or scaly skin) because the sweat and sebaceous glands have been impacted by the RT, or to moist desquamation, where blistering, peeling, and sloughing of the skin occur. Damage to the hair follicles and sweat glands can be permanent at higher doses. Necrosis is rare and involves damage to the deeper layers of the skin that may include the dermis and subcutaneous tissue.
   c) NCI has a five-point scale of color stages or skin patterns; however, the patient's

subjective feeling is not considered in this scale (NCI CTEP, 2010). Further assessment could include subjective pain (0–10 scale), sensation (burning, prickly, or pruritus), and interference with ADL.

d) Assessment should include visual inspection of treatment fields and exit sites.

4. Acute effects

a) The major acute side effects to the skin while receiving RT are erythema, dry desquamation, moist desquamation, and ulceration. The overall goal is to keep the skin intact by minimizing scratching and rubbing and by keeping the skin moisturized. If moist desquamation develops, the goal is to support epithelial recovery and avoid superinfections.

b) Interventions

(1) During treatment planning, special positioning devices may be used to reduce skin folds by moving tissue out of the treatment field.

(2) All surgical wounds should be healed before initiating RT.

(3) Few well-designed randomized studies have been conducted to evaluate skin care products. The different methodologic approaches used make comparison across studies difficult (Gosselin et al., 2010). Few standardized protocols are available on skin care products (D'haese, Van Roy, Bate, Bijdekerke, & Vinh-Hung, 2010; Moore-Higgs & Amdur, 2001; Pazdur, Coia, Hoskins, & Wagman, 2003).

(4) Recommendations from four reviews of the literature noted that patients could use hydrophilic agents (agents that absorb water) and continue to bathe using soap and water, and that further study of products was warranted (Bolderston et al., 2006; Maddocks-Jennings, Wilkinson, & Shillington, 2005; McQuestion, 2006; Wickline, 2004).

(5) Many products are available for patients to use to manage erythema, yet few have been studied systematically to show a definitive benefit, and therefore their effectiveness has not been established. Two common products have not demonstrated a benefit in managing radiodermatitis:

(a) Biafine® (Ortho Dermatologics): Radiation Therapy Oncology Group (RTOG) 97-13 demonstrated no prophylactic capability (Fisher et al., 2000).

(b) Aloe vera gels: No skin differences were seen with aloe vera gels

(Heggie et al., 2002; Williams et al., 1996).

(6) Calendula and hyaluronic acid are likely to be effective in reducing the incidence of radiodermatitis (Baney et al., 2011); however, a recent phase III study demonstrated no difference between hyaluronic acid and a simple emollient in the treatment of radiodermatitis (Kirova et al., 2011).

(7) The effectiveness of hydrocolloid and hydrogel dressings for the management of moist desquamation has also not been established (Baney et al., 2011).

(8) Historically, use of topical agents (e.g., lotions, deodorants) prior to RT has been discouraged due to the potential buildup of the product and the chemical composition. A 1997 study found that only a small amount (1%–5%) of skin dose increased when products were used prior to treatment (Burch, Parker, Vann, & Arazie, 1997).

5. Long-term effects

a) Major late side effects: Telangiectasias, fibrosis, and necrosis can occur after receiving therapy because of physiologic changes in the wound healing process. The goal is to improve skin texture and elasticity.

b) Interventions

(1) Keep the skin moist and supple with moisturizing lotions.

(2) Use sunblock.

6. Documentation

a) Use the NCI CTCAE scale when documenting the skin reaction. It is a vital component of nursing care that reflects changes over time, responses to interventions, and wound healing.

b) Include patients' subjective feelings about pain, pruritus, or burning.

c) Document any serous drainage (e.g., type, amount, odor) and topical fungal or other infections.

7. Patient and family education outcomes

a) Teach overall general skin care (Haas, 2004).

(1) Gently wash the skin with tepid water, using a soft washcloth (no scrubbing) and nondeodorant soap. Studies have demonstrated that Dove® (Unilever) is a mild, nonirritating soap (Frosch & Klingman, 1979; Roy, Fortin, & Larochelle, 2001). Avoid removing any temporary marks that may be placed at the time of simulation before tattooing occurs. Pat dry.

(2) Wear loose-fitting, natural-fiber clothing (e.g., silk, 100% cotton).

(3) Avoid perfumed skin products and powders.

(4) Use only recommended skin care products, and avoid applying makeup to the treatment fields.

(5) Avoid scratching the skin. Seek advice from healthcare professional for possible steroid cream if documented folliculitis is present.

(6) Use an electric razor instead of wet shaving.

(7) Protect skin from wind, sun, and extreme temperatures. Sunblock with sun protection factor (SPF) 30 with UVA/UVB protection is recommended for irradiated skin. Skin that has received prior irradiation is more sensitive to the sun.

(8) Avoid putting anything hot or cold, such as heating pads or ice packs, directly on the treated skin.

(9) Being in a hot tub, swimming pool, or lake should be avoided, as the water may exacerbate a skin reaction (McQuestion, 2006).

(10) Avoid adhesive tape or bandage within the treatment fields; consider form-fitting dressings if needed.

(11) Try using gentle detergents to wash clothes, and avoid starching clothes that are worn over treatment areas.

b) Teach the patient and family members when to expect skin reactions, as well as the duration and resolution of the reactions.

c) Teach the patient and family members how to care for all stages of skin breakdown and to report any signs of infection.

References

Archambeau, J. (1987). Relative radiation sensitivity of the integumentary system dose response of the epidermal, microvascular, and dermal population. *Advances in Radiation Biology, 12,* 147–203.

Archambeau, J.O., Pezner, R., & Wasserman, T. (1995). Pathophysiology of irradiated skin and breast. *International Journal of Radiation Oncology, Biology, Physics, 31,* 1171–1185. doi:10.1016/0360-3016(94)00423-I

Baney, T., McQuestion, M., Bell, K., Bruce, S., Feight, D., Weis-Smith, L., & Haas, M. (2011). ONS PEP resource: Radiodermatitis. In L.H. Eaton, J.M. Tipton, & M. Irwin (Eds.), *Putting evidence into practice: Improving oncology patient outcomes, volume 2* (pp. 57–75). Pittsburgh, PA: Oncology Nursing Society.

Bolderston, A., Lloyd, N.S., Wong, R.K.S., Holden, L., Robb-Blenderman, L., & Supportive Care Guidelines Group of Cancer Care Ontario Program in Evidence-Based Care. (2006). The

prevention and management of acute skin reactions related to radiation therapy: A systematic review and practice guideline. *Supportive Care in Cancer, 14,* 802–817. doi:10.1007/s00520-006-0063-4

Bonner, J.A., Harari, P.M., Giralt, J., Cohen, R.B., Jones, C.U., Sur, R.K., … Ang, K.K. (2010). Radiotherapy plus cetuximab for locoregionally advanced head and neck cancer: 5-year survival data from a phase 3 randomised trial, and relation between cetuximab-induced rash and survival. *Lancet Oncology, 11,* 21–28. doi:10.1016/S1470-2045(09)70311-0

Broughton, G., II, Janis, J.E., & Attinger, C.E. (2006). The basic science of wound healing. *Plastic and Reconstructive Surgery, 117*(Suppl. 7), 12S–34S. doi:10.1097/01.prs.0000225430.42531.c2

Burch, S.E., Parker, S.A., Vann, A.M., & Arazie, J.C. (1997). Measurement of 6-MV x-ray surface dose when topical agents are applied prior to external beam irradiation. *International Journal of Radiation Oncology, Biology, Physics, 38,* 447–451. doi:10.1016/S0360-3016(97)00095-3

Chao, K.S.C., Perez, C.A., & Brady, L.W. (Eds.). (2002). *Radiation oncology: Management decisions* (2nd ed.). Philadelphia, PA: Lippincott Williams & Wilkins.

Cohen, J.L., Jorizzo, J.L., & Kircik, L.H. (2007). Use of a topical emulsion for wound healing. *Journal of Supportive Oncology, 5*(10, Suppl. 5), 1–9.

D'haese, S., Van Roy, M., Bate, T., Bijdekerke, P., & Vinh-Hung, V. (2010). Management of skin reactions during radiotherapy in Flanders (Belgium): A study of nursing practice before and after the introduction of a skin care protocol. *European Journal of Oncology Nursing, 14,* 367–372. doi:10.1016/j.ejon.2009.10.006

Fisher, J., Scott, C., Stevens, R., Marconi, B., Champion, L., Freedman, G.M., … Wong, G. (2000). Randomized phase III study comparing best supportive care to Biafine as a prophylactic agent for radiation-induced skin toxicity for women undergoing breast irradiation: Radiation Therapy Oncology Group (RTOG) 97-13. *International Journal of Radiation Oncology, Biology, Physics, 48,* 1307–1310. doi:10.1016/S0360-3016(00)00782-3

Frosch, P.J., & Klingman, A.M. (1979). The soap chamber test: A new method for assessing the irritancy of soaps. *Journal of the American Academy of Dermatology, 1,* 35–41.

Gosselin, T.K., Schneider, S.M., Plambeck, M.A., & Rowe, K. (2010). A prospective randomized, placebo-controlled skin care study in women diagnosed with breast cancer undergoing radiation therapy. *Oncology Nursing Forum, 37,* 619–626. doi:10.1188/10.ONF.619-626

Haas, M.L. (2004). Radiation therapy. In C.G. Varricchio (Ed.), *A cancer source book for nurses* (8th ed., pp. 131–147). Sudbury, MA: Jones and Bartlett.

Heggie, S., Bryant, G.P., Tripcony, L., Keller, J., Rose, P., Glendenning, M., & Heath, J. (2002). A phase III study on the efficacy of topical aloe vera gel on irradiated breast tissue. *Cancer Nursing, 25,* 442–451.

Kirova, Y.M., Fromantin, I., De Rycke, Y., Fourquet, A., Morvan, E., Padiglione, S., … Bollet, M.A. (2011). Can we decrease the skin reaction in breast cancer patients using hyaluronic acid during radiation therapy? Results of a phase III randomised trial. *Radiotherapy and Oncology, 100,* 205–209. doi:10.1016/j.radonc.2011.05.014

Maddocks-Jennings, W., Wilkinson, J.M., & Shillington, D. (2005). Novel approaches to radiotherapy-induced skin reactions: A literature review. *Complementary Therapies in Clinical Practice, 11,* 224–231. doi:10.1016/j.ctcp.2005.02.001

McQuestion, M. (2006). Evidence-based skin care management in radiation therapy. *Seminars in Oncology Nursing, 22,* 163–173. doi:10.1016/j.soncn.2006.04.004

Moore-Higgs, G.J., & Amdur, R.J. (2001). Sustained integrity of protective mechanisms (skin, oral, immune system). In D.W. Bruner, G. Moore-Higgs, & M. Haas (Eds.), *Outcomes in radiation therapy: Multidisciplinary management* (pp. 493–518). Sudbury, MA: Jones and Bartlett.

National Cancer Institute Cancer Therapy Evaluation Program. (2010). *Common terminology criteria for adverse advents* [v.4.03]. Retrieved from http://evs.nci.nih.gov/ftp1/CTCAE/CTCAE_4.03_2010-06-14_QuickReference_8.5x11.pdf

Pazdur, R., Coia, L.R., Hoskins, W.J., & Wagman, L.G. (Eds.). (2003). *Cancer management: A multidisciplinary approach* (7th ed.). Melville, NY: Oncology Group.

Porock, D., Kristjanson, L., Nikoletti, S., Cameron, F., & Pedler, P. (1998). Predicting the severity of radiation skin reactions in women with breast cancer. *Oncology Nursing Forum, 25,* 1019–1029.

Roy, I., Fortin, A., & Larochelle, M. (2001). The impact of skin washing with water and soap during breast irradiation: A randomized study. *Radiotherapy and Oncology, 58,* 333–339. doi:10.1016/S0167-8140(00)00322-4

Wickline, M.M. (2004). Prevention and treatment of acute radiation dermatitis: A literature review. *Oncology Nursing Forum, 31,* 237–244. doi:10.1188/04.ONF.237-247

Williams, M.S., Burk, M., Loprinzi, C.L., Hill, M., Schomberg, P.J., Nearhood, K., … Eggleston, W.D. (1996). Phase III double-blind evaluation of an aloe vera gel as a prophylactic agent for radiation-induced skin toxicity. *International Journal of Radiation Oncology, Biology, Physics, 36,* 345–349. doi:10.1016/S0360-3016(96)00320-3

D. Pain
   1. Pathophysiology: Cancer pain can be acute or chronic (more than three months in duration) and can occur as a result of the cancer or its treatment. Pain can be classified as nociceptive or neuropathic based on its underlying pathophysiologic mechanism (Miaskowski et al., 2005).
     a) *Nociceptive* pain occurs as a result of tissue injury.
       (1) Radiation-induced causes of nociceptive pain include mucositis, skin reactions, enteritis, and proctitis.
       (2) Disease-related causes of nociceptive pain include bone metastasis and obstruction of a hollow viscus.
     b) *Neuropathic* pain results from nerve injury.
       (1) Radiation-induced causes of neuropathic pain include cervical, brachial, or lumbosacral plexopathies and polyneuropathies.
       (2) Disease- and treatment-related causes of neuropathic pain include epidural spinal cord compression, tumor-induced plexopathies, and postherpetic neuralgia.
   2. Pain occurs in approximately 50% of patients who are receiving treatment for cancer (Caraceni & Portenoy, 1999) and in 80%–90% of patients during the terminal phases of the disease (Potter, Hami, Bryan, & Quigley, 2003).
   3. Assessment is the cornerstone of effective pain management. All patients with cancer should be screened for pain at each encounter with the healthcare system. If the patient reports pain during the universal screening procedure, a comprehensive pain assessment should be conducted to evaluate for persistent and breakthrough pain and to diagnose the cause of the pain (Miaskowski et al., 2005). Ongoing assessments should be performed to determine the effectiveness of the pain management plan.
     a) Comprehensive pain assessment—Determines the cause of the patient's pain
       (1) Persistent pain: Constant pain that lasts for long periods of time
         (a) Onset
         (b) Description
         (c) Location
         (d) Intensity/severity (rated using a 0 [no pain] to 10 [worst pain imaginable] numeric rating scale)
         (e) Aggravating and relieving factors
         (f) Previous and current treatments and their effectiveness
         (g) Associated symptoms, such as fatigue, insomnia, depression, or changes in appetite (Miaskowski et al., 2005)
       (2) Breakthrough pain: Sudden, severe flare-ups of pain that come and go (Lossignol & Dumitrescu, 2010)
         (a) Presence of breakthrough pain
         (b) Frequency and duration of the episodes of breakthrough pain
         (c) Intensity
         (d) Occurrence of the painful episode—Spontaneous, incident
         (e) Previous and current treatments and their effectiveness
       (3) Physical examination
         (a) General examination
         (b) Focused neurologic examination
       (4) Appropriate diagnostic tests—Pain medication should be administered to facilitate the diagnostic workup.
     b) Ongoing pain assessments—Should determine whether the pain management plan is effective. Assessments include evaluation of
       (1) Pain intensity
       (2) Pain relief
       (3) The impact of pain on functional status and quality of life

(4) The patient's level of adherence with the pain management plan.

4. Documentation

a) Document the results of universal screening for pain at each patient visit.

b) Document the findings from the comprehensive pain assessment in the patient's medical record.

c) Document ratings of pain intensity at each visit.

d) Document plan

e) Evaluation of side effects of interventions

f) Evaluation of patient's level of adherence with the pain management plan or factors interfering with same (e.g., finances, misconceptions)

5. Collaborative management

a) Use appropriate combinations of nonopioid, opioid, and coanalgesics, depending on the cause and the severity of the patient's pain (Aiello-Laws et al., 2009; Green et al., 2010; Miaskowski et al., 2005; Raphael, Ahmedzai, et al., 2010).

(1) Nonopioid analgesics (e.g., acetaminophen, NSAIDs)

(a) Indicated for mild to moderate pain

(b) Have a narrow therapeutic window and a ceiling effect

(2) Opioid analgesics

(a) Indicated for moderate to severe pain

(b) Doses and schedules should be adjusted to produce maximal analgesia with minimal side effects.

(3) Coanalgesics are medications that do not have a primary indication for pain but produce analgesia. These medications often are used in the management of neuropathic pain.

b) Chronic persistent pain should be managed with a long-acting opioid that is administered on a regular schedule. Breakthrough pain should be managed with a short-acting opioid that is administered as needed (Lossignol & Dumitrescu, 2010).

c) Side effects of nonopioid, opioid, and coanalgesics should be monitored and managed to improve adherence with the pain management plan.

d) Nonpharmacologic strategies should be used to supplement pharmacologic strategies in the management of cancer pain (Raphael, Hester, et al., 2010).

(1) Relaxation

(2) Distraction

(3) Guided imagery

e) Pain from bone metastasis may be treated with RT or radiopharmaceuticals (e.g., ^{89}Sr,

[153]Sm) (Miaskowski et al., 2005). Analgesic regimens may require adjustment following the administration of these therapies.

6. Patient and family education

a) Discuss concerns about and differences in tolerance, physical dependence, and psychological addiction.

b) Teach patients how to aggressively manage the side effects of analgesic medication to improve adherence with the pain management plan (Miaskowski et al., 2001).

(1) Constipation

(2) Sedation

(3) Nausea

(4) Pruritus

c) Teach patients how to use a pain management diary to record changes in pain intensity and medication use (West et al., 2003).

d) Teach patients how to communicate unrelieved pain to clinicians (West et al., 2003).

References

Aiello-Laws, L., Reynolds, J., Deizer, N., Peterson, M., Ameringer, S., & Bakitas, M. (2009). Putting evidence into practice: What are the pharmacologic interventions for nociceptive and neuropathic cancer pain in adults? *Clinical Journal of Oncology Nursing, 13,* 649–655. doi:10.1188/09.CJON.649-655

Caraceni, A., & Portenoy, R.K. (1999). An international survey of cancer pain characteristics and syndromes. IASP Task Force on Cancer Pain. International Association for the Study of Pain. *Pain, 82,* 263–274. doi:10.1016/S0304-3959(99)00073-1

Green, E., Zwaal, C., Beals, C., Fitzgerald, B., Harle, I., Jones, J., ... Wiernikowski, J. (2010). Cancer-related pain management: A report of evidence-based recommendations to guide practice. *Clinical Journal of Pain, 26,* 449–462. doi:10.1097/AJP.0b013e3181dacd62

Lossignol, D.A., & Dumitrescu, C. (2010). Breakthrough pain: Progress in management. *Current Opinion in Oncology, 22,* 302–306. doi:10.1097/CCO.0b013e32833a873a

Miaskowski, C., Cleary, J., Burney, R., Coyne, P., Finley, R., Foster, R., ... Zahrbock, C. (2005). *Guideline for the management of cancer pain in adults and children* (Vol. 3). Glenview, IL: American Pain Society.

Miaskowski, C., Dodd, M.J., West, C., Paul, S.M., Tripathy, D., Koo, P., & Schumacher, K. (2001). Lack of adherence with the analgesic regimen: A significant barrier to effective cancer pain management. *Journal of Clinical Oncology, 19,* 4275–4279.

Potter, J., Hami, F., Bryan, T., & Quigley, C. (2003). Symptoms in 400 patients referred to palliative care services: Prevalence and patterns. *Palliative Medicine, 17,* 310–314. doi:10.1191/0269216303pm760oa

Raphael, J., Ahmedzai, S., Hester, J., Urch, C., Barrie, J., Williams, J., ... Sparkes, E. (2010). Cancer pain: Part 1: Pathophysiology; oncological, pharmacological, and psychological treatments: A perspective from the British Pain Society endorsed by the UK Association of Palliative Medicine and the Royal College of General Practitioners. *Pain Medicine, 11,* 742–764. doi:10.1111/j.1526-4637.2010.00840.x

Raphael, J., Hester, J., Ahmedzai, S., Barrie, J., Farquhar-Smith, P., Williams, J., … Sparkes, E. (2010). Cancer pain: Part 2: Physical, interventional and complimentary therapies; management in the community; acute, treatment-related and complex cancer pain: A perspective from the British Pain Society endorsed by the UK Association of Palliative Medicine and the Royal College of General Practitioners. *Pain Medicine, 11,* 872–896. doi:10.1111/j.1526-4637.2010.00841.x

West, C.M., Dodd, M.J., Paul, S.M., Schumacher, K., Tripathy, D., Koo, P., & Miaskowski, C. (2003). The PRO-SELF©: Pain Control Program—An effective approach for cancer pain management. *Oncology Nursing Forum, 30,* 65–73. doi:10.1188/03.ONF.65-73

E. Distress/coping
   1. Definitions
      a) *Emotional distress* is a negative emotional state of mind, most frequently expressed as anxiety or depression.
         (1) NCCN defines distress in cancer as "a multifactorial unpleasant emotional experience of a psychological (cognitive, behavioral, emotional), social, and/or spiritual nature that may interfere with the ability to cope effectively with cancer, its physical symptoms and its treatment. Distress extends along a continuum, ranging from common normal feelings of vulnerability, sadness, and fears to problems that can become disabling, such as depression, anxiety, panic, social isolation, and existential and spiritual crisis" (NCCN, 2010, p. DIS-2).
         (2) *Anxiety* can be defined as vague uneasy and unpleasant feelings of potential harm or distress (Gobel, 2004).
         (3) *Depression* can be defined as a feeling of gloom, emptiness, numbness, or despair (Barsevick & Much, 2004). It is frequently associated with feelings of helplessness and hopelessness.
         (4) Emotional distress can range from mild to severe. It can be disabling and may be accompanied by other symptoms, such as sleep difficulties. When distress is severe, patients may meet criteria for psychiatric disorders, such as major depressive disorder or generalized anxiety disorder.
      b) *Coping* is the "constantly changing cognitive and behavioral efforts to manage specific external and/or internal demands that are appraised as taxing or exceeding the resources of the person" (Lazarus & Folkman, 1984, p. 141).
   2. Outcomes of distress
      a) In a study assessing emotional distress and other symptoms before and within two weeks of RT, significant associations were found among emotional distress, depression, fatigue and diagnosis, physical distress, functional disability, and quality of sleep (Smets et al., 1998).
      b) Suicidal thoughts can be part of distress. Among patients with cancer in general, the incidence of suicide is twice that of the populace (NCCN, 2010).
      c) Depression has been strongly linked to mortality and is possibly related to cancer progression (Hjerl et al., 2003; Onitilo, Nietert, & Egede, 2006; Satin, Linden, & Phillips, 2009; Spiegel & Giese-Davis, 2003).
   3. Course and prevalence
      a) A literature search using MEDLINE® and PsycLIT (now part of PsycINFO) databases over the period of 1980 to 2002 identified studies on psychological functioning in patients treated with EBRT, assessing a variety of cancer sites, treatment goals (curative or palliative), and adjuvant therapies (Stiegelis, Ranchor, & Sanderman, 2004).
         (1) About 10%–20% of patients experienced feelings of anxiety prior to RT, but depressive symptoms were not common.
         (2) Feelings of anxiety were substantial at the time of the first treatment, ranging from 21% to 54%. While anxiety declined during the course of treatment, depressive symptoms rose, ranging from 12% to 31%.
         (3) After RT, rates of anxiety and depression were inconsistent across studies and varied widely. Patients with depressive symptoms varied from 8% to greater than 40%.
         (4) Examination of results from longitudinal studies showed improvements in psychological functioning over time. (See Stiegelis et al., 2004, for full details.)
      b) In a longitudinal study of 12 symptoms assessed by a checklist during RT in 1,129 patients with cancer, emotional distress was the fourth most frequent symptom, following fatigue, drowsiness, and sleep problems at baseline. At five weeks follow-up in 415 patients, distress was the fifth most frequently reported symptom (Hickok, Morrow, Roscoe, Mustian, & Okunieff, 2005).
      c) A study of coping strategies assessed 276 patients up to two years following RT (Sehlen, Song, et al., 2003). Coping was assessed with the Freiburg Questionnaire Coping with Disease.

(1) *Active problem-orientated coping* and *distractions* were the most important coping strategies. Only *active problem-orientated* and *depressive* coping showed a significant decrease across time.

(2) Women had higher scores on the coping scales. Marital status had a significant influence on active problem-orientated coping and spirituality, whereas age, children, education, tumor/metastases status, and curative/palliative treatment had no influence on coping styles.

(3) *Depressive* coping and *minimizing importance* at baseline were associated with high psychosocial distress and low quality of life at the two-year follow-up.

4. Risk factors of emotional distress

   a) Sociodemographic variables

      (1) Sex: Women treated with RT report higher levels of emotional distress than men (Iqbal & Siddiqui, 2002; Krischer & Xu, 2008; Sehlen, Hollenhorst, et al., 2003; Voigtmann et al., 2010).

      (2) Social status: Marriage and social support may protect against distress during RT (Chen et al., 2009; de Leeuw et al., 2000; Krischer & Xu, 2008; Sehlen, Hollenhorst, et al., 2003). Patients with breast cancer were at greater risk for distress when they had more children (dependents) at home (Deshields, Tibbs, Fan, & Taylor, 2006).

      (3) Age: Results are mixed regarding age as a risk factor. Some studies have found younger age to be a risk factor of distress, particularly among patients with breast cancer (Chen et al., 2009; Epping-Jordan et al., 1999; Hopwood, Sumo, Mills, Haviland, & Bliss, 2010; Mose et al., 2001), whereas other studies assessing mixed cancers have not found age to be a predictor of distress (Kamer et al., 2007; Sehlen, Hollenhorst, et al., 2003; Turner, Muers, Haward, & Mulley, 2007).

      (4) Education: Most studies have found lower educational levels to be associated with emotional distress (Hopwood et al., 2010; Iqbal & Siddiqui, 2002; Kamer et al., 2007; Krischer & Xu, 2008).

   b) Cancer characteristics

      (1) Stage of disease

         (a) The 1980–2002 review by Stiegelis et al. (2004) concluded that results for stage of disease are inconsistent, although most studies found no significant association with psychological functioning.

         (b) However, in a large sample of mixed cancer types (N = 265), patients at an advanced tumor stage had a 4.8-fold higher risk for stress compared with patients at early stages (Sehlen, Hollenhorst, et al., 2003).

      (2) Cancer site

         (a) Stiegelis et al. (2004) found that only a few authors studied cancer site as a risk factor and found that results were inconsistent.

         (b) RT studies since 2002 indicate that emotional distress is lower among patients with breast and prostate cancer compared to patients with other cancers.

            i. Patients with CNS cancers reported the most severe difficulties with feeling distressed at baseline compared to patients with a range of cancer sites, including prostate, breast, and head and neck (Hickok et al., 2005).

            ii. Patients with breast and prostate cancer were at lower risk for distress than patients with other cancers during RT (Krischer & Xu, 2008).

            iii. Mean depression score was significantly higher among patients with lung cancer versus those with prostate or head and neck cancer, but no differences were seen for anxiety (Fischer, Villines, Kim, Epstein, & Wilkie, 2010).

   c) Cancer treatment

      (1) In general, there is a lack of evidence that treatment modality or radiation type contribute to emotional distress (Epping-Jordan et al., 1999; Kobayashi et al., 2009; Stiegelis et al., 2004; Voigtmann et al., 2010). However, patients with prostate cancer receiving EBRT may have greater distress than those who received brachytherapy or prostatectomy (Hervouet et al., 2005).

      (2) Patients treated palliatively with RT reported more anxiety than patients treated curatively (Stiegelis et al., 2004).

   d) Physical and mental well-being
     (1) Poor physical functioning and symptoms have been associated with emotional distress among RT-treated patients with cancer (de Leeuw et al., 2000; Jim, Andrykowski, Munster, & Jacobsen, 2007; Stiegelis et al., 2004).
     (2) Pretreatment distress and substance abuse disorders have been predictors for emotional distress (Chen et al., 2009; de Leeuw et al., 2000; Sehlen, Hollenhorst, et al., 2003).
   e) Coping style: Similar to Sehlen, Song, et al.'s (2003) study, other RT studies have found associations between coping style and emotional distress (de Leeuw et al., 2000; Fischer et al., 2010). Avoidance and catastrophization were associated with greater distress.
   f) Risk factors of distress among cancer patients in general identified by the NCCN (2010) distress management guidelines are a history of psychiatric disorder or depression, substance abuse, cognitive impairment, severe comorbid illnesses, social problems, and communication barriers. Risk factors for greater distress are past psychiatric disorder, alcohol or substance abuse, younger age, being female, living alone, having young children, and prior physical or sexual abuse.
 5. Clinical assessment
   a) Few empirically tested, clinically relevant, and easy-to-use assessment tools for emotional distress are available in the outpatient radiation oncology setting.
     (1) One RT-specific validation study (Leopold et al., 1998) found a 10-minute structured interview, the Primary Care Evaluation of Mental Disorders (PRIME-MD), to be a reliable method for oncologists to identify depressive and anxiety disorders.
       (a) A diagnosis of a depressive or anxiety disorder by PRIME-MD was made in 59 of the 122 patients (48%).
       (b) In comparison to one of the most commonly used diagnostic depression instruments, the Structured Clinical Interview for DSM Disorders (*Diagnostic and Statistical Manual of Mental Disorders*), the sensitivity of the PRIME-MD in detecting any diagnosis was 77% and the specificity was 93%.
     (2) The preliminary version of the Stress Index RadioOncology was found to be valid, reliable, and feasible in the clinical setting, but it has only been published in German (Sehlen, Fahmüller, et al., 2003).
     (3) Among RT-treated patients with head and neck cancer, three screening instruments—the Beck Depression Inventory, the Hospital Anxiety and Depression Scale, and the Center for Epidemiologic Studies Depression Scale—were found to be concordant with diagnostic structured interviews (Katz, Kopek, Waldron, Devins, & Tomlinson, 2004).
     (4) The Screening Inventory of Psychosocial Problems is a short, validated, self-reported questionnaire to identify psychosocial problems, including physical complaints, psychological complaints, and social and sexual problems, among patients with cancer treated with RT (Braeken, Lechner, Houben, Van Gils, & Kempen, 2010).
   b) Additional tools for the assessment of emotional distress are available, and more comprehensive reviews can be found elsewhere (Barsevick & Much, 2004; Bruner & Diefenbach, 2001; Gobel, 2004; NCCN, 2010).
     (1) Spielberger State-Trait Anxiety Inventory
     (2) Impact of Event Scale
     (3) Medical Outcomes Study–Depression Scale
     (4) NCCN distress thermometer
   c) Despite available measures, research suggests that screening for distress is less than optimal (Jacobsen & Ransom, 2007; Mitchell, Kaar, Coggan, & Herdman, 2008). Screening for distress should occur at the initial visit, at appropriate intervals, and as clinically indicated, especially when changes occur in disease status (NCCN, 2010).

d) Documentation from oncology nurses should include the following.
  (1) Risk factors for distress described previously
  (2) For those at risk, screening for distress and psychosocial needs (NCCN, 2010)
  (3) A treatment plan to address the needs identified and implementation of that plan (NCCN, 2010)
  (4) Referral to services (social worker, psychologist, psychiatrist, mental health nurse practitioner, clergy) as needed for psychosocial care
  (5) Reevaluation at prescribed intervals and as clinically indicated (e.g., a change in disease status such as recurrence or progression) (NCCN, 2010)
  (6) The ONS *Radiation Therapy Patient Care Record* (Catlin-Huth, Haas, & Pollock, 2002): Emotional alterations—Coping
    (a) 0—Effective
    (b) 1—Ineffective
6. Clinical interventions
  a) Quality care standard
    (1) The Institute of Medicine identified psychosocial care as a standard for quality care that must be incorporated into routine care of all patients with cancer in all settings (Adler & Page, 2008).
    (2) Standards of care for distress management (NCCN, 2010)
  b) Clinical practice guidelines
    (1) Evidence-supported interventions for the treatment of distress related to cancer have been developed by
      (a) Association of Community Cancer Centers (www.accc-cancer.org)
      (b) Australian National Breast Cancer Centre and the National Cancer Control Initiative (www.nhmrc.gov.au/publications/synopses/cp90syn.htm)
      (c) NCCN (www.nccn.org)
      (d) Research-Tested Intervention Programs from NCI in collaboration with other organizations (http://rtips.cancer.gov/rtips/index.do).
    (2) In addition, literature reviews are available that detail evidence-based practices for patients with cancer in general (Dy et al., 2008; Jacobsen & Jim, 2008).
      (a) However, a number of limitations were noted in the literature (Jacobsen & Jim, 2008).
        i. Absence of patients with certain demographic, disease,

and treatment characteristics in studies
        ii. Inconsistent findings
        iii. Poor methodologic quality or poor reporting of methods
        iv. Lack of research on patients experiencing clinically significant levels of anxiety and depression
  c) Evidence-based recommendations of psychosocial interventions for patients treated with RT (Jacobsen & Jim, 2008)
    (1) Relaxation techniques and supportive therapies are effective in preventing or relieving anxiety and depression (Decker, Cline-Elsen, & Gallagher, 1992; Evans & Connis, 1995; Pruitt et al., 1993).
    (2) Two RT-specific studies among patients with breast cancer have been published since 2008. Both suggested that cognitive-behavioral therapies may help reduce distress, but the methodologic rigor of the studies was not determined (Schnur et al., 2009; Yoo, Lee, & Yoon, 2009).
  d) Complementary and alternative medicine (CAM) for emotional distress among patients with cancer undergoing RT
    (1) Thomas et al. (2010) reviewed potential CAM therapies shown to be effective in decreasing emotional distress related to RT. Potential treatments included music therapy, relaxation techniques, massage, meditation, yoga, healing touch, art therapy, laughter therapy, acupuncture, and nutritional and antioxidant supplements. The methodologic quality of the reviewed studies was not addressed.
    (2) One study found no evidence to support that aromatherapy reduces emotional distress among patients with cancer treated with RT (Graham, Browne, Cox, & Graham, 2003).
  e) Medical management
    (1) Psychotherapy and pharmacotherapy combined are more effective than either alone in treating emotional distress, as well as in preventing the relapse of distress in patients with cancer in general (Twillman & Manetto, 1998). Patients should receive appropriate referrals.
    (2) Pharmacotherapy alone (For more comprehensive lists, drug interactions, and evidence-based management, see

Barsevick & Much, 2004; Bruner & Diefenbach, 2001; Gobel, 2004.)

(a) Benzodiazepines (e.g., diazepam, alprazolam)—Most commonly used for acute and chronic anxiety

(b) SSRIs (e.g., paroxetine, fluoxetine)—Most commonly used for depression caused by cancer

   i. In general, medications for depression among patients with cancer have shown effectiveness (Dy et al., 2008).

   ii. Some SSRIs may be contraindicated for certain patients (e.g., patients with breast cancer taking tamoxifen [Jin et al., 2005]).

(c) Tricyclic antidepressants (e.g., amitriptyline, doxepin)

(d) Lithium

(e) Monoamine oxidase inhibitors (e.g., phenelzine, tranylcypromine)

(3) Family and couples therapy (NCCN, 2010)

f) Oncology nursing role: The nursing challenge with such a complex, multifaceted problem as distress is finding strategies that are realistic within the primarily outpatient RT department.

(1) Education

(a) Discuss with the patient and family the potential for the variety of challenges presented by cancer, such as distress.

(b) Instruct the patient and family that open communication is the best way of dealing with distress, and the patient should inform his or her nurse, doctor, and family of this symptom.

(c) Reassure the patient and family that strategies do exist to help emotional distress.

(d) Several self-care guides for dealing with emotional distress exist and can be copied and given to the patient. They include

   i. Relaxation and guided imagery (Gobel, 2004)

   ii. Depression (Barsevick & Much, 2004)

   iii. Taking antidepressant medications (Barsevick & Much, 2004)

   iv. Side effects of antidepressant medications (Barsevick & Much, 2004)

   v. Depression self-care data log (Barsevick & Much, 2004).

(2) Resources

(a) The Internet is a rich resource for cancer-related information. All sites do not contain the same level of accuracy, so before making recommendations to a patient, the nurse should be aware of what the Web site contains.

(b) ACS

   i. General Web site: www.cancer.org; or refer patients to the local office by telephone

   ii. ACS Cancer Survivors Network: http://csn.cancer.org

(c) Mental Health America (formerly known as the National Mental Health Association): www.nmha.org

(d) NCI Cancer Topics: www.cancer.gov/cancertopics

(e) National Institute of Mental Health: www.nimh.nih.gov/index.shtml

(f) NCCN: www.nccn.org

(3) Outcomes

(a) The patient will be assessed for distress at each outpatient visit.

(b) The patient will demonstrate awareness of treatment services for distress in the treatment center and in the community.

(c) The patient and family will demonstrate adequate knowledge about distress through communication or seeking medical assistance and support.

(d) The patient will demonstrate adaptive coping.

(e) The patient will report a decrease in distress.

(f) The patient will be able to function mentally and emotionally.

7. Treatment seeking and use

a) Need for services

(1) Only 10%–25% of patients with cancer who are at high risk for psychosocial problems will eventually use psychosocial oncology services (Cwikel & Behar, 1999; Holland, 1997).

(2) In a study of 117 RT patients, 33% preferred professional psychosocial support from their oncologist, and 41% preferred support from their oncologist and from a psychotherapist or social worker. Interest in professional psychosocial

support correlated with the amount of distress but not with sociodemographic variables (de Vries et al., 1998).

(3) In another RT study, mental disorders were diagnosed in 51% of the patients assessed. The diagnostician regarded 32% of patients as needing psychotherapeutic treatment, compared with 43% of the patients who were motivated to accept at least one of the psychotherapeutic treatments offered (Fritzsche, Liptai, & Henke, 2004).

(4) Among patients with breast cancer starting RT, 36% reported needs for additional emotional support, and 75% said they would be willing to accept support if it were offered to them (Frick, Tyroller, & Panzer, 2007).

b) Major barriers to implementation of effective strategies to improve coping

(1) Lack of screening (Jacobsen & Ransom, 2007; Mitchell et al., 2008), although screening may not appropriately identify patients who want supportive services (Faller, Olshausen, & Flentje, 2003)

(2) Lack of knowledge of the multifaceted nature of cancer distress

(3) Outmoded attitudes of patients, staff, and institutions about psychological issues and patient difficulty in accepting help (Frick et al., 2007)

(4) Stigmatizing labels for those who access psychological therapy (Bruner & Diefenbach, 2001)

(5) Possible differences in perceived needs between patients and staff (Fritzsche et al., 2004).

References

Adler, N.E., & Page, N.E.K. (Eds.). (2008). *Cancer care for the whole patient: Meeting psychosocial health needs.* Washington, DC: National Academies Press.

Barsevick, A.M., & Much, J.K. (2004). Depression. In C.H. Yarbro, M.H. Frogge, & M. Goodman (Eds.), *Cancer symptom management* (3rd ed., pp. 668–692). Sudbury, MA: Jones and Bartlett.

Braeken, A.P., Lechner, L., Houben, R.M., Van Gils, F.C., & Kempen, G.I. (2010). Psychometric properties of the Screening Inventory of Psychosocial Problems (SIPP) in Dutch cancer patients treated with radiotherapy. *European Journal of Cancer Care, 20*, 305–314. doi:10.1111/j.1365-2354.2010.01182.x

Bruner, D.W., & Diefenbach, M. (2001). Distress/coping. In D.W. Bruner, G. Moore-Higgs, & M. Haas (Eds.), *Outcomes in radiation therapy: Multidisciplinary management* (pp. 563–589). Sudbury, MA: Jones and Bartlett.

Catlin-Huth, C., Haas, M., & Pollock, V. (Eds.). (2002). *Radiation therapy patient care record: A tool for documenting nursing care.* Pittsburgh, PA: Oncology Nursing Society.

Chen, A.M., Jennelle, R.L.S., Grady, V., Tovar, A., Bowen, K., Simonin, P., ... Vijayakumar, S. (2009). Prospective study of psychosocial distress among patients undergoing radiotherapy for head and neck cancer. *International Journal of Radiation Oncology, Biology, Physics, 73*, 187–193. doi:10.1016/j.ijrobp.2008.04.010

Cwikel, J.G., & Behar, L.C. (1999). Organizing social work services with adult cancer patients: Integrating empirical research. *Social Work in Health Care, 28*(3), 55–76.

Decker, T.W., Cline-Elsen, J., & Gallagher, M. (1992). Relaxation therapy as an adjunct in radiation oncology. *Journal of Clinical Psychology, 48*, 388–393.

de Leeuw, J.R., de Graeff, A., Ros, W.J., Blijham, G.H., Hordijk, G.J., & Winnubst, J.A. (2000). Prediction of depressive symptomatology after treatment of head and neck cancer: The influence of pre-treatment physical and depressive symptoms, coping, and social support. *Head and Neck, 22*, 799–807. doi:10.1002/1097-0347(200012)22:8<799::AID-HED9>3.0.CO;2-E

de Vries, A., Söllner, W., Steixner, E., Auer, V., Schiessling, G., Stzankay, A., ... Lukas, P. (1998). [Subjective psychological stress and need for psychosocial support in cancer patients during radiotherapy treatment]. *Strahlentherapie und Onkologie, 174*, 408–414.

Deshields, T., Tibbs, T., Fan, M.Y., & Taylor, M. (2006). Differences in patterns of depression after treatment for breast cancer. *Psycho-Oncology, 15*, 398–406. doi:10.1002/pon.962

Dy, S.M., Lorenz, K.A., Naeim, A., Sanati, H., Walling, A., & Asch, S.M. (2008). Evidence-based recommendations for cancer fatigue, anorexia, depression, and dyspnea. *Journal of Clinical Oncology, 26*, 3886–3895. doi:10.1200/JCO.2007.15.9525

Epping-Jordan, J.E., Compas, B.E., Osowiecki, D.M., Oppedisano, G., Gerhardt, C., Primo, K., & Krag, D.N. (1999). Psychological adjustment in breast cancer: Processes of emotional distress. *Health Psychology, 18*, 315–326. doi:10.1037/0278-6133.18.4.315

Evans, R.L., & Connis, R.T. (1995). Comparison of brief group therapies for depressed cancer patients receiving radiation treatment. *Public Health Reports, 110*, 306–311.

Faller, H., Olshausen, B., & Flentje, M. (2003). [Emotional distress and needs for psychosocial support among breast cancer patients at start of radiotherapy]. *Psychotherapie, Psychosomatik, Medizinische Psychologie, 53*, 229–235. doi:10.1055/s-2003-38864

Fischer, D.J., Villines, D., Kim, Y.O., Epstein, J.B., & Wilkie, D.J. (2010). Anxiety, depression, and pain: Differences by primary cancer. *Supportive Care in Cancer, 18*, 801–810. doi:10.1007/s00520-009-0712-5

Frick, E., Tyroller, M., & Panzer, M. (2007). Anxiety, depression and quality of life of cancer patients undergoing radiation therapy: A cross-sectional study in a community hospital outpatient centre. *European Journal of Cancer Care, 16*, 130–136. doi:10.1111/j.1365-2354.2006.00720.x

Fritzsche, K., Liptai, C., & Henke, M. (2004). Psychosocial distress and need for psychotherapeutic treatment in cancer patients undergoing radiotherapy. *Radiotherapy and Oncology, 72*, 183–189. doi:10.1016/j.radonc.2004.03.015

Gobel, B.H. (2004). Anxiety. In C.H. Yarbro, M.H. Frogge, & M. Goodman (Eds.), *Cancer symptom management* (3rd ed., pp. 651–667). Sudbury, MA: Jones and Bartlett.

Graham, P.H., Browne, L., Cox, H., & Graham, J. (2003). Inhalation aromatherapy during radiotherapy: Results of a placebo-controlled double-blind randomized trial. *Journal of Clinical Oncology, 21*, 2372–2376. doi:10.1200/JCO.2003.10.126

Hervouet, S., Savard, J., Simard, S., Ivers, H., Laverdière, J., Vigneault, E., ... Lacombe, L. (2005). Psychological functioning associated with prostate cancer: Cross-sectional comparison of patients treated with radiotherapy, brachytherapy, or surgery. *Journal of Pain and Symptom Management, 30,* 474–484. doi:10.1016/j.jpainsymman.2005.05.011

Hickok, J.T., Morrow, G.R., Roscoe, J.A., Mustian, K., & Okunieff, P. (2005). Occurrence, severity, and longitudinal course of twelve common symptoms in 1129 consecutive patients during radiotherapy for cancer. *Journal of Pain and Symptom Management, 30,* 433–442. doi:10.1016/j.jpainsymman.2005.04.012

Hjerl, K., Andersen, E.W., Keiding, N., Mouridsen, H.T., Mortensen, P.B., & Jørgensen, T. (2003). Depression as a prognostic factor for breast cancer mortality. *Psychosomatics, 44,* 24–30.

Holland, J.C. (1997). Preliminary guidelines for the treatment of distress. *Oncology, 11*(11A), 109–114.

Hopwood, P., Sumo, G., Mills, J., Haviland, J., & Bliss, J.M. (2010). The course of anxiety and depression over 5 years of follow-up and risk factors in women with early breast cancer: Results from the UK Standardisation of Radiotherapy Trials (START). *Breast, 19,* 84–91. doi:10.1016/j.breast.2009.11.007

Iqbal, A., & Siddiqui, K.S. (2002). The incidence of anxiety and its correlates in cancer patients receiving radiotherapy. *Pakistan Journal of Medical Sciences, 18,* 187–191.

Jacobsen, P.B., & Jim, H.S. (2008). Psychosocial interventions for anxiety and depression in adult cancer patients: Achievements and challenges. *CA: A Cancer Journal for Clinicians, 58,* 214–230. doi:10.3322/CA.2008.0003

Jacobsen, P.B., & Ransom, S. (2007). Implementation of NCCN distress management guidelines by member institutions. *Journal of the National Comprehensive Cancer Network, 5,* 99–103.

Jim, H.S., Andrykowski, M.A., Munster, P.N., & Jacobsen, P.B. (2007). Physical symptoms/side effects during breast cancer treatment predict posttreatment distress. *Annals of Behavioral Medicine, 34,* 200–208. doi:10.1080/08836610701566969

Jin, Y., Desta, Z., Stearns, V., Ward, B., Ho, H., Lee, K.H., … Flockhart, D.A. (2005). CYP2D6 genotype, antidepressant use, and tamoxifen metabolism during adjuvant breast cancer treatment. *Journal of the National Cancer Institute, 97,* 30–39. doi:10.1093/jnci/dji005

Kamer, S., Ozsaran, Z., Celik, O., Bildik, O., Yalman, D., Bölükbaşi, Y., & Haydaroğlu, A. (2007). Evaluation of anxiety levels during intracavitary brachytherapy applications in women with gynecological malignancies. *European Journal of Gynaecological Oncology, 28,* 121–124.

Katz, M.R., Kopek, N., Waldron, J., Devins, G.M., & Tomlinson, G. (2004). Screening for depression in head and neck cancer. *Psycho-Oncology, 13,* 269–280. doi:10.1002/pon.734

Kobayashi, M., Ohno, T., Noguchi, W., Matsuda, A., Matsushima, E., Kato, S., & Tsujii, H. (2009). Psychological distress and quality of life in cervical cancer survivors after radiotherapy: Do treatment modalities, disease stage, and self-esteem influence outcomes? *International Journal of Gynecological Cancer, 19,* 1264–1268. doi:10.1111/IGC.0b013e3181a3e124

Krischer, M.M., & Xu, P. (2008). Determinants of psychological functioning in patients undergoing radiotherapy: A descriptive study. *Journal of Psychosocial Oncology, 26*(4), 1–13. doi:10.1080/07347330802359552

Lazarus, R.S., & Folkman, S. (1984). *Stress, appraisal, and coping.* New York, NY: Springer.

Leopold, K.A., Ahles, T.A., Walch, S., Amdur, R.J., Mott, L.A., Wiegand-Packard, L., & Oxman, T.E. (1998). Prevalence of mood disorders and utility of the PRIME-MD in patients undergoing radiation therapy. *International Journal of Radiation Oncology, Biology, Physics, 42,* 1105–1112. doi:10.1016/S0360-3016(98)00346-0

Mitchell, A.J., Kaar, S., Coggan, C., & Herdman, J. (2008). Acceptability of common screening methods used to detect distress and related mood disorders—Preferences of cancer specialists and non-specialists. *Psycho-Oncology, 17,* 226–236. doi:10.1002/pon.1228

Mose, S., Budischewski, K.M., Rahn, A.N., Zander-Heinz, A.C., Bormeth, S., & Böttcher, H.D. (2001). Influence of irradiation on therapy-associated psychological distress in breast carcinoma patients. *International Journal of Radiation Oncology, Biology, Physics, 51,* 1328–1335. doi:10.1016/S0360-3016(01)01711-4

National Comprehensive Cancer Network. (2010). *NCCN Clinical Practice Guidelines in Oncology: Distress management* [v.1.2011]. Retrieved from http://www.nccn.org/professionals/physician_gls/pdf/distress.pdf

Onitilo, A.A., Nietert, P.J., & Egede, L.E. (2006). Effect of depression on all-cause mortality in adults with cancer and differential effects by cancer site. *General Hospital Psychiatry, 28,* 396–402. doi:10.1016/j.genhosppsych.2006.05.006

Pruitt, B.T., Waligora-Serafin, B., McMahon, T., Byrd, G., Besselman, L., Kelly, G.M., … Cuellar, D. (1993). An educational intervention for newly-diagnosed cancer patients undergoing radiotherapy. *Psycho-Oncology, 2,* 55–62. doi:10.1002/pon.2960020108

Satin, J.R., Linden, W., & Phillips, M.J. (2009). Depression as a predictor of disease progression and mortality in cancer patients: A meta-analysis. *Cancer, 115,* 5349–5361. doi:10.1002/cncr.24561

Schnur, J.B., David, D., Kangas, M., Green, S., Bovbjerg, D.H., & Montgomery, G.H. (2009). A randomized trial of a cognitive-behavioral therapy and hypnosis intervention on positive and negative affect during breast cancer radiotherapy. *Journal of Clinical Psychology, 65,* 443–455. doi:10.1002/jclp.20559

Sehlen, S., Fahmüller, H., Herschbach, P., Aydemir, U., Lenk, M., & Dühmke, E. (2003). [Psychometric properties of the Stress Index RadioOncology (SIRO)—A new questionnaire measuring quality of life of cancer patients during radiotherapy]. *Strahlentherapie und Onkologie, 179,* 261–269. doi:10.1007/s00066-003-1057-5

Sehlen, S., Hollenhorst, H., Schymura, B., Herschbach, P., Aydemir, U., Firsching, M., & Dühmke, E. (2003). Psychosocial stress in cancer patients during and after radiotherapy. *Strahlentherapie und Onkologie, 179,* 175–180. doi:10.1007/s00066-003-1018-z

Sehlen, S., Song, R., Fahmüller, H., Herschbach, P., Lenk, M., Hollenhorst, H., … Dühmke, E. (2003). Coping of cancer patients during and after radiotherapy—A follow-up of 2 years. *Onkologie, 26,* 557–563. doi:10.1159/000074151

Smets, E.M., Visser, M.R., Willems-Groot, A.F., Garssen, B., Oldenburger, F., van Tienhoven, G., & de Haes, J.C. (1998). Fatigue and radiotherapy: Experience in patients undergoing treatment. *British Journal of Cancer, 78,* 899–906.

Spiegel, D., & Giese-Davis, J. (2003). Depression and cancer: Mechanisms and disease progression. *Biological Psychiatry, 54,* 269–282. doi:10.1016/S0006-3223(03)00566-3

Stiegelis, H.E., Ranchor, A.V., & Sanderman, R. (2004). Psychological functioning in cancer patients treated with radiotherapy. *Patient Education and Counseling, 52,* 131–141. doi:10.1016/S0738-3991(03)00021-1

Thomas, J., Beinhorn, C., Norton, D., Richardson, M., Sumler, S.S., & Frenkel, M. (2010). Managing radiation therapy side effects with complementary medicine. *Journal of the Society for Integrative Oncology, 8,* 65–80. doi:10.2310/7200.2009.0023

Turner, N.J., Muers, M.F., Haward, R.A., & Mulley, G.P. (2007). Psychological distress and concerns of elderly patients treated with palliative radiotherapy for lung cancer. *Psycho-Oncology, 16,* 707–713. doi:10.1002/pon.1109

Twillman, R.K., & Manetto, C. (1998). Concurrent psychotherapy and pharmacotherapy in the treatment of depression and anxiety in cancer patients. *Psycho-Oncology, 7,* 285–290. doi:10.1002/(SICI)1099-1611(199807/08)7:4<285::AID-PON362>3.0.CO;2-G

Voigtmann, K., Köllner, V., Einsle, F., Alheit, H., Joraschky, P., & Herrmann, T. (2010). Emotional state of patients in radiotherapy and how they deal with their disorder. *Strahlentherapie und Onkologie, 186,* 229–235. doi:10.1007/s00066-010-2109-2

Yoo, M.S., Lee, H., & Yoon, J.A. (2009). [Effects of a cognitive-behavioral nursing intervention on anxiety and depression in women with breast cancer undergoing radiotherapy]. *Journal of Korean Academy of Nursing, 39,* 157–165. doi:10.4040/jkan.2009.39.2.157

F. Sexual dysfunction
   1. Pathophysiology
      a) General: Three phases of the sexual response cycle—desire, arousal, and orgasm—can be affected by cancer and cancer therapies (Wilmoth & Bruner, 2002).
         (1) *Sexual desire* is an interest in sexual activity and is affected by factors such as anger, pain, body image, disease processes, and medications.
         (2) *Sexual arousal* is the perception of being "turned on" sexually. Subsequent to arousal, vasodilation and vasocongestion occur, leading to penile erection in men and vaginal lubrication in women. Impairment may result from surgery that cut through the vessels, or RT may cause sclerosis of the vessels necessary for these functions.
         (3) *Orgasm* is the peak of sexual pleasure, usually characterized by strong feelings of pleasure and a series of involuntary contractions of the muscles of the genitals. It is mediated by the sympathetic nervous system. Therapies such as surgery, RT, and chemotherapy may have an adverse effect on the nerves involved in this portion of the sexual response cycle (Wilmoth & Bruner, 2002).
      b) Acute
         (1) RT denudes the vaginal epithelium in females and the urethral epithelium in males and females, leading to inflammation. These changes account for the majority of acute RT effects experienced during sexual intercourse (Shield, 1995).
         (2) Disease may affect libido, or decreased libido may be related to decreased or ablated ovarian or testicular function that can occur at doses as low as 6 Gy (Howell & Shalet, 1998).
      c) Late
         (1) Narrowing and obliteration of the small pelvic vessels and circumferential fibrosis of the perivaginal tissue contribute to vaginal stenosis in women treated with pelvic RT and are more pronounced in those receiving brachytherapy (Grigsby et al., 1995), as brachytherapy increases the surface dose to the vagina.
         (2) The vaginal epithelium may appear thin, pale, and atrophic over time and may be traumatized by intercourse or masturbation. Diminished or lack of vaginal lubrication following arousal may cause dyspareunia.
         (3) Radiation-induced erectile dysfunction is multifactorial, but arterial damage seems to be the main cause (Incrocci, Slob, & Levendag, 2002). It currently is undetermined which structures are responsible for radiation-induced erectile dysfunction because of inconclusive data and lacking research (van der Wielen, Mulhall, & Incrocci, 2007).
         (4) Men may experience dyspareunia immediately after ejaculation.
   2. Prevalence
      a) General: Sexual dysfunction does not occur in all patients with cancer (Hendren et al., 2005). However, almost half (more than 45%) of patients treated for cancer experience altered sexual function (Baker, Denniston, Smith, & West, 2005) that may decrease their quality of life (Galbraith, Arechiga, Ramirez, & Pedro, 2005; Kendirci, Bejma, & Hellstrom, 2006) and affect their significant other (Galbraith et al., 2005; Kadmon, Ganz, Rom, & Woloski-Wruble, 2008).
      b) Pelvic cancer: Some degree of sexual dysfunction has been reported in most patients treated for pelvic cancers (gynecologic, prostate, bladder, rectal) with RT, depending on the site, volume treated, and dose (Bruner, 2001).

c) Breast cancer: A recent literature review indicated that women with breast cancer who are treated with chemotherapy are at higher risk for sexual dysfunction than those who have not had chemotherapy. Chemotherapy is associated with dysfunctions related to arousal, lubrication, orgasm, and dyspareunia, whereas radiation to the breast is associated with feeling medically "invaded" but is less likely to be associated with decreased sexual desire as chemotherapy (Emilee, Ussher, & Perz, 2010). Women treated with EBRT in combination with lumpectomy for breast cancer may experience disruption in sexual activity, most likely a result of temporary effects of skin discomfort and fatigue (Bruner & Berk, 2004). However, an advantage of partial mastectomy (breast conservation) over immediate breast reconstruction after mastectomy was documented in terms of maintaining pleasure and frequency of breast caressing during sexual activity (Schover et al., 1995).

d) Head and neck cancer: One study of sexual functioning in 55 patients with head and neck cancer following RT with or without surgery found that 58% were no longer having intercourse, although 85% were still interested in sex. The majority reported arousal problems, and 58% had orgasmic problems, yet 49% were satisfied with their current sexual functioning (Monga, Tan, Ostermann, & Monga, 1997).

e) Cervical cancer: In comparison to surgery, RT generally has been associated with higher rates of sexual dysfunction in women treated for cervical carcinoma (Schover, Fife, & Gershenson, 1989; Seibel, Freeman, & Graves, 1980). However, one report indicated that surgery accounted for the majority of risk of vaginal stenosis, as well as insufficient lubrication and reduced vaginal elasticity, when compared to RT (Bergmark, Avall-Lundqvist, Dickman, Henningsohn, & Steineck, 1999). Women treated with RT had worse scores across domains of sexual functioning (sexual interest, satisfaction, lubrication, dyspareunia) compared to aged-matched controls (Jensen et al., 2003). Women aged 50 and older may be at greater risk for vaginal stenosis (Brand, Bull, & Cakir, 2006).

f) Endometrial cancer: Little research has been conducted to report the degree of sexual dysfunction after RT for endometrial can-

cer. Vaginal stenosis has been reported in up to 72% of women treated with intracavitary radiation for endometrial cancer and 88% of women treated for cervical cancer (Bruner et al., 1993).

g) Prostate cancer: In a systematic review, erectile dysfunction after RT was 43% compared to 86% after androgen deprivation therapy and 58% after radical prostatectomy (Wilt et al., 2008). Reduced or absent semen production can also occur with RT of the prostate.

h) Bladder cancer: Very little research has been conducted on sexual dysfunction after treatment for bladder cancer. In a rare study of sexual function in males treated with RT for bladder cancer, 71% felt their sex life was worse following RT, but only 56% were concerned about the deterioration (Little & Howard, 1998).

i) Testicular cancer: RT for testicular cancer has been associated with reduced or absent semen volume (60%), reduced erectile potential (48%), premature ejaculation (40%), reduced intensity of orgasm (38%), loss of sexual desire (17%), and an inability to ejaculate (5%), yet only 8% of the men treated with RT reported a decrease in sexual satisfaction from prior to therapy (Arai, Kawakita, Okada, & Yoshida, 1997).

j) Anorectal cancer: The ability to have an orgasm after multimodality therapy (preoperative RT followed by surgery) has been reported to be absent in 50% of both male and female patients. Orgasm may be absent in 45%–57% of patients after treatment for locally advanced primary or recurrent rectal cancer treatments (Mannaerts et al., 2001). In long-term follow-up, patients with anal carcinoma who were treated with RT were found to have acceptable overall quality-of-life scores but poor sexual function scores (Das et al., 2010). Men in homosexual relationships have an increased risk for anorectal cancer, and treatment for the disease may significantly interfere with both male and female homosexual relationships (Frisch, Smith, Grulich, & Johansen, 2003; Goldstone, Winkler, Ufford, Alt, & Palefsky, 2001).

k) Penile cancer: The risk of male dyspareunia or penile pain when having intercourse either vaginally or rectally increases with treatment such as EBRT, which may cause thinning of penile skin, or laser treatment (Nishimoto & Mark, 2010; Windahl, Skeppner, Andersson, & Fugl-Meyer, 2004).

3. Assessment

a) Risk factors: Pretreatment sexual activity appears to be the best predictor of post-treatment sexual function (Andersen, Cyranowski, & Espindle, 1999). Pretreatment dysfunction needs to be assessed because of greater risk of sexual problems following RT.

b) Sexual history: For a comprehensive sexual history assessment tool, see Bruner and Berk, 2004.

   (1) Age: Changes occur frequently with advancing age as a result of comorbidities (Burns-Cox & Gingell, 1997).

   (2) Cultural/ethnic background: Sexual values and norms vary widely among cultures (Meston, Trapnell, & Gorzalka, 1996; Wyatt et al., 1998).

   (3) History of sexual activity, including sexual orientation, age at first intercourse, number of partners, marital discord, and problems with desire, arousal, or orgasm

   (4) History of sexual abuse: An estimated 366,470 women and 36,440 men are forcibly raped or sexually assaulted in the United States each year (Maguire, 2008). It has been estimated that 16% of women treated for gynecologic malignancies have been sexually abused (Bergmark et al., 1999).

   (5) Frequency of sexual activity over the past six months

   (6) Satisfaction with sexual ability and frequency

   (7) Medications that may interfere with sexual function (e.g., antihypertensives, antidepressants)

   (8) Female issues

      (a) Dyspareunia

      (b) Vaginal dryness

   (9) Male issues

      (a) Erectile ability

      (b) Retrograde ejaculation

      (c) Dyspareunia

c) Physical examination

   (1) Female

      (a) Check skin over vulva and around anus for breakdown, lesions, or inflammation.

      (b) Check for vaginal stenosis.

      (c) Check for vaginal discharge or bleeding.

   (2) Male

      (a) Check skin over the penis and scrotum for breakdown, lesions, or inflammation.

      (b) Check anal area for breakdown, fissures, or lesions.

d) Documentation (in addition to previously discussed) (Catlin-Huth, Haas, & Pollock, 2002)

   (1) Sexual alteration

      (a) 0—Absent

      (b) 1—Present

   (2) Vaginal drainage

      (a) 0—Absent

      (b) 1—Present

4. Acute effects and evidence-based management

  a) Psychological—Prepare the patient and partner for the possible treatment effects on sexual function.

  b) Behavioral

   (1) Discuss the need for the patient to manage symptoms (e.g., pain) before trying to engage in sexual activity.

   (2) Encourage communication between the patient and partner concerning fears regarding continued sexual function.

  c) Medical

   (1) A structured review of the literature found topical estrogens and benzydamine to have the strongest evidence of treatment benefit for acute radiation-induced vaginal changes (Denton & Maher, 2003).

   (2) The structured literature review also found evidence to support the use of vaginal dilators to maintain vaginal patency (Denton & Maher, 2003).

   (3) The use of dilators should begin as soon as the patient can tolerate it to prevent adhesions (fibrous tissue) from forming.

      (a) The patient can begin during RT if she can tolerate it.

      (b) A condom stuffed with cotton balls and tied at the bottom, used with ample lubricant, may make the experience more tolerable.

5. Long-term effects and evidence-based management

  a) Psychological

   (1) Support the patient and partner with concerns regarding sexual function.

   (2) Refer patients with history of sexual abuse or marital problems to a social worker, family therapist, or sex counselor.

  b) Behavioral

   (1) Encourage communication between the patient and partner concerning fears regarding continued sexual function.

   (2) Teach proper positioning for continued sexual activity that would prevent discomfort depending on the therapy

or problem (see Bruner & Berk, 2004, for pictorial suggestions for positioning).

c) Medical

(1) Women need to continue to perform vaginal dilation with a penis, vaginal dilator, or vaginal vibrator at least three times per week for life.

(2) Vaginal dryness can be managed with water-soluble lubricants (Bruner & Berk, 2004).

(3) A Cochrane review found that phosphodiesterase type-5 (PDE5) inhibitors (e.g., sildenafil, tadalafil, vardenafil) are an effective treatment for erectile dysfunction following RT for prostate cancer (Miles et al., 2007). However, following treatment with concurrent androgen deprivation therapy and RT, less than 25% of men treated with sildenafil had improvement in erectile function (Bruner et al., 2011). The primary contraindications include heart failure, uncontrolled hypertension, current use of nitrates (e.g., use of nitroglycerin); current use of cimetidine, ketoconazole, itraconazole, erythromycin, or ritonavir; moderate to severe renal insufficiency or end-stage renal disease; or severe hepatic impairment. The most common side effects are headache, flushing, dyspepsia, and nasal congestion. The risk of at least one side effect is about 30% across all PDE5 inhibitors. Most side effects are mild, and only about 4% of men discontinue the drug because of adverse events (Tsertsvadze et al., 2009).

(4) Refer men to a urologist. For men who are not candidates for oral medications to improve erections, other potential treatments include penile implants, injectable medications, or vacuum devices. Positive outcomes have

been reported with some erectile aids (Litwin et al., 1999).

(5) Refer women to a urologist or sex therapist.

(6) PDE5 inhibitors improve genital vasocongestion but have shown little or no improvement in female self-report of sexual function (Chivers & Rosen, 2010), although this has not been tested in women with sexual dysfunction related to cancer therapies.

(7) Fertility issues after RT are beyond the scope of this outline, and readers are referred elsewhere (Dohle, 2010; Georgescu, Goldberg, du Plessis, & Agarwal, 2008).

6. Patient and family education

a) Teach the patient and partner about the potential impact on sexual function caused by pelvic irradiation (see Schover, 1999). The expected outcome is that they will be able to verbalize an understanding of potential sexual dysfunction and will discuss issues with their nurse or physician.

b) Teach the patient and partner methods to minimize sexual discomfort or dysfunction (see Bruner and Berk, 2004, for more indepth instructions). The expected outcome is that the patient (and partner) will comply with methods to minimize sexual dysfunction.

c) Teach women to use a vaginal dilator to prevent vaginal stenosis after an intracavitary implant (Bruner & Berk, 2004). The expected outcome is that the patient will maintain vaginal patency.

d) Teach men how to use erectile aids, if needed. The expected outcome is that the patient will maintain erectile function.

e) Discuss with the patient and partner about when to resume intercourse and/or masturbation after therapy. The expected outcome is that the patient will not act too soon and risk incurring pain or performance anxiety, but also that he or she will not wait too long and build up a fear of returning to normal function.

f) Teach the patient and partner to report continued sexual dysfunction to the nurse or physician.

g) Assure the patient that, if needed, he or she can be referred to specialists in sexual dysfunction, such as a urologist, psychologist, or sex therapist, if physical, psychological, or relationship problems persist.

(1) The American Association of Sexuality Educators, Counselors, and Thera-

pists (AASECT), a nonprofit, interdisciplinary professional organization, includes sex educators, counselors, and therapists, as well as physicians, nurses, social workers, psychologists, allied healthcare professionals, clergy members, lawyers, sociologists, marriage and family counselors and therapists, family planning specialists, and researchers.

(2) The AASECT directory lists members by state (www.aasect.org/directory.asp).

h) Related Web sites

(1) ACS's information on sexual side effects in women and men: www.cancer.org/Treatment/TreatmentsandSideEffects/PhysicalSideEffects/index

(2) For a list of links to cancer site–specific and general sex education Web pages: www.bigeye.com/sexeducation/index.html

i) Suggested readings

(1) Alterowitz, R., & Alterowitz, B. (1999). *The lovin' ain't over: The couple's guide to better sex after prostate disease.* Westbury, NY: Health Education Literary Publisher.

(2) Katz, A. (2007). *Breaking the silence on cancer and sexuality: A handbook for healthcare providers.* Pittsburgh, PA: Oncology Nursing Society.

(3) Katz, A. (2009). *Woman cancer sex.* Pittsburgh, PA: Hygeia Media.

(4) Katz, A. (2010). *Man cancer sex.* Pittsburgh, PA: Hygeia Media.

(5) Shaw, G.M. (2011). *Having children after cancer: How to make informed choices before and after treatment and build the family of your dreams.* Berkeley, CA: Celestial Arts.

References

Andersen, B.L., Cyranowski, J.M., & Espindle, D. (1999). Men's sexual self-schema. *Journal of Personality and Social Psychology, 76,* 645–661. doi:10.1037/0022-3514.76.4.645

Arai, Y., Kawakita, M., Okada, Y., & Yoshida, O. (1997). Sexuality and fertility in long-term survivors of testicular cancer. *Journal of Clinical Oncology, 15,* 1444–1448.

Baker, F., Denniston, M., Smith, T., & West, M.M. (2005). Adult cancer survivors: How are they faring? *Cancer, 104,* 2565–2576. doi:10.1002/cncr.21488

Bergmark, K., Avall-Lundqvist, E., Dickman, P.W., Henningsohn, L., & Steineck, G. (1999). Vaginal changes and sexuality in women with a history of cervical cancer. *New England Journal of Medicine, 340,* 1383–1389. doi:10.1056/NEJM199905063401802

Brand, A.H., Bull, C.A., & Cakir, B. (2006). Vaginal stenosis in patients treated with radiotherapy for carcinoma of the cervix.

International Journal of Gynecological Cancer, 16, 288–293. doi:10.1111/j.1525-1438.2006.00348.x

Bruner, D.W. (2001). Maintenance of body image and sexual function. In D.W. Bruner, G. Moore-Higgs, & M. Haas (Eds.), *Outcomes in radiation therapy: Multidisciplinary management* (pp. 611–636). Sudbury, MA: Jones and Bartlett.

Bruner, D.W., & Berk, L. (2004). Altered body image and sexual health. In C.H. Yarbro, M.H. Frogge, & M. Goodman (Eds.), *Cancer symptom management* (3rd ed., pp. 596–603). Sudbury, MA: Jones and Bartlett.

Bruner, D.W., James, J.L., Bryan, C.J., Pisansky, T.M., Rotman, M., Corbett, T., ... Berk, L. (2011). Randomized, double-blinded, placebo-controlled crossover trial of treating erectile dysfunction with sildenafil after radiotherapy and short-term androgen deprivation therapy: Results of RTOG 0215. *Journal of Sexual Medicine, 8,* 1228–1238. doi:10.1111/j.1743-6109.2010.02164.x

Bruner, D.W., Lanciano, R., Keegan, M., Corn, B., Martin, E., & Hanks, G. (1993). Vaginal stenosis and sexual function following intracavitary radiation for the treatment of cervical and endometrial carcinoma. *International Journal of Radiation Oncology, Biology, Physics, 27,* 825–830. doi:10.1016/0360-3016(93)90455-5

Burns-Cox, N., & Gingell, C. (1997). The andropause: Fact or fiction? *Postgraduate Medical Journal, 73,* 553–556.

Catlin-Huth, C., Haas, M., & Pollock, V. (Eds.). (2002). *Radiation therapy patient care record: A tool for documenting nursing care.* Pittsburgh, PA: Oncology Nursing Society.

Chivers, M.L., & Rosen, R.C. (2010). Phosphodiesterase type 5 inhibitors and female sexual response: Faulty protocols or paradigms? *Journal of Sexual Medicine, 7*(2, Pt. 2), 858–872. doi:10.1111/j.1743-6109.2009.01599.x

Das, P., Cantor, S.B., Parker, C.L., Zampieri, J.B., Baschnagel, A., Eng, C., ... Crane, C.H. (2010). Long-term quality of life after radiotherapy for the treatment of anal cancer. *Cancer, 116,* 822–829. doi:10.1002/cncr.24906

Denton, A.S., & Maher, J. (2003). Interventions for the physical aspects of sexual dysfunction in women following pelvic radiotherapy. *Cochrane Database of Systematic Reviews* 2003, Issue 1. Art. No.: CD003750. doi:10.1002/14651858.CD003750

Dohle, G.R. (2010). Male infertility in cancer patients: Review of the literature. *International Journal of Urology, 17,* 327–331. doi:10.1111/j.1442-2042.2010.02484.x

Emilee, G., Ussher, J.M., & Perz, J. (2010). Sexuality after breast cancer: A review. *Maturitas, 66,* 397–407. doi:10.1016/j.maturitas.2010.03.027

Frisch, M., Smith, E., Grulich, A., & Johansen, C. (2003). Cancer in a population-based cohort of men and women in registered homosexual partnerships. *American Journal of Epidemiology, 157,* 966–972. doi:10.1093/aje/kwg067

Galbraith, M.E., Arechiga, A., Ramirez, J., & Pedro, L.W. (2005). Prostate cancer survivors' and partners' self-reports of health-related quality of life, treatment symptoms, and marital satisfaction 2.5–5.5 years after treatment [Online exclusive]. *Oncology Nursing Forum, 32,* E30–E41. doi:10.1188/05.ONF.E30-E41

Georgescu, E.S., Goldberg, J.M., du Plessis, S.S., & Agarwal, A. (2008). Present and future fertility preservation strategies for female cancer patients. *Obstetrical and Gynecological Survey, 63,* 725–732. doi:10.1097/OGX.0b013e318186aaea

Goldstone, S.E., Winkler, B., Ufford, L.J., Alt, E., & Palefsky, J.M. (2001). High prevalence of anal squamous intraepithelial lesions and squamous-cell carcinoma in men who have sex with men as seen in a surgical practice. *Diseases of the Colon and Rectum, 44,* 690–698.

Grigsby, P.W., Russell, A., Bruner, D., Eifel, P., Koh, W.-J., Spanos, W., … Sullivan, J. (1995). Late injury of cancer therapy on the female reproductive tract. *International Journal of Radiation Oncology, Biology, Physics, 31,* 1281–1299. doi:10.1016/0360-3016(94)00426-L

Hendren, S.K., O'Connor, B.I., Liu, M., Asano, T., Cohen, Z., Swallow, C.J., … McLeod, R.S. (2005). Prevalence of male and female sexual dysfunction is high following surgery for rectal cancer. *Annals of Surgery, 242,* 212–223.

Howell, S., & Shalet, S. (1998). Gonadal damage from chemotherapy and radiotherapy. *Endocrinology and Metabolism Clinics of North America, 27,* 927–943.

Incrocci, L., Slob, A.K., & Levendag, P.C. (2002). Sexual (dys)function after radiotherapy for prostate cancer: A review. *International Journal of Radiation Oncology, Biology, Physics, 52,* 681–693. doi:10.1016/S0360-3016(01)02727-4

Jensen, P.T., Groenvold, M., Klee, M.C., Thranov, I., Petersen, M.A., & Machin, D. (2003). Longitudinal study of sexual function and vaginal changes after radiotherapy for cervical cancer. *International Journal of Radiation Oncology, Biology, Physics, 56,* 937–949. doi:10.1016/S0360-3016(03)00362-6

Kadmon, I., Ganz, F.D., Rom, M., & Woloski-Wruble, A.C. (2008). Social, marital, and sexual adjustment of Israeli men whose wives were diagnosed with breast cancer. *Oncology Nursing Forum, 35,* 131–135. doi:10.1188/08.ONF.131-135

Kendirci, M., Bejma, J., & Hellstrom, W.J.G. (2006). Update on erectile dysfunction in prostate cancer patients. *Current Opinion in Urology, 16,* 186–195. doi:10.1097/01.mou.0000193407.05285.d8

Little, F.A., & Howard, G.C. (1998). Sexual function following radical radiotherapy for bladder cancer. *Radiotherapy and Oncology, 49,* 157–161. doi:10.1016/S0167-8140(98)00109-1

Litwin, M.S., Flanders, S.C., Pasta, D.J., Stoddard, M.L., Lubeck, D.P., & Henning, J.M. (1999). Sexual function and bother after radical prostatectomy or radiation for prostate cancer: Multivariate quality-of-life analysis from CaPSURE. Cancer of the Prostate Strategic Urologic Research Endeavor. *Urology, 54,* 503–508. doi:10.1016/S0090-4295(99)00172-7

Maguire, K. (Ed.). (2008). *Sourcebook of criminal justice statistics.* Retrieved from http://www.albany.edu/sourcebook/pdf/t31062008.pdf

Mannaerts, G.H., Schijven, M.P., Hendrikx, A., Martijn, H., Rutten, H.J., & Wiggers, T. (2001). Urologic and sexual morbidity following multimodality treatment for locally advanced primary and locally recurrent rectal cancer. *European Journal of Surgical Oncology, 27,* 265–272. doi:10.1053/ejso.2000.1099

Meston, C.M., Trapnell, P.D., & Gorzalka, B.B. (1996). Ethnic and gender differences in sexuality: Variations in sexual behavior between Asian and non-Asian university students. *Archives of Sexual Behavior, 25,* 33–72. doi:10.1007/BF02437906

Miles, C., Candy, B., Jones, L., Williams, R., Tookman, A., & King, M. (2007). Interventions for sexual dysfunction following treatments for cancer. *Cochrane Database of Systematic Reviews 2007,* Issue 4. Art. No.: CD005540. doi:10.1002/14651858.CD005540

Monga, U., Tan, G., Ostermann, H., & Monga, T. (1997). Sexuality in the head and neck cancer patient. *Archives of Physical Medicine and Rehabilitation, 78,* 298–304.

Nishimoto, P.W., & Mark, D.D. (2010). Altered sexuality patterns. In C.G. Brown (Ed.), *A guide to oncology symptom management* (pp. 423–455). Pittsburgh, PA: Oncology Nursing Society.

Schover, L.R. (1999). Counseling cancer patients about changes in sexual function. *Oncology, 13,* 1585–1591.

Schover, L.R., Fife, M., & Gershenson, D. (1989). Sexual dysfunction and treatment for early stage cervical cancer. *Cancer, 63,* 204–212. doi:10.1002/1097-0142(19890101)63:1<204::AID-CNCR2820630133>3.0.CO;2-U

Schover, L.R., Yetman, R.J., Tuason, L.J., Meisler, E., Esselstyn, C.B., Hermann, R.E., … Dowden, R.V. (1995). Partial mastectomy and breast reconstruction. A comparison of their effects on psychosocial adjustment, body image, and sexuality. *Cancer, 75,* 54–64. doi:10.1002/1097-0142(19950101)75:1<54::AID-CNCR2820750111>3.0.CO;2-I

Seibel, M.M., Freeman, M.G., & Graves, W.L. (1980). Carcinoma of the cervix and sexual function. *Obstetrics and Gynecology, 55,* 484–487.

Shield, P.W. (1995). Chronic radiation effects: A correlative study of smears and biopsies from the cervix and vagina. *Diagnostic Cytopathology, 13,* 107–119.

Tsertsvadze, A., Fink, H.A., Yazdi, F., MacDonald, R., Bella, A.J., Ansari, M.T., … Wilt, T.J. (2009). Oral phosphodiesterase-5 inhibitors and hormonal treatments for erectile dysfunction: A systematic review and meta-analysis. *Annals of Internal Medicine, 151,* 650–661. doi:10.1059/0003-4819-151-9-200911030-00150

van der Wielen, G.J., Mulhall, J.P., & Incrocci, L. (2007). Erectile dysfunction after radiotherapy for prostate cancer and radiation dose to the penile structures: A critical review. *Radiotherapy and Oncology, 84,* 107–113. doi:10.1016/j.radonc.2007.07.018

Wilmoth, M.C., & Bruner, D.W. (2002). Integrating sexuality into cancer nursing practice. *Oncology Nursing: Patient Treatment and Support, 9*(1), 1–14.

Wilt, T.J., MacDonald, R., Rutks, I., Shamliyan, T.A., Taylor, B.C., & Kane, R.L. (2008). Systematic review: Comparative effectiveness and harms of treatments for clinically localized prostate cancer. *Annals of Internal Medicine, 148,* 435–448.

Windahl, T., Skeppner, E., Andersson, S.O., & Fugl-Meyer, K.S. (2004). Sexual function and satisfaction in men after laser treatment for penile carcinoma. *Journal of Urology, 172,* 648–651. doi:10.1097/01.ju.0000132891.68094.87

Wyatt, G.E., Desmond, K.A., Ganz, P.A., Rowland, J.H., Ashing-Giwa, K., & Meyerowitz, B.E. (1998). Sexual functioning and intimacy in African American and white breast cancer survivors: A descriptive study. *Women's Health, 4,* 385–405.

G. Nutritional issues
   1. Pathophysiology
      a) Effect of RT on healthy tissue can cause changes in normal physiologic function, which may eventually decrease a patient's nutritional status by interfering with the ingestion, digestion, or absorption of nutrients (Huhmann & Cunningham, 2005). Side effects depend on the radiation dose, duration, and treatment site and may be greater if radiation is given in conjunction with other antineoplastic therapies such as chemotherapy (Charney & Cranganu, 2010).
      b) Patients with aerodigestive tract tumors, including the head and neck, lungs, esophagus, pelvic regions, colorectal area, or pancreas, are most at risk for developing nutrition-related side effects (Luthringer, 2006). Examples from various tumor sites include the following.

(1) CNS (brain, spinal column)
  (a) Acute: Nausea, vomiting, fatigue, loss of appetite
  (b) Chronic: Dysphagia, weight loss, hyperglycemia, lethargy
(2) Head and neck areas (larynx, pharynx, tonsils, tongue, nasopharynx, salivary glands, hypopharynx, sinuses, oral cavity, oropharynx, lips)
  (a) Acute: Mucositis, sore mouth and throat, dysphagia, odynophagia, xerostomia, dysgeusia, dysosmia, anorexia, weight loss, fatigue, dental problems
  (b) Chronic: Cachexia, xerostomia, dysgeusia, dental caries, ulcers, osteoradionecrosis, trismus, dysphagia, odynophagia, anorexia, thickened saliva, dysosmia (olfactory dysfunction)
(3) Thorax areas (esophagus, lung)
  (a) Acute: Anorexia, dysphagia, gastric reflux, nausea, esophagitis, odynophagia
  (b) Chronic: Fibrosis, stenosis, perforations, fistula
(4) Abdominal and pelvic areas (cervical, prostate, pancreatic, uterine, colon, rectal, reproductive organs, testicles, liver, GI system)
  (a) Acute: Anorexia, nausea, vomiting, early satiety, pain, changes in urinary frequency, changes in bowel function (e.g., diarrhea, constipation, cramping, gas, bloating), acute colitis and enteritis, choleretic enteropathy, proctitis, and tenesmus
  (b) Chronic: Diarrhea, maldigestion, malabsorption, chronic colitis and enteritis, ulcer, stricture, obstruction, perforation, fistula, proctitis, tenesmus

c) Acute side effects begin approximately the second or third week of treatment. Symptoms peak about two-thirds of the way through treatment and may continue three to six weeks after treatment is completed. Taste and saliva changes caused by head and neck radiation can take months to improve and may never return to baseline (Luthringer, 2006).

d) Chronic radiation injury is also likely to adversely affect nutrition. Chronic indications, however, may not occur for months to years after treatment and can be irreversible.

2. Incidence
  a) CNS: As many as 40%–80% of patients undergoing RT will experience nausea and/or vomiting (Feyer et al., 2005).
  b) Head and neck areas
    (1) Taste impairment/changes
      (a) During an RT course of 60–70 Gy over six to eight weeks, measureable taste impairment can occur as early as the first or second week of treatment, with even greater alterations in taste during the third and fourth weeks of treatment and lasting throughout the entire course of RT. Patients reported a 50% taste loss involving all four tastes, up to an accumulated 30 Gy (Redda & Allis, 2006; Silverman, 2003). Almost all patients report a loss of taste at a dose of 60 Gy or within the first month of RT (Redda & Allis, 2006).
      (b) A dose this high has been previously seen to cause permanent taste loss in 90% of patients (Madeya, 1996), but with more specialized technologies, such as conformal RT and IMRT, many patients report an improvement in taste acuity within six months after completing RT (Redda & Allis, 2006).
      (c) Taste changes have been reported in 14% of patients with head and neck cancer before RT and in 84% of patients by the fifth week of treatment (Capra, Ferguson, & Reid, 2001; Larsson, Hedelin, Johansson, & Athlin, 2005; Tong, Isenring, & Yates, 2009). Zinc sulfate supplementation (220 mg, twice a day) may be helpful to some patients experiencing dysgeusia following their treatment (Silverman, 2003).
    (2) Forty percent to 60% of patients with head and neck cancer experienced swallowing difficulties because of RT (Capra et al., 2001; Jensen, Pedersen, Reibel, & Nauntofte, 2003; Larsson et al., 2005).
    (3) Xerostomia is also a common side effect of RT to the head and neck area, often reported as early as the second week of treatment or with an accumulated dose of 20 Gy. In one study (Jensen et al., 2003), xerostomia was reported in 25% of 74 patients with head and neck can-

cer before RT and in 80% of patients by the fourth week of RT. Diminished salivary flow may persist for more than five years after radiation (Shiboski, Hodgson, Ship, & Schiødt, 2007).

    (4) In another retrospective series of 204 consecutive patients who underwent RT for head and neck cancer at University of Texas MD Anderson Cancer Center in 2002 (Elting, Cooksley, Chambers, & Garden, 2007), mucositis incidence was 91% overall, with 66% of patients reporting severe mucositis (grade 3 or 4). The incidence was greater in patients receiving chemotherapy as well as RT, at 98%.

  c) Thoracic areas: Irradiation of thoracic malignancies commonly causes esophagitis. Therefore, patients may complain of dysphagia or odynophagia two to three weeks after the initiation of therapy. Symptoms may continue for the duration of therapy and for up to 16 weeks after the completion of therapy (Larsson et al., 2005; Werner-Wasik, Yu, Marks, & Shultheiss, 2004). Anorexia is also a very common side effect, occurring most often in patients receiving concurrent chemoradiation (Charney & Cranganu, 2010).

  d) Abdominal and pelvic areas: In patients receiving RT to the lower abdominal and pelvic regions, 3%–11% have reported nutrition problems (Capra et al., 2001). The incidence of nutrition problems is often higher among patients receiving both chemotherapy and RT (Charney & Cranganu, 2010). Chronic radiation enteritis is a possible side effect of radiation to this area and can interfere with digestion and absorption of nutrients. It can affect up to 50% of patients following pelvic RT (Abayomi, Kirwan, & Hackett, 2009).

3. Assessment

  a) Risk factors

    (1) Poor or inadequate dietary intake prior to treatment

    (2) Weight loss of 5% or more in one month or 10% or more in six months prior to treatment

    (3) Evident protein-energy malnutrition prior to treatment

    (4) Alcohol and tobacco use or substance abuse prior to or during treatment

    (5) Vitamin and mineral supplementation—Megadoses of vitamins and minerals in the form of supplements are discouraged, as they may decrease the effectiveness of cancer therapy (Deng et al., 2009).

    (6) Herbal supplement use may delay cancer treatment or interact with certain types of cancer treatment (Deng et al., 2009) by altering metabolism rates of certain medications, including chemotherapy. In fact, decreased levels of chemotherapeutic agents have been noted in the blood of patients who were taking herbal supplements while on chemotherapy (Meijerman, Beijnen, & Schellens, 2006).

    (7) Medical history—Concurrent illnesses/diseases (e.g., diabetes, coronary artery disease, dementia, depression, renal disease, HIV, previous cancer, an underlying GI pathology such as ulcerative colitis or Crohn disease)

    (8) Social situations—Poverty, diminished self-care ability or lack of caretaker, living alone, lack of adequate housing, lack of equipment to store and prepare meals (e.g., refrigerator, stove, oven, microwave)

    (9) Concurrent therapies (e.g., aggressive chemotherapy, dialysis) (Charney & Cranganu, 2010)

    (10) Tumor site—Tumor that obstructs food from passing through the digestive tract normally, tumor that obstructs ducts where digestive enzymes are secreted, loss of pancreatic enzymes for nutrient absorption after Whipple procedure for pancreatic cancer, loss of intestinal absorptive capacity after bowel resection for bowel or colorectal cancer, decreased gastric volume after gastrectomy

  b) Clinical manifestations of RT affecting nutrition (NCI, 2010) (see Table 9)

    (1) CNS: Headaches, seizures, altered mental status, nausea, vomiting, fatigue, hyperglycemia, anorexia

    (2) Head and neck areas: Xerostomia, taste changes, weight loss, dysphagia, odynophagia, pain, decrease in the width of mouth opening (trismus), sore mouth and throat, sore tongue, dysosmia, changes in saliva production, chewing problems, mouth sores, anorexia, increased phlegm production, salivary gland fibrosis, osteoradionecrosis, mucosal atrophy, ulceration

    (3) Thoracic areas: Dysphagia, odynophagia, indigestion, early satiety, weight loss, pain, shortness of breath, gastric reflux, regurgitation, esophagitis

Table 9. Common Effects of Radiation Therapy on Nutritional Intake

Site of Radiation Therapy	Effect on Nutritional Intake
Central nervous system (brain, spinal column)	Headache Seizures Altered mental status Nausea Vomiting Fatigue Hyperglycemia—related to steroids Anorexia Dysphagia (difficult swallowing) Odynophagia (painful swallowing) Dysosmia/hyposmia/anosmia (olfactory dysfunction—altered, diminished, or lack of sense of smell)
Head and neck region (larynx, pharynx, tonsils, tongue, nasopharynx, salivary glands, oropharynx, sinuses, mouth, throat, lips)	Xerostomia (dry mouth) Dysgeusia/hypogeusia/ageusia (altered, diminished, or lack of taste) Dysosmia/hyposmia/anosmia Sore mouth and throat Mucositis/thrush (mucosal inflammation and ulceration) Dysphagia/odynophagia Trismus (decrease in the width of mouth opening) Salivary gland fibrosis Thick saliva or phlegm Chewing difficulty Weight loss Fatigue Anorexia Pain Osteoradionecrosis
Thoracic region (esophagus, lung, and breasts if treatment field involves esophagus)	Dysphagia/odynophagia Indigestion/reflux Early satiety Pain Shortness of breath Regurgitation Esophagitis (inflammation or ulceration in the esophagus) Weight loss
Abdomen and pelvic region (cervical, prostate, pancreatic, uterine, colon, rectal, reproductive organs, testicles, liver, gastrointestinal system)	Nausea Vomiting Early satiety Regurgitation Malabsorption/maldigestion Enteritis/gastritis Changes in urinary frequency/burning sensation with urine (causing individuals to avoid fluid intake in order to avoid painful urination) Lactose intolerance Fatigue Changes in bowel function, including diarrhea, constipation, cramping, gas and bloating, colitis and enteritis Enterofistula (in severe toxicity to radiation therapy)

Note. Based on information from National Cancer Institute, 2010.

Created by Maria C. Romano, MS, RD, CDN.

(4) Abdomen and pelvis: Nausea, vomiting, early satiety, regurgitation, malabsorption, maldigestion, enteritis, gastritis, changes in urinary frequency, burning sensation with urine (causing individuals to avoid fluid intake in order to avoid painful urination), lactose intolerance, fatigue, changes in bowel function including diarrhea, constipation, cramping, gas, and bloating, colitis and enteritis

c) Physical examination

(1) Baseline data
    (a) Physical examination (e.g., height/weight, body mass index [BMI], muscle tone, skin, nails, lips, overall appearance, performance status)
    (b) Vital signs
    (c) Laboratory data (e.g., Chem-7, white blood cell count, liver function tests, prealbumin*, hemoglobin, transferrin, hematocrit, electrolytes)
    *Prealbumin is a better indicator of dietary changes or dietary insufficiency than albumin because of its shorter half-life of two to three days. In addition, albumin, an acute-phase visceral protein, can be inaccurate due to states of dehydration (it will be falsely high) or edema/fluid retention/anasarca, as is commonly seen in hepatic or biliary cancers (it will be falsely low) (Pronsky, 2006).
    (d) Patient-Generated Subjective Global Assessment (PG-SGA)—Ottery (2001) modified this for use in the oncology population. It remains the gold standard for assessment of the patient's quality of life during cancer treatment.
        i. 0—Minimal impact on nutritional status (stage A)
        ii. 1—Mild impact; monitor/reassess on a regular basis.
        iii. 2—Moderate impact (stage B); request a nutrition consult.
        iv. 3—Potentially severe impact; request a nutrition consult.
        v. 4—Potentially life threatening (stage C); request a nutrition consult.
    (e) Interpretation of total scores—Ottery (2001) recommended
        i. 0–1: No intervention; reassess on a regular basis.
        ii. 2–3: Patient/family teaching by nurse, dietitian, or other clinician; pharmacologic intervention as needed; laboratory assessment may be warranted.
        iii. 4–8: Dietitian intervention necessary, together with nurse or physician, to manage nutritional impact symptoms
        iv. 9 or higher: Critical need for improved symptom management and/or nutritional intervention
(2) Examination
    (a) General appearance—Muscle tone, fit of clothing
    (b) Karnofsky performance status: www.hospicepatients.org/karnofsky.html (Hospice Patients Alliance, n.d.)
    (c) Oral cavity: Infections, dental condition/dentition, inflammation of oral mucosa, appearance of oral ulcers, consistency of saliva, tongue mobility, mastication ability, and disfiguration of face, mouth, or throat (usually resulting from surgical resection or tumor site)
    (d) Nutritional intake: Fluids, solids, calories, and protein
    (e) Skin turgor
    (f) Edema/ascites
    (g) Scored PG-SGA
    (h) Request a nutrition consult by a registered dietitian based on PG-SGA score.
4. Documentation (NCI CTEP, 2010)
    a) Weight loss (NCI CTEP, 2010)
        (1) 1—5% to less than 10% from baseline; intervention not indicated
        (2) 2—10% to less than 20% from baseline; nutritional support indicated
        (3) 3—20% or more from baseline
    b) Anorexia (NCI CTEP, 2010)
        (1) 1—Loss of appetite without alteration in eating habits
        (2) 2—Oral intake altered without significant weight loss or malnutrition; oral nutrition supplements indicated
        (3) 3—Associated with significant weight loss or malnutrition (e.g., inadequate oral caloric or fluid intake); IV fluids, tube feeding, or total parenteral nutrition (TPN) indicated
        (4) 4—Life-threatening consequences; urgent intervention indicated
        (5) 5—Death
    c) Nausea (NCI CTEP, 2010)
        (1) 1—Loss of appetite without alteration in eating habits
        (2) 2—Oral intake decreased without significant weight loss, dehydration, or malnutrition
        (3) 3—Inadequate oral caloric or fluid intake; tube feeding, TPN, or hospitalization indicated
    d) Vomiting (NCI CTEP, 2010)

      (1) 1—One to two episodes (separated by five minutes) in 24 hours

      (2) 2—Three to five episodes (separated by five minutes) in 24 hours

      (3) 3—Six or more episodes (separated by five minutes) in 24 hours; tube feeding, TPN, or hospitalization indicated

      (4) 4—Life-threatening consequences; urgent intervention indicated

      (5) 5—Death

e) Diarrhea (NCI CTEP, 2010)

      (1) 1—Increase of less than four stools per day over baseline; mild increase in ostomy output compared to baseline

      (2) 2—Increase of four to six stools per day over baseline; moderate increase in ostomy output compared to baseline

      (3) 3—Increase of more than seven stools per day over baseline; incontinence; hospitalization indicated; severe increase in ostomy output compared to baseline; limiting self-care ADL

      (4) 4—Life-threatening consequences; urgent intervention indicated

      (5) 5—Death

f) Salivary duct inflammation (NCI CTEP, 2010)

      (1) 1—Slightly thickened saliva; slightly altered taste (e.g., metallic)

      (2) 2—Thick, ropy, sticky saliva; markedly altered taste; alteration in diet indicated; secretion-induced symptoms limiting instrumental ADL

      (3) 3—Acute salivary gland necrosis; severe secretion-induced symptoms (e.g., thick saliva/oral secretions or gagging); tube feeding or TPN indicated; limiting self-care ADL; disabling

      (4) 4—Life-threatening consequences; urgent intervention indicated

      (5) 5—Death

g) Taste disturbance (NCI CTEP, 2010)

      (1) 1—Slightly altered; no change in diet

      (2) 2—Markedly altered with change in diet; noxious or unpleasant taste; loss of taste

h) Constipation (NCI CTEP, 2010)

      (1) 1—Occasional or intermittent symptoms; occasional use of stool softeners, laxatives, dietary modification, or enema

      (2) 2—Persistent symptoms with regular use of laxatives or enemas; limiting instrumental ADL

      (3) 3—Obstipation with manual evacuation indicated; limiting self-care ADL

      (4) 4—Life-threatening consequences; urgent intervention indicated

      (5) 5—Death

i) Dyspepsia and/or heartburn (NCI CTEP, 2010)

      (1) 1—Mild symptoms; intervention not indicated

      (2) 2—Moderate symptoms; medical intervention indicated

      (3) 3—Severe symptoms; surgical intervention indicated

j) Dysphagia (NCI CTEP, 2010)

      (1) 1—Symptomatic; able to eat regular diet

      (2) 2—Symptomatic and altered eating/swallowing

      (3) 3—Severely altered eating/swallowing; tube feeding, TPN, or hospitalization indicated

      (4) 4—Life-threatening consequences; urgent intervention indicated

      (5) 5—Death

k) Esophagitis (NCI CTEP, 2010)

      (1) 1—Asymptomatic; clinical or diagnostic observations only; intervention not indicated

      (2) 2—Symptomatic; altered eating/swallowing; oral supplements indicated

      (3) 3—Severely altered eating/swallowing; tube feeding, TPN, or hospitalization indicated

      (4) 4—Life-threatening consequences; urgent operative intervention indicated

      (5) 5—Death

l) Oral pain (NCI CTEP, 2010)

      (1) 1—Mild pain

      (2) 2—Moderate pain; limiting instrumental ADL

      (3) 3—Severely altered GI function; TPN or hospitalization indicated; elective operative intervention indicated

      (4) 4—Life-threatening consequences; urgent intervention indicated

      (5) 5—Death

5. Collaborative management
   a) Early nutritional intervention is key. Preventing cancer-induced weight loss and other symptoms helps to promote better tolerance to treatment and a better quality of life. Adequate screening, nutrition intervention, and diet-related patient education performed proactively can prevent or decrease the RT-related nutritional symptoms.
   b) Instruct the patient on consuming a high-calorie/high-protein diet to maintain weight. If weight loss occurs, also encourage commercial nutrition supplements to maintain proper nutritional intake or fruit and yogurt smoothies made with a powdered whey protein supplement.
   c) Instruct the patient about the importance of exercise to prevent muscle atrophy or lean tissue loss, to enhance tolerance of cancer treatments, and to stimulate appetite.
   d) Instruct the patient and caregiver on bland, moist, soft, nonacidic, low-lactose, and low-residue foods, especially if the patient is experiencing difficulty tolerating foods without mentioned side effects.
   e) Consult with a clinical dietitian and speech pathologist for patients at risk for aspiration.
   f) Encourage the use of enteral nutrition, also referred to as tube feeding, when indicated. If oral intake is not possible or inadequate, enteral feeding is the preferred method of nutrition support because it continues to use the gut, promoting more efficient metabolism and utilization of nutrients, maintaining gut integrity and preventing translocation of bacteria (Abou-Assi, Khurana, & Schubert, 2005; Schattner & Chike, 2006; Wildhaber, Yang, Spencer, Drongowski, & Teitelbaum, 2005).
      (1) Enteral nutrition is indicated for patients who are unable to ingest adequate calories, protein, vitamins, minerals, and fluids by mouth, yet have a functional GI tract. Indications for enteral nutrition include states of hypermetabolism, as in sepsis, burns, or trauma, neurologic disease, such as stroke or dysphagia, GI disease, oncologic disease, psychiatric disease, and organ system failure.
      (2) Contraindications for enteral nutrition are a malfunctioning GI tract, mechanical obstruction distal to the lowest possible area of enteral access, prolonged or paralytic ileus, severe GI hemorrhage, intractable vomiting or diarrhea, GI fistulas in locations that cannot be bypassed by an enteral tube, malabsorptive conditions, hemodynamic instability, a high-output GI tract, and/or a clinical prognosis that is not consistent with aggressive nutrition therapy (Gupta & Martindale, 2005).
   g) Parenteral nutrition is the last resort to maintain intake or infusion of nutrients. If TPN is truly indicated, consult a registered dietitian and then observe for refeeding syndrome. Refeeding syndrome is characterized by fluid retention leading to cardiac decompensation and rapid drop in serum levels of phosphorus, magnesium, and potassium (Gupta & Martindale, 2005; Hearing, 2004).
   h) Counseling early in the patient's course of treatment is necessary. The importance of maintaining good nutrition, curtailing further weight loss, and discussing anticipated eating difficulties all should be reviewed with the patient and family.
   i) Encourage oral health examination (see section V.B—Head and neck) as well as meticulous oral hygiene.
   j) Encourage the importance of eating small, frequent meals.
   k) Monitor hydration closely and replace electrolytes as needed.
   l) Suggest probiotic supplementation and psyllium fiber (pectin-containing) supplementation to prevent diarrhea in patients receiving radiation to the abdomen or pelvis (Muehlbauer et al., 2009).
   m) Consult a registered dietitian for patients with evidence of protein-energy malnutrition prior to the start of their therapies, as soon as a patient begins showing signs of possible protein-energy malnutrition, if side effects of therapies are severe or prolonged, or if the patient is receiving or will receive chemotherapy or RT for cancer of the head, neck, face, abdomen, or pelvic area (see Figure 17). These patients may experience increased toxicities of treatment that will affect their ability to achieve or maintain adequate nutritional intake, causing a possible interruption in their treatment schedule and possible rapid deterioration without early intervention from the registered dietitian.
   n) Anticipate the need to start appetite stimulants early. Pharmacologic management can include the following.
      (1) Megestrol acetate—Progestin that stimulates appetite, caloric intake, sen-

---

Figure 17. When to Consult a Registered Dietitian

Nutrition Consult Criteria
- Weight loss
  - Greater than 5% in one month
  - Greater than 10% in six months
- BMI less than 19
- NPO for more than three days
- Pressure sores/decubitus ulcers/open wounds
- Nausea/vomiting for more than three days
- Chronic/severe constipation
- Chronic/severe diarrhea
- Cachexia
- Failure to thrive
- Severe food allergy/intolerance
- Small bowel obstruction/ileus
- Malabsorption/maldigestion
- Status post surgery to the head, face, or neck, including the oral cavity
- Status post gastrointestinal surgery (e.g., Whipple, gastrectomy, bowel resection, esophagectomy, ostomy)
- Decreased appetite/poor PO intake (more than three days) related to any of the following
  - Chemotherapy/radiation therapy side effects
  - Dysphagia
  - Poor PO tolerance
  - Refusing PO
  - Mucositis/esophagitis
  - Dry mouth
  - Altered taste
  - Early satiety
  - Drug-nutrient interaction
  - Ascites/fluid overload/anasarca
  - Poor dentition/difficulty chewing
  - Anorexia
  - Head and neck surgery
  - Nausea/vomiting
- Patient is receiving or will receive chemotherapy and/or radiation therapy to the head, neck, face, abdomen, or pelvis.
- Patient has been diagnosed with cancer to any area of the gastrointestinal tract.
- Patient is currently receiving or would benefit from enteral nutrition support.
- Patient is currently receiving or would benefit from parenteral nutrition support.

BMI—body mass index; NPO—nothing by mouth; PO—oral
Note. Created by Maria C. Romano, MS, RD, CDN.

---

sations of well-being, and weight gain but mostly as fat; is dose dependent (800 mg/day). Possible side effects include hypogonadism (impotence, muscle loss), decreased glucose tolerance, hypertension, Cushing syndrome, alopecia, peripheral edema, breakthrough vaginal bleeding, adrenal insufficiency, and GI effects (nausea/vomiting/diarrhea, gas, dry mouth) (Amen, 2010). Studies suggest improved effectiveness in patients with better digestive function; therefore, targeted nutritional strategies such as digestive enzymes

or elemental diets may be useful. Doses greater than 800 mg/day are not indicated in patients with breast cancer who have a history of blood clots because of the possibility of thrombotic events (NCI, 2010).

(2) Dronabinol—Cannabinoid that is designed to increase appetite, improve mood, and decrease nausea. It is commonly used with good success in advanced HIV disease. Appetite is maintained long term. No adverse GI side effects, no development of tolerance to therapeutic effects/no toxicity, and no addiction. Side effects seem to be age-related and may include lethargy or decreased alertness. Decreasing dose may eliminate or lessen adverse effects. Dose is 2.5 mg twice a day (Loprinzi & Jatoi, 2010).

(3) Corticosteroids (dexamethasone)—Short-lived appetite stimulant that provides no real weight gain. Side effects include muscle loss/weakness, increased anxiety, suppressed immunity, redistribution of fat, easy bruising, fragile skin, osteoporosis, fluid retention, high blood sugar, electrolyte disturbances, insomnia, and gastric irritation (nausea/vomiting) (Yavuzsen, Davis, Walsh, LeGrand, & Lagman, 2005).

(4) Cyproheptadine—Histamine and serotonin antagonist approved in the United States for treatment of allergic disorders. Studies have been conducted in patients with cancer, AIDS, dry mouth, drowsiness, and urination difficulties. Limited efficacy has been shown with a mild stimulatory effect on appetite but no true prevention of weight loss (Loprinzi & Jatoi, 2010). Sedation is a frequent adverse effect that may limit usefulness in patients with cancer.

(5) Hydrazine sulfate—Evaluated because of its ability to inhibit gluconeogenesis by inhibiting phosphoenolpyruvate kinase. It has been widely used for the treatment of cancer-related anorexia or cachexia. It is well tolerated but has not been shown to stimulate appetite or weight gain in advanced cancer (Loprinzi & Jatoi, 2010).

(6) Anabolic agents—Testosterone derivatives that are well studied in patients with AIDS but not so much in patients with cancer. They are not safe to use

in some cancers. Anabolic agents include androgens (or anabolic steroids) and growth hormones. Anabolic steroids have been shown to be less effective than megestrol acetate as an appetite stimulant, but they may have a selective effect that induces lean body mass increases along with body fat decreases, contributing to a decrease in overall weight (Lesser et al., 2008). Recombinant human growth hormone use in critically ill adults has previously been associated with high mortality rates (Kotler, 2000). As a result, the alternative approach of ghrelin use is being studied. Ghrelin has the ability to induce the release of growth hormone, and preliminary studies show administration of multiple doses of parenteral ghrelin therapy is safe in patients with advanced cancer (Lundholm et al., 2010; Strasser et al., 2008).

(7) Metoclopramide—Treats early satiety and nausea by increasing GI motility, thereby speeding up gastric emptying and increasing appetite. Patients with dysmotility will benefit the most, usually at 10 mg, four times a day; side effects (often diarrhea and hyperactivity of the GI tract) respond to dose reduction (Loprinzi & Jatoi, 2010).

6. Patient and family education: Sessions in which behavioral topics are covered may vary according to the patient's readiness, skills, resources, and need for lifestyle changes.

a) Dry mouth or thick saliva (NCI, 2010)
(1) Perform frequent oral care every two hours.
(2) Drink 8–12 cups of liquid a day to help loosen mucus.
(3) Use a straw to drink liquids.
(4) Include soft, moist, bland-tasting, room-temperature foods. Consider use of pureed fruits and vegetables, as well as ice pops or shaved ice.

(5) Use broths, soups, gravies, or sauces to moisten foods. Consider drizzling oil over foods to increase moisture.
(6) Avoid citrus or dry foods and alcohol or alcohol-containing products.
(7) Suck on sugarless sour candy.
(8) Use artificial saliva or other mouth lubricants. Consider using olive oil or flaxseed oil to coat the oral mucosa, especially before bed.
(9) Make a saltwater rinse (¼ teaspoon baking soda and ½ teaspoon salt dissolved in 1 cup of warm water); use mixture at room temperature at least four to five times per day.

b) Taste changes or loss of taste (NCI, 2010)
(1) Use plastic utensils to reduce metallic taste.
(2) Experiment with cold or cool-temperature foods that have less taste or aroma.
(3) Try unflavored nutrition supplements intended for tube feeding, such as Osmolite® or Jevity® (Abbott Nutrition) or Isosource® (Nestlé Nutrition).
(4) Try tart or spicy foods, if oral mucosa is not distressed.
(5) If the oral mucosa is not irritated, eat a few pineapple chunks to get rid of bad taste or to change taste sensations between eating different foods.
(6) Use sugar-free lemon drops, gum, or mints (if oral mucosa is intact and not inflamed) to decrease metallic or bitter taste in the mouth.
(7) Eat meat with something sweet, such as cranberry sauce, jelly, or applesauce.

c) Dysphagia (American Dietetic Association, 2004; NCI, 2010)
(1) Add gravy, broth, or sauces to foods to increase moisture and facilitate swallowing. Consider drizzling oil onto foods to increase calorie content, as well as moisture content. Can also try drizzling Benecalorie® (Nestlé Nutrition) calorie supplement on foods for the same purpose.
(2) Eat semisolid or soft foods, avoiding rough-textured foods, or consider commercial baby foods or blended foods. Warm foods before blending for best results, adding high-calorie, high-protein foods to maximize nutrient density without increasing total food volume (e.g., light cream, grated cheese, cooked eggs, cottage cheese, ricotta cheese).

(3) Accept the importance of nutrition supplements or milkshake recipes for calorie and protein intake. If preparing milkshakes or smoothies at home as opposed to purchasing a premade nutrition supplement, be sure to add a protein source such as whey protein powder (Beneprotein® made by Nestlé Nutrition), peanut butter, or plain yogurt.

(4) If dysphagia occurs with thin liquids, encourage thickening products such as gelatin, tapioca, commercial thickeners, pureed vegetables, instant potato mix, flour, or baby rice cereal.

(5) If aspiration is a risk, sit upright when eating and drinking and practice safe swallowing positioning as per a speech language pathologist's recommendations.

(6) If dysphagia is related to brain metastases, referral to a speech language pathologist may help to prevent secondary aspiration risk.

(7) If dysphagia is severely limiting the patient's ability to achieve or maintain adequate protein-energy intake, or if aspiration risk is very high, consider placement of a feeding tube for tube feeds that will better meet the patient's nutritional needs.

d) Diarrhea (Meier, Burri, & Steuerwald, 2003; Muehlbauer et al., 2009; NCI, 2010)

(1) Avoid raw fruits and vegetables, whole grain bread and cereals, nuts, popcorn, skins, and seeds in the presence of radiation enteritis.

(2) Follow a bland diet. Try pectin-containing foods such as potatoes, applesauce, oatmeal, bananas, cooked carrots, and rice.

(3) Do not drink large quantities of fruit juice or sweetened fruit drinks.

(4) Replace fluid losses with one cup of water for each episode of diarrhea. Avoid caffeine, alcohol, and lactose fluids.

(5) Consume foods and beverages high in sodium and potassium, such as soups, bananas, potatoes, and bouillon broths.

(6) May want to use products containing glutamine, such as GlutaSolve® or Impact® Glutamine (Nestlé Nutrition), which can improve gut integrity and lessen the effects of intestinal toxicity from certain chemotherapeutic agents.

(7) Limit spicy or greasy foods, which can exacerbate diarrhea.

(8) Limit the use of sugar-free candies or gums made with sorbitol (sugar alcohol) (Muehlbauer et al., 2009).

(9) Eliminate milk and milk products until the source of the problem is determined.

(10) Limit gas-forming or fibrous foods such as dried beans, cruciferous vegetables, soda, and chewing gum, which may contribute to frequent stools, especially in the presence of radiation enteritis.

(11) Consider probiotic supplementation such as Culturelle® (Amerifit) or increased intake of pasteurized plain yogurt containing live cultures.

(12) Consider a clear liquid, low-residue oral nutritional supplement such as Resource® Breeze (Nestlé Nutrition) or an elemental oral nutrition supplement such as Peptamen® OS (Nestlé Nutrition) to promote absorption of nutrients without exacerbating diarrhea.

e) Gas and bloating (Muehlbauer et al., 2009; NCI, 2010)

(1) Avoid gas-producing beverages (carbonated products), additives (artificial sweeteners), and foods (broccoli, cabbage, cauliflower, beans, lentils, and eggs).

(2) Use an enzyme product to help digest the carbohydrates in gas-producing foods.

(3) Eat five to six small meals a day

(4) Increase water intake as much as possible to prevent excessive gas formation.

f) Nausea and vomiting (NCI, 2010)

(1) Schedule a light meal before or after treatment and/or carry food to eat after treatment.

(2) Try dry foods, such as crackers, toast, or breadsticks, every few hours during the day.

(3) Choose foods that do not have a strong odor, and avoid eating in a room that has cooking odors.

(4) Avoid foods that are overly sweet, fatty, fried, or spicy. Bland, soft, easy-to-digest foods are always preferred.

(5) Sit up or recline for one hour after eating.

(6) Eat cool or room-temperature foods instead of hot foods.

(7) Sip ginger ale, ginger tea, or chamomile tea 30 minutes before eating to promote belching and prevent nausea.

(8) Consider a clear liquid, low-residue oral nutritional supplement such as Resource Breeze that can be sipped or frozen into ice pops to increase calorie and protein intake without exacerbating nausea.

g) Sore mouth and throat (American Dietetic Association, 2004)

(1) Use prescribed anesthetic mouth rinses or gels containing diphenhydramine, Maalox® (Novartis Consumer Health), and viscous lidocaine to numb the mouth and throat 20 minutes before meals.

(2) Consume ice chips or a frozen ice pop before eating to numb the mouth before meals.

(3) Consider nutrition supplements and milkshake recipes if unable to consume solid foods in adequate quantities. For homemade milkshakes or smoothies, add a protein source such as whey protein powder, peanut butter, or plain yogurt.

(4) Drink nectars instead of apple, grape, or other acidic juices.

(5) Stew all foods (including fruits, vegetables, and meats) with plenty of liquid and then puree and cool before eating.

(6) Eat small, frequent meals of high-calorie, high-protein liquids or high-calorie, high-protein foods, texture as tolerated (pureed, soft, moist), for the term of the treatment.

(7) Avoid spicy, rough, tart, or acidic foods, or foods that can scratch or scrape the oral mucosa.

(8) Restrict the use of dentures for mealtimes only, if at all, to prevent unnecessary irritation to the gums.

h) Fat malabsorption

(1) Use medium-chain triglyceride oil (MCT Oil® [Nestlé Nutrition]) or a medium-chain triglyceride oil–containing supplement such as Optimental® (Abbott Nutrition) or Peptamen® (Nestlé Nutrition) if necessary.

(2) Eat a low-fat diet while maintaining sufficient calorie intake through the previously mentioned supplements or through small, frequent meals of low-fat foods.

(3) If fat malabsorption is related to pancreatic insufficiency, discuss pancreatic enzyme replacement therapy with the doctor.

(4) Begin peripheral parenteral nutrition or TPN if intestinal function is so impaired that enteral provision of nutrients is unsafe or impossible to achieve or if severe malnutrition cannot be corrected by enteral nutrition support.

i) Anorexia/cachexia (American Dietetic Association, 2004; NCI, 2010)

(1) Estimated nutritional needs

(a) 20 kcal/kg—Initial refeeding of patients who are malnourished or depleted

(b) 21–25 kcal/kg—Obese patients for maintenance

(c) 25–30 kcal/kg—Maintenance/standard

(d) 30–35 kcal/kg—Malnourished and/or extensive treatment or bone marrow transplant

(e) 35–45 kcal/kg—Depleted and/or hypermetabolic state

(2) For protein needs

(a) 0.5–0.8 g/kg—Renal compromise

(b) 0.8–1 g/kg—Recommended dietary allowance for adults

(c) 1–1.5 g/kg—Most patients with cancer

(d) 1.5 g/kg—Bone marrow transplant recipients

(e) 1.5–2 g/kg—Patients with cancer who are depleted of protein or cachectic

(3) Encourage small, frequent meals of high-calorie, high-protein foods.

(4) Encourage liquids between meals, not during.

(5) Encourage high-protein foods or enhance protein content of diet.

(6) Use specialized commercial nutrition supplements containing omega-3 fatty acids and essential amino acids to promote weight gain, build muscle, and support immune function.

(7) Nutrient-dense supplements

(a) Ensure®, Ensure Plus®, Ensure Clinical Strength®, Glucerna 1.5®, Jevity 1.5, TwoCal® HN (Abbott Nutrition)

(b) Boost®, Boost Plus®, Boost Glucose Control®, Fibersource® HN, Isosource HN and 1.5 Cal, Nutren 1.5®, Nutren 2.0®, Carnation® Instant Breakfast® Lactose Free Plus and VHC (very high calorie), Nutren® 2.0, Peptamen OS and OS 1.5

(c) Impact® (Nestlé Nutrition)

(d) Clear liquid nutrition supplements including Enlive!® (Abbott Nutrition) or Resource Breeze

(e) Protein and calorie additives, such as Resource and Resource Bene-protein, or a generic whey protein powder.

(f) Fortified milk and yogurts

j) Expected clinical outcomes of ideal/goal values (Pronsky, 2006)

  (1) Albumin: 3.5–5 mg/dl

  (2) Prealbumin: 18–38 mg/dl

  (3) Hemoglobin: 12.1–15.6 g/dl (for women) or 14.6–17.5 g/dl (for men)

  (4) Hematocrit: 34%–45% (for women) or 41%–51% (for men)

  (5) Complete metabolic profile within normal limits

  (6) Maintain weight at or above 85% usual body weight

k) Web sites

  (1) ACS: www.cancer.org. Contents include tips for symptom management of nutrition-related problems.

  (2) American Dietetic Association: www.eatright.org. Contents include evidence-based nutrition recommendations, recipes, journal articles on nutrition-related studies, and a database of nutrition professionals for patient referral as needed.

  (3) American Institute for Cancer Research: www.aicr.org. Contents include recipes, information for cancer prevention and cancer survivors, serving size finder, and research updates.

  (4) A Dietitian's Cancer Story: www.cancerrd.com. Contents include recipes, menus, information about soy, and nutritional strategies to use during treatment or recovery.

  (5) NCI: www.cancer.gov. Contents include Eating Hints: Recipes and Tips for Better Nutrition During Treatment, recipes and nutrition for patients with cancer (PDQ® document)—versions for patients and healthcare professionals, nutritional implications of cancer therapies, nutritional suggestions for symptom management, and a table on herbs and possible food-drug interactions.

  (6) Oncology Nutrition Dietetic Practice Group of the American Dietetic Association: www.oncologynutrition.org. Contents include evidence-based research information and nutrition tips.

  (7) Support for People with Oral and Head and Neck Cancer: www.spohnc.org. A patient-friendly Web site offering support to those with oral, head, or neck cancer. Patients are able to order educational materials free of charge and seek additional information about available clinical trials and current press releases related to their own cancer diagnosis.

l) Cookbooks

  (1) American Cancer Society. (2005). *American Cancer Society's healthy eating cookbook: A celebration of food, friends, and healthy living* (3rd ed.). Atlanta, GA: Author.

  (2) Bloch, A., Cassileth, B.R., Holmes, M.D., & Thomson, C.A. (Eds.). (2004). *Eating well, staying well during and after cancer.* Atlanta, GA: American Cancer Society.

  (3) Clegg, H., & Miletello, G. (2006). *Eating well through cancer: Easy recipes and recommendations during and after treatment.* Nashville, TN: Favorite Recipes Press.

  (4) Eldridge, B., & Hamilton, K. (2004). *Management of nutrition impact symptoms in cancer and educational handouts.* Chicago, IL: American Dietetic Association.

  (5) Ghosh, K., Carson, L., & Cohen, E. (2002). *Betty Crocker's living with cancer cookbook: Easy recipes and tips through treatment and beyond.* New York, NY: Hungry Minds.

  (6) Luthringer, S.L., & Kogut, V.J. (2011). *Nutrition and cancer: Practical tips and tasty recipes.* Pittsburgh, PA: Hygeia Media.

  (7) Support for People with Oral and Head and Neck Cancer. (2008). *We have walked in your shoes—A guide to oral, head, and neck cancer.* Locust Valley, NY: Author. (Publication possible through the support of Bristol-Myers Squibb and ImClone Systems)

  (8) Weihofen, D.L., Robbins, J., & Sullivan, P.A. (2002). *Easy-to-swallow, easy-to-chew cookbook: Over 150 tasty and nutritious recipes for people who have difficulty swallowing.* New York, NY: John Wiley & Sons.

  (9) Wilson, J.R. (2003). *I-can't-chew cookbook: Delicious soft-diet recipes for people with chewing, swallowing, or dry-mouth disorders.* Alameda, CA: Hunter House.

References

Abayomi, J., Kirwan, J., & Hackett, A. (2009). The prevalence of chronic radiation enteritis following radiotherapy for cervical or endometrial cancer and its impact on quality of life. *European Journal of Oncology Nursing, 13*, 262–267. doi:10.1016/j.ejon.2009.02.007

Abou-Assi, S.G., Khurana, V., & Schubert, M.L. (2005). Gastric and postpyloric total enteral nutrition. *Current Treatment Options in Gastroenterology, 8*, 145–152.

Amen, K. (2010). Food in the fight against cancer: The evidence on cancer-related anorexia. *American Nurse Today, 5*(4). Retrieved from http://www.americannursetoday.com/article.aspx?id=6486&fid=6462

American Dietetic Association. (2004). *Management of nutrition impact symptoms in cancer and educational handouts.* Chicago, IL: Author.

Capra, S., Ferguson, M., & Ried, K. (2001). Cancer: Impact of nutrition intervention outcome—Nutrition issues for patients. *Nutrition, 17*, 769–772. doi:10.1016/S0899-9007(01)00632-3

Charney, P., & Cranganu, A. (2010). Nutrition screening and assessment in oncology. In M. Marian & S. Roberts (Eds.), *Clinical nutrition for oncology patients* (pp. 21–44). Sudbury, MA: Jones and Bartlett.

Deng, G.E., Frenkel, M., Cohen, L., Cassileth, B.R., Abrams, D.I., Calpodice, J.L., ... Sagar, S. (2009). Evidence-based clinical practice guidelines for integrative oncology: Complementary therapies and botanicals. *Journal of the Society for Integrative Oncology, 7*, 85–120. doi:10.2310/7200.2009.0019

Elting, L.S., Cooksley, C.D., Chambers, M.S., & Garden, A.S. (2007). Risk, outcomes, and costs of radiation-induced oral mucositis among patients with head-and-neck malignancies. *International Journal of Radiation Oncology, Biology, Physics, 68*, 1110–1120. doi:10.1016/j.ijrobp.2007.01.053

Feyer, P.C., Maranzano, E., Molassiotis, A., Clark-Snow, R.A., Roila, F., Warr, D., & Olver, I. (2005). Radiotherapy-induced nausea and vomiting (RINV): Antiemetic guidelines. *Supportive Care in Cancer, 13*, 122–128. doi:10.1007/s00520-004-0705-3

Gupta, N., & Martindale, R.G. (2005). Parenteral versus enteral nutrition. In G. Cresci (Ed.), *Nutrition support for the critically ill patient: A guide to practice* (pp. 193–208). Boca Raton, FL: Taylor and Francis.

Hearing, S.D. (2004). Refeeding syndrome. *BMJ, 328*, 908–909. doi:10.1136/bmj.328.7445.908

Hospice Patients Alliance. (n.d.). Karnofsky performance scale index. Retrieved from http://www.hospicepatients.org/karnofsky.html

Huhmann, M.B., & Cunningham, R.S. (2005). Importance of nutritional screening in treatment of cancer-related weight loss. *Lancet Oncology, 6*, 334–343. doi:10.1016/S1470-2045(05)70170-4

Jensen, S.B., Pedersen, A.M., Reibel, J., & Nauntofte, B. (2003). Xerostomia and hypofunction of the salivary glands in cancer therapy. *Supportive Care in Cancer, 11*, 207–225. doi:10.1007/s00520-002-0407-7

Kotler, D.P. (2000). Cachexia. *Annals of Internal Medicine, 133*, 622–634.

Larsson, M., Hedelin, B., Johansson, I., & Athlin, E. (2005). Eating problems and weight loss for patients with head and neck cancer: A chart review from diagnosis until one year after treatment. *Cancer Nursing, 28*, 425–435.

Lesser, G.J., Case, D., Ottery, F., McQuellon, R., Choksi, J.K., Sanders, G., ... Shaw, E.G. (2008). A phase III randomized study comparing the effects of oxandrolone (Ox) and meges-trol acetate (Meg) on lean body mass (LBM), weight (wt) and quality of life (QOL) in patients with solid tumors and weight loss receiving chemotherapy [Abstract No. 9513]. *Journal of Clinical Oncology, 26*(Suppl.). Retrieved from http://www.asco.org/ASCOv2/Meetings/Abstracts?&vmview=abst_detail_view&confID=55&abstractID=32583

Loprinzi, C.L., & Jatoi, A. (2010). Pharmacologic management of cancer anorexia/cachexia. Retrieved from http://www.uptodate.com/contents/pharmacologic-management-of-cancer-anorexia-cachexia

Lundholm, K., Gunnebo, L., Körner, U., Iresjö, B.M., Engström, C., Hyltander, A., ... Bosaeus, I. (2010). Effects by daily long term provision of ghrelin to unselected weight-losing cancer patients: A randomized double-blind study. *Cancer, 116*, 2044–2052. doi:10.1002/cncr.24917

Luthringer, S. (2006). Nutritional implications of radiation therapy. In L. Elliot, L. Molseed, P.D. McCallum, & B. Grant (Eds.), *The clinical guide to oncology nutrition* (2nd ed., pp. 88–93). Chicago, IL: American Dietetic Association.

Madeya, M.L. (1996). Oral complications from cancer therapy: Part 1—Pathophysiology and secondary complications. *Oncology Nursing Forum, 23*, 801–807.

Meier, R., Burri, E., & Steuerwald, M. (2003). The role of nutrition in diarrhoea syndromes. *Current Opinion in Clinical Nutrition and Metabolic Care, 6*, 563–567.

Meijerman, I., Beijnen, J.H., & Schellens, J.H.M. (2006). Herb-drug interactions in oncology. Focus on mechanisms of induction. *Oncologist, 11*, 742–752.

Muehlbauer, P., Thorpe, D., Davis, A.B., Drabot, R.C., Kiker, E.S., & Rawlings, B. (2009). ONS PEP resource: Diarrhea. In L.H. Eaton & J.M. Tipton (Eds.), *Putting evidence into practice: Improving oncology patient outcomes* (pp. 125–134). Pittsburgh, PA: Oncology Nursing Society.

National Cancer Institute. (2010). Nutrition in cancer care (PDQ®) [Health professional version]. Retrieved from http://www.cancer.gov/cancertopics/pdq/supportivecare/nutrition/healthprofessional

National Cancer Institute Cancer Therapy Evaluation Program. (2010). *Common terminology criteria for adverse events* [v.4.03]. Bethesda, MD: National Cancer Institute.

Ottery, F. (2001). *Nutritional oncology: Planning a winning strategy.* Online presentation given June 28, 2001, in a live chat. Retrieved from http://www.cancersource.com/ppt/22311ppt/Ross_files/frame.htm

Pronsky, Z.M. (2006). *Food medication interactions* (14th ed.). Birchrunville, PA: Food-Medication Interactions.

Redda, M.G.R., & Allis, S. (2006). Radiotherapy-induced taste impairment. *Cancer Treatment Reviews, 32*, 541–547. doi:10.1016/j.ctrv.2006.06.003

Schattner, M., & Chike, M. (2006). Nutrition support of the patient with cancer. In M.E. Shils, M. Shike, C.A. Ross, B. Caballero, & R.J. Cousins (Eds.), *Modern nutrition in health and disease* (10th ed., pp. 1291–1313). Philadelphia, PA: Lippincott Williams & Wilkins.

Shiboski, C.H., Hodgson, T.A., Ship, J.A., & Schiødt, M. (2007). Management of salivary hypofunction during and after radiotherapy. *Oral Surgery, Oral Medicine, Oral Pathology, Oral Radiology, and Endodontology, 103*(Suppl. 1), S66.e1–S66.e19.

Silverman, S., Jr. (2003). Complications of treatment. In S. Silverman Jr. (Ed.), *Oral cancer* (5th ed., pp. 113–128). Hamilton, Ontario, Canada: BC Decker.

Strasser, F., Lutz, T.A., Maeder, M.T., Thuerlimann, B., Bueche, D., Tschöp, M., ... Cerny, T. (2008). Safety, tolerability and pharmacokinetics of intravenous ghrelin for cancer-related anorexia/cachexia: A randomised, placebo-controlled, double-blind, double-crossover study. *British Journal of Cancer, 98,* 300–308. doi:10.1038/sj.bjc.6604148

Tong, H., Isenring, E., & Yates, P. (2009). The prevalence of nutrition impact symptoms and their relationship to quality of life and clinical outcomes in medical oncology patients. *Supportive Care in Cancer, 17,* 83–90. doi:10.1007/s00520-008-0472-7

Werner-Wasik, M., Yu, X., Marks, L.B., & Schultheiss, T.E. (2004). Normal-tissue toxicities of thoracic radiation therapy: Esophagus, lung, and spinal cord as organs at risk. *Hematology/Oncology Clinics of North America, 18,* 131–160. doi:10.1016/S0889-8588(03)00150-3

Wildhaber, B.E., Yang, H., Spencer, A.U., Drongowski, R.A., & Teitelbaum, D.H. (2005). Lack of enteral nutrition—Effects on the intestinal immune system. *Journal of Surgical Research, 123,* 8–16. doi:10.1016/j.jss.2004.06.015

Yavuzsen, T., Davis, M.P., Walsh, D., LeGrand, S., & Lagman, R. (2005). Systematic review of the treatment of cancer-associated anorexia and weight loss. *Journal of Clinical Oncology, 23,* 8500–8511. doi:10.1200/JCO.2005.01.8010

V. Site-specific management

A. Brain and CNS
1. Categories (Louis et al., 2007)
   a) Tumors of the neuroepithelium
      (1) Astrocytic tumors: Derived from astrocytes that undergo abnormal growth and cellular transformation. Astrocytes provide physical and biochemical support, insulation of the receptive surface of neurons, and interactions with capillary endothelial cells in the establishment and maintenance of the blood-brain barrier (Snell, 2010). Tumors are divided histopathologically into four World Health Organization (WHO) grades differentiating benign and malignant features.
         (a) Grade I astrocytoma—slow-growing tumor; most common is pilocytic astrocytoma.
            i. Histologic presence is prominent for Rosenthal fibers and low or absent mitotic activity (Berger, Leibel, Bruner, Finlay, & Levin, 2002).
            ii. Molecular genetics—Chromosome 17q deletions are the most common, in up to 30% of tumors, thereby inactivating tumor suppressor genes and promoting oncogenesis (Kanu et al., 2009; Louis, 2006).
            iii. Ten-year survival is greater than 95% in children and teens following gross total resection and decreases to 87% for adults ages 20–44 and 67% for those age 45 and older (Central Brain Tumor Registry of the United States [CBTRUS], 2010). Routine follow-up is required to monitor for potential recurrence.
         (b) Grade II astrocytoma—Unencapsulated infiltrating and slow-growing mass; most common is well-differentiated astrocytoma.
            i. Pathologically characterized by a strong immunoreactivity to glial fibrillary acidic protein (GFAP)
            ii. Fifty percent of these tumors become more aggressive, transforming to a grade III or IV astrocytoma (Kanu et al., 2009; Louis, 2006).
            iii. Molecular genetics
               • Fifty percent of cases have *TP53* mutations (Kanu et al., 2009; Louis, 2006).
               • Increased platelet-derived growth factor, vascular endothelial growth factor, and EGFR
               • Loss of chromosome 22q and gain of chromosome 7q are common in up to 50% of tumors (Kanu et al., 2009; Louis, 2006).
            iv. Ten-year survival is greater than 75% in children and teens, near 45% for adults ages 20–44, slightly greater than 25% for adults ages 45–54, and 10% or less for those age 55 and older (CBTRUS, 2010).
         (c) Grade III astrocytoma—Diffusely infiltrating mass with areas of cysts and hemorrhage; most common is anaplastic astrocytoma.
            i. Pathologically characterized by hypercellularity, pleomorphism, mitosis, and vascular proliferation
            ii. Molecular genetics (Kanu et al., 2009; Louis, 2006)
               • Deletion of cyclin-dependent kinase (CDK) 2A in 50% of tumors and amplification of CDK4 in 10%–15% of tumors (Kanu et al., 2009; Louis, 2006)
               • Deletion of p16 in 50% of tumors (Kanu et al., 2009; Louis, 2006)
               • *TP53* mutation in up to 40% of tumors (Kanu et al., 2009; Louis, 2006)

- Other common changes: Deletion of mutation of *PTEN* (only 10%), murine double minute 2 (MDM2) overexpression (5%–10%), and EGFR amplification (10%–15%) (Kanu et al., 2009; Louis, 2006)

iii. Ten-year survival is 25% for children and teens, 36% for adults ages 20–44, 13.7% for adults ages 45–54, and 5.8% for adults ages 55–64 (CB-TRUS, 2010).

(d) Grade IV astrocytoma—Fast-growing aggressive infiltrative tumor; most common is a glioblastoma multiforme (GBM), primary or secondary (from transformation).

i. Pathologically characterized by nuclear atypia, mitotic activity, vascular proliferation, and necrosis

ii. Molecular genetics (Kanu et al., 2009; Louis, 2006) distinguished by primary or secondary development
- Deletion of *TP53*—10% in primary GBM; 60% in secondary GBM (Kanu et al., 2009; Louis, 2006)
- Amplification of EGFR—40%–60% in primary GBM; rare for secondary (Kanu et al., 2009; Louis, 2006)
- Deletion or mutation of chromosome 10—60%–95% of primary GBM (Kanu et al., 2009; Louis, 2006)
- Deletion of *PTEN*—44% of primary GBM (Kanu et al., 2009; Louis, 2006)
- Deletion of chromosome 1p—31% of secondary GBM (Kanu et al., 2009; Louis, 2006)
- Deletion of 7q—9%–12% of secondary GBM (Kanu et al., 2009; Louis, 2006)
- Changes in MDM2, CDK2A, and CDK4 similar to those observed for grade III astrocytoma

iii. Ten-year survival is 10% for those ages 0–44. Five-year survival is slightly greater than 15% for patients ages 0–44, 5% for those ages 45–54, and less than 3% for those age 55 and older (CBTRUS, 2010).

iv. Other distinctively aggressive astrocytomas characterized by unique pathologic characteristics include gliosarcoma and gliomatosis cerebri.
- Gliosarcoma is composed of neoplastic glial cells and spindle-cell sarcomatous elements and presents similarly to GBM but with a worse prognosis. Surgical resection and RT may improve outcome; chemotherapy efficacy is yet to be defined. Gliosarcomas have a greater propensity for temporal lobe location with a tendency to locate peripherally for dural invasion to the skull and falx cerebri. Also, 15%–30% have extracranial metastasis as well as metastasis to visceral organs (Kozak, Mahadevan, & Moody, 2009).
- Gliomatosis cerebri is characterized by a diffusely infiltrating mass into underlying brain architecture involving more than two cerebral hemispheres. Because of the diffuse involvement, surgical resection is not usually optimal; thus, therapy involves RT and chemotherapy (Sanson, Napolitano, Cartalat-Carel, & Taillibert, 2005).

(2) Oligodendroglial tumors: Derived from oligodendrocytes, whose principal function is the production and maintenance of the CNS myelin (Snell, 2010)

(a) Classified as WHO grade I, II, or III. Most are grade II well-differentiated or grade III anaplastic classifications (Louis et al., 2007).

(b) Pathologically characterized by a well-circumscribed unencapsulated white matter tumor with cystic involvement. Hemorrhage and necroses usually are absent, even in

anaplastic cases. Calcification is frequently observed in 70%–90% of cases (Kanu et al., 2009; Louis, 2006).

(c) Molecular genetics: First identified brain tumor for which molecular genetic analysis had practical ramifications (Kanu et al., 2009; Louis, 2006).

    i. Loss-of-heterozygosity analysis on chromosomes 1p and 19q, suggesting a synergistic effect of both genetic alterations in tumor growth in 40%–80% of cases (Giordana et al., 2004; Kanu et al., 2009; Louis, 2006).

    ii. Loss of heterozygosity on chromosome 10q is associated with poor survival (Thiessen et al., 2003).

    iii. Ten-year survival for WHO grade II tumors is greater than 88% for children and teens, greater than 55% for adults ages 20–44, approaching 50% for adults ages 55–64, and 25% for those age 65 and older. Ten-year survival decreases for WHO grade III anaplastic ligodendrogliomas to 50% for adults ages 20–44, 36.5% for adults ages 45–54, and approaching 15% for those age 55 and older (CBTRUS, 2010).

(3) Ependymomas: Abnormal tumor growth of the ependymal cells that line the ventricular walls and spinal cord. Ependymomas commonly present with hydrocephalus secondary to obstruction of the fourth ventricle. Depending on its location, it is difficult to completely excise (Packer, Friedman, Kun, & Fuller, 2002).

(a) Pathologic characteristics range from well-differentiated grade II with rare mitoses, mild cellular pleomorphism, presence of perivascular pseudorosettes, and minimal or no necrosis to anaplastic grade III with high cell density, mitotic activity, cellular pleomorphism, vascular proliferation, and extensive necrosis (Leeds, Kumar, & Jackson, 2002; McGuire, Sainani, & Fisher, 2009; Packer et al., 2002).

(b) Locations

    i. 60% of intracranial ependymomas are located in the posterior fossa; 90% of those are in the fourth ventricle (McGuire et al., 2009).

    ii. Tumors occurring in the first two decades of life typically present in the fourth ventricle, whereas those developing in midlife typically present in the spinal cord.

    iii. Myxopapillary ependymomas exclusively occur in the spinal cord, usually in the conus medullaris or filum terminum.

    iv. Subependymomas are rare benign tumors of the fourth ventricle or foramen of Monro.

(c) Molecular genetics—Most common is deletion of chromosome 22 inactivating tumor suppressor genes and promoting oncogenesis in 25%–50% of tumors (James, Smith, & Jenkins, 2002).

(d) Ten-year survival is greater than 80% for adults ages 20–64 and less than 35% for adults age 75 and older (CBTRUS, 2010).

(4) Mixed oligoastrocytoma: Characterized by a cellular lineage of both astrocytes and oligodendrocytes; either cell line may be the predominant type.

(a) Ranges from grade II to anaplastic grade III.

(b) Molecular genetics—Presents with *TP53* mutations (astrocytic line) and chromosome losses of 1p and 19q (oligodendrogliomas).

(5) Choroid plexus tumors: Composed of cuboid epithelial cells, which provide a continuous layer with ependymal cells, which produce cerebrospinal fluid (CSF). The cuboid epithelial lining acts as a brain-CSF barrier preventing toxic substances from entering the ventricular system (Snell, 2010).

(a) Ninety percent of tumors occur in children younger than five years old, primarily at the atrium of the lateral ventricle, with the rest occurring in young adults, primarily at the fourth ventricle (Snell, 2010).

(b) Histologically characterized by cellular atypia, brisk mitotic activity, and extensive necrosis

(c) Genetics and molecular genetics: Observed in those with Li-Fraumeni syndrome, an autosomal dominant disorder characterized by multiple primary neoplasms in children and young adults, including soft tissue sarcomas, osteosarcomas, breast cancer, brain tumors, leukemia, and adrenocortical carcinoma.
   i. Related to *TP53* germ-line mutations
   ii. Also observed with von Hippel-Lindau disease (VHL), which is inherited through an autosomal dominant trait and characterized by the development of capillary hemangioblastomas of the CNS and retina, clear cell renal carcinoma, pheochromocytoma, pancreatic tumors, and inner ear tumors. VHL is caused by germline mutations of the *VHL* tumor suppressor gene (Kleihues & Cavenee, 2000).

(d) Five-year survival rates: Choroid plexus papillomas have greater than 80% five-year survival and choroid plexus carcinomas have 40% (NCI, 2010; Wolff, Sajedi, Brant, Coppes, & Egeler, 2002).

(6) Other neuroepithelial tumors: Tumors of uncertain origin, including astroblastoma, chordoid glioma of the third ventricle, and angiocentric glioma (Louis et al., 2007)
   (a) Astroblastoma is a rare tumor (Kim, Park, & Lee, 2004; Thiessen et al., 2003).
      i. Occurs primarily in children and young adults
      ii. Usually well demarcated and characterized by perivascular pseudorosettes, frequent vas-

cular sclerosis, and focal tumor necrosis. It has a strong positive reaction to GFAP.
      iii. Tumors range from low-grade to anaplastic astroblastoma.
      iv. Gross total resection of the tumor improves survival.
   (b) Chordoid glioma is a rare tumor located at the third ventricle (Iwami et al., 2009). It is characterized by a strong positive GFAP reaction and a lack of chromosomal or genetic aberrations.
   (c) Angiocentric glioma is a rare subcortical tumor of the temporal or parietal lobe (Preusser et al., 2007).
      i. Astrocytic and ependymal differentiation
      ii. It is characterized by a strong positive GFAP reaction and a lack of chromosomal or genetic aberrations.

(7) Neuronal and mixed neuronal-glial tumors: Includes gangliocytoma, ganglioma, malignant ganglioma, dysplastic gangliocytoma, desmoplastic infantile ganglioma, and dysembryoplastic neuroepithelial tumors (Louis et al., 2007)

(8) Pineal tumors: Rare tumors of the pineal gland located in the posterior portion of the third ventricle. These tumors comprise less than 1% of intracranial tumors (Louis et al., 2007).

(9) Embryonal tumors: Rapidly growing masses from embryonic or fetal cells. These include medulloblastoma, CNS primitive neuroectodermal tumor, and atypical teratoid/rhabdoid tumor (Louis et al., 2007).
   (a) Medulloblastoma arises from immature neuronal precursors in the cerebellum (Huse & Holland, 2010).
      i. Characterized by small, round blue cells with increased mitotic activity (Huse & Holland, 2010)
      ii. It may be low grade or anaplastic (Louis et al., 2007).
   (b) CNS primitive neuroectodermal tumor is a neural crest tumor (Maris, 2010).
      i. Derives from cells that have not matured into neurons
      ii. Can be supra- or infratentorial or within the autonomic nervous system

(c) Atypical teratoid/rhabdoid tumor is a rare aggressive tumor (Parwani, Stelow, Pambuccian, Burger, & Ali, 2005).

    i. Characterized by large, round plasmocytoid and rhabdoid cells

    ii. Variants may have small, round primitive neuronal cells and bizarre multinucleated giant cells.

    iii. Histology consists of apoptotic bodies, numerous mitoses, and necrosis.

b) Tumors of the cranial and paraspinal nerves

  (1) Schwannoma: Benign tumor of the peripheral nerve sheath; common example is a vestibular schwannoma (acoustic neuroma).

  (2) Neurofibroma: Benign tumor

c) Tumors of the meninges

  (1) Meningioma: Tumor arising from the lining of the brain, usually arachnoid (Alexiou, Gogou, Markoula, & Kyritsis, 2010).

    (a) Associated with slow growth

    (b) Multiple meningiomas may be present in patients with neurofibromatosis type 2.

    (c) Increasing incidence with age, especially older than 65 years of age (CBTRUS, 2010; NCI, 2010)

    (d) Pathological characteristics

      i. WHO grade 1: Most common of meningiomas and is predominately fibroblastic and microcystic

      ii. WHO grade II: Atypical, chordoid, and clear cell

      iii. WHO grade III: Anaplastic with rhabdoid and papillary histologic features

  (2) Hemangiopericytoma is a sarcomatous lesion that develops most commonly in blood vessels along the base of the skull. It also commonly spreads systemically.

  (3) Hemangioblastoma is a benign vascular tumor associated with VHL disease.

d) Lymphomas and hematopoietic neoplasms

  (1) Primary central nervous system lymphoma (PCNSL)—Usually from a non-Hodgkin B-cell lineage. Immunodeficiency is a risk factor for development of PCNSL with a significant increase in frequency in the early 1990s as a complication of HIV infection (Gerstner & Batchelor, 2007).

  (2) Plasmacytoma usually occurs in vertebrae and skull bones.

  (3) Granulocytic sarcoma, previously known as chloroma, is a rare neoplasm composed of immature myeloid cells at an extramedullary site, most commonly seen secondary to acute or chronic myeloid leukemia or myelodysplastic syndrome within 6–12 months from primary diagnosis (Vela-Chávez, Arrecillas-Zamora, Quintero-Cuadra, & Fend, 2009).

e) Germ cell tumors: May respond best to radiation, although neoadjuvant chemotherapy may have a role (Siker et al., 2008).

f) Pituitary tumors may originate from adenoma (benign) or carcinoma (malignant) lines.

g) Metastatic tumors: The most common causation of tumor formation in the brain, yet may occur within the spinal cord and CSF space (Kalkanis & Linskey, 2010). Histology of primary cancer is the most important risk factor for the development of metastases. Although metastatic disease may occur as a result from any cancer, the most common causes include the following (listed in order of incidence).

  (1) Brain metastasis—Up to 85% arise from lung, breast, melanoma, colorectal, and renal cell carcinoma (NCI, 2010; Robinson, Kalkanis, Linskey, & Santaguida, 2010).

    (a) 80% are located in the cerebral hemispheres near arterial borders (NCI, 2010).

    (b) 15% are located in the cerebellum (NCI, 2010).

    (c) 3% are located in the basal ganglia (NCI, 2010).

  (2) Intramedullary spinal metastasis—Up to 75% arise from breast, lung, and prostate cancer and lymphomas (NCI, 2010).

  (3) Leptomeningeal metastasis—Most commonly associated with leukemia and lymphoma but also occurs with breast and GI carcinomas (NCI, 2010).

2. Incidence and epidemiology

  a) An estimated 22,340 new brain and CNS cases (12,260 male, 10,080 female) with 13,110 deaths occurred in the United States in 2011 (Siegel, Ward, Brawley, & Jemal, 2011).

b) The incidence of brain tumors increases with age (CBTRUS, 2010).

   (1) Meningiomas and GBM are the two most common CNS tumors diagnosed in adults older than age 45.

   (2) The incidence per 100,000 of GBM diagnosis for ages 45–54 is 3.73, increasing to 8.16 for people ages 55–64, 13.10 for ages 65–74, 14.49 for ages 75–84, and 8.4 for those age 85 and older (CBTRUS, 2010).

   (3) Five-year survival rate for people ages 65–74 with GBM is 1.3% and 0.6% for those age 75 and older. Ten-year survival rate decreases to 0.6% for ages 65–74 and is not available for those older (CBTRUS, 2010).

c) The only environmental factor unequivocally associated with the increased risk of developing primary CNS tumors is prior exposure to ionizing radiation (Ohgaki & Kleihues, 2005). Debate is ongoing regarding the association of cell phone use and glioma development (Ahlbom et al., 2009; Khurana, Teo, Kundi, Hardell, & Carlberg, 2009).

d) Some epidemiologic case-controlled studies have found reduced glioma risks in patients with history of allergic disease such as asthma, hay fever, and eczema (Schoemaker et al., 2010).

e) Further study is searching for possible gene-environment interactions (genetic variants) in glioma development (Schoemaker et al., 2010).

3. Treatment standard of care—Dependent on tumor pathology and sensitivity to RT

  a) Combined-modality therapy—Malignant CNS tumors (WHO grade III–IV) require combined-modality therapy with optimal surgical resection followed by fractionated conformal partial brain RT and concurrent/adjuvant chemotherapy (NCCN, 2010; Siker et al., 2008).

   (1) Daily administration of temozolomide during RT has been shown to increase survival at 28 months to 14.6 months compared to 12.1 months with RT alone (Stupp et al., 2009).

   (2) Combined therapy has been found to be superior for survival comparisons (hazard ratio 0.6, 95% CI 0.5–0.7, p < 0.0001): 27.2% with combined therapy versus 10.9% with RT alone at two years, 16% versus 4.4% at three years, 12.1% versus 3% at four years, and 9.8% versus 1.9% at five years (Stupp et al., 2009).

   (3) Benefit was observed in all clinical subgroups, including those aged 60–70 years. *MGMT* methylation was the strongest predictor.

   (4) Intratumoral therapies that deliver therapies locally to the tumor cavity and limit systemic effects with varying impact on outcomes of tumor control or quality of life

     (a) Chemotherapy-coated polymer wafers, usually carmustine, are placed along the borders of the surgical cavity (Affronti et al., 2009; NCCN, 2010).

     (b) Convection delivery systems have been used to deliver radioactive iodine or toxins (Adkison, Thomadsen, & Howard, 2008; Kunwar et al., 2010; Reardon et al., 2008).

  b) Single RT modality—Treatment for benign CNS tumors (WHO grade I–II) generally includes optimal surgical resection as indicated followed by fractionated conformal partial brain RT as a single modality (NCCN, 2010; Siker et al., 2008).

  c) RT treatment that varies from these standards is specified within section 4 below.

4. Routinely irradiated CNS tumors (CBTRUS, 2010; Siker et al., 2008)

  a) Malignant glioma—Accounts for approximately half of all primary brain tumors in adults (Kanu et al., 2009; Siker et al., 2008); 4.1% of spinal tumors are malignant gliomas (CBTRUS, 2010).

   (1) GBM (WHO grade IV)—Accounts for 17% of all CNS tumors (CBTRUS, 2010) and approximately 75% of all high-grade gliomas (Siker et al., 2008).

   (2) Anaplastic glioma (WHO grade III)—Accounts for 5% of all CNS tumors (CBTRUS, 2010) and approximately 25% of all high-grade gliomas (Siker et al., 2008). Includes anaplastic astrocytoma, anaplastic oligodendroglioma, and anaplastic mixed oligoastrocytoma.

  b) Low-grade glioma—Accounts for approximately 20% of glioma cases and 10% of all primary brain tumors in adults (Kanu et al., 2009).

   (1) Diffusely infiltrating glioma (WHO grade II)—Accounts for 6% of all CNS tumors (Kanu et al., 2009). Gross total surgical resection is difficult because of the infiltrative nature of this disease and is unlikely to be curative. Postoperative radiation improves me-

dian five-year progression-free survival to 44% compared to 37% for those undergoing observation only (Stieber & Mehta, 2007).

    (2) Pilocytic astrocytoma (WHO grade I)—Accounts for 1.7% of all CNS tumors; accounts for 1.4% of spinal tumors. Postoperative radiation is appropriate for subtotal surgical resection (Kanu et al., 2009).

c) Brain stem glioma—Accounts for 11.2% of all pediatric brain tumors and 1.7% of adult CNS tumors (Packer et al., 2002).

    (1) Diffuse intrinsic pontine—WHO grade II–IV glioma

    (2) Exophytic cervicomedullary—Primarily a low-grade glioma

    (3) Focal midbrain or intrinsic pontine—Primarily a low-grade glioma

d) Ependymoma—Accounts for 1.9% of primary brain tumors, 5% of intracranial gliomas, and 33.6% of spinal tumors (CBTRUS, 2010). WHO grade II–III with potential to disseminate the CSF. Craniospinal irradiation is used for disseminated disease.

e) Medulloblastoma—Accounts for 1% of all adult primary brain tumors (CBTRUS, 2010); CSF dissemination is common. Multiple variants exist, which are used to create risk categories for treatment recommendations. All risk categories require craniospinal irradiation and chemotherapy.

f) PCNSL—Accounts for 2.4% of all primary brain tumors (CBTRUS, 2010). Requires whole brain RT as adjuvant to optimal chemotherapy.

g) Meningioma—Accounts for 33.8% of primary brain tumors in adults and 6.1% of spinal tumors (CBTRUS, 2010).

    (1) WHO grade I (90% of cases; NCI, 2010)—Postoperative radiation is appropriate for subtotal resection or recurrent disease.

    (2) WHO grade II and III—Postoperative radiation is recommended for all patients after maximal resection.

h) Craniopharyngioma—Accounts for 0.7% of adult primary brain tumors (CBTRUS, 2010). More common in children or adults in their fifth decade of life. Because gross total resection is difficult, postoperative radiation is usually required. SRS may be considered for very small lesions (less than 2 cm). Cystic lesions also may be treated with endocavitary irradiation with a β-emitter (^{186}Re, ^{32}P, ^{198}Au, or ^{90}Y) (Derrey et al., 2008).

i) Vestibular schwannoma (also called acoustic neuroma)—Accounts for 5.6% of adult primary brain tumors and 40.5% of spinal nerve sheath tumors (Kanu et al., 2009; Louis, 2006). Small lesions may be treated with SRS with less morbidity than surgery, including preservation of facial function and hearing.

j) Hemangioblastoma—Accounts for 1% of all CNS tumors in adults and 2.6% of spinal tumors (Kanu et al., 2009; Louis, 2006). Radiosurgery is appropriate for unresectable locations.

k) Hemangiopericytoma—Accounts for less than 1% of all CNS tumors (Kanu et al., 2009; Louis, 2006). Postoperative radiation is appropriate for all cases.

l) CNS metastasis—Occurs in approximately 20%–40% of people with systemic cancer (Robinson et al., 2010). Incidence is increasing because of improved survival, an aging population, and earlier detection. Treatment standard of care pertains to the number, size, and location of lesions.

    (1) A solitary lesion may be treated with surgical excision followed by whole brain RT, which is superior to either modality used alone (Gaspar et al., 2010).

    (2) For patients with one to four lesions and good performance status, whole brain RT plus SRS boost is superior to whole brain RT alone in terms of local control and maintaining functional status (Linskey et al., 2010)

    (3) SRS alone is a reasonable treatment option but carries a higher risk of distant brain recurrence and thus requires careful, active surveillance to ensure early identification of recurrences and appropriate salvage therapy (Linskey et al., 2010).

5. Symptoms of CNS irradiation

a) Acute effects: Toxicities that occur during the onset of treatment and manifest up to six weeks after treatment (Siker et al., 2008)

    (1) Focal symptoms—Transient worsening of pretreatment deficits localized to tumor placement within the brain parenchyma or spine

        (a) Pathophysiology: A multifactorial process from tumor and therapy effects that results in localized peritumoral edema from both vasogenic and cytotoxic edema

i. Vasogenic edema—Tumor effects from gliomas or brain metastases resulting in the disruption of the blood-brain barrier (BBB), allowing passage of fluid into the extracellular space of the brain parenchyma (Wen et al., 2006). Production of angiogenic factors, such as vascular endothelial growth factor, promotes tumor angiogenesis of permeable vessels that increases the surrounding edema. RT causes further injury to vascular endothelial structures, increasing leakiness and edema, hypoxia, and reactive gliosis (Siker et al., 2008).

ii. Cytotoxic edema—Cytotoxic effects from RT produce cellular swelling, which increases intracellular compartments and leads to cellular death (Forman, 2002).

iii. Localized peritumoral edema from radiation-induced injury is dependent on multiple factors including total dose, doses per fraction, treatment volume, and specific target cell population (Siker et al., 2008).

iv. More prevalent with partial brain RT than whole brain RT because of the higher dose provided in partial brain irradiation.

v. Disruption of the BBB and edema often occur as early T2 signal abnormality on MRI.

(b) Assessment: Neurologic symptoms and deficits will be based on the region of the brain affected.

i. Perform a thorough neurologic and physical examination—See Table 10 for the parameters of a normal neurologic examination.

ii. See Table 11 for localized symptoms according to brain structure involvement.

(c) Documentation: According to facility requirements; see Figure 18 for standard documentation sources.

(d) Collaborative management

i. Steroid therapy—Used for the management of focal symptoms caused by localized peritumoral edema. Steroids reduce capillary permeability.

- May initiate use of dexamethasone or methylprednisolone therapy or increase current dose to alleviate focal symptoms.
- Steroids reduce capillary permeability as soon as one hour after a single dose.
- Dexamethasone often is used because of its relatively little mineralocorticoid activity (Siker et al., 2008; Wen et al., 2006).
- Dexamethasone is a strong inducer of the CYP3A4 pathway; thus, drug interactions will need monitoring for dose adjustment. Likewise, hepatic microsomal enzyme inducers can increase the metabolism of glucocorticoids, requiring dose adjustments.

ii. Associated symptoms—Symptoms not fully alleviated by steroid therapy may require additional management.

- Pain medications or antiepileptic medications may be used in management for headaches, restless legs, muscular spasms, sleep disorders, and mood disorders.
- Monitor new medications for tolerance and side effects.
- Consider initiation of nonpharmacologic interventions, such as relaxation techniques, as appropriately indicated.

(e) Patient and family education: Educate regarding the many side effects of corticosteroid therapy.

i. Provide written and verbal instructions for recognizing the signs and symptoms of peritumoral edema.

ii. Provide written and verbal instructions for the use of steroid and antiepileptic medication

Table 10. Components of Neurologic Assessment

Component	Subcomponents	Assessment
Mental status	Level of consciousness	Alert, full consciousness
		Lethargy
		Obtunded
		Stupor
		Coma
	Orientation	Person
		Place
		Time
		Recent events
	Affect	"Normal"
		Abnormal ranging from flat to manic
Cranial nerves (CNs)	Olfactory (CN I)	Smell
	Optic (CN II)	Central and peripheral vision
	Oculomotor (CN III)	Pupillary constriction and eye movement
	Trochlear (CN IV)	Medial eye movement
	Trigeminal (CN V)	Sensory function of face and jaw clenching
	Abducens (CN VI)	Lateral eye movement
	Facial (CN VII)	Motor function of face and taste: Anterior two-thirds of tongue
	Acoustic (CN VIII)	Hearing and sense of balance
	Glossopharyngeal (CN IX)	Gag and taste: Posterior one-third of tongue
	Vagus (CN X)	Swallowing and palate elevation
	Spinal accessory (CN XI)	Neck and shoulder shrug
	Hypoglossal (CN XII)	Tongue movement
Speech	Expressive	Speech fluency
	Receptive	Following commands
Peripheral function of extremities	Motor	Hand grips, dorsi/plantar flexion, and individual muscular movements
	Sensory	Light touch, temperature discrimination
	Proprioception	Recognizing limb position
	Vibratory sense	Recognizing vibration
	Deep tendon reflexes	Absent, hyper- or hyporeflexive
Coordination	Point-to-point	Finger to nose, heel to shin
	Rapid alternating movements	Rapid hand or feet tapping
Gait	Walking	Normal and tandem gaits
Balance	Romberg	Standing with eyes closed

Note. Based on information from Snell, 2010; Wilson-Pauwels et al., 2010.

with particular emphasis on the importance of maintaining the medication schedule and risks involved in abrupt, unsupervised cessation of either drug, which could result in withdrawal side effects (Wen et al., 2006). Both medications require supervised tapering according to individual symptom responses to achieve desired outcomes.

iii. Instruct the patient and family about the side effects of prolonged steroid use. Common side effects include the following (Wen et al., 2006).
- Dermatologic effects— Acne, impaired wound

Table 11. Localized Symptoms Frequently Observed, Based on Primary and Metastatic Tumor Location

Structure	Normal Function	Symptom
Cerebral Cortex		
Frontal		
• Anterior precentral	Motor activity assembled from past experience	Difficulty performing skilled movements
• Posterior precentral-motor strip	Individual movements of different parts of the body	Paralysis of contralateral body parts, Jacksonian epileptic seizure, muscle spasm
• Frontal eye field	Scanning eye movements independent of visual stimuli	Both eyes deviate to the affected side, inability to turn eyes to opposite side
• Olfactory area	Cranial nerve (CN) I—emotional and autonomic response to smell	Altered or absent sense of smell
• Broca area	Motor area of speech, located in dominant hemisphere (left side for majority of the population)	Expressive aphasia; global aphasia if associated with Wernicke area
• Prefrontal	Personality, attention, sequential processes, executive function, emotional states, self-awareness, appetite	Loss of initiative, poor judgment, emotional changes, loss of social inhibition
Parietal		
• Primary somatic sensory	Interprets sensory input from body parts	Contralateral sensory disturbance
• Somesthetic association	Integrates touch, pressure, and proprioception	Contralateral astereognosis
Occipital		
• Primary visual area	Receives fibers from the retina and macula	Visual field defects
• Secondary visual area	Visual information of past visual experiences	Contralateral inability to recognize objects
Temporal		
• Primary auditory area	Reception of sounds from cochlea	Bilateral hearing loss (greater in contralateral ear)
• Secondary auditory area	Interpretation of sounds	Acoustic verbal agnosia
• Wernicke area	Receptive understanding of written and spoken language in dominant hemisphere	Receptive aphasia; global aphasia if associated with Broca area
Limbic System/Central Brain		
• Thalamus	Receives sensory information and relays to cerebral cortex	Contralateral impairment of light touch, tactile localization, discrimination; loss of appreciation of joint movements
– Pineal gland	Endocrine gland influencing (mainly inhibitory) pituitary, adrenal, gonads, pancreas, parathyroid	Severe alteration of reproductive function
– Hypothalamus	Emotional states, sleep, body temperature, appetite, genital function; function in pituitary hormone release; fat, carbohydrate, water metabolism	Genital hypoplasia; diabetes insipidus; obesity; sleep disturbances; irregular pyrexia; emaciation
• Hippocampal formation	Integration of memory and emotional behaviors	Inability to form memory; amnesia
– Optic chiasm	Visual information relay: optic nerve to optic tracts	Bilateral blindness
• Lateral and third ventricle	Cerebrospinal fluid circulation	Hydrocephalus
• Basal ganglia	Integrates global sensory and motor input	Severe motor or sensory symptoms
• Corpus callosum	Transfers information across hemispheres	Altered memory and contralateral sensory discrimination
• Internal capsule	Connects cerebral cortex to brain stem and spinal cord	Widespread effects on contralateral body

(Continued on next page)

Table 11. Localized Symptoms Frequently Observed, Based on Primary and Metastatic Tumor Location *(Continued)*

Structure	Normal Function	Symptom
Cerebellum	Receives afferent information from cerebral cortex, muscles, tendons, and joints on voluntary movements; receives balance information from the vestibular nerve; cerebellar output information influences motor activity; functions as a coordinator of precise movements by continually comparing the output from the motor area of the cerebral cortex with the proprioceptive information from the site of muscle action	Altered gait (wide-based, stiff-legged), ipsilateral dysdiadochokinesia (difficulty with rapid alternating movements), dysarthria (altered articulation), prolonged deep tendon reflexes, nystagmus, hypotonia; tremor with fine motor movements, vermis syndrome (head and trunk muscle incoordination, tendency to fall forward or backward)
Brain Stem		
• Medulla oblongata	Corticospinal tracts from spinal cord to the brain Foramen magnum of skull CN IX–XII location: • CN IX—glossopharyngeal • CN X—vagus • CN XI—spinal accessory • CN XII—hypoglossal	Increased intracranial pressure—headache, stiff neck, vital function failure, and paralysis of CN IX–XII • CN IX—poor gag reflex, loss of taste (posterior tongue) • CN X—dysphagia, asymmetry of soft palate elevation, hoarseness • CN XI—affected side weakness head turn and shoulder raising • CN XII—tongue deviates toward affected side; atrophy of tongue Herniation—increased intracranial pressure causes downward displacement of the medulla and cerebellar tonsils through foramen magnum
• Pons	Continues corticospinal tracts; CN V–VIII location: • CN V—trigeminal • CN VI—abducens • CN VII—facial • CN VIII—vestibulocochlear	Ipsilateral CN paralysis: • CN V—facial sensory deficit to light touch • CN VI—decreased lateral gaze, nystagmus • CN VII—facial weakness • CN VIII—impaired hearing Contralateral hemiparesis
• Midbrain	Continues corticospinal tracts (red nucleus, substantia nigra) CN II–IV location: • CN II—optic • CN III—oculomotor • CN IV—trochlear	• CN II—dilated nonreactive pupil • CN III—ipsilateral paralysis of muscles producing upward, downward, inward gaze • CN IV—contralateral paralysis of superior oblique muscle Hydrocephalus—blocked cerebral aqueduct
Spinal cord	Contains cervical, thoracic, lumbar, and sacral afferent and efferent nerves for motor and sensory functions	Ipsilateral dysfunction in motor or sensory areas (dermatome charts useful). In rare cases, radiation-induced Lhermitte syndrome may occur.

Note. Based on information from Snell, 2010; Wilson-Pauwels et al., 2010.

healing, hirsutism, thin and fragile skin, atrophy, petechiae, and bruising
• Endocrine system—Increased blood sugar (requires close monitoring of diabetic patients), cushingoid state, growth retardation, menstrual irregularities, and decreased carbohydrate tolerance
• Fluid and electrolyte disturbances—Sodium retention, potassium loss, hypertension, and moon face
• GI system—Stomach irritation and abdominal distension. Instruct the patient in the use of antacids to be given with steroid dose to prevent peptic ulcers.
• Infection—Increased susceptibility, especially to *Candida* and *Pneumocystis*; also may mask signs of infection, such as fever

---

Figure 18. Standardized Documentation Sources

- National Cancer Institute *Common Terminology Criteria for Adverse Events* for treatment-related side effects
- Performance status
  - Karnofsky performance scale: 0 (death) to 100 (perfect health*)
  - Eastern Cooperative Oncology Group scale: 0 (perfect health*) to 5 (death)

* Perfect health: The ability to perform full activities of daily living and no restrictions on activities.

Figure 19. Organizations and Web Sites That Provide Multiple Programs for Support of People With Central Nervous System Cancers

- American Brain Tumor Association: www.abta.org
- American Cancer Society: www.cancer.org
- National Brain Tumor Society: www.braintumor.org
- National Cancer Institute: www.cancer.gov

- Musculoskeletal system—Proximal steroid myopathy (especially in thigh muscles, then upper arms) and osteoporosis
- Nervous system—Mood swings, restlessness, insomnia, vertigo, psychoses, headaches, euphoria, intracerebral hemorrhage, cataracts, and increased intraocular pressure

   iv. Long-term steroid use affects the patient's quality of life and self-image as a result of fluid retention, weight gain, leg weakness, insomnia, diabetes, and delayed wound healing.

   v. Provide literature regarding support programs; see Figure 19 for more information.

(2) Headache

   (a) Pathophysiology: Headache results from increases in edema caused by BBB disruption, capillary permeability, and increased intracranial pressure from primary tumor, metastatic growth, or treatment-related effects that distort nerve endings in the pain-sensitive dura (Armstrong & Gilbert, 2000; Lovely, 2004).

   (b) Risk factors

     i. Incidence increases with higher RT doses per fraction. Prevalence is higher with whole brain RT than in partial brain RT because of the greater volume treated (Stieber & Mehta, 2007).

     ii. Steroid prophylaxis may reduce occurrence (Armstrong & Gilbert, 2000).

     iii. Edema may occur if steroids are tapered quickly (Ryken et al., 2010; Stewart-Amidei, 2005).

     iv. Headaches may develop as a presenting symptom or during the course of the disease, particularly in the early morning. Headaches may recur more commonly in patients for whom headache was a presenting symptom; therefore, these patients should be evaluated for disease progression (Lovely, 2004).

   (c) Assessment (Camp-Sorrell, 2006)

     i. Perform a thorough neurologic and physical examination—See Table 10 for the parameters of a normal neurologic examination.

     ii. Obtain headache history.

- Current cancer treatment plan and history
- History of presenting symptoms, including precipitating factors, headache frequency, duration, intensity, location, time of day, initial presentation, and changes in symptoms over time
- Associated symptoms, including nausea, vomiting, syncope, visual changes, and fatigue
- Prodromal signs, including feeling tired, clumsy, or thirsty, and light or sound sensitivity
- Pharmacologic and non-pharmacologic interventions that have been tried and the results
- Any recent changes in medications, specifically steroid therapy

     iii. Sudden severe headache may indicate late signs of increased intracranial pressure and may be associated with a widening pulse pressure, bradycardia, and severe hypertension (Lovely, 2004).

(d) Documentation: According to facility requirements; see Figure 18 for standard documentation sources.

(e) Collaborative management

  i. Steroid therapy—Consider initiation or increase in current dose of dexamethasone or methylprednisolone. See information under focal symptoms.

  ii. Pain medications, such as nonsteroidal medications, may provide symptomatic relief.

  iii. Nonpharmacologic interventions, such as relaxation techniques, may be useful.

(f) Patient and family education

  i. Development of new or worsening headaches needs to be reported to the healthcare team, including precipitating and alleviating factors, frequency, duration, intensity, location, and associated symptoms.

  ii. Provide written and verbal instructions for the use of steroid therapy and any additional pharmacologic agents, such as nonsteroidal medications. Refer to previous section on steroid management under focal symptoms.

  iii. Provide literature regarding support programs; see Figure 19 for more information.

(3) Seizures—Sudden excessive abnormal electrical stimulation in the brain that alters neurologic function, including motor, sensory, and autonomic visceral function and mental status (Armstrong, Baumgartner, & Min, 2006); may constitute the presenting symptom for diagnosis or disease progression and recurrence in 30%–90% of patients (Lovely, 2004)

(a) Pathophysiology (Lee et al., 2010; Wen et al., 2006)

  i. The mechanism of how brain tumors cause seizures is not well understood but may be related to focal irritation.

  ii. Tumor locations more frequently associated with seizures include temporal lobes, frontal lobes and their motor cortices, and parietal lobes and their sensory cortices (Lovely, 2004).

  iii. Low-grade primary brain tumors presenting with seizures usually are larger than those presenting with other symptoms, whereas high-grade primary tumors presenting with seizures are likely to be smaller than those presenting with other symptoms.

(b) Incidence

  i. Seizures occur more often in patients with primary tumors than metastases. Seizures are more likely to occur in those with low-grade primary brain tumors than those with high-grade tumors.

  ii. Seizures are a presenting symptom in 30%–50% of patients with primary brain tumors (Lee et al., 2010) and 15%–20% of patients with brain metastases (Maschio et al., 2010). In both groups, a similar proportion of patients will eventually develop seizures after diagnosis.

(c) Assessment (Armstrong et al., 2006)

  i. Perform a thorough neurologic and physical examination—See Table 10 for the parameters of a normal neurologic examination.

  ii. Obtain seizure history.

   • Current cancer treatment plan and history

   • History of presenting symptoms, including precipitating factors, frequency, duration, intensity, location, time of day, initial presentation, and changes in symptoms over time

   • Precipitating signs or aura, including sensing unusual odor, tastes, or sounds, visual disturbances, or feelings of flushing

   • Associated symptoms, including nausea, headache, or weakness

- Pharmacologic and non-pharmacologic interventions that have been tried and the results
- Any recent changes in medications, specifically steroid therapy

iii. Obtain laboratory profiles such as blood chemistries, liver function tests, complete blood counts, and appropriate drug levels if on antiepileptic drugs (AEDs).

iv. Obtain neuroradiologic tests to rule out hemorrhage, tumor progression or new lesion, and increased cerebral edema.

v. May need to rule out infectious source through CSF collection; only perform lumbar puncture if absence of increased intracranial pressure is confirmed. Assess craniotomy site for potential source of infection if applicable.

vi. Obtain electroencephalogram within 24 hours of event or if altered mental status persists.

(d) Documentation: According to facility requirements; see Figure 18 for standard documentation sources.

(e) Collaborative management
 i. Multiple studies have demonstrated that prophylactic AEDs are not effective in preventing seizures in those newly diagnosed with brain tumors (Lee et al., 2010) and are not recommended by the American Academy of Neurology (Glantz et al., 2000).

 ii. AEDs are appropriate to initiate in patients who experience a seizure.

iii. Multiple older AEDs (phenytoin, carbamazepine, oxcarbazepine, phenobarbital, mysoline) are cytochrome P450 enzyme inducers; thus, drug interactions require monitoring for dose adjustments, such as corticosteroids and various chemotherapies (Wen et al., 2006).

iv. Multiple newer AEDs, such as levetiracetam, gabapentin, pregabalin, and lamotrigine, are not enzyme inducers.

v. One recent prospective study of patients with brain metastases demonstrated safety and efficacy with use of monotherapy of levetiracetam, oxcarbazepine, and topiramate to reduce seizure frequency with few side effects (Maschio et al., 2010).

vi. Monitor AED therapy with serum drug levels for agents with narrow pharmacologic therapeutic index; in addition, monitor blood chemistries, liver function, and complete blood counts (Armstrong & Gilbert, 2000).

vii. Refer to a neurologist for refractory seizure management.

(f) Patient and family education
 i. Patients with primary brain tumors are at increased risk for developing dermatologic reactions to AEDs, higher than 20%, which includes development of Stevens-Johnson syndrome (Wen et al., 2006).

 ii. All reactions need to be reported to the healthcare team, as 20% of patients with primary brain tumors on AED therapy have reported severe reactions warranting AED discontinuation (Wen et al., 2006).

iii. If the patient is on an enzyme-inducing AED, alert the patient and family to potential drug interactions and monitoring parameters.

iv. Provide information regarding the importance for drug adherence, as AEDs should not be stopped abruptly.

v. Advise regarding state-mandated driving regulations and restrictions for patients who have had any seizure activity within the past six months; note that some states have mandatory healthcare reporting.

vi. Provide literature regarding support programs; see Figure 19 for more information.

(4) Nausea and vomiting (Murphy-Ende, 2006)

(a) Pathophysiology—A multifactorial process involving neural structures and neurotransmitters, which can be affected by tumor location and treatment

i. The vomiting center lies within the lateral reticular formation of the medulla, near the floor of the fourth ventricle, and is activated by several mechanisms: cerebral cortex, vestibular apparatus, chemoreceptor trigger zone, and visceral and vagal afferent pathways of the GI tract. Tumor location, increases in intracranial pressure or cerebral edema, and disruption of these structures can activate the complex processes involved in nausea and vomiting.

ii. Neurotransmitters are sensitive to many chemical toxins within the blood and CNS: dopamine, serotonin, neurokinin-1 (NK1), muscarinic, substance P, and histamine. Disruption of the BBB and the normal receptor-transmitter actions will cause nausea and vomiting.

iii. Although several cancer therapies for patients with brain tumors may not be considered highly emetogenic, persistent nausea or nausea with emesis may exist, requiring additional support; anticipatory nausea may ensue as a result of the overwhelming persistence of previous uncontrolled nausea.

(b) Risk factors

i. Tumor location near or adjacent to the vomiting center, fourth ventricle, medulla, or known increased cerebral edema affecting those locations

ii. RT targets containing the neural structures of the vomiting center

(c) Assessment

i. Perform a thorough neurologic and physical examination—See Table 10 for the parameters of a normal neurologic examination.

ii. Obtain history (Friend et al., 2009).

- Current cancer treatment plan and history

- History of presenting symptoms, including precipitating factors, onset and duration, descriptors of the vomitus, prior experiences with nausea and vomiting, smell/odor sensitivities, and interference with daily life

- Associated symptoms including increased salivation, diaphoresis, retching, dysphagia, thirst, tachycardia, diarrhea, loss of appetite, and anxiety

- Assessment for other symptoms, including cachexia, anemia, endocrine dysfunction, pain, fluid and electrolyte disturbances, seizures, and infection

- Pharmacologic and non-pharmacologic interventions that have been tried and the results

- Any recent changes in medications, including steroid therapy and AEDs

iii. Obtain laboratory profiles such as blood chemistries, liver function tests, complete blood counts, and appropriate drug levels if on AEDs.

(d) Documentation: According to facility requirements; see Figure 18 for standard documentation sources.

(e) Collaborative management

i. Administer serotonin receptor (5-HT$_3$) antagonist and maximize dose as necessary.

    ii. Initiate or adjust dosage of steroid therapy.

    iii. Use of an NK1 receptor antagonist may be beneficial for concurrent chemotherapy administration.

    iv. Consider adding cannabinoids to daily regimen; these agents are safe with low toxicity profile in patients with primary brain tumors (Allen, Vredenburgh, Dryman, Carter, & Freeman, 2009).

    v. Benzodiazepines may be useful for those with anticipatory nausea; however, the sedative side effect can alter the patient's mental status.

    vi. Additional pharmacologic agents include phenothiazines and anticholinergics, but sedative side effects will need monitoring in this patient population.

    vii. Nonpharmacologic interventions such as relaxation therapy, diversion or attention distraction, hypnosis, and imagery may be beneficial.

(f) Patient and family education

    i. Instruct patient to journal episodes of nausea and emesis to assess for precipitating factors and adjust interventions as necessary.

    ii. Provide information regarding side effects of pharmacologic agents and be aware of drug interactions.

    iii. Provide literature regarding support programs; see Figure 19 for more information.

(5) Acute alopecia

(a) Pathophysiology: Hair follicles and glands are more susceptible to radiation damage because of the relatively rapid growth and proliferation. Radiation causes premature conversion of hair follicle cells from the anagen (active) phase to the telogen (resting) phase, which results in new hairs being shed at an increased rate (Rannan-Eliya, Rannan-Eliya, Graham, Pizer, & McDowell, 2007; Trüeb, 2009).

(b) Incidence (Roberge, Parker, Niazi, & Olivares, 2005)

    i. Temporary alopecia occurs with doses as low as 5 Gy.

    ii. Whole brain RT of 30 Gy (300 cGy/fraction) can result in permanent vertex alopecia caused by dose accumulation.

    iii. Patchy alopecia occurs after partial brain RT in scalp areas receiving approximately 45 Gy (180–200 cGy/fraction).

    iv. Higher doses (45 Gy or greater) may produce permanent alopecia or delayed regrowth for more than a year.

(c) Assessment: Scalp evaluation for complications of acute side effects of brain irradiation

    i. Dry scalp

    ii. Radiation dermatitis

    iii. Hyperpigmentation

    iv. Alopecia

(d) Documentation: According to facility requirements; see Figure 18 for standard documentation sources.

(e) Collaborative management (Roberge et al., 2005)

    i. Gently wash hair with mild shampoo one to two times a week. Use a water-soluble lubricant on scalp.

    ii. Use a soft-bristle brush on hair to diminish follicular injury.

    iii. Avoid sun exposure to the scalp by wearing a hat or covering; may apply a sunscreen with SPF 30 or greater.

    iv. Check behind auricle for moist desquamation, as radiation dose may concentrate in skin folds.

    v. Avoid hair dyes and permanents.

    vi. Consider surgical reconstructive intervention, particularly in the pediatric population (Rannan-Eliya et al., 2007).

(f) Patient and family education (Rannan-Eliya et al., 2007; Roberge et al., 2005)

    i. Instruct the patient about the areas in which radiation alopecia is expected to occur related to the calculated scalp dose.

    ii. Alopecia is expected to begin two to three weeks after initiation of treatment; regrowth takes three to six months after completion of treatment.

iii. Hair regrowth may be of a different color or consistency.

iv. Some hair loss may be permanent, depending on RT dose (e.g., whole brain RT 30 Gy or partial brain RT 45 Gy).

v. Provide literature regarding wigs (types, where to purchase, insurance reimbursement, wig alternatives) and reconstructive interventions if appropriate; see Figure 19 for more information.

b) Subacute effects: Toxicities that develop from six-week to six-month period following RT (Siker et al., 2008)

(1) Fatigue

(a) Pathophysiology: Treatment-related effects from the immune system's (HPA axis) release of cytokines cause muscular wasting, which leads to fatigue. Central and peripheral mechanisms also contribute to fatigue (Cope, 2006; Mitchell, Beck, Hood, Moore, & Tanner, 2009).

i. Central mechanisms originate in the CNS, including brain chemistry, spinal cord innervation, and nerve cell disruption.

ii. Peripheral mechanisms at the neuromuscular junction, muscle, or cellular level occur during physical activity.

(b) Incidence: Although fatigue may begin during RT, it usually persists after completion of therapy, which may be due to central mechanisms and damage to the HPA axis provoking cytokine release (Lovely, 2004). Other factors include

i. Concurrent and continuing administration of chemotherapy

ii. Long-term use of steroid therapy

iii. Neuroendocrine organs within the RT target volume.

(c) Assessment

i. Perform a thorough neurologic and physical examination—see Table 10 for the parameters of a normal neurologic examination.

ii. Obtain history (Mitchell et al., 2009).

• Current cancer treatment plan and history

• History of presenting symptoms, including precipitating factors, duration and intensity of fatigue, time of day that fatigue is noticed, and interference with daily life

• Associated symptoms including sleep disturbances, depression, loss of appetite, cognitive disturbances, and changes in ADL

• Assessment for other symptoms including cachexia, anemia, endocrine dysfunction, pain, fluid and electrolyte disturbances, and infection

• Pharmacologic and nonpharmacologic interventions that have been tried and the results

• Any recent changes in medications, specifically steroid therapy

iii. Obtain laboratory profiles such as blood chemistries, liver function tests, complete blood counts, and appropriate drug levels if on AEDs.

(d) Documentation: According to facility requirements; see Figure 18 for standard documentation sources.

(e) Collaborative management (Mitchell et al., 2009)

i. Correct underlying diagnoses, including anemia, electrolyte imbalances, or infection.

ii. Initiate steroid taper if associated with long-term use; may need to use a mineralocorticoid supplement if adrenal insufficiency is present.

iii. May consider methylphenidate or other stimulant medications, which have been useful to improve fatigue in some cases.

iv. Nonpharmacologic interventions, such as relaxation therapy or exercise, may be beneficial for some.

(f) Patient and family education

i. Teach patients and caregivers to schedule and pace daily activities with frequent rest intervals to promote balancing of metabolic demands, also referred to as energy conservation and activity management.

ii. Promote exercise tailored to individual ability, tolerance, and associated symptoms. While daily walking is beneficial, monitoring during exercise activities may be required. Consider physical or occupational therapy consults for individuals with seizure disorders, motor weakness, paresis, or paresthesias to provide exercise and safety recommendations.

iii. Promote adequate and restful sleep.

iv. Instruct on the best times of the day to take medications for maximum health function, such as steroids, AEDs, and stimulants.

v. Encourage a balanced diet with adequate fluid intake.

vi. Attention-restoring activities and alternative therapies such as relaxation, massage, healing touch, polarity therapy, and haptotherapy may be beneficial.

(2) Cranial neuropathies: Predominantly visual and auditory

   (a) Pathophysiology (Armstrong, Hancock, & Gilbert, 2000)

      i. Focal irritation to ocular apparatus or cochlea causes temporary visual (changes in acuity) or auditory (ringing) disturbances.

      ii. Inflammation to the external ear canal causes increased cerumen production, resulting in difficulties hearing.

   (b) Risk factors: RT field proximity to the optic chiasm, optic nerves, optic globes, acoustic nerve, and cochlear areas increases risk (Stieber & Mehta, 2007).

      i. Damage to the lacrimal gland with dry eye and corneal injury

      ii. Cataract formation may occur with doses exceeding 35 Gy.

      iii. Damage to the optic chiasm and nerves is dose dependent

at 0.3% for dose fractions below 2 Gy versus 4% for dose fractions at 2 Gy or higher (Stieber & Mehta, 2007).

iv. For single-fraction SRS, injury to optic apparatus causing optic neuropathy is dose dependent. Occurrence is 78% for doses above 14 Gy, 27% for dose of 10–15 Gy, and minimal incidence with doses below 10 Gy (Stieber & Mehta, 2007).

v. Most cranial neuropathies are temporary and reported at 13% incidence, with only 8% being permanent, for doses up to 40 Gy (Stieber & Mehta, 2007).

(c) Assessment

   i. Perform a thorough neurologic and physical examination—See Table 10 for the parameters of a normal neurologic examination.

   ii. For visual acuity disturbances
- Current cancer treatment plan and history
- History of presenting symptoms, including precipitating factors, time of day that disturbance is worse or better, interference with daily life, and light sensitivity
- Assessment for scleral and conjunctival irritation
- Consideration of infectious processes
- May need to consider neuroradiographic evaluations to rule out hemorrhage, tumor progression or new lesion, and increasing cerebral edema
- Pharmacologic and nonpharmacologic interventions that have been tried and the results
- Any recent changes in medications, specifically steroid therapy

   iii. For auditory disturbances
- Current cancer treatment plan and history
- History of presenting symptoms, including precipitating factors, time of day that disturbance is worse or bet-

ter, interference with daily life, and sound sensitivity
- Assessment of ear canal for infection, desquamation, and cerumen impaction
- Weber and Rinne tests for conductive and sensorineural hearing loss (SNHL)
- Consideration of infectious processes
- Pharmacologic and non-pharmacologic interventions that have been tried and the results
- Any recent changes in medications, specifically steroid therapy

iv. Obtain laboratory profiles such as blood chemistries, liver function tests, complete blood counts, and appropriate drug levels if on AEDs

(d) Documentation: According to facility requirements; see Figure 18 for standard documentation sources.

(e) Collaborative management
i. Visual acuity disturbances
- Refer patient to have corrective lenses adjusted to promote safety with gait, driving, and performing other ADL.
- Adjust medications, particularly steroid therapy, as appropriate.
- Consider neuro-ophthalmology referral if disturbance persists.

ii. Auditory disturbances
- Remove cerumen blockage if appropriate, and institute routine management of cerumen.
- Treat infection if underlying cause.
- Consider formal auditory testing and evaluation if disturbance persists for recommendations of surgical options or hearing aid use.

(f) Patient and family education
i. Provide information that these disturbances are usually of a short duration.
ii. Instruct the patient to inform providers if symptoms persist or worsen over time.

(3) Somnolence syndrome (Kelsey & Marks, 2006)
(a) Pathophysiology: Radiation-induced brain injury characterized by somnolence ranging from mild drowsiness to overwhelming exhaustion, low-grade fever, nausea, vomiting, and headache. Symptoms typically occur one to four months after completion of RT.
(b) Incidence: Typically encountered after whole brain RT in children; although occurance is rare, it also is reported in adults.
(c) Assessment
i. Perform a thorough neurologic and physical examination—See Table 10 for the parameters of a normal neurologic examination.
ii. Consider neuroradiographic evaluations to rule out hemorrhage, tumor progression or new lesion, and increased cerebral edema.
iii. Obtain laboratory profiles such as blood chemistries, liver function tests, complete blood counts, and appropriate drug levels if on AEDs.
(d) Documentation: According to facility requirements; see Figure 18 for standard documentation sources.
(e) Collaborative management: Symptoms are transient and resolve within several weeks. Corticosteroid therapy may be useful.
(f) Patient and family education
i. Provide information that these disturbances usually are of a short duration.
ii. Instruct the patient to inform providers if symptoms persist or worsen over time.

c) Late effects—Usually irreversible and progressive sequelae to RT occurring from six months to years after treatment. Possible etiology is white matter damage from vascular injury, demyelination, and necrosis. Vascular injury involves damage to the endothelium leading to platelet aggregation and thrombus formation, followed by endothelial proliferation and intraluminal collagen formation (Siker et al., 2008).

(1) Radiation necrosis

    (a) Pathophysiology: Severe brain injury to white matter resulting in perivascular necrosis. Radiation necrosis mimics recurrent tumor on MRI and CT imaging with the shared characteristics of location close to original tumor site, contrast enhancement, edema, growth over time, and exertion of mass effect (Leeds et al., 2002).

    (b) Incidence: Extensive review of the literature has recently been undertaken to determine dose-volume predictors of developing radiation necrosis (Lawrence et al., 2010).

        i. For partial brain RT, a dose-response relationship exists. At 2 Gy per fraction, incidence of necrosis is 5% at average 72 Gy (range 60–84) and 10% at average 90 Gy (range 84–102).

        ii. For twice-daily fractionation, a steep increase in toxicity occurs with dose higher than 62.5 Gy.

        iii. For large fraction size (greater than 2.5 Gy), the incidence and severity of toxicity are unpredictable.

        iv. Factors affecting the risk of developing radiation necrosis include total dose, dose per fraction, and volume of brain treated. Suggested risk factors include chemotherapy, dose variance within the volume treated, shorter overall treatment time, older age, and diabetes mellitus.

        v. Median appearance is one to two years following therapy.

    (c) Assessment: Clinically observed as reappearance or worsening of initial symptoms and neurologic deficits (Siker et al., 2008); see Table 10 for neurologic assessment and Table 11 on focal symptoms for details.

    (d) Documentation: According to facility requirements; see Figure 18 for standard documentation sources.

    (e) Collaborative management

        i. Initial treatment is corticosteroid therapy (Leeds et al., 2002; Siker et al., 2008).

        ii. Surgical excision of mass lesions or drainage of cystic lesions can significantly improve neurologic symptoms if conservative management fails (Foroughi et al., 2010).

        iii. Hyperbaric oxygen therapy is a potential therapeutic option for treatment of radiation necrosis (Cihan, Uzun, Yildiz, & Dönmez, 2009).

          • Indicated for radiation necrosis in head and neck cancers and soft tissue injury; however, evidence-based guidelines for indication in radiation injuries to the CNS have not been established.

          • Anecdotal case studies of hyperbaric oxygen therapy for CNS injuries have been reported.

    (f) Patient and family education

        i. Neurologic symptoms or changes need to be reported immediately to the healthcare team.

        ii. Instruct regarding management of side effects and risks of corticosteroid therapy.

        iii. Explore support services needed for worsening functional deficits (i.e., speech, physical, or occupational therapy) and provide literature regarding support programs (see Figure 19).

(2) Radiation myelopathy

    (a) Pathophysiology: A rare radiation-induced severe spinal cord injury that may result in pain, paresthesias, paralysis, sensory deficits, Brown-Séquard syndrome, or bowel/bladder incontinence. Most cases occur within three years af-

ter therapy but rarely before six months after treatment.

(b) Incidence: Extensive review of the literature has recently been undertaken to determine dose-volume predictors of developing radiation necrosis (Kirkpatrick, van der Kogel, & Schultheiss, 2010).

   i. With conventional fractionation of 1.8–2 Gy to full-thickness spinal cord, the estimated risk of myelopathy (defined as CTCAE grade 2 or higher) is less than 1% at 54 Gy and less than 10% at 61 Gy.

   ii. Reirradiation data suggest partial repair of radiation-induced subclinical damage at approximately six months after treatment and increasing over two years.

   iii. Risk effect with concurrent chemotherapy is unknown.

(c) Assessment

   i. Perform neurologic and physical examination.

   ii. Neuroimaging demonstrates MRI features: Hypointensity on T1 weighted images, hyperintensity on T2 weighted images, and hyperintensity on T1 gadolinium diethylenetriamine penta-acetic acid (also known as Gd-DTPA) contrasted images (Michalski, 2008).

(d) Documentation: According to facility requirements, see Figure 18 for standard documentation sources.

(e) Collaborative management

   i. The patient may require specialized pain management.

   ii. Include urology evaluation for management of bladder incontinence.

   iii. Initiate a bowel management program.

(f) Patient and family education

   i. Provide education regarding neurologic symptoms, including back or extremity pain, weakness, numbness or tingling, and bowel or bladder incontinence, which need to be reported immediately to the healthcare team, as these could be symptoms of spinal cord compression (SCC) requiring emergent intervention.

   ii. Assess for safety issues in the home environment if the patient has altered extremity strength or sensation.

   iii. Provide specialized instruction as needed for management of pain and bowel or bladder incontinence (i.e., urinary catheterization, bowel regimen, epidural catheter for pain control).

   iv. Explore support services needed for worsening functional deficits and provide literature regarding support programs (see Figure 19).

(3) Cranial neuropathies: Radiation-induced optic neuropathy (RION) and SNHL

(a) Pathophysiology

   i. RION—Usually presents as painless visual loss, with vasculature injury believed to be the most significant contributing cause. Field of visual loss depends on location of injury. Visual symptoms generally develop within three years of RT (Mayo et al., 2010).

   ii. SNHL—Damage to the cochlea or acoustic nerve producing clinically significant increase in bone conduction threshold at the key human speech frequencies (0.5–4 kHz). After fractionated RT, this rarely occurs as early as three months, with a median latency of 1.5–2 years (Bhandare et al., 2010).

(b) Incidence

   i. Mayo et al. (2010) recently performed an extensive review of the literature to determine dose-volume predictors of developing RION.

     • Total dose and fraction size are the most important treatment-related risk factors.

     • Age older than 70 years is a patient-related risk factor (Mayo et al., 2010).

   ii. Incidence of RION for conventionally fractionated RT

is near zero with doses up to 50 Gy, unusual for doses less than 55 Gy, 3%–7% with doses of 55–60 Gy, and 7%–20% for doses above 60 Gy (Mayo et al., 2010).

   iii. Bhandare et al. (2010) recently reviewed the literature to determine dose-volume predictors of developing radiation-induced SNHL after treatment of head and neck cancer and vestibular schwannoma. The mean dose to the cochlea should be limited to 45 Gy or less for conventionally fractionated RT to minimize risk.

(c) Assessment
   i. For RION: Visual acuity, visual fields
   ii. For SNHL: Pure-tone audiometry and speech discrimination

(d) Documentation: According to facility requirements; see Figure 18 for standard documentation sources.

(e) Collaborative management
   i. Referral to neuro-ophthalmologist or low-vision ophthalmologist for RION
   ii. Referral to otolaryngology or auditory specialists for SNHL
   iii. Referral to disability specialists for special needs regarding low vision, blindness, or deafness

(f) Patient and family education
   i. Provide information regarding support for patients and family, as this is a long-term disability and special needs may be required (see Figure 19).
   ii. Consider home safety evaluation for visual and auditory assistive devices.

   iii. An occupational therapy driving evaluation for visual losses may be needed to assess for safety.

(4) Neuroendocrinopathies
   (a) Pathophysiology: HPA damage and organ dysfunction may induce neuroendocrinopathies such as panhypopituitarism, hypothyroidism, adrenal insufficiency, and sex hormone dysfunction (Agha et al., 2005; Johannesen, Lien, Hole, & Lote, 2003).

   (b) Incidence and risk factors
     i. Involvement of pituitary gland within RT field increases long-term risk of diabetes insipidus.
      • In one study with 25 of 33 patients whose RT field overlapped the thyroid or pituitary axis, 76% had endocrine dysfunction a median of 60 months after treatment completion that included hypothyroidism, hypogonadism, menopause, and adrenocorticotropic hormone (ACTH) deficiency (Johannesen et al., 2003).
      • In another large study of patients whose RT did not involve the pituitary areas, 41% developed deficiencies in growth hormones, ACTH, gonadotropin, and thyroid-stimulating hormone (TSH) and hypopituitarism, 25% of subjects had multiple deficiencies, and 7% experienced panhypopituitarism (Agha et al., 2005).
     ii. Pediatric patients are susceptible to long-term neuroendocrine deficiencies.

   (c) Assessment
     i. Perform a thorough neurologic and physical examination—See Table 10 for the parameters of a normal neurologic examination.
     ii. Consider neuroradiographic evaluations to rule out hemorrhage, tumor progression or new lesion, and increased cerebral edema.

iii. Obtain laboratory profiles, such as endocrine function tests, blood chemistries, liver function tests, complete blood counts, and appropriate drug levels if on AEDs.

(d) Documentation: According to facility requirements; see Figure 18 for standard documentation sources.

(e) Collaborative management

i. Administer replacement therapies for endocrine disorders, and monitor for medication adjustments.

ii. Perform reproductive assessment and planning for patients of childbearing years.

iii. Refer to neuroendocrinologist for long-term follow-up.

(f) Patient and family education

i. Provide information regarding support for the patient and family, as this is a long-term disability and special needs may be required (see Figure 19).

ii. Provide information regarding potential effects on reproductive abilities and sexual functioning.

(5) Neurocognitive impairment: Cognitive function is the result of healthy brain performance (Jansen, Miaskowski, Dodd, Dowling, & Kramer, 2005) and entails several cognitive domains that relay information for optimal performance through subcortical pathways. These domains include attention, executive function, information processing speed, visuospatial skill, motor function, language, and memory. Neurocognitive impairment, frequently referred to as cognitive impairment or dysfunction, is defined as a decline in function in either one or more cognitive domains (Lezak, Howieson, & Loring, 2004).

(a) Pathophysiology: Precise mechanisms of neurocognitive impairments observed beyond tumor location are not fully understood but are most likely multifactorial. Some of these factors may include the following.

i. Cellular DNA damage from RT to the cerebral cortex and subcortical pathways used in cognitive function (Ahles & Saykin, 2007; Stieber & Mehta, 2007)

ii. Structural damage to axons and myelin in the cerebral white matter from RT (Stieber & Mehta, 2007)

iii. Cytokine release in response to prolonged inflammation of the HPA axis (Ahles & Saykin, 2007; Wefel, Witgert, & Meyers, 2008)

(b) Risk factors

i. Whole brain RT has been associated with increased risk (Li, Bentzen, Li, Renschler, & Mehta, 2008).

ii. Total dose of partial RT and field location have been associated with cognitive decline (Meyers, Geara, Wong, & Morrison, 2000; Meyers & Kayl, 2002).

• Doses as low as 18 Gy have resulted in neurocognitive deficits in pediatric patients (Stieber & Mehta, 2007).

• Hippocampal stem cells promoting neurogenesis for memory function may be sensitive to radiation dose as low as 5 Gy (Stieber & Mehta, 2007).

• Specific areas of cognitive impairments from RT may include slowed information processing speed, alterations in executive function, impaired memory, impaired sustained attention, and dysfunction of motor coordination (Meyers & Kayl, 2002).

iii. Associated factors

• Cognitive decline occurs with aging (Meyers & Kayl, 2002); neuropsychological measurement batteries have established age-based norms (Lezak et al., 2004).

• Presence of apolipoprotein E ε4 gene has been associated with cognitive decline in long-term cancer survivors; areas of specific decline pertained to visual memory and visuospatial skills (Ahles & Saykin, 2007; Ahles et al., 2003).

- Premorbid intelligence and educational attainment may offer a protective component in the development of cognitive impairment (Lezak et al., 2004).
- Individuals undergoing concurrent RT and high-dose chemotherapy may be at higher risk for developing cognitive impairment (Meyers & Kayl, 2002).

(c) Assessment

i. Perform a thorough neurologic and physical examination (see Table 10).

ii. Global neurocognitive assessment can be performed for trending change over time with instruments such as the Mini-Mental State Examination. However, global cognitive assessments are limited in discerning mild cognitive impairments (Allen, 2011).

iii. Subjective cognitive instruments assess the patient's perspective of cognitive function (Allen, 2011). Some of these include the Attentional Function Index, Cognitive Failures Questionnaire, Functional Assessment of Cancer Therapy–Cognitive, Patient's Assessment of Own Functioning Inventory, and Perception of Cognition Questionnaire.

iv. Consider neuroradiographic evaluations to rule out vascular-related dementia.

v. Obtain laboratory profiles such as blood chemistries, liver function tests, and complete blood counts.

(d) Documentation: According to facility requirements; see Figure 18 for standard documentation sources.

(e) Collaborative management

i. Monitoring for changes in subjective and global cognitive function measures is useful over time.

ii. Consider referral to a neuropsychologist for a complete neuropsychological evaluation if changes are observed. A baseline evaluation of cognitive function early in the diagnosis is helpful in order to objectively monitor for changes over time.

iii. Consider pharmacologic and nonpharmacologic interventions (Allen, 2011).

- Although methylphenidate and other stimulants have been suggested as being useful in improving cognitive impairment, study limitations warrant further research.
- Cognitive training programs also have demonstrated some benefit in improving cognitive function, yet need further research.
- Use of erythropoietin-stimulating agents for cognitive function is not recommended because of FDA warnings.

(f) Patient and family education

i. Monitor for signs of cognitive change over time; have the patient or family contact the healthcare team if changes are observed.

ii. Refer to a neuropsychologist for a complete neuropsychological evaluation if changes are observed. Follow recommendations, which may include the following.

- Monitor effects of stimulants and make appropriate dose adjustments; monitor for associated side effects.
- Provide information on available cognitive training programs.

iii. Provide information regarding support for the patient and family, as this is a long-term disability and special needs may be required (see Figure 19).

(6) Post-RT vasculopathy

(a) Pathophysiology: Inflammation to intracranial and extracranial vessels creates vascular irregularities (Grisold, Oberndorfer, & Struhal, 2009; Johannesen et al., 2003).

(b) Incidence: In a long-term follow-up 6–25 years after total irradiation doses of 45–59.4 Gy, adult survivors of primary brain tumors were observed to have hemorrhagic foci (24%), large confluent areas of white matter changes (52%), and lacunar white matter lesions (55%) (Johannesen et al., 2003). Although white matter changes were found in all subjects, increasing age influenced the severity of lesions.

(c) Assessment
  i. Perform a thorough neurologic and physical examination (see Table 10).
  ii. Assess onset of symptoms such as headache, syncope, and other stroke-like symptoms.
  iii. Consider neuroradiographic evaluations to determine the type of vascular impairment and associated cerebral edema.
  iv. Obtain laboratory profiles such as coagulation profiles, blood chemistries, liver function tests, and complete blood counts.

(d) Documentation: According to facility requirements; see Figure 18 for standard documentation sources.

(e) Collaborative management
  i. Treatment is aimed at correction of the underlying cause and correction of coagulopathies.
  ii. Manage associated symptoms, such as steroid therapy for cerebral edema.

(f) Patient and family education
  i. Provide information regarding support for the patient and family for long-term disability and special needs that may be required (see Figure 19).
  ii. Provide information regarding persistent risk for recurrent vascular events and monitoring of recurrent events of stroke symptoms.

References

Adkison, J., Thomadsen, B., & Howard, S.P. (2008). Systemic iodine 125 activity after GliaSite brachytherapy: Safety considerations. *Brachytherapy, 7*, 43–46. doi:10.1016/j.brachy.2007.11.001

Affronti, M.L., Heery, C.R., Herndon, J.E., II, Rich, J.N., Reardon, D.A., Desjardins, A., ... Friedman, H.S. (2009). Overall survival of newly diagnosed glioblastoma patients receiving carmustine wafers followed by radiation and concurrent temozolomide plus rotational multiagent chemotherapy. *Cancer, 115*, 3501–3511. doi:10.1002/cncr.24398

Agha, A., Sherlock, M., Brennan, S., O'Connor, S.A., O'Sullivan, E., Rogers, B., ... Thompson, C.J. (2005). Hypothalamic-pituitary dysfunction after irradiation of nonpituitary brain tumors in adults. *Journal of Clinical Endocrinology and Metabolism, 90*, 6355–6360. doi:10.1210/jc.2005-1525

Ahlbom, A., Feychting, M., Green, A., Kheifets, L., Savitz, D.A., & Swerdlow, A.J. (2009). Epidemiologic evidence on mobile phones and tumor risk: A review. *Epidemiology, 20*, 639–652. doi:10.1097/EDE.0b013e3181b0927d

Ahles, T.A., & Saykin, A.J. (2007). Candidate mechanisms for chemotherapy-induced cognitive changes. *Nature Reviews Cancer, 7*, 192–201. doi:10.1038/nrc2073

Ahles, T.A., Saykin, A.J., Noll, W.W., Furstenberg, C.T., Guerin, S., Cole, B., & Mott, L.A. (2003). The relationship of APOE genotype of neuropsychological performance in long-term cancer survivors treated with standard dose chemotherapy. *Psycho-Oncology, 12*, 612–619. doi:10.1002/pon.742

Alexiou, G.A., Gogou, P., Markoula, S., & Kyritsis, A.P. (2010). Management of meningiomas. *Clinical Neurology and Neurosurgery, 112*, 177–182. doi:10.1016/j.clineuro.2009.12.011

Allen, D. (2011). Cognitive impairment. In L.H. Eaton, J.M. Tipton, & M. Irwin (Eds.), *Putting evidence into practice: Improving oncology patient outcomes, volume 2* (pp. 15–22). Pittsburgh, PA: Oncology Nursing Society.

Allen, D.H., Vredenburgh, J.J., Dryman, B., Carter, K., & Freeman, M.W. (2009). Toxicity profile for use of dronabinol in adult patients with primary malignant gliomas to manage CINV [Abstract 405]. *Neuro-Oncology, 11*, 657.

Armstrong, T., Baumgartner, K., & Min, S. (2006). Seizures. In D. Camp-Sorrell & R.A. Hawkins (Eds.), *Clinical manual for the oncology advanced practice nurse* (2nd ed., pp. 967–975). Pittsburgh, PA: Oncology Nursing Society.

Armstrong, T., & Gilbert, M. (2000). Metastatic brain tumors: Diagnosis, treatment, and nursing interventions. *Clinical Journal of Oncology Nursing, 4*, 217–225.

Armstrong, T., Hancock, C., & Gilbert, M. (2000). Symptom management of the patient with a brain tumor at the end of life [Abstract]. *Oncology Nursing Forum, 27*, 616.

Berger, M., Leibel, S., Bruner, J., Finlay, J., & Levin, V. (2002). Primary cerebral tumors. In V. Levin (Ed.), *Cancer in the nervous system* (2nd ed., pp. 75–148). New York, NY: Oxford University Press.

Bhandare, N., Jackson, A., Eisbruch, A., Pan, C.C., Flickinger, J.C., Antonelli, P., & Mendenhall, W. (2010). Radiation therapy and hearing loss. *International Journal of Radiation Oncology, Biology, Physics, 76*(Suppl. 3), S50–S57. doi:10.1016/j.ijrobp.2009.04.096

Camp-Sorrell, D. (2006). Headache. In D. Camp-Sorrell & R.A. Hawkins (Eds.), *Clinical manual for the oncology advanced practice nurse* (2nd ed., pp. 937–944). Pittsburgh, PA: Oncology Nursing Society.

Central Brain Tumor Registry of the United States. (2010). *CBTRUS statistical report: Primary brain and central nervous system tumors diagnosed in the United States in 2004-2006*. Hinsdale, IL: Author.

Cihan, Y.B., Uzun, G., Yildiz, Ş., & Dönmez, H. (2009). Hyperbaric oxygen therapy for radiation-induced brain necrosis in a patient with primary central nervous system lymphoma. *Journal of Surgical Oncology, 100*, 732–735. doi:10.1002/jso.21387

Cope, D. (2006). Fatigue. In D. Camp-Sorrell & R.A. Hawkins (Eds.), *Clinical manual for the oncology advanced practice nurse* (2nd ed., pp. 1127–1132). Pittsburgh, PA: Oncology Nursing Society.

Derrey, S., Blond, S., Reyns, N., Touzet, G., Carpentier, P., Gauthier, H., & Dhellemmes, P. (2008). Management of cystic craniopharyngiomas with stereotactic endocavitary irradiation using colloidal 186: A retrospective study of 48 consecutive patients. *Neurosurgery, 63,* 1045–1052. doi:10.1227/01.NEU.0000335786.10968.2F

Forman, A. (2002). Altered mental status. In V. Levin (Ed.), *Cancer in the nervous system* (2nd ed., pp. 543–556). New York, NY: Oxford University Press.

Foroughi, M., Kemeny, A.A., Lehecka, M., Wons, J., Kajdi, L., Hatfield, R., & Marks, S. (2010). Operative intervention for delayed symptomatic radionecrotic masses developing following stereotactic radiosurgery for cerebral arteriovenous malformations—Case analysis and literature review. *Acta Neurochirurgica, 152,* 803–815. doi:10.1007/s00701-009-0581-1

Friend, P.J., Johnston, M.P., Tipton, J.M., McDaniel, R.W., Barbour, L.A., Starr, P., … Ripple, M.L. (2009). ONS PEP resource: Chemotherapy-induced nausea and vomiting. In L.H. Eaton & J.M. Tipton (Eds.), *Putting evidence into practice: Improving oncology patient outcomes* (pp. 71–83). Pittsburgh, PA: Oncology Nursing Society.

Gaspar, L.E., Mehta, M.P., Patchell, R.A., Burri, S.H., Robinson, P.D., Morris, R.E., … Kalkanis, S.N. (2010). The role of whole brain radiation therapy in the management of newly diagnosed brain metastases: A systematic review and evidence-based clinical practice guideline. *Journal of Neuro-Oncology, 96,* 17–32. doi:10.1007/s11060-009-0060-9

Gerstner, E., & Batchelor, T. (2007). Primary CNS lymphoma. *Expert Review of Anticancer Therapy, 7,* 689–700. doi:10.1586/14737140.7.5.689

Giordana, M.T., Ghimenti, C., Leonardo, E., Balteri, I., Iudicello, M., & Duò, D. (2004). Molecular genetic study of a metastatic oligodendroglioma. *Journal of Neuro-Oncology, 66,* 265–271. doi:10.1023/B:NEON.0000014519.61604.da

Glantz, M., Cole, B., Forsyth, P., Recht, L., Wen, P., Chamberlain, M., … Cairncross, J. (2000). Practice parameter: Anticonvulsant prophylaxis in patients with newly diagnosed brain tumors. Report of the Quality Standards Subcommittee of the American Academy of Neurology. *Neurology, 54,* 1886–1893.

Grisold, W., Oberndorfer, S., & Struhal, W. (2009). Stroke and cancer: A review. *Acta Neurologica Scandinavica, 119,* 1–16. doi:10.1111/j.1600-0404.2008.01059.x

Huse, J.T., & Holland, E.C. (2010). Targeting brain cancer: Advances in the molecular pathology of malignant glioma and medulloblastoma. *Nature Reviews Cancer, 10,* 319–331. doi:10.1038/nrc2818

Iwami, K., Arima, T., Oooka, F., Fukumoto, M., Takagi, T., & Takayasu, M. (2009). Chordoid glioma with calcification and neurofilament expression: Case report and review of the literature. *Surgical Neurology, 71,* 115–120. doi:10.1016/j.surneu.2007.07.03210.1016/j.surneu.2007.07.032

James, C.D., Smith, J.S., & Jenkins, R.B. (2002). Genetic and molecular basis of primary central nervous system tumors. In V.A. Levin (Ed.), *Cancer in the nervous system* (2nd ed., pp. 239–251). New York, NY: Oxford University Press.

Jansen, C., Miaskowski, D., Dodd, M., Dowling, G., & Kramer, J. (2005). Potential mechanisms for chemotherapy-induced impairments in cognitive function. *Oncology Nursing Forum, 32,* 1151–1163. doi:10.1188/05.ONF.1151-1163

Johannesen, T.B., Lien, H.H., Hole, K.H., & Lote, K. (2003). Radiological and clinical assessment of long-term brain tumor survivors after radiotherapy. *Radiotherapy and Oncology, 69,* 169–176. doi:10.1016/S0167-8140(03)00192-0

Kalkanis, S.N., & Linskey, M.E. (2010). Evidence-based clinical practice parameter guidelines for the treatment of patients with metastatic brain tumors: Introduction. *Journal of Neuro-Oncology, 96,* 7–10. doi:10.1007/s11060-009-0065-4

Kanu, O.O., Hughes, B., Di, C., Lin, N., Fu, J., Bigner, D.D., … Adamson, C. (2009). Glioblastoma multiforme oncogenomics and signaling pathways. *Clinical Medicine Insights: Oncology, 3,* 39–52.

Kelsey, C.R., & Marks, L.B. (2006). Somnolence syndrome after focal radiation therapy to the pineal region: Case report and review of the literature. *Journal of Neuro-Oncology, 78,* 153–156. doi:10.1007/s11060-005-9073-1

Khurana, V.G., Teo, C., Kundi, M., Hardell, L., & Carlberg, M. (2009). Cell phones and brain tumors: A review including the long-term epidemiologic data. *Surgical Neurology, 72,* 205–214. doi:10.1016/j.surneu.2009.01.019

Kim, D.S., Park, S.Y., & Lee, S.P. (2004). Astroblastoma: A case report. *Journal of Korean Medical Science, 19,* 772–777. doi:10.3346/jkms.2004.19.5.772

Kirkpatrick, J.P., van der Kogel, A.J., & Schultheiss, T.E. (2010). Radiation dose-volume effects in the spinal cord. *International Journal of Radiation Oncology, Biology, Physics, 76*(Suppl. 3), S42–S49. doi:10.1016/j.ijrobp.2009.04.095

Kleihues, P., & Cavenee, W.K. (Eds.). (2000). *World Health Organization classification of tumours. Pathology and genetics of tumours of the nervous system.* Lyon, France: IARC Press.

Kozak, K.R., Mahadevan, A., & Moody, J.S. (2009). Adult gliosarcoma: Epidemiology, natural history, and factors associated with outcome. *Neuro-Oncology, 11,* 183–191. doi:10.1215/15228517-2008-076

Kunwar, S., Chang, S., Westphal, M., Vogelbaum, M., Sampson, J., Barnett, G., … Puri, R.K. (2010). Phase III randomized trial of CED of IL13-PE38QQR vs Gliadel wafers for recurrent glioblastoma. *Neuro-Oncology, 12,* 871–881. doi:10.1093/neuonc/nop054

Lawrence, Y.R., Li, X.A., el Naqa, I., Hahn, C.A., Marks, L.B., Merchant, T.E., … Dicker, A. (2010). Radiation dose-volume effects in the brain. *International Journal of Radiation Oncology, Biology, Physics, 76*(Suppl. 3), S20–S27. doi:10.1016/j.ijrobp.2009.02.091

Lee, J.W., Wen, P.Y., Hurwitz, S., Black, P., Kesari, S., Drappatz, J., … Broomfield, E.B. (2010). Morphological characteristics of brain tumors causing seizures. *Archives in Neurology, 67,* 336–342. doi:10.1001/archneurol.2010.2

Leeds, N., Kumar, A., & Jackson, E. (2002). Diagnostic imaging. In V.A. Levin (Ed.), *Cancer in the nervous system* (2nd ed., pp. 3–59). New York, NY: Oxford University Press.

Lezak, M.D., Howieson, D.B., & Loring, D.W. (2004). *Neuropsychological assessment* (4th ed.). New York, NY: Oxford University Press.

Li, J., Bentzen, S.M., Li, J., Renschler, M., & Mehta, M.P. (2008). Relationship between neurocognitive function and quality of life after whole-brain radiotherapy in patients with brain metastasis. *International Journal of Radiation Oncology, Biology, Physics, 71,* 64–70. doi:10.1016/j.ijrobp.2007.09.059

Linskey, M.E., Andrews, D.W., Asher, A.L., Burri, S.H., Kondziolka, D., Robinson, P.D., … Kalkanis, S.N. (2010). The role of stereotactic radiosurgery in the management of patients with newly diagnosed brain metastases: A systematic review and evidence-based clinical practice guideline. *Journal of Neuro-Oncology, 96,* 45–68. doi:10.1007/s11060-009-0073-4

Louis, D.N. (2006). Molecular pathology of malignant gliomas. *Annual Review of Pathology, 1,* 97–117. doi:10.1146/annurev.pathol.1.110304.100043

Louis, D.N., Ohgaki, H., Wiestler, O.D., Cavenee, W.K., Burger, P.C., Jouvet, A., … Kleihues, P. (2007). The 2007 WHO classification of tumours of the central nervous system. *Acta Neuropathologica, 114,* 97–109. doi:10.1007/s00401-007-0243-4

Lovely, M.P. (2004). Symptom management of brain tumor patients. *Seminars in Oncology Nursing, 20,* 273–283. doi:10.1016/j.soncn.2004.07.007

Maris, J.M. (2010). Recent advances in neuroblastoma. *New England Journal of Medicine, 362,* 2201–2211. doi:10.1056/NEJMra0804577

Maschio, M., Dinapoli, L., Gomellini, S., Ferraresi, V., Sperati, F., Vidiri, A., … Jandolo, B. (2010). Antiepileptics in brain metastases: Safety, efficacy and impact on life expectancy. *Journal of Neuro-Oncology, 98,* 109–116. doi:10.1007/s11060-009-0069-0

Mayo, C., Martel, M.K., Marks, L.B., Flickinger, J., Nam, J., & Kirkpatrick, J. (2010). Radiation dose-volume effects of optic nerves and chiasm. *International Journal of Radiation Oncology, Biology, Physics, 76*(Suppl. 3), S28–S35. doi:10.1016/j.ijrobp.2009.07.1753

McGuire, C.S., Sainani, K.L., & Fisher, P.G. (2009). Incidence patterns for ependymoma: A surveillance, epidemiology, and end results study. *Journal of Neurosurgery, 110,* 725–729. doi:10.3171/2008.9.JNS08117

Meyers, C.A., Geara, F., Wong, P.F., & Morrison, W.H. (2000). Neurocognitive effects of therapeutic irradiation for base of skull tumors. *International Journal of Radiation Oncology, Biology, Physics, 46,* 51–55. doi:10.1016/S0360-3016(99)00376-4

Meyers, C., & Kayl, A. (2002). Neurocognitive function. In V.A. Levin (Ed.), *Cancer in the nervous system* (2nd ed., pp. 557–571). New York, NY: Oxford University Press.

Michalski, J.M. (2008). Spinal cord. In E.C. Halperin, C.A. Perez, & L.W. Brady (Eds.), *Perez and Brady's principles and practice of radiation oncology* (5th ed., pp. 765–777). Philadelphia, PA: Lippincott Williams & Wilkins.

Mitchell, S.A., Beck, S.L., Hood, L.E., Moore, K., & Tanner, E.R. (2009). ONS PEP resource: Fatigue. In L.H. Eaton & J.M. Tipton (Eds.), *Putting evidence into practice: Improving oncology patient outcomes* (pp. 155–174). Pittsburgh, PA: Oncology Nursing Society.

Murphy-Ende, K. (2006). Nausea and vomiting. In D. Camp-Sorrell & R.A. Hawkins (Eds.), *Clinical manual for the oncology advanced practice nurse* (2nd ed., pp. 465–471). Pittsburgh, PA: Oncology Nursing Society.

National Cancer Institute. (2010). Adult brain tumors treatment (PDQ®). Retrieved from http://cancer.gov/cancertopics/pdq/treatment/adultbrain/HealthProfessional

National Comprehensive Cancer Network. (2010). *NCCN Clinical Practice Guidelines in Oncology: Central nervous system cancer* [v.1.2010]. Retrieved from http://www.nccn.org/professionals/physician_gls/PDF/cns.pdf

Ohgaki, H., & Kleihues, P. (2005). Epidemiology and etiology of gliomas. *Acta Neuropathologica, 109,* 93–108. doi:10.1007/s00401-005-0991-y

Packer, R.J., Friedman, H.S., Kun, L.E., & Fuller, G.N. (2002). Tumors of the brain stem, cerebellum, and fourth ventricle. In V.A. Levin (Ed.), *Cancer in the nervous system* (2nd ed., pp. 171–192). New York, NY: Oxford University Press.

Parwani, A.V., Stelow, E.B., Pambuccian, S.E., Burger, P.C., & Ali, S.Z. (2005). Atypical teratoid/rhabdoid tumor of the brain: Cytopathologic characteristics and differential diagnosis. *Cancer, 105,* 65–70. doi:10.1002/cncr.20872

Preusser, M., Hoischen, A., Novak, K., Czech, T., Prayer, D., Hainfellner, J., … Hans, V. (2007). Angiocentric glioma: Report of clinico-pathologic and genetic findings in 8 cases. *American Journal of Surgical Pathology, 31,* 1709–1718. doi:10.1097/PAS.0b013e31804a7ebb

Rannan-Eliya, Y.F., Rannan-Eliya, S., Graham, K., Pizer, B., & McDowell, H.P. (2007). Surgical interventions for the treatment of radiation-induced alopecia in pediatric practice. *Pediatric Blood and Cancer, 49,* 731–760. doi:10.1002/pbc.20689

Reardon, D.A., Zalutsky, M.R., Akabani, G., Coleman, R.E., Friedman, A.H., Herndon, J.E., II, … Bigner, D.D. (2008). A pilot study: ^{131}I-antitenascin monoclonal antibody 81c6 to deliver a 44-Gy resection cavity boost. *Neuro-Oncology, 10,* 182–189. doi:10.1215/15228517-2007-053

Roberge, D., Parker, W., Niazi, T.M., & Olivares, M. (2005). Treating the contents and not the container: Dosimetric study of hair-sparing whole brain intensity modulated radiation therapy. *Technology in Cancer Research and Treatment, 4,* 567–570.

Robinson, P.D., Kalkanis, S.N., Linskey, M.E., & Santaguida, P.L. (2010). Methodology used to develop the AANS/CNS management of brain metastases evidence-based clinical practice parameter guidelines. *Journal of Neuro-Oncology, 96,* 11–16. doi:10.1007/s11060-009-0059-2

Ryken, T.C., McDermott, M., Robinson, P.D., Ammirati, M., Andrews, D.W., Asher, A.L., … Kalkanis, S.N. (2010). The role of steroids in the management of brain metastases: A systematic review and evidence-based clinical practice guideline. *Journal of Neuro-Oncology, 96,* 103–114. doi:10.1007/s11060-009-0057-4

Sanson, M., Napolitano, M., Cartalat-Carel, S., & Taillibert, S. (2005). [Gliomatosis cerebri]. *Revue Neurologique, 161,* 173–181.

Schoemaker, M.J., Robertson, L., Wigertz, A., Jones, M.E., Hosking, F.J., Feychting, M., … Swerdlow, A. (2010). Interaction between 5 genetic variants and allergy in glioma risk. *American Journal of Epidemiology, 171,* 1165–1173.

Siegel, R., Ward, E., Brawley, O., & Jemal, A. (2011). Cancer statistics, 2011. *CA: A Cancer Journal for Clinicians, 61,* 212–236. doi:10.3322/caac.20121

Siker, M.L., Donahue, B.R., Volgelbaum, M.A., Toma, W.A., Gilbert, M.R., & Mehta, M.P. (2008). Primary intracranial neoplasms. In E.C. Halperin, C.A. Perez, & L.W. Brady (Eds.), *Perez and Brady's principles and practice of radiation oncology* (5th ed., pp. 717–750). Philadelphia, PA: Lippincott Williams & Wilkins.

Snell, R. (2010). *Clinical neuroanatomy* (7th ed.). Philadelphia, PA: Lippincott Williams & Wilkins.

Stewart-Amidei, C. (2005). Managing symptoms and side effects during brain tumor illness. *Expert Review of Neurotherapeutics, 5*(Suppl. 6), S71–S76. doi:10.1586/14737175.5.6.S71

Stieber, V.W., & Mehta, M.P. (2007). Advances in radiation therapy for brain tumors. *Neurologic Clinics, 25,* 1005–1033. doi:10.1016/j.ncl.2007.07.005

Stupp, R., Hegi, M.E., Mason, W.P., van den Bent, M.J., Taphoorn, M.J., Janzer, R.C., … Mirimanoff, R.O. (2009). Effects of radiotherapy with concomitant and adjuvant temozolomide versus radiotherapy alone on survival in glioblastoma in a randomised phase III study: 5-year analysis of the EORTC-NCIC trial. *Lancet Oncology, 10,* 459–466. doi:10.1016/S1470-2045(09)70025-7

Thiessen, B., Maguire, J.A., McNeil, K., Huntsman, D., Martin, M.A., & Horsman, D. (2003). Loss of heterozygosity for loci on chromosome arms 1p and 10q in oligodendroglial tumors: Relationship to outcome and chemosensitivity. *Journal of Neuro-Oncology, 64,* 271–278. doi:10.1023/A:1025689004046

Trüeb, R.M. (2009). Chemotherapy-induced alopecia. *Seminars in Cutaneous Medicine and Surgery, 28,* 11–14. doi:10.1016/j.sder.2008.12.001

Vela-Chávez, T.A., Arrecillas-Zamora, M.D., Quintero-Cuadra, L.Y., & Fend, F. (2009). Granulocytic sarcoma of the breast without development of bone marrow involvement: A case report. *Diagnostic Pathology, 4,* 2. doi:10.1186/1746-1596-4-2

Wefel, J.S., Witgert, M.E., & Meyers, C.A. (2008). Neuropsychological sequelae of non-central nervous system cancer and cancer therapy. *Neuropsychology Review, 18,* 121–131. doi:10.1007/s11065-008-9058-x

Wen, P.Y., Schiff, D., Kesari, S., Drappatz, J., Gigas, D.C., & Doherty, L. (2006). Medical management of patients with brain tumors. *Journal of Neuro-Oncology, 80,* 313–332. doi:10.1007/s11060-006-9193-2

Wilson-Pauwels, L., Stewart, P., Akesson, E., & Spacey, S. (2010). *Cranial nerves: Function and dysfunction* (3rd ed.). Shelton, CT: People's Medical Publishing House.

Wolff, J.E.A., Sajedi, M., Brant, R., Coppes, M.J., & Egeler, R.M. (2002). Choroid plexus tumours. *British Journal of Cancer, 87,* 1086–1091. doi:10.1038/sj.bjc.6600609

B. Head and neck
  1. Incidence: Head and neck cancers account for approximately 5% of all cancers. In 2011, an estimated 52,140 people in the United States were diagnosed with cancers of the oral cavity, pharynx, or larynx. The estimated number of deaths in 2011 from these specific cancers is approximately 11,460 (Siegel, Ward, Brawley, & Jemal, 2011). New cases are 2.5 times more common in men than in women. Approximately 90% of oral cancers occur in patients 45 years or older (Carr, 2011; Siegel et al., 2011).
  2. Sites
    a) Head and neck squamous cell cancers develop from membranes lining the upper aerodigestive tract (Edge et al., 2010).
    b) Six major sites exist for head and neck cancer: the oral cavity, the pharynx (nasopharynx, oropharynx, and hypopharynx), the larynx, the paranasal sinuses, the salivary glands, and the thyroid gland (Edge et al., 2010).
    c) Regional lymph node status is the primary prognostic indicator for all head and neck cancers and must be assessed to accurately stage the disease. Survival is significantly worse if lymph nodes past the first echelon or in the supraclavicular region are positive for cancer (Edge et al., 2010).
  3. Squamous cell carcinoma
    a) Predominant histopathology of head and neck cancers (Edge et al., 2010)
    b) The full etiology of squamous cell carcinoma of the head and neck region remains unknown, but it is clearly linked to exposure to tobacco and alcohol. Oral and environmental irritants are risk factors for the disease (Carper, 2007).
    c) Human papillomavirus (HPV) is recognized to play a role in the pathogenesis of a subset of head and neck squamous cell carcinomas. HPV-positive tumors may be associated with a better prognostic outcome. Fakhry et al. (2008) reported in their prospective trial of 96 patients with advanced-stage head and neck cancer that patients with HPV-positive tumors were associated with the Caucasian race, had better performance status, and were less likely to have 20 or more pack-years of exposure to cigarettes.
  4. Treatment for head and neck cancer
    a) Treatment is dependent on the tumor location and stage. Stage I and II head and neck cancers often can be cured with single-modality treatment. Most patients are diagnosed with locally advanced disease and are best managed in a multidisciplinary setting. Surgery, radiation, chemotherapy, and more recently biologic therapy often are employed in various combinations to eradicate tumor and maintain function and quality of life. The use of higher radiation doses, sophisticated delivery techniques, and radiosensitizing chemotherapy have improved survival and local control (Burri & Lee, 2009).
    b) Aggressive treatment resulting in tumor control comes with increased acute and late toxicities. Nursing management of radiation toxicities enhances outcomes for both survival and quality of life.
  5. Head and neck cancer and treatment symptoms
    a) Mucositis, stomatitis, pharyngitis, esophagitis (upper one-third of esophagus)
      (1) Pathophysiology: *Mucositis* is the inflammation and potential ulceration of the mucous membranes that occurs secondary to cytotoxic cancer treatment, including both chemotherapy and radiation. *Mucositis* is a general term; terms such as *stomatitis, pharyngitis, esophagitis,* and others may be used to discuss mucositis found in specific structures. Although the pathogenesis of mucositis is not completely understood, it is a complex process involving biologic and chemical interactions (Eilers & Million, 2007). Damage to mucosal tissues can contribute to potential adverse outcomes, including treatment breaks, dehydra-

tion, narcotic use, weight loss, hospitalization, and increased cost (Narayan et al., 2008). Sonis et al. (2004) described the biologic phases of mucositis. These phases include

(a) Initiation: DNA and non-DNA damage, direct cellular injury to basal epithelial cells, and generation of reactive oxygen species

(b) Primary damage response: Damage to genes is followed by upregulation of genes that results in the production of a range of destructive proteins and molecules such as the proinflammatory cytokines. This upregulation leads to apoptosis and tissue injury.

(c) Signal amplification: Substances from the damage response phase provide a positive feedback loop that drives the destructive process forward.

(d) Ulceration: The oral epithelium breaks down and ulcerates. Infections may occur at this stage, as it frequently corresponds with neutropenia and an increase in gram-negative organisms. Infections may be viral, bacterial, or fungal (e.g., candidiasis).

(e) Healing: Biologically dynamic phase with signaling from the submucosal extracellular matrix, stimulating the migration, differentiation, and proliferation of the healing epithelium (Harris, Eilers, Harriman, Cashavelly, & Maxwell, 2008; Scully, Sonis, & Diz, 2006).

(2) Incidence and risk factors

(a) Trotti et al. (2003) performed a systematic literature review to better understand the incidence and clinical and economic consequences of acute mucositis in the head and neck population. These authors found a mean mucositis incidence of 80%, with severe mucositis in 56% of patients receiving altered fractionation compared to 34% of patients who received conventional radiation (Trotti et al., 2003). Incidence of mucositis lesions is related to the field, radiation dose per fraction, and individual variables (Avritscher, Cooksley, & Elting, 2004; Epstein,

Wan, Chrisman, Dale, & Jackson, 2007). Palazzi et al. (2008) studied 149 patients with head and neck cancer and found the incidence of severe symptoms (mucositis, dysphagia, pain, and skin toxicity) to range from 12% to 40%. Severe symptoms were worse in patients receiving RT in combination with chemotherapy. Symptoms may begin as early as within one week and typically resolve within four to eight weeks (Epstein et al., 2007; Narayan et al., 2008). Some late effects, including chronic open wounds, mucosal scarring, and loss of mucosal compliance, may occur (Rosenthal & Trotti, 2009).

(b) Patient risk factors (Eilers & Million, 2007; Rosenthal & Trotti, 2009)

　i. Age (children and older adults)

　ii. Sex (women are at higher risk for severe mucositis)

　iii. Poor oral health and hygiene

　iv. Decreased salivary flow

　v. High levels of cytokines

　vi. Low BMI (less than 20 for men, less than 19 for women)

　vii. Decreased renal function

　viii. Smoking

　ix. Previous cancer treatment

　x. Blood or stem cell transplantation

(c) Treatment risk factors (Eilers & Million, 2007; Rosenthal & Trotti, 2009)

　i. Radiation site

　ii. Use of hyperfractionation or accelerated RT (greater than 20 Gy)

　iii. Use of chemotherapy with RT

(3) Assessment

(a) Many mucositis assessment and grading tools are available. Ideally, the same tool that is tested for interrater reliability should be used throughout a patient's treatment course. The tool should address physical and functional aspects of the assessment. The Oral Assessment Guide for nurses is one such tool (see Table 12). Patient-reported symptom inventories also are available and avoid interrater variability and accurately capture the patient's symptom burden (Rosenthal et al., 2008). The goal of assessment is to track changes over time and to tailor interventions to specific findings.

(b) A baseline oral assessment and dental evaluation should occur before treatment begins. Poor oral hygiene and poor dentition should be addressed before initiation of treatment to prevent worsening of problems during and after treatment.

(c) Oral assessment and intervention should occur weekly or more frequently if the patient experiences mouth lesions, pain, weight loss, taste alterations, salivary changes, voice changes, or dysphagia (Palazzi et al., 2008). Weekly weights are included in assessments.

Table 12. Oral Assessment Guide

Category	Tools for Assessment	Methods of Measurement	Numeric and Descriptive Ratings		
			1	2	3
Voice	Auditory	Converse with patient	Normal	Deeper or raspy	Difficulty talking or painful
Swallow	Observation	Ask patient to swallow. To test gag reflex, gently place blade on back of tongue and depress. Observe result.	Normal swallow	Some pain on swallow	Unable to swallow
Lips	Visual observation/palpation	Observe and feel tissue.	Smooth, pink, and moist	Dry or cracked	Ulcerated or bleeding
Tongue	Visual observation and/or palpation	Feel and observe appearance of tissue.	Pink, moist, and papillae present	Coated or loss of papillae with a shiny appearance with or without redness	Blistered or cracked
Saliva	Tongue blade	Insert blade into mouth, touching the center of the tongue and the floor of the mouth.	Watery	Thick or ropy	Absent
Mucous membranes	Visual observation	Observe appearance of tissue.	Pink and moist	Reddened or coated (increased whiteness) without ulcerations	Ulcerations with or without bleeding
Gingiva	Tongue blade and visual observation	Gently press tissue with tip of blade.	Pink and stippled and firm	Edematous with or without redness	Spontaneous bleeding or bleeding with pressure
Teeth or dentures (or denture-bearing area)	Visual observation	Observe appearance of teeth or denture-bearing area.	Clean and no debris	Plaque or debris in localized areas (between teeth if present)	Plaque or debris generalized along gum line or denture-bearing area

Note. Table courtesy of June Eilers, PhD, APRN-CNS, BC, The Nebraska Medical Center. Used with permission.

(d) Physical examination: Examine lips, tongue, gingiva, and oral cavity for color, moisture, integrity, and presence of lesions, ulcers, or infection.

(e) Functional examination: Obtain patient report of difficulties with eating, swallowing, or talking.

(4) Documentation

(a) According to the Oral Assessment Guide (see Table 12): Every aspect should be scored. A score of 8 is normal, scores of 9–16 indicate mild to moderate mucositis, and scores of 17–24 indicate moderate to severe mucositis.

(b) Additional documentation may include grading of mucous membrane assessment, presence or absence of thrush, severity of dysphagia or odynophagia, and a complete pain assessment.

(c) The NCI CTEP common toxicity grading developed in 1998 has been widely adopted for reporting mucositis toxicity. This grading scale has been updated, and version 4.03 was published in 2010.

(5) Oral mucositis grading (NCI CTEP, 2010)

(a) 1—Asymptomatic or mild symptoms; intervention not indicated

(b) 2—Moderate pain; not interfering with oral intake; modified diet indicated

(c) 3—Severe pain; interfering with oral intake

(d) 4—Life-threatening consequences; urgent intervention indicated

(e) 5—Death

(6) Collaborative management of mucositis, stomatitis, pharyngitis, and esophagitis

(a) Prevention

 i. No current FDA-approved interventions exist for prevention of radiation-induced mucositis.

 ii. Recommendations for basic oral care (Eilers & Million, 2007; Harris et al., 2008; Rosenthal & Trotti, 2009)

 • Schedule dental evaluation for care of existing teeth; perform necessary dental extraction before radiation begins. Refer to section

on xerostomia for recommendations on long-term use of fluoride. Patients may describe prescription-strength fluoride gel as irritating to oral mucositis. When prescription-strength fluoride is irritating to mucositis, it should be held until mucositis heals.

• Wearing fluoride dental guards (without fluoride) during treatment may reduce the severity of mucositis (not evidence-based). This will physically add distance between buccal or lingual tissues and dental work, decreasing the incidence of "scatter" lesions. If patients find that the guards take up too much space in their mouth, the same benefit can be achieved by using damp gauze between dental work and the cheek or tongue.

• Avoid irritants such as alcohol, cigarettes, alcohol-based mouthwashes, spicy foods, and rough items.

• Brush teeth and prosthetics with a soft toothbrush after each meal and at bedtime. Use a toothpaste containing fluoride. Floss teeth if this is part of the patient's normal routine. Patients should discontinue flossing when thrombocytopenic (platelets less than 50,000) or neutropenic (absolute neutrophil count less than 1,000) as necessary.

• Frequently use bland mouth rinses (normal saline with or without sodium bicarbonate), lasting one to two minutes (see section IV.G—Nutritional issues).

• Maintain hydration and a diet high in calories and protein. Supplemental nutrition drinks (Ensure®, Boost®, Carnation Instant Breakfast®) may be required.

- Use water-based moisturizers (such as Aquaphor® [Beiersdorf Inc.]) to protect lips.
  iii. Limit treatment intensification to those patients most likely to benefit and in whom it would not risk the probability of curing the cancer.
  iv. Use radiosensitizing agents that do not worsen mucositis, such as cisplatin.
  v. Interventions that may have some benefit for prevention but require further research include amifostine, antibiotic pastille or paste, benzydamine, calcium phosphate (Caphosol®, EUSA Pharma), glutamine, growth factors, honey, hydrolytic enzymes, ice chips, low-level-laser therapy, povidone, and zinc sulfate (Eilers & Million, 2007). Amifostine is FDA-approved to decrease xerostomia (Rosenthal & Trotti, 2009). The salivary preservation may have an indirect effect; however, no current recommendation advises use of this agent to prevent mucositis. It should be noted that amifostine toxicity includes nausea, vomiting, and hypotension. Benzydamine is a topical nonsteroidal agent not currently FDA-approved in the United States but is available in Canada and the European Union. A phase III trial showed that benzydamine reduced the incidence of mucositis at 50 Gy. It has not been recommended, howev-

er, because most patients are treated at doses greater than 60 Gy, and a large phase III, randomized placebo trial in the United States was closed early because an interim analysis concluded that continuation was futile (Eilers & Million, 2007; Rosenthal & Trotti, 2009).

(b) Interventions for mouth and throat tenderness
   i. Continue recommendations for basic oral care. In a study of self-care behaviors among 49 patients with head and neck cancer, frequent rinsing and oral analgesics were found to be the most effective interventions (Wong et al., 2006). These findings were supported by Ogama et al. (2010), who found that frequency of oral care correlates with appetite and quality of life.
   ii. Perform more frequent mouth assessments to evaluate possible infection. Bacterial and fungal infections should be treated with appropriate medications. Oral ketoconazole or fluconazole are preferred over topical nystatin (Rosenthal & Trotti, 2009).
   iii. Assess weight and hydration biweekly. A feeding tube may be necessary if aspiration, inadequate hydration, or rapid weight loss is a concern.
   iv. Minimize use of dentures.
   v. Pain management is imperative. Patients will likely require both systemic and topical analgesics. Drug dose, frequency, and duration should be adjusted frequently to provide adequate pain relief.
      - Systemic: Recommendations should be made based on the patient's ability to swallow, the level of pain, and the agent's compatibility with other medications. Patients with neutropenia should be reminded that anti-inflammatory medication or acetaminophen

could mask a fever. Transdermal pain medication or delivery of pain medication through a feeding tube is an option for patients who cannot swallow or who are at risk for aspiration.

- Topical: Topical agents should be used if patients are able to achieve pain control with the agent. Many of these agents have demonstrated only minor benefits in small studies. Patients should be warned of the potential for worsening damage with numbing agents. Agents available include viscous lidocaine and various "magic mouthwash" recipes. These mouthwashes have not been shown to be superior to bland rinses (Harris et al., 2008). The following agents have been FDA approved as medical devices: Gelclair® (EKR Therapeutics, Inc.), MuGard™ (Access Pharmaceuticals, Inc.), and Caphosol (Rosenthal & Trotti, 2009). Sucralfate is not recommended because of insufficient evidence (Harris et al., 2008; Rosenthal & Trotti, 2009).
- Investigational approaches. Topical recombinant human epidermal growth factor (rhEGF)—Hong et al. (2009) used rhEGF on 11 patients who developed severe mucositis after head and neck irradiation and found that all patients showed significant improvement. Further studies are needed to determine optimal dosage and schedule.

(7) Patient and family education

(a) Instruct the patient and family about the oral care regimen and need for routine follow-up with a dentist. Elements of oral care regimen:

  i. Brush teeth four times a day with a soft toothbrush.

  ii. Floss daily, if flossed previously.

  iii. Rinse the mouth four times a day with a bland rinse and increase as needed for comfort.

  iv. Remove and clean dental appliances each time the mouth is cleaned.

  v. Avoid irritants (e.g., tobacco; alcohol; rough, spicy, or acidic foods and fluids).

  vi. Encourage a soft pureed or liquid diet including oral liquid supplements.

  vii. Refer for dietary counseling.

  viii. Monitor for pain and consult with physician about use of topical and systemic analgesics if indicated.

  ix. Monitor for signs of fungal, viral, or bacterial infections and consult with physician about use of medications if indicated.

  x. Monitor weight, fluid, and nutrition status and consult with physician about placement of a feeding tube or use of IV hydration if indicated.

  xi. Instruct the patient on swallowing and jaw exercises to maintain swallowing function and prevent jaw tightening.

(b) Instruct the patient to perform oral assessment daily and symptoms to monitor and report to the healthcare provider. Provide written instruction and education. Verify understanding with return explanation and demonstration (Harris, Eilers, Cashavelly, Maxwell, & Harriman, 2009).

b) Dysphagia

(1) Pathophysiology: *Dysphagia*, or difficult or painful swallowing (painful swallowing is known by the more specific term *odynophagia*), is a common symptom that patients with head and neck tumors experience. The normal swallowing mechanism is characterized by the oral preparatory, oral, pharyngeal, and esophageal phases. The completion of swallowing involves an involuntary reflex that must be triggered, and this is frequently affected by therapy (Rosenthal, Lewin, & Eisbruch, 2006). Swallowing can be dis-

rupted in the following ways (Gould & Lewis, 2006; Nguyen, Smith, & Sallah, 2007; Rosenthal et al., 2006).

(a) Size or location of tumor interrupts or damages the coordinated process needed to swallow.

(b) Surgical resection impedes the swallowing process. Flap reconstructions may cause difficulty with sensation, mobility, and lack of secretions. Tracheostomy placement also may interfere with swallowing in all phases.

(c) Oral mucositis/esophagitis (acute effect) develops. Thick, ropy secretions interfere with swallowing and lead to gagging, regurgitation, and increased risk for aspiration.

(d) Late effects from RT and chemotherapy can lead to fibrosis, vascular and nerve injury, and submandibular lymphedema.

(2) Incidence and risk factors: The literature reports that a wide range of patients are affected by dysphagia. Some authors report that all patients are affected to some degree, with up to 50% experiencing significant dysphagia (Rosenthal et al., 2006). Trotti et al. (2003) reported an incidence of 56% in a review of published studies that included 660 patients. High-dose radiation and concurrent chemotherapy treatments are known to cause higher rates of dysphagia. The literature has stated that dysphagia is underreported (Rosenthal et al., 2006; Trotti et al., 2003).

(a) Incidence is dependent upon tumor size, tumor location, radiation dose, and use of concurrent chemotherapy.

  i. Tumor size and location—At highest risk are patients with T3 and T4 lesions. Locations of highest risk are the hypopharynx and larynx (Rosenthal et al., 2006).

  ii. Acute side effect from radiation and chemotherapy—Palazzi et al. (2008) found concomitant chemotherapy to be the only significant variable to predict dysphagia.

  iii. Long-term effects—Although the literature indicates underreporting and lack of adequate

measurement tools, Caudell et al. (2009) found 38.5% of patients to have long-term dysphagia in a study of 122 patients treated for locally advanced head and neck cancer. Smith, Goldman, Beitler, and Wadler (2004) found significant differences in long-term effects in patients treated with greater than 74.4 Gy compared to patients treated with 60 Gy. In this study, 78% of patients in the first group required gastrostomy feedings at 12 months compared to only 18% in the 60 Gy group.

(b) Patient risk factors (Lazarus, 2009; Rosenthal et al., 2006)

  i. Increased age

  ii. Dysphagia at presentation

  iii. T3 or T4 lesion (associated with severe late toxicity)

  iv. Involvement of pharynx, hypopharynx, and larynx

(c) Treatment risk factors

  i. Use of concomitant chemotherapy

  ii. Radiation to the pharynx, larynx, and hypopharynx: Late effect of fibrosis to the pharyngeal constrictor muscles is associated with more challenging swallowing and poor swallowing outcome.

  iii. High-dose radiation (doses greater than 60 Gy) (Rancati et al., 2010)

  iv. Severe mucositis

  v. Lack of access to collaborative management for dysphagia before, during, and after treatment

(3) Assessment

(a) Perform baseline and ongoing oral assessment. Evaluate range of motion of lips, tongue, and jaw. Assess cough reflex and gag reflex.

(b) Modified barium swallow is recognized as the gold standard for swallowing evaluation. Patients should receive serial examinations to ensure continued safe alimentation (Rosenthal et al., 2006).

(c) Nutrition assessment—Evaluate laboratory values and physical indications of dehydration and malnutrition. Evaluate the patient's current intake. Obtain dietitian consult prior to therapy; follow up throughout treatment and thereafter.

(d) Pain assessment—Painful swallowing may be related to infection, tumor infiltration, or inflammation from radiation.

(e) Swallowing (nonradiologic), pain, and weight assessments should be evaluated weekly during treatment.

(4) Documentation

(a) Consensus in the literature finds inadequate evaluation of dysphagia and aspiration risk. The CTCAE (version 4.03, NCI CTEP, 2010) is an accepted grading system.

   i. 1—Symptomatic; able to eat regular diet

   ii. 2—Symptomatic and altered eating/swallowing

   iii. 3—Severely altered eating/swallowing; tube feeding, TPN, or hospitalization indicated.

   iv. 4—Life-threatening consequences; urgent intervention indicated

   v. 5—Death

(b) Additional documentation may include complete pain assessment and response to interventions and presence of absence of thrush.

(5) Collaborative management

(a) Acute side effects—Goals are to optimize comfort, swallowing safety, hydration, and nutrition.

   i. Pain management—Treatment of painful oral lesions, xerostomia, and infection will improve swallowing. See previous recommendations for pain management.

   ii. Swallowing therapy and direct swallowing exercises are effective when initiated early and improve patient quality of life (Nguyen et al., 2007). Swallowing exercises designed to strengthen musculature, increase the precision of movements, and maintain range of motion are most beneficial for prevention of long-term dysfunction. Patients are recommended to swallow volumes and viscosities of food as maximally tolerated, even if a feeding tube is present. Swallowing pathologists should be consulted for the optimal exercise regimen and patient education (Lazarus, 2009; Rosenthal et al., 2006). Although some studies have not shown decreased tongue strength or ability to maintain oral nutrition, other studies have shown improved quality of life for patients who were randomized to perform swallowing exercises (Lazarus, 2009).

   iii. Prophylactic gastrostomy tube placement is controversial. Gastrostomy tube placement is necessary when the patient is aspirating or cannot maintain hydration and nutrition. Periods of nothing-by-mouth (NPO) should be avoided whenever possible because of the association with poor swallowing outcomes (Rosenthal et al., 2006). Chen et al. (2010) evaluated the role of prophylactic gastrostomy tube prior to chemoradiation for head and neck cancer. They concluded that gastrostomy tube placement was effective at preventing acute weight loss and the need for IV hydration, but it was associated with significantly higher rates of esophageal toxicity. The benefits should be balanced with the risks.

   iv. Assess the patient at least biweekly or if new complaints emerge during manifestation of acute side effects.

   v. Consult with a dietitian for appropriate dietary interventions, such as eating small, frequent meals, increasing calories and protein, and ensuring proper texture of diet, or recommendation of a feeding tube (Gould & Lewis, 2006).

   vi. Techniques that may be effective to decrease the severity of dysphagia: Use of IMRT to reduce radiation dose to critical structures, use of amifostine, use of cetuximab (head and neck cancer) or rituximab (non-Hodgkin lymphoma) as radiosensitizers, and limiting the radiation dose to the larynx (Nguyen et al., 2007; Rosenthal et al., 2006).

(b) Long-term risk for dysphagia—By optimizing swallowing technique during therapy, most patients will be able to maintain nutrition without the need for a gastrostomy tube long term. Caudell et al. (2009) identified three factors that, if present 12 months after the completion of therapy, indicate long-term issues with dysphagia: percutaneous endoscopic gastrostomy tube dependence, aspiration, and presence of pharyngoesophageal stricture. Optimal swallowing interventions include the following.

　i. Good oral hygiene—Evaluate for good dentition and properly fitting dentures or prosthesis; encourage comfort measures for xerostomia, meticulous oral hygiene, and fluoride treatments; promote and encourage good nutrition.

　ii. Evaluation by swallowing pathologist—Patients with post-treatment dysphagia should be evaluated annually or when symptoms change. Evaluation may detect specific problems with dysphagia and encourage preventive measures for safe eating and decreasing fibrosis.

　iii. Long-term follow-up should include an assessment for changes in nutrition intake, for symptoms of aspiration, and for compliance with exercises or swallowing techniques recommended by the swallowing pathologist. Radiographic swallowing studies and follow-up with the swallowing pathologist should be ordered upon changes in nutrition or complaint of dysphagia.

(6) Patient and family education

(a) Instruct the patient and family on maintaining adequate nutrition, caloric and protein intake, and the need for follow-up with the oncologist, swallowing pathologist, and other professionals as needed.

(b) Instruct the patient on symptoms of dysphagia and aspiration and which symptoms to monitor and report to the healthcare provider.

(c) Instruct the patient to swallow as much as possible during treatment, perform swallowing exercises daily as ordered, and strive for swallowing recovery as quickly as possible (Lazarus, 2009; Rosenthal et al., 2006).

(d) Instruct the patient to follow the recommendations for oral care as outlined previously with special attention to pain assessment, need for analgesia, signs of thrush, weight, and fluid and nutrition status.

c) Xerostomia

(1) Pathophysiology: *Xerostomia* is defined as an individual's subjective feeling of dry mouth and salivary gland hypofunction (Orellana, Lagravère, Boychuk, Major, & Flores-Mir, 2006). Within the oral cavity are major and minor salivary glands. The major salivary glands include the parotid, submandibular, and sublingual glands. Saliva produced from the major glands keeps the mucous membranes of the mouth moist, lubricates food during mastication, begins the digestion of starches, serves as an intrinsic "mouthwash," enhances the ability to taste, and regulates the acidity in the oral cavity to prevent tooth decay. The more than 600 minor salivary glands in the oral cavity are located in the palate, lips, cheeks, tonsils, and tongue. Minor salivary glands coat the oral cavity to keep it moist (Moore & Agur, 2002). Many factors can contribute to xerostomia. Radiation to the oral cavity can result in lifelong survivorship struggles with xerostomia.

(a) Xerostomia has been reported after one week or approximately 10 Gy of radiation to the oral cavity. Severity of xerostomia is directly related to radiation dosimetry, total radiation dose, volume irradiated, fraction size, and duration of treatment. The incidence of xerostomia is much smaller for patients

in whom one or both parotids were spared from radiation (Blanco & Chao, 2006; Bruce, 2004).

(b) Radiation changes to the vascular supply and nerves supplying the salivary glands result in loss of acinar cells, alteration in duct epithelium, fibrosis, and fatty degeneration (Blanco & Chao, 2006; Bruce, 2004).

(c) Changes in the oral cavity as a result of salivary gland hypofunction include that saliva viscosity increases and impairs mouth lubrication; buffering is compromised and flora is more pathogenic; plaque levels accumulate; and the patient develops increased risk for dental caries and progressive periodontal disease (Blanco & Chao, 2006).

(2) Incidence and risk factors

(a) Every patient receiving 35 Gy to a major saliva gland will experience the effects of xerostomia. The use of IMRT, amifostine, pilocarpine, or pretreatment salivary gland transfer may reduce the damage to the glands (Blanco & Chao, 2006).

(b) Xerostomia is exacerbated by surgical excision of the salivary gland, oral infection, low humidity climate, and medications. Drug classes implicated to cause xerostomia include antidepressants, anxiolytics, antipsychotics, antihistamines, antihypertensives, diuretics, anticholinergic compounds, and analgesics (Bruce, 2004; Maher, 2004).

(3) Assessment

(a) Quality-of-life issues with prolonged xerostomia may include complaints of dryness, thirst, and burning; dental caries; difficulty with dentures; fissures; problems with chewing and swallowing leading to decreased nutrition intake; alterations in voice; increased problems with kissing; sleep disturbances; and increased risk for oral infections (Blanco & Chao, 2006; Bruce, 2004).

(b) Physical examination

i. Inspect the oral cavity. The mouth may appear dry with furrowing of the tongue. Debris may adhere to the surface. Oral secretions may be thick, ropy, or absent. Assess for signs of infection or irritation from dentures or prosthesis (Maher, 2004).

ii. Monitor weight. Weight loss may occur because of difficulty eating or swallowing.

(4) Documentation: Dry mouth (NCI CTEP, 2010)

(a) 1—Symptomatic (e.g., dry or thick saliva) without significant dietary alteration; unstimulated saliva flow greater than 0.2 ml/min

(b) 2—Moderate symptoms; oral intake alterations (e.g., copious water, other lubricants, diet limited to purees and/or soft, moist foods); unstimulated saliva 0.1–0.2 ml/min

(c) 3—Inability to adequately aliment orally; tube feeding or TPN indicated; unstimulated saliva less than 0.1 ml/min

(5) Collaborative management

(a) Prevention and treatment options

i. IMRT—Radiation treatment using IMRT protects the parotid glands, reduces the incidence and severity of xerostomia, and does not increase local failure rate of tumor. Doses less than 26–30 Gy significantly preserve salivary gland function. Study results have shown that 17%–30% of patients developed grade 2 xerostomia as a late toxicity after IMRT compared to 60%–70% with conventional radiation techniques (Chao et al., 2001; Münter et al., 2004).

ii. Radiation protectant—Brizel et al. (2000) reported a randomized study of 315 patients, half of whom received only radiation and half of whom received radiation and amifostine. At one-year follow-up, chronic xerostomia occurred in 34% of patients who received amifostine and in 57% of those who did not receive amifostine. Antonadou, Pepelassi, Synodinou, Puglisi, and Throuvalas (2002) reported on their study of 50 patients with head and neck cancer receiving radiation and carboplatin. Half of the patients received amifostine. Eighteen months after treatment completion, 27% of the patients who received amifostine experienced grade 2 xerostomia compared to 73.9% of the control group. The use of amifostine within the head and neck population is controversial. The benefit of salivary gland protection with IMRT has led some to question the need to use amifostine. Side effects from amifostine include nausea, hypotension, allergic reactions, and skin reactions at the injection site. Rades et al. (2004) reported that 14 of 39 (41%) patients with head and neck cancer receiving radiation discontinued IV amifostine because of severe adverse events. Participants in their phase III study were given either 200 or 340 mg/m^2. Prior to the five-minute IV infusion, participants received 1,000 ml IV fluids to reduce the risk of hypotension.

iii. Pilocarpine is a cholinergic drug that acts at the level of receptors that have the potential to increase saliva from residual salivary glands. Scarantino et al. (2006) summarized multiple studies in the 1990s, concluding that pilocarpine increased salivary output and resulted in signifi-cant subjective improvement in oral moisture and comfort in head and neck patients following radiation. It showed effectiveness in increasing salivary flow and reducing the symptom of xerostomia. Scarantino et al. (2006) reported on the RTOG 97-09 phase III study. The randomized, double-blinded study revealed that patients randomized to pilocarpine demonstrated a significant improvement in unstimulated salivary flow at the end of head and neck RT. It should be used with caution in patients with other comorbidities, and if ineffective after several months, the drug should be discontinued.

iv. Acupuncture for chronic xerostomia—Two proposed mechanisms support the use of acupuncture to relieve radiation-induced xerostomia: Acupuncture stimulates the autonomic nervous system, resulting in increased activity of the parasympathetic nervous system. This stimulation enhances release of neuropeptides that increase blood flow to salivary glands, which results in an increase of saliva production and possibly regeneration of tissue. The second mechanism may involve stimulation of minor salivary glands present in nonirradiated tissue (Wong, Jones, Sagar, Babjak, & Whelan, 2003). Wong et al. (2003) and Cho et al. (2008) both reported therapeutic efficacy of acupuncture on radiation-induced xerostomia. Both studies delivered acupuncture using different techniques.

v. Caphosol is a topical oral agent of supersaturated calcium phosphate rinse indicated for dry mouth that has been clinically proven to shorten the duration and severity of mucositis and relieve dry mouth when used with fluoride. Kizhner, Xu, and Krespi (2011) supported that Caphosol may lessen the complication of halitosis from xerostomia.

  vi. Additional enhancement therapies: Fox (2004) reported additional saliva enhancement therapies. They include bromhexine, anethole trithione, yohimbine, interferon alpha, primrose oil, gamma-linolenic acid, LongoVital® (Cederroth), infliximab, and cevimeline. Studies on these therapies have been with Sjögren syndrome or antidepressant therapy. No evidence exists to support they are effective with radiation-induced xerostomia.

(b) Therapeutic self-care measures (Bruce, 2004; Carr, 2011; Maher, 2004)

  i. Encourage the patient to increase fluid intake of nonacidic juices or water. This will promote comfort and support hydration and calories. The use of a portable water bottle is often a necessity in providing relief for xerostomia.

  ii. Instruct the patient to perform mouth care before and after meals and at bedtime to refresh the mouth and make eating more comfortable. Sodium bicarbonate toothpaste and swabs will help to thin the saliva and partially correct the acidic effect from the altered saliva.

  iii. The patient should avoid mouthwashes with alcohol. Normal saline mouth rinse is recommended.

  iv. Soft, moist foods are easier to consume. The patient should avoid dry and sticky foods.

  v. Commercial artificial saliva substitutes and lubricants may provide temporary relief. They are often costly.

  vi. Suggest adding humidity to the environment, especially the bedroom.

  vii. Use of sugar-free hard candy (lemon or sour flavors) and gum may increase saliva production.

  viii. Cigarette smoking and alcohol consumption will enhance xerostomia. Educate the patient about cessation and obtaining support for addiction.

  ix. Recommendations, without evidence, include drinking papaya juice (liquefies thick saliva), rinsing and expectorating a solution of meat tenderizer and water (dissolves thick saliva), and smearing olive oil on the tongue before bedtime.

  x. Instruct the patient to avoid potential injury to mucosa; for example, suction equipment may cause injury to mucosa in mouth.

d) Compromised dental integrity

  (1) Pathophysiology—Radiation to the oral cavity increases the risk for compromised dentition. Xerostomia, changes to dental collagen, trismus, oral infection, and osteoradionecrosis are the leading causes for poor dentition following radiation to the oral cavity (Sandow, 2009).

    (a) Xerostomia—Radiation-induced damage to salivary glands reduces the ability of saliva to remineralize teeth, compromises the cleaning and buffering capability of the oral cavity, and increases colonization of bacteria (Sandow, 2009).

    (b) Changes to dental collagen—Principal component of the human tooth is dentin, and 90% of dentin is collagen. Radiogenic destruction of collagen within the dental pulp contributes to fibrosis of the tooth and decreased vascularity, thereby impairing metabolism of the tooth (Springer et al., 2005).

    (c) Trismus, osteoradionecrosis, and oral cavity infections affect preservation of teeth after radiation (Sandow, 2009).

  (2) Incidence and risk factors

    (a) Treatment-related risks for compromised dental integrity include radiation dose greater than 55 Gy, RT field that includes molars, teeth in close proximity to tumor,

and radiation treatments initiated less than 14 days after extractions (Schiødt & Hermund, 2002).

(b) Oral cavity risks for compromised dental integrity include teeth that have nonrestorable fractures, extensive caries, indications for root canals, or periodontal disease (Sandow, 2009).

(c) Patient characteristics that increase risk for compromised dental integrity include poor oral hygiene, low dental awareness, lack of cooperation, heavy smoking, heavy alcohol consumption, and lack of dental insurance (Schiødt & Hermund, 2002).

(3) Assessment

(a) Oral cavity assessment needs to be performed by a dentist. The dentist needs to identify existing oral disease and potential risk for oral disease (Schiødt & Hermund, 2002).

(b) Assist the patient in obtaining dental support. The nurse should have a dental referral list and involve social services if the patient lacks financial or insurance support.

(4) Collaborative management

(a) Educate the patient and dentist about management of oral disease before RT. Confirm that the patient has seen the dentist and that teeth with unfavorable prognosis or teeth located in a high-dose field are extracted a minimum of 14 days before RT is initiated (Sandow, 2009).

(b) Confirm fluoride carriers are fabricated and delivered before the onset of mucositis. The dentist will recommend sodium fluoride gel. The nurse reinforces recommendation of daily fluoride application

for the remainder of the patient's life (Sandow, 2009).

(c) See earlier section on mucositis for recommendations on oral care during acute toxicity of treatment.

(d) See earlier section on management of xerostomia for suggested self-care.

(e) As part of survivorship care, confirm that the patient continues with aggressive oral hygiene and dental evaluations.

e) Taste changes

(1) Pathophysiology: Taste buds are the anatomic structures that house the receptor cells that subserve the sense of taste. The taste buds are located principally on the tongue but also are found on the palate, pharynx, epiglottis, and larynx. The tongue is covered with specialized structures called *papillae*, which contain taste buds. Each taste bud contains 50–100 taste receptor cells, which have a constant rate of turnover and a life span of approximately 10–11 days. If the nerve fiber that innervates a taste bud is cut or injured, the taste bud will degenerate (Sandow, Hejrat-Yazdi, & Heft, 2006). Four main taste categories can be distinguished: sweet, salty, sour, and bitter. Irradiation of the taste buds typically leads to partial (hypogeusia) or complete (ageusia) inability to taste or abnormal taste (dysgeusia) (Maes et al., 2002). A fifth category of taste has been identified but is not often used in the Western culture. Savoriness (*umami*) is the name for the distinctive taste sensation produced by the free glutamates commonly found in fermented and aged food (Yamaguchi & Ninomiya, 2000).

(2) Incidence and risk factors

(a) Taste changes are dependent on radiation dose. Changes have been reported to occur two to three days after the onset of radiation with doses as small as 2–4 Gy. Taste bud degeneration typically occurs six to seven days after irradiation (Sandow et al., 2006). Maes et al. (2002) reported a study of 73 patients who received radiation for head and neck cancer. They found loss of taste after radiation to be most pronounced after two months. Bitter and salty qualities were most impaired. Gradual recovery occurred during the first year of treatment. Partial taste loss persisted one to two years after treatment and was responsible for slight to moderate discomfort.

(b) Risk factors that may lead to worsening of symptoms include concomitant chemotherapy, biologic therapies, surgery, xerostomia, damage to nerves involving taste, oral infection, antibiotic therapy, dental or gum problems, changes in smell, and nausea and vomiting (Cancer.Net Editorial Board, 2009).

(3) Assessment

(a) Clinical manifestations

   i. The patient reports taste changes.

   ii. Ask the patient to be specific about the type of taste change experienced. Can the patient taste sweet, salty, sour, and bitter?

   iii. Note foods that are avoided or not eaten.

(b) Physical examination

   i. Monitor weight.

   ii. Examine mouth.

(4) Documentation: Dysgeusia (taste disturbances) (NCI CTEP, 2010)

(a) 1—Altered taste, but no change in diet

(b) 2—Altered taste with change in diet; noxious or unpleasant taste; loss of taste

(5) Collaborative management of taste changes: Therapeutic measures (Cancer.Net Editorial Board, 2009) include the following.

(a) Choose foods that smell and taste good, even if food is unfamiliar.

(b) Eliminate cooking smells by using an exhaust fan, cooking on an outdoor grill, or buying precooked foods. Cold or room-temperature foods have less of an aroma.

(c) Try using plastic utensils and glass cookware to lessen metallic taste.

(d) Sugar-free mint gum or hard candies can mask bitter or metallic taste in the mouth.

(e) If red meat does not taste good, try other protein sources such as poultry, eggs, fish, peanut butter, beans, or dairy products.

(f) Try marinating meats or flavoring foods with fruit juices, sweet wines, salad dressings, or other sauces.

(g) Specific foods may remind patients of when they experienced nausea and vomiting. These foods should be avoided when experiencing taste alterations.

(h) Rinsing the mouth with salt and baking soda before meals may help neutralize taste in the mouth (½ teaspoon of salt and ½ teaspoon of baking soda in 1 cup of warm water).

(i) Keep the mouth clean and healthy.

(j) Ripamonti et al. (1998) reported a randomized study finding that zinc sulfate improved taste with patients receiving radiation for head and neck cancer. No other studies have been repeated to support this evidence.

(6) Patient and family education

(a) Instruct the patient and family about taste changes, including when they may occur and how long they may last.

(b) Teach the patient and family measures on how to cope with taste changes.

   i. Explain that taste changes may be long-lasting. Return of taste is individualized.

   ii. Nutritional intake should be monitored to prevent weight loss.

   iii. Patients may have to avoid certain taste improvement recommendations during mucositis (e.g., using lemon and certain spices) but may attempt these measures after mucositis has resolved.

f) Changes in voice quality

(1) Pathophysiology: Speech sounds are produced when the airflow passes through vibrating vocal cords and resonates through the oral and nasal cavities, and intact tongue and lips articulate necessary sounds. Location of tumor and/or treatment can disrupt the structures necessary for speech production and affect the voice's intelligibility (Nguyen, Sallah, Karlsson, & Antoine, 2002). Edematous larynx cartilage may lead to impaired

mobility of vocal cords resulting in temporary hoarseness, but total dose of radiation will influence long-term quality-of-life issues with voice quality.

(2) Incidence and risk factors

   (a) Changes in voice quality are dependent on radiation dose. Dornfeld et al. (2007) reported decreased quality of speech when doses higher than 66 Gy were delivered to the aryepiglottic folds, pre-epiglottic space, false vocal cords, and lateral pharyngeal wall.

   (b) Risk factors include tumor location (patients with larynx cancer often present with hoarseness), initial biopsy procedure, smoking history, and older age. Postradiation xerostomia, fibrosis, and edema will affect voice quality (Carrara-de Angelis, Feher, Barros, Nishimoto, & Kowalski, 2003).

(3) Assessment

   (a) Clinical manifestations—Note voice quality before, during, and after treatment. Assess level of hoarseness.

   (b) Physical examination—Indirect laryngoscopy reveals vocal cord edema, erythema, and paralysis.

   (c) Psychosocial assessment—Ascertain whether voice quality has affected the patient's telephone use, socialization, or job security.

(4) Documentation: Hoarseness and aphonia assessment (NCI CTEP, 2010)

   (a) 1—Mild or intermittent voice change; fully understandable; self-resolves.

   (b) 2—Moderate or persistent voice changes; may require occasional repetition but understandable on telephone; medical evaluation indicated.

   (c) 3—Severe voice changes including predominantly whispered speech.

   (d) Aphonia assessment: Grade 3—Voicelessness, unable to speak

(5) Collaborative management

   (a) Avoid straining the voice to minimize irritation to the vocal cords.

   (b) Avoid use of alcohol, tobacco, and spicy and acidic foods. Spicy and acidic foods may contribute to gastric reflux disease, which may affect voice quality.

   (c) Warm saline gargle can be soothing and can clear thick mucus.

   (d) Increase humidification of air, especially when sleeping.

   (e) Consult for pain management if needed.

   (f) Occasionally, steroids or alpha-adrenergic agents may be necessary if edema becomes severe. In rare instances, a tracheostomy is necessary because of airway compromise (Haas & Kuehn, 2001).

   (g) Consult with a speech pathologist for optimal instructions and exercises to enhance voice quality.

(6) Patient and family education

   (a) Instruct the patient and family on measures to preserve voice and soothe throat.

   (b) Instruct the patient and family regarding symptoms of airway obstruction and how to obtain emergency care.

   (c) Refer the patient and family to social worker or community support network if voice changes have affected social interactions, job security, or financial stability.

g) Hearing changes

(1) Pathophysiology: Hearing changes are defined as an altered perception in the ability to hear. SNHL occurs when the inner ear and cochlea are included in the RT field. Patients can develop transient serous otitis media during or immediately following radiation treatments. Permanent SNHL can occur when doses to the cochlea are greater than 50 Gy (Pan et al., 2005).

(2) Incidence and risk factors

   (a) At highest risk for hearing loss are patients treated for cancers of the nasopharynx, parotid gland, paranasal sinuses, skin cancer of the ear, or brain cancer (Pan et al., 2005).

   (b) Additional risks for hearing loss include preexisting hearing loss, older age, hypertension, diabetes mellitus, and treatment with cisplatin (Pan et al., 2005).

(3) Assessment (Yueh, Shapiro, MacLean, & Shekelle, 2003)

   (a) Clinical manifestations: The patient reports decreased hearing acuity or tinnitus.

   (b) Physical examination

i. Simple evaluation may include the whispered voice test, in which the examiner whispers words from behind the patient at various distances. An additional simple screening may include determining the patient's ability to hear the sound of an examiner's fingers rubbing together near each ear.

ii. Inspect the ear canal and, using an otoscope, note the presence of ear wax and debris. A tuning fork may be used to assess for air and bone conduction.

iii. The tympanic membrane should appear opalescent. If the membrane appears bulging, erythematous, or punctured or if drainage or blood is present, an otolaryngologist needs to perform further evaluation.

(4) Documentation of hearing impairment when patients are not enrolled in a monitoring program (NCI CTEP, 2010)
 (a) 1—Subjective change in hearing in the absence of documented hearing loss
 (b) 2—Hearing loss but hearing aid or intervention not indicated; limiting instrumental ADL
 (c) 3—Hearing loss with hearing aid or intervention indicated; limiting self-care ADL
 (d) 4—Decrease in hearing to profound bilateral loss (absolute threshold greater than 80 dB HL [decibel hearing level] at 2 kilohertz and above); nonserviceable hearing

(5) Collaborative management
 (a) Administer pseudoephedrine, as directed, if fluid has accumulated in the middle ear.
 (b) Administer antibiotics, as directed, for ear infections.
 (c) Arrange for immediate evaluation with an otolaryngologist if any sudden, acute hearing loss occurs. Recommend evaluation with otolaryngologist or audiologist for subtle changes in hearing during survivorship.
 (d) Arrange for removal of cerumen by trained staff in otolaryngology.

(6) Patient and family education
 (a) Instruct the patient and family to monitor for hearing changes.
 (b) Advise the patient to report any sudden, acute changes in hearing immediately or subtle changes in hearing during survivorship.

h) Osteoradionecrosis
 (1) Pathophysiology: *Osteoradionecrosis* is a severe delayed injury caused by failure of bone healing. A theory for the pathogenesis of osteoradionecrosis is that damage to bone is caused by radiation-induced fibrosis. Cells in bone are damaged as a result of inflammation, free radicals, and chronic activation of fibroblasts by a series of growth hormones. The mandible within an RT field is at highest risk. Progression often occurs six months to five years after radiation, and the bone does not heal spontaneously (Delanian, Depondt, & Lefaix, 2005; Lyons & Ghazali, 2008; Reuther, Schuster, Mende, & Kübler, 2003).

 (2) Incidence and risk factors
 (a) Mandibular osteoradionecrosis has widely varied incidences in the literature but is unavoidable in 5%–15% of cases. Most cases occur after the mandible has received more than 60 Gy (Delanian et al., 2005; Wahl, 2006).
 (b) Treatment-related risk factors include total radiation dose, dose per fraction, irradiated volume, use of brachytherapy, concomitant chemotherapy, and surgical intervention surrounding or including the mandible (Delanian et al., 2005). Ben-David et al. (2006) reported an incidence of less than 2% in 176 patients when radiation was delivered with IMRT. Incidence was reported with two-year follow-up. Longer follow-up is needed.
 (c) Risk factors for osteoradionecrosis include poor oral hygiene, local biopsy sites, bone proximity to the tumor, intercurrent illnesses such as microvascular or endocrine diseases, and time lapse (less than 14 days) between preradiation extractions and commencement of RT. Even though smoking and alcohol consumption are common with head and neck cancer,

no evidence supports that smoking or drinking alcohol causes osteoradionecrosis (Delanian et al., 2005; Wahl, 2006).

(3) Assessment
  (a) Evaluation of risk factors
  (b) Clinical manifestations
    i. Oral, jaw, or facial pain
    ii. Mandibular fracture
  (c) Physical examination
    i. Assess the oral cavity, especially the condition of the teeth and buccal mucosa.
    ii. Assess for infection, nonhealing wounds, and condition of the mandible.

(4) Documentation of osteoradionecrosis of the jaw (NCI CTEP, 2010)
  (a) 1—Asymptomatic; clinical or diagnostic observation only; intervention not indicated
  (b) 2—Symptomatic; medical intervention indicated (e.g., topical agents); limiting instrumental ADL
  (c) 3—Severe symptoms; limiting self-care ADL; elective operative intervention indicated
  (d) 4—Life-threatening consequences; urgent intervention indicated
  (e) 5—Death

(5) Collaborative management (acute and long term)
  (a) Prevention
    i. Consult with a dentist prior to radiation to optimize oral health and repair poorly fitting oral/dental prosthesis. Postradiation dental extractions may cause osteoradionecrosis; recommend that all nonrestorable teeth be extracted at least 14 days before RT commences.
    ii. Prophylactic antibiotics have never been shown to prevent osteoradionecrosis. Antibiotics should be prescribed to treat oral infections.
    iii. Hyperbaric oxygen shows no benefit for those diagnosed with osteoradionecrosis. However, Wahl (2006) reported that prophylactic hyperbaric oxygen before and after aggressive dental procedures in areas treated with more than 60 Gy decreases the risk of developing osteoradionecrosis. Wahl (2006) summarized that hyperbaric oxygen therapy is time consuming and costly. Typical protocol calls for 30 hours of pre-extraction treatment in 20 90-minute sessions in a hyperbaric chamber, followed by 15 hours of postextraction treatment in 10 90-minute sessions. Cost will vary depending on the billing policies of the facility where the hyperbaric oxygen is delivered. In 2011, the cost of 45 hours of hyperbaric oxygen treatments ranged from $5,000 to $11,250.
    iv. Additional treatment recommendations include pentoxifylline (vasodilator that inhibits fibrosis) and tocopherol (vitamin E) to reduce damage caused by free radicals. Medications should be prescribed one week before planned extractions and continue for eight weeks afterward (Lyons & Ghazali, 2008).
    v. Continue meticulous oral care and use of fluoride to prevent dental caries.
    vi. Instruct the patient to minimize oral irritants.
    vii. Maintain good nutritional status.
    viii. Patient is aware of lifelong recommendation that dentist be informed of treatment with radiation to the oral cavity. Radiation oncologist should be consulted before any aggressive dental procedures (e.g., extraction) regarding the need for hyperbaric oxygen.
  (b) Intervention when osteoradionecrosis occurs (Delanian et al., 2005; Lyons & Ghazali, 2008)
    i. Medical only—Pentoxifylline 400 mg twice daily and tocopherol 1,000 IU once daily. If unresponsive, add clodronate 1,600 mg daily.
    ii. Medical and surgical—Initiate pentoxifylline, tocopherol, and clodronate three months

before surgery; resection of mandible; consider extending antioxidants after surgery.

    iii. Surgery when pathologic fracture is present or imminent; requires vascularized composite tissue transfer

    iv. Reuther et al. (2003) reported a benefit when hyperbaric oxygen therapy was added to surgical procedures to promote revascularization of tissue (will not heal dead bone).

(6) Patient and family education

    (a) Instruct the patient and family about osteoradionecrosis, including risk factors, signs and symptoms, and measures of prevention.

    (b) Instruct the patient and family to continue meticulous mouth care and routine evaluations by dentistry.

i) Trismus

(1) Pathophysiology: *Trismus*, or limited jaw opening, may develop because of tumor invasion of the masticatory muscles and/or the temporomandibular joint (TMJ), may result after radiation if masticatory muscles or the TMJ is included in the field of radiation, or because of a combination of both. The limited jaw opening interferes with oral hygiene, speech, nutritional intake, examination of the oropharynx, and dental treatment and causes discomfort or pain to the patient (Kent et al., 2008; Vissink, Jansma, Spijkervet, Burlage, & Coppes, 2003). Quality of life is affected when patients are embarrassed to eat in public and need a longer time to eat a simple meal.

(2) Incidence and risk factors

    (a) Kent et al. (2008) reported that limitations in jaw opening have been reported in 6%–86% of patients receiving radiation to the TMJ or masseter/pterygoid muscles, with a frequency or severity that is somewhat unpredictable.

    (b) Risk increases over time. It often starts to develop three to six months after RT has completed and frequently becomes a lifelong problem. Additional risk factors include the location of tumor growth, surgical procedures, and

the configuration and dose of the radiation (Vissink et al., 2003).

    (c) Patients are also at risk when they are resistant to mouth stretching exercises. Melchers et al. (2009) reported study results with exercise adherence with the use of the TheraBite® Jaw Motion Rehabilitation System™ (Atos Medical Inc.). Internal motivation to exercise, the perceived effect, self-discipline, pain, anxiety, and having exercise goals influenced exercise adherence.

(3) Assessment

    (a) Clinical manifestations

        i. Patient reports difficulty opening mouth.

        ii. Patient reports difficulty chewing.

    (b) Physical examination: Ability to open mouth is limited. Assessment for trismus is performed by measuring the amount of millimeters a patient can open the mouth.

(4) Trismus documentation (NCI CTEP, 2010)

    (a) 1—Decreased range of motion without impaired eating

    (b) 2—Decreased range of motion requiring small bites, soft foods, or purees

    (c) 3—Decreased range of motion with inability to adequately aliment or hydrate orally

(5) Collaborative prevention and management

    (a) Measures to prevent trismus (caused from muscle fibrosis) should be initiated before patient starts RT. Consult with a physical therapist or speech therapist for evaluation and recommendations. Mouth exercises and the use of stacked tongue blades or

a clothespin may be beneficial (Kent et al., 2008). Many devices to improve trismus are on the market. Some include the TheraBite, Jaw Dynasplint™ System (Dynasplint Systems, Inc.), and the OraStretch™ press jaw motion rehabilitation system (CranioMandibular Rehab, Inc.). No evidence exists to support that any one device is more effective than another.

(b) Consult with dietitian when trismus interferes with the patient's nutritional intake.

(6) Patient and family education

(a) Inform the patient and family regarding risks for trismus and to report changes in mouth mobility.

(b) Instruct the patient and family about mouth and chewing exercises to prevent fibrosis.

j) Shoulder mobility

(1) Pathophysiology: Shoulder mobility usually is associated with neck dissection procedures but can be a complication from postradiation neck fibrosis. The spinal accessory nerve is the principal motor innervation to the trapezius muscle. The trapezius muscle provides passive support to the shoulder complex and is a stabilizer of the scapula. Changes in the trapezius muscle alter the alignment of the scapula and disrupt the normal motion of the shoulder complex. Long-term shoulder discomfort and neck tightness can lead to chronic pain and difficulties in dressing, writing, driving, lifting, and reaching for objects. These challenges can affect ADL, social activities, recreation, and employment (McNeely, Parliament, Courneya, & Haykowsky, 2004).

(2) Incidence and risk factors: McNeely, Parliament, Courneya, Seikaly, et al. (2004) found that although selective neck dissections have been associated with less shoulder pain and dysfunction compared with radical procedures, a variable degree of shoulder dysfunction still occurs in 29%–39%.

(3) Assessment: Accurate and thorough assessment should be performed by a physical therapist. Range of motion should be assessed for the combined motion of the joints of the shoulder complex. Active shoulder movements include flexion, abduction, and external rotation. Passive shoulder movements include flexion, abduction, external rotation, internal rotation, and horizontal abduction.

(4) Documentation: The Shoulder Pain and Disability Index, or SPADI, is a valid instrument that produces a score that averages the pain and disability of the shoulder. It is self-administered and requires 5–10 minutes to complete (McNeely, Parliament, Courneya, Seikaly, et al., 2004).

(5) Intervention: McNeely, Parliament, Courneya, and Haykowsky (2004) and McNeely, Parliament, Courneya, Seikaly, et al. (2004) reported improved outcomes with physical therapy. The recommendations included passive range of motion, joint mobilization, and stretching of the major and minor pectoralis muscles. Exercises progressed to include isometric scapular strengthening and strengthening the biceps, triceps, and shoulder external rotators.

k) Hypothyroidism

(1) Pathophysiology: Treatment for head and neck malignancies often includes irradiation of the cervical neck nodes, which results in a moderate to high radiation dose to all or part of the thyroid gland. Thyroid dysfunction can occur because of direct radiation damage to the thyroid gland (Bhandare, Kennedy, Malyapa, Morris, & Mendenhall, 2007).

(2) Incidence and risk factors: Tell et al. (2004) reported the risk for developing hypothyroidism after radiation for head and neck cancer was 20% at 5 years and 27% at 10 years. Bilateral neck radiation treatment places patients at higher risk. Time for development can be as early as 3 months to 10 years after treatment.

(3) Assessment

(a) The TSH blood test is the screening tool to monitor thyroid function for patients who received locoregional radiation for nonthyroid head and neck cancer. Patients should be tested before the RT begins to screen for preexisting thyroid abnormalities. All pa-

tients receiving radiation to the head and neck region should undergo frequent serum TSH screening beginning six months after RT has completed. TSH serum level should be repeated one year after completion of RT and every year afterward. Patients who develop symptoms or have problems with medication adjustment should be tested more often based on the managing practitioner's judgment (Colevas et al., 2001; Tell et al., 2004).

(b) Symptoms—Patients may complain of fatigue, cold intolerance, muscle cramps, hair changes, and weight gain. If it is left untreated, depression, slow mentation, pericardial or pleural effusions, decreased GI mobility, decreased wound healing, and acceleration of atherosclerosis may occur (Tell et al., 2004).

(4) Documentation (NCI CTEP, 2010)

(a) 1—Asymptomatic; clinical or diagnostic observations only; intervention not indicated

(b) 2—Symptomatic; thyroid replacement indicated; limiting instrumental ADL

(c) 3—Severe symptoms; limiting self-care ADL; hospitalization indicated

(d) 4—Life-threatening consequences; urgent intervention indicated

(e) 5 Death

(5) Interventions

(a) Symptoms of hypothyroidism are similar to symptoms of recovery from treatment. The patient and family need to be taught about delayed effects of radiation to the thyroid and report symptoms to the nurse or physician.

(b) Management of medication for hypothyroidism is most often the role of the medical oncologist or primary care physician. The nurse needs to document that the patient is compliant with follow-up and monitoring.

l) Increased risk of stroke

(1) Pathophysiology: Long-term complication after radiation to the neck is an increased risk of vascular stenosis and thromboembolism resulting in a high-er risk of ischemic stroke. The pathogenesis of radiation-induced vascular disease is an acceleration of the atherosclerotic process due to endothelial cell damage, fibrosis of the intima-media layer, and the development of atheromatous plaques. These occlusive changes lead to ischemia of the carotid artery (Dorresteijn et al., 2002).

(2) Incidence and risk factors

(a) Dorresteijn et al. (2002) reported increased risk of stroke after radiation to the neck. The 15-year cumulative risk was 12%.

(b) Dorresteiijn et al. (2002) reported that patients with a history of smoking, hypertension, diabetes, and hypercholesterolemia had increased risk of stroke after radiation to the neck.

(3) Assessment

(a) Clinical manifestations: Follow-up visits should include an assessment of changes in neurologic symptoms.

(b) Lifestyle assessment: Current cigarette smoking patterns should be followed.

(c) Physical examination: Assessment of hypertension, hypercholesterolemia, and routine performance of carotid ultrasound may be worthwhile (Dorresteijn et al., 2002).

(4) Documentation: Risk for ischemic stroke has been demonstrated to be a lifelong risk. Changes in neurologic status, hypertension and diabetes screening, cigarette smoking patterns, and screening for hypercholesterolemia should be followed for changes during follow-up visits after radiation to the neck (Dorresteijn et al., 2002).

(5) Collaborative management and patient and family education

(a) The patient and family should be educated about the increased risk for ischemic stroke. Smoking cessation is recommended.

(b) The patient and family should be educated about lifestyle prevention measures and the rationale for increased screening of hypertension, diabetes, and hypercholesterolemia. Medication management of hypertension, diabetes, and hypercholesterolemia may be necessary.

(c) Managing practitioner screens carotid arteries through ultrasound or CT scan of neck. Referral to vascular surgeon may be necessary to investigate therapeutic interventions.

m) Lhermitte sign/transient radiation myelopathy

(1) Pathology: Lhermitte sign, or *transient radiation myelopathy*, is characterized by electric shock–like sensation spreading into both arms, down the dorsal spine, and into the legs, on flexion of the neck. The probable cause is the temporary interference with the turnover of myelin, leading to focal demyelination (Lewanski, Sinclair, & Stewart, 2000).

(2) Incidence and risk factors (Lewanski et al., 2000)

(a) Incidence is rare; it usually appears within four months of treatment completion and resolves after six months of treatment completion.

(b) Cervical doses greater than 50 Gy in total or more than 2 Gy per fraction are the only significant variables. Radiation planning for head and neck cancer will stop treating the cervical spine after 45 Gy.

(c) Cisplatin given with radiation may increase the risk of transient radiation myelopathy.

(3) Assessment: Patient complains of intermittent electric shock–like sensation traveling from the neck to both arms. Often stimulated when patient puts chin to chest.

(4) Management (Lewanski et al., 2000)

(a) Patient should be managed conservatively because no specific treatment exists.

(b) Soft neck collar may restrict unnecessary flexion of the spine and limit symptoms.

(c) Neither steroids nor hyperbaric oxygen have proved to be of value.

(d) Educate the patient and caregivers about Lhermitte sign and reassure that for vast majority of patients, the symptoms resolve after six months. The patient should inform the clinician if symptoms worsen or do not resolve within six months after treatment.

n) Psychosocial distress and coping (see section IV.E—Distress/coping)

o) Skin reactions (see section IV.C—Skin reactions)

References

Antonadou, D., Pepelassi, M., Synodinou, M., Puglisi, M., & Throuvalas, N. (2002). Prophylactic use of amifostine to prevent radiochemotherapy-induced mucositis and xerostomia in head-and-neck cancer. *International Journal of Radiation Oncology, Biology, Physics, 52,* 739–747. doi:10.1016/S0360-3016(01)02683-9

Avritscher, E.B., Cooksley, C.D., & Elting, L.S. (2004). Scope and epidemiology of cancer therapy-induced oral and gastrointestinal mucositis. *Seminars in Oncology Nursing, 20,* 3–10.

Ben-David, M.A., Diamante, M., Radawski, J.D., Vineberg, K.A., Stroup, C., Murdoch-Kinch, C.A., … Eisbruch, A. (2006). Lack of osteoradionecrosis of the mandible after intensity-modulated radiotherapy for head and neck cancer: Likely contributions of both dental care and improved dose distributions. *International Journal of Radiation Oncology, Biology, Physics, 68,* 396–402. doi:10.1016/j.ijrobp.2006.11.059

Bhandare, N., Kennedy, L., Malyapa, R.S., Morris, C.G., & Mendenhall, W.M. (2007). Primary and central hypothyroidism after radiotherapy for head-and-neck tumors. *International Journal of Radiation Oncology, Biology, Physics, 68,* 1131–1139. doi:10.1016/j.ijrobp.2007.01.029

Blanco, A., & Chao, C. (2006). Management of radiation-induced head and neck injury. In W. Small Jr. & G.E. Woloschak (Eds.), *Radiation toxicity: A practical guide* (pp. 23–41). New York, NY: Springer.

Brizel, D.M., Wasserman, T.H., Henke, M., Strnad, V., Rudat, V., Monnier, A., … Sauer, R. (2000). Phase III randomized trial of amifostine as a radioprotector in head and neck cancer. *Journal of Clinical Oncology, 18,* 3339–3345.

Bruce, S.D. (2004). Radiation-induced xerostomia: How dry is your patient? *Clinical Journal of Oncology Nursing, 8,* 61–67. doi:10.1188/04.CJON.61-67

Burri, R.J., & Lee, N.Y. (2009). Concurrent chemotherapy and radiotherapy for head and neck cancer. *Expert Review of Anticancer Therapy, 9,* 293–302. doi:10.1586/14737140.9.3.293

Cancer.Net Editorial Board. (2009, April). Taste changes. Retrieved from http://www.cancer.net/patient/All+About+Cancer/Treating+Cancer/Managing+Side+Effects/Taste+Changes

Carper, E. (2007). Head and neck cancers. In M.L. Haas, W.P. Hogle, G.J. Moore-Higgs, & T.K. Gosselin-Acomb (Eds.), *Radiation therapy: A guide to patient care* (pp. 84–117). St. Louis, MO: Elsevier Mosby.

Carr, E. (2011). Head and neck malignancies. In C.H. Yarbro, D. Wujcik, & B.H. Gobel (Eds.), *Cancer nursing: Principles and practice* (7th ed., pp. 1334–1368). Sudbury, MA: Jones and Bartlett.

Carrara-de Angelis, E., Feher, O., Barros, A.P., Nishimoto, I.N., & Kowalski, L.P. (2003). Voice and swallowing in patients enrolled in a larynx preservation trial. *Archives of Otolaryngology—Head and Neck Surgery, 129,* 733–738. doi:10.1001/archotol.129.7.733

Caudell, J.J., Schaner, P.E., Meredith, R.F., Locher, J.L., Nabell, L.M., Carroll, W.R., ... Bonner, J.A. (2009). Factors associated with long-term dysphagia after definitive radiotherapy for locally advanced head-and-neck cancer. *International Journal of Radiation Oncology, Biology, Physics, 73,* 410–415. doi:10.1016/j.ijrobp.2008.04.048

Chao, K.S., Majhail, N., Huang, C.J., Simpson, J.R., Perez, C.A., Haughey, B., & Spector, G. (2001). Intensity-modulated radiation therapy reduces late salivary toxicity without compromising tumor control in patients with oropharyngeal carcinoma: A comparison with conventional techniques. *Radiotherapy and Oncology, 61,* 275–280. doi:10.1016/S0167-8140(01)00449-2

Chen, A.M., Li, B.Q., Lau, D.H., Farwell, D.G., Luu, Q., Stuart, K., ... Vijayakumar, S. (2010). Evaluating the role of prophylactic gastrostomy tube placement prior to definitive chemoradiotherapy for head and neck cancer. *International Journal of Radiation Oncology, Biology, Physics, 78,* 1026–1032. doi:10.1016/j.ijrobp.2009.09.036

Cho, J.H., Chung, W.K., Kang, W., Choi, S.M., Cho, C.K., & Son, C.G. (2008). Manual acupuncture improved quality of life in cancer patients with radiation-induced xerostomia. *Journal of Alternative and Complementary Medicine, 14,* 523–526. doi:10.1089/acm.2007.0793

Colevas, A.D., Read, R., Thornhill, J., Adak, S., Tishler, R., Busse, P., ... Posner, M. (2001). Hypothyroidism incidence after multimodality treatment for stage III and IV squamous cell carcinomas of the head and neck. *International Journal of Radiation Oncology, Biology, Physics, 51,* 599–604. doi:10.1016/S0360-3016(01)01688-1

Delanian, S., Depondt, J., & Lefaix, J.L. (2005). Major healing of refractory mandible osteoradionecrosis after treatment combining pentoxifylline and tocopherol: A phase II trial. *Head and Neck, 27,* 114–123. doi:10.1002/hed.20121

Dornfeld, K., Simmons, J.R., Karnell, L., Karnell, M., Funk, G., Yao, M., ... Buatti, J.M. (2007). Radiation doses to structures within and adjacent to the larynx are correlated with long-term diet- and speech-related quality of life. *International Journal of Radiation Oncology, Biology, Physics, 68,* 750–757. doi:10.1016/j.ijrobp.2007.01.047

Dorresteijn, L.D., Kappelle, A.C., Boogerd, W., Klokman, W.J., Balm, A.J., Keus, R.B., ... Bartelink, H. (2002). Increased risk of ischemic stroke after radiotherapy on the neck in patients younger than 60 years. *Journal of Clinical Oncology, 20,* 282–288. doi:10.1200/JCO.20.1.282

Edge, S.B., Byrd, D.R., Compton, C.C., Fritz, A.G., Greene, F.L., & Trotti, A., III. (Eds.). (2010). *AJCC cancer staging manual* (7th ed.). New York, NY: Springer.

Eilers, J., & Million, R. (2007). Prevention and management of oral mucositis in patients with cancer. *Seminars in Oncology Nursing, 23,* 201–212. doi:10.1016/j.soncn.2007.05.005

Epstein, J.B., Wan, L., Chrisman, P., Dale, B.A., & Jackson, D. (2007). Use of mucosal fluid collection to assess oral mucositis in patients receiving head and neck radiation therapy: A feasibility study. *Journal of Applied Research, 7,* 50–57.

Fakhry, C., Westra, W.H., Li, S., Cmelak, A., Ridge, J.A., Pinto, H., ... Gillison, M.L. (2008). Improved survival of patients with human papillomavirus-positive head and neck squamous cell carcinoma in a prospective clinical trial. *Journal of the National Cancer Institute, 100,* 261–269. doi:10.1093/jnci/djn011

Fox, P.C. (2004). Salivary enhancement therapies. *Caries Research, 38,* 241–246. doi:10.1159/000077761

Gould, L., & Lewis, S. (2006). Care of head and neck cancer patients with swallowing difficulties. *British Journal of Nursing, 15,* 1091–1096.

Haas, M., & Kuehn, E. (2001). Head and neck cancers. In D.W. Bruner, G. Moore-Higgs, & M. Haas (Eds.), *Outcomes in radiation therapy: Multidisciplinary management* (pp. 195–213). Sudbury, MA: Jones and Bartlett.

Harris, D.J., Eilers, J.G., Cashavelly, B.J., Maxwell, C.L., & Harriman, A. (2009). ONS PEP resource: Mucositis. In L.H. Eaton & J.M. Tipton (Eds.), *Putting evidence into practice: Improving oncology patient outcomes* (pp. 201–213). Pittsburgh, PA: Oncology Nursing Society.

Harris, D.J., Eilers, J., Harriman, A., Cashavelly, B.J., & Maxwell, C. (2008). Putting evidence into practice: Evidence-based interventions for the management of oral mucositis. *Clinical Journal of Oncology Nursing, 12,* 141–152. doi:10.1188/08.CJON.141-152

Hong, J.P., Lee, S.W., Song, S.Y., Ahn, S.D., Shin, S.S., Choi, E.K., & Kim, J.H. (2009). Recombinant human epidermal growth factor treatment of radiation-induced severe oral mucositis in patients with head and neck malignancies. *European Journal of Cancer Care, 18,* 636–641. doi:10.1111/j.1365-2354.2008.00971.x

Kent, M.L., Brennan, M.T., Noll, J.L., Fox, P.C., Burri, S.H., Hunter, J.C., & Lockhart, P.B. (2008). Radiation-induced trismus in head and neck cancer patients. *Supportive Care in Cancer, 16,* 305–309. doi:10.1007/s00520-007-0345-5

Kizhner, V., Xu, D., & Krespi, Y.P. (2011, February 16). A new tool measuring oral malodor quality of life. *European Archives of Oto-Rhino-Laryngology, 268,* 1227–1232. doi:10.1007/s00405-011-1518-x

Lazarus, C.L. (2009). Effects of chemoradiotherapy on voice and swallowing. *Current Opinion in Otolaryngology and Head and Neck Surgery, 17,* 172–178. doi:10.1097/MOO.0b013e32832af12f

Lewanski, C.R., Sinclair, J.A., & Stewart, J.S. (2000). Lhermitte's sign following head and neck radiotherapy. *Clinical Oncology, 12,* 98–103.

Lyons, A., & Ghazali, N. (2008). Osteoradionecrosis of the jaws: Current understanding of its pathophysiology and treatment. *British Journal of Oral and Maxillofacial Surgery, 46,* 653–660. doi:10.1016/j.bjoms.2008.04.006

Maes, A., Huygh, I., Weltens, C., Vandevelde, G., Delaere, P., Evers, G., & Van den Bogaert, W. (2002). De Gustibus: Time scale of loss and recovery of tastes caused by radiotherapy. *Radiotherapy and Oncology, 63,* 195–201. doi:10.1016/S0167-8140(02)00025-7

Maher, K. (2004). Xerostomia. In C.H. Yarbro, M.H. Frogge, & M. Goodman (Eds.), *Cancer symptom management* (3rd ed., pp. 215–229). Sudbury, MA: Jones and Bartlett.

McNeely, M.L., Parliament, M., Courneya, K.S., & Haykowsky, M. (2004). Resistance exercise for post neck dissection shoulder pain: Three case reports. *Physiotherapy Theory and Practice, 20,* 41–56. doi:10.1080/09593980490425094

McNeely, M.L., Parliament, M., Courneya, K.S., Seikaly, H., Jha, N., Scrimger, R., & Hanson, J. (2004). A pilot study of a randomized controlled trial to evaluate the effects of progressive resistance exercise training on shoulder dysfunction caused by spinal accessory neurapraxia/neurectomy in head and neck cancer survivors. *Head and Neck, 26,* 518–530. doi:10.1002/hed.20010

Melchers, L.J., Van Weert, E., Beurskens, C.H., Reintsema, H., Slagter, A.P., Roodenberg, J.L., & Dijkstra, P.U. (2009). Exercise adherence in patients with trismus due to head and neck oncology: A qualitative study into the use of the Therabite®. *International Journal of Oral and Maxillofacial Surgery, 38,* 947–954. doi:10.1016/j.ijom.2009.04.003

Moore, K.L., & Agur, A.M.R. (2002). *Essential clinical anatomy* (2nd ed.). Philadelphia, PA: Lippincott Williams & Wilkins.

Münter, M.W., Karger, C.P., Hoffner, S.G., Hof, H., Thilmann, C., Rudat, V., … Debus, J. (2004). Evaluation of salivary gland function after treatment of head-and-neck tumors with intensity-modulated radiotherapy by quantitative pertechnetate scintigraphy. *International Journal of Radiation Oncology, Biology, Physics, 58,* 175–184. doi:10.1016/S0360-3016(03)01437-8

Narayan, S., Lehmann, J., Coleman, M.A., Vaughan, A., Yang, C.C., Enepekides, D., … Vijayakumar, S. (2008). Prospective evaluation to establish a dose response for clinical oral mucositis in patients undergoing head-and-neck conformal radiotherapy. *International Journal of Radiation Oncology, Biology, Physics, 72,* 756–762. doi:10.1016/j.ijrobp.2008.01.060

National Cancer Institute Cancer Therapy Evaluation Program. (2010). *Common terminology criteria for adverse events* [v.4.03]. Retrieved from http://evs.nci.nih.gov/ftp1/CTCAE/About.html

Nguyen, N.P., Sallah, S., Karlsson, U., & Antoine, J.E. (2002). Combined chemotherapy and radiation therapy for head and neck malignancies: Quality of life issues. *Cancer, 94,* 1131–1141. doi:10.1002/cncr.10257

Nguyen, N.P., Smith, H.J., & Sallah, S. (2007). Evaluation and management of swallowing dysfunction following chemoradiation for head and neck cancer. *Current Opinion in Otolaryngology and Head and Neck Surgery, 15,* 130–133. doi:10.1097/MOO.0b013e32801da0e8

Ogama, N., Suzuki, S., Umeshita, K., Kobayashi, T., Kaneko, S., Kato, S., & Shimizu, Y. (2010). Appetite and adverse effects associated with radiation therapy in patients with head and neck cancer. *European Journal of Oncology Nursing, 14,* 3–10. doi:10.1016/j.ejon.2009.07.004

Orellana, M.F., Lagravère, M., Boychuk, D.G., Major, P.W., & Flores-Mir, C. (2006). Prevalence of xerostomia in population-based samples: A systematic review. *Journal of Public Health Dentistry, 66,* 152–158. doi:10.1111/j.1752-7325.2006.tb02572.x

Palazzi, M., Tomatis, S., Orlandi, E., Guzzo, M., Sangalli, C., Potepan, P., … Olmi, P. (2008). Effects of treatment intensification on acute local toxicity during radiotherapy for head and neck cancer: Prospective observational study validated CTCAE, version 3.0, scoring system. *International Journal of Radiation Oncology, Biology, Physics, 70,* 330–337. doi:10.1016/j.ijrobp.2007.06.022

Pan, C.C., Eisbruch, A., Lee, J.S., Snorrason, R.M., Ten Haken, R.K., & Kileny, P.R. (2005). Prospective study of inner ear radiation dose and hearing loss in head-and-neck cancer patients. *International Journal of Radiation Oncology, Biology, Physics, 61,* 1393–1401. doi:10.1016/j.ijrobp.2004.08.019

Rades, D., Fehlauer, F., Bajrovic, A., Mahlmann, B., Rickter, E., & Alberti, W. (2004). Serious adverse effects of amifostine during radiotherapy in head and neck cancer patients. *Radiotherapy and Oncology, 70,* 261–264. doi:10.1016/j.radonc.2003.10.005

Rancati, T., Schwarz, M., Allen, A.M., Feng, F., Popovtzer, A., Mittal, B., & Eisbruch, A. (2010). Radiation dose-volume effects in the larynx and pharynx. *International Journal of Radiation Oncology, Biology, Physics, 76*(3, Suppl. 1), S64–S69. doi:10.1016/j.ijrobp.2009.03.079

Reuther, T., Schuster, T., Mende, U., & Kübler, A. (2003). Osteoradionecrosis of the jaws as a side effect of radiotherapy of head and neck tumour patients—A report of a thirty year retrospective review. *International Journal of Oral and Maxillofacial Surgery, 32,* 289–295. doi:10.1054/ijom.2002.0332

Ripamonti, C., Zecca, E., Brunelli, C., Fulfaro, F., Villa, S., Balzarini, A., … De Conno, F. (1998). A randomized, controlled clinical trial to evaluate the effects of zinc sulfate on cancer patients with taste alterations caused by head and neck irradiation. *Cancer, 82,* 1938–1945. doi:10.1002/(SICI)1097-0142(19980515)82:10<1938::AID-CNCR18>3.0.CO;2-U

Rosenthal, D.I., Lewin, J.S., & Eisbruch, A. (2006). Prevention and treatment of dysphagia and aspiration after chemoradiation for head and neck cancer. *Journal of Clinical Oncology, 24,* 2636–2643. doi:10.1200/JCO.2006.06.0079

Rosenthal, D.I., Mendoza, T.R., Chambers, M.S., Burkett, V.S., Garden, A.S., Hessell, A.C., … Cleeland, C.S. (2008). The M.D. Anderson Symptom Inventory–Head and Neck module, a patient-reported outcome instrument, accurately predicts the severity of radiation-induced mucositis. *International Journal of Radiation Oncology, Biology, Physics, 72,* 1355–1361. doi:10.1016/j.ijrobp.2008.02.072

Rosenthal, D.I., & Trotti, A. (2009). Strategies for managing radiation-induced mucositis in head and neck cancer. *Seminars in Radiation Oncology, 19,* 29–34. doi:10.1016/j.semradonc.2008.09.006

Sandow, P. (2009). Dental prophylaxis and care. In P.M. Harari, N.P. Connor, & C. Grau (Eds.), *Functional preservation and quality of life in head and neck radiotherapy* (pp. 269–276). Berlin, Germany: Springer.

Sandow, P.L., Hejrat-Yazdi, M., & Heft, M.W. (2006). Taste loss and recovery following radiation therapy. *Journal of Dental Research, 85,* 608–611. doi:10.1177/154405910608500705

Scarantino, C., LeVeque, F., Swann, R.S., White, R., Schulsinger, A., Hodson, D.I., … Lee, N. (2006). Effect of pilocarpine during radiation therapy: Results of RTOG 97-09, a phase III randomized study in head and neck cancer patients. *Journal of Supportive Oncology, 4,* 252–258.

Schiødt, M., & Hermund, N.U. (2002). Management of oral disease prior to radiation therapy. *Supportive Care in Cancer, 10,* 40–43.

Scully, C., Sonis, S., & Diz, P.D. (2006). Oral mucositis. *Oral Diseases, 12,* 229–241. doi:10.1111/j.1601-0825.2006.01258.x

Siegel, R., Ward, E., Brawley, O., & Jemal, A. (2011). Cancer statistics, 2011. *CA: A Cancer Journal for Clinicians, 61,* 212–236. doi:10.3322/caac.20121

Smith, R.V., Goldman, S.Y., Beitler, J.J., & Wadler, S.S. (2004). Decreased short- and long-term swallowing problems with altered radiotherapy dosing used in an organ-sparing protocol for advanced pharyngeal carcinoma. *Archives of Otolaryngology—Head and Neck Surgery, 130,* 831–836. doi:10.1001/archotol.130.7.831

Sonis, S.T., Elting, L.S., Keefe, D., Peterson, D.E., Schubert, M., Hauer-Jensen, M., … Rubenstein, E.B. (2004). Perspectives on cancer therapy-induced mucosal injury: Pathogenesis, measurement, epidemiology, and consequences for patients. *Cancer, 100,* 1995–2025. doi:10.1002/cncr.20162

Springer, I.N., Niehoff, P., Warnke, P.H., Böcek, G., Kovács, G., Suhr, M., … Açil, Y. (2005). Radiation caries—Radiogenic destruction of dental collagen. *Oral Oncology, 41,* 723–728. doi:10.1016/j.oraloncology.2005.03.011

Tell, R., Lundell, G., Nilsson, B., Sjödin, H., Lewin, F., & Lewensohn, R. (2004). Long-term incidence of hypothyroidism after radiotherapy in patients with head-and-neck cancer. *International Journal of Radiation Oncology, Biology, Physics, 60,* 395–400. doi:10.1016/j.ijrobp.2004.03.020

Trotti, A., Bellm, L.A., Epstein, J.B., Frame, D., Fuchs, H.J., Gwede, C.K., … Zilberberg, M.D. (2003). Mucositis incidence, severity and associated outcomes in patients with head and neck cancer receiving radiotherapy with or without chemotherapy: A systematic literature review. *Radiotherapy and Oncology, 66,* 253–262. doi:10.1016/S0167-8140(02)00404-8

Vissink, A., Jansma, J., Spijkervet, F.K., Burlage, F.R., & Coppes, R.P. (2003). Oral sequelae of head and neck radiotherapy. *Critical Reviews in Oral Biology and Medicine, 14,* 199–212. doi:10.1177/154411130301400305

Wahl, M.J. (2006). Osteoradionecrosis prevention myths. *International Journal of Radiation Oncology, Biology, Physics, 64,* 661–669. doi:10.1016/j.ijrobp.2005.10.021

Wong, P.C., Dodd, M.J., Miaskowski, C., Paul, S.M., Bank, K.A., Shiba, G.H., & Facione, N. (2006). Mucositis pain induced by radiation therapy: Prevalence, severity, and use of self-care behaviors. *Journal of Pain and Symptom Management, 32,* 27–37. doi:10.1016/j.jpainsymman.2005.12.020

Wong, R.K.W., Jones, G.W., Sagar, S.M., Babjak, A.-F., & Whelan, T. (2003). A phase I–II study in the use of acupuncture-like transcutaneous nerve stimulation in the treatment of radiation-induced xerostomia in head-and-neck cancer patients treated with radical radiotherapy. *International Journal of Radiation Oncology, Biology, Physics, 57,* 472–480. doi:10.1016/S0360-3016(03)00572-8

Yamaguchi, S., & Ninomiya, K. (2000). Umami and food palatability. *Journal of Nutrition, 130*(Suppl. 4S), 921S–925S.

Yueh, B., Shapiro, N., MacLean, C.H., & Shekelle, P.G. (2003). Screening and management of adult hearing loss in primary care: Scientific review. *JAMA, 289,* 1976–1985. doi:10.1001/jama.289.15.1976

C. Breast
   1. Purpose/goal: RT is prescribed as a single-modality treatment used in the adjuvant setting either after chemotherapy or surgery. The goal of adjuvant RT is to destroy any cancer cells left behind within the breast, the chest wall, and the nodes draining into lymphatics in order to reduce the chance of local recurrence and improve overall survival (Buchholz & Haffty, 2008; Haffty, Buchholz, & Perez, 2008; Wazer & Arthur, 2008).
   2. Techniques
      a) EBRT
         (1) EBRT is a local therapy in which high doses of radiation are delivered over a longer period of time from a linear accelerator delivering radiation through medial and lateral tangential beams.
         (2) Tangential beam arrangement helps to minimize the amount of radiation delivered to the normal lung tissue and cardiac tissue for left-sided breast cancers.
         (3) Standard therapy
            (a) Most patients diagnosed with ductal carcinoma in situ and early-stage invasive cancer receive 2 Gy per fraction to a total dose of 50 Gy in 25 fractions. An additional 10 Gy in five fractions is delivered to the volume of breast surrounding the excision site, known as a *bed boost* (Hunt, Robb, Strom, & Ueno, 2001), although different fractionation schedules may be prescribed. For patients with close surgical margins, the operative bed may receive a boost up to 14 Gy in seven fractions (Hunt et al., 2001).
            (b) The regional lymph nodes are at risk in patients diagnosed with locally advanced breast carcinoma. For patients who have undergone breast-conserving surgery, the RT fields should be modified to include these node-bearing regions in addition to the glandular breast (Hunt et al., 2001).
            (c) For patients who received neoadjuvant chemotherapy and subsequent surgery for locally advanced breast cancers, treatment fields should encompass the original extent of disease (Hunt et al., 2001).
               i. In addition to the glandular breast, the treatment field should be expanded to include the ipsilateral supraclavicular fossa and the axilla and/or internal mammary lymph nodes, which can involve the use of multiple adjacent treatment fields (Hunt et al., 2001).
               ii. Multiple adjacent treatment fields must be carefully matched to avoid geographic overdosage (hot spots) or geographic underdosage (cold spots) (McBride & Withers, 2008).
               iii. Geographic overdosage can result in decreased range of motion, fibrosis, telangiectasia, and even necrosis (Hunt et al., 2001).
               iv. Geographic underdosage can result in locoregional recurrence following RT when an area of tissue harboring residual disease receives a subtherapeutic dose of radiation (Hunt et al., 2001).
            (d) Postmastectomy RT may be indicated based on tumor size, lymph node involvement, or for a close or positive posterior margin.

    i. Postmastectomy RT has an important role in reducing the risk of recurrence in patients diagnosed with locally advanced breast cancer (Buchholz & Haffty, 2008).

    ii. The entire volume of the mastectomy flaps must be included in the treatment field, including the entire length of the mastectomy scar and any clips, as well as drain sites (Hunt et al., 2001).

    iii. A dose of 50 Gy in 25 fractions is administered with a boost to the mastectomy flaps (Hunt et al., 2001).

    iv. For negative margins, 10 Gy in five fractions is given, and for patients with close or positive margins, 14–16 Gy in seven or eight fractions is given (Hunt et al., 2001).

b) Accelerated, hypofractionated whole breast RT

(1) Accelerated, hypofractionated whole breast RT (or "Canadian hypofractionation") includes a dose-fractionation scheme administering 42.5 Gy in 16 fractions.

(2) After 10 years of follow-up, local recurrence was comparable to standard therapy (6.2% recurrence rate for those who received Canadian fractionation versus 6.7% in patients who received standard therapy of 50 Gy in 25 fractions over 35 days) (Hopwood et al., 2010; Whelan et al., 2010).

(3) Patients treated with the accelerated, hypofractionated regimen had invasive breast cancer, negative axillary nodes, and negative surgical margins (Hopwood et al., 2010; Whelan et al., 2010).

(4) Those excluded were patients with node-positive breast cancer, tumors larger than 5 cm, breast width of 25 cm or more at the posterior border of the medial and lateral tangential beams, high-grade tumors, and ductal carcinoma in situ (Hopwood et al., 2010; Whelan et al., 2010).

(5) Boost irradiation was not used in the Whelan et al. (2010) trial but was administered in both of the Standardisation of Breast Radiotherapy (or START) trials A and B (Hopwood et al., 2010; Whelan et al., 2010).

c) Brachytherapy

(1) Brachytherapy, also known as accelerated partial breast irradiation (APBI), uses a high dose of RT delivered to the operative cavity and an additional 1–2 cm of adjacent tissue surrounding the operative cavity (Anné & Curran, 2010; Chronowski & Buchholz, 2007; Lehman & Hickey, 2010; Sanders, Scroggins, Ampil, & Li, 2007).

(2) Because a higher dose of radiation is delivered, therapy can be completed in a shorter period of time.

(3) In addition to a shorter overall treatment time, the amount of normal breast tissue that is treated is decreased, which can minimize both early and late reactions, such as skin toxicity, fatigue, and damage to surrounding organs such as the heart and lung while not compromising local control or cosmesis (Chronowski & Buchholz, 2007; Lehman & Hickey, 2010; Sanders et al., 2007).

(4) APBI techniques

    (a) Interstitial APBI (Anné & Curran, 2010; Chronowski & Buchholz, 2007; Lee & Harris, 2009; Lehman & Hickey, 2010; Sanders et al., 2007)

        i. Interstitial APBI uses LDR therapy.

        ii. Approximately 10–20 afterloading catheters are inserted through the surgical cavity at 1 cm intervals and fixed in place at the skin at the point of insertion and exit.

        iii. The radioactive source remains in the patient for the duration of treatment and provides a consistent dose delivery.

        iv. A total of 45–50 Gy is delivered over three to five days.

        v. Acute side effects
- Edema
- Erythema
- Fatigue
- Infection
- Pain
- Tenderness
- Hyperpigmentation

        vi. Late side effects
- Breast tenderness
- Fibrosis
- Skin thickening

- Telangiectasias
- Fat necrosis

(b) Intraoperative APBI (Anné & Curran, 2010; Chronowski & Buchholz, 2007; Sanders et al., 2007; Zeiss, 2010)

    i. Intraoperative APBI uses a high dose of low-energy (50 kV) x-rays to precisely deliver RT in the operative cavity.

    ii. The Intrabeam® System (Carl Zeiss Meditec) is currently under clinical evaluation. The TARGeted Intraoperative radioTherapy, or TARGiT, Trial is an international phase III randomized clinical trial comparing the delivery of targeted intraoperative RT with the Intrabeam System with conventional EBRT for the treatment of early-stage breast cancer. The purpose of the study is to determine whether one single fraction with the Intrabeam System is as effective as conventional EBRT in decreasing the risk of local recurrence and long-term changes within the breast.

    iii. The Intrabeam System allows patients to receive RT in the operating room at the time of breast-conserving surgery. Before the surgeon closes the incision, the Intrabeam applicator tip is placed directly into the operative cavity once the cancer has been removed. The spherical applicators range in size from 1.5 to 5 cm in diameter, which allows for precise conformation to the size of the operative bed. Low-energy radiation in a single fraction is delivered locally to the operative bed. The low-energy x-rays are rapidly absorbed over 1–2 cm. The radiation is delivered over 20–35 minutes. The Intrabeam applicator is removed and the surgeon then closes the incision.

(c) Intracavitary APBI (Anné & Curran, 2010; Bensaleh, Bezak, & Borg, 2009; Chronowski & Buchholz, 2007; Lehman &

Hickey, 2010; Pollock, 2007; Sanders et al., 2007)

    i. Intracavitary APBI uses HDR therapy.

    ii. At the time of breast-conserving surgery (open technique), a deflated single-entry multiple lumen balloon catheter or strut-adjusted volume implant (SAVI®, Cianna Medical, Inc.) device is placed into the operative cavity.

    iii. If the catheter is placed after surgery (closed technique), cavity evaluation is done to evaluate the cavity for the correct size of catheter. Under ultrasound guidance, the catheter is placed into the operative cavity.

    iv. The catheter exits the skin at a single point either through the surgical incision or a separate puncture site made by a trocar under ultrasound guidance.

    v. Once the catheter has been placed, saline and radiographic contrasts are instilled into the balloon catheter to position the breast tissue and to ensure the catheter fits snuggly in place. The SAVI device does not require the use of saline or contrast.

    vi. A small portion of the catheter remains outside of the breast and is secured to a gauze pad to prevent movement of the catheter.

    vii. CT scan or ultrasound is used to ensure proper geometry.

    viii. The use of a single-entry multiple-lumen catheter allows for a more flexible dose distribution.

ix. The catheter is attached to the HDR afterloading unit.

x. The HDR loading unit positions a ^{192}Ir radioactive source at either a single position or multiple positions within the catheter.

xi. After completion of each treatment, the radioactive source is removed.

xii. After each treatment, the site is cleansed with antibiotic solution, a thin layer of antibiotic ointment around the catheter is applied, and the exit site is covered with sterile gauze. The end of the catheter should contour to the patient's body to prevent excessive motion (Contura, n.d.).

xiii. A total dose of 34 Gy in 10 fractions given twice daily over five days is prescribed, with a minimum of six hours between each fraction.

xiv. After the final fraction, the catheter is removed through the same incision in which it was placed, and the incision is covered with a small dressing.

xv. Acute side effects
- Erythema
- Fatigue
- Infection
- Pain
- Tenderness
- Seroma formation

xvi. Late side effects
- Breast tenderness
- Fibrosis
- Fat necrosis

xvii. Patient eligibility
- Selection criteria from the American Brachytherapy Society (Hologic, 2010) include age 50 or older, unifocal invasive ductal carcinoma, tumor size less than or equal to 3 cm, negative microscopic surgical margins, and no lymph node involvement.
- Selection criteria from the American Society of Breast Surgeons and the American College of Radiation Oncology (Hologic, 2010) include age 45 or older, ductal carcinoma in situ or invasive ductal carcinoma, tumor size 3 cm or smaller, negative microscopic surgical margins, and negative sentinel lymph node.
- Characteristics of "suitable" patients according to ASTRO (Hologic, 2010) include age 60 or older, unifocal invasive ductal carcinoma or other favorable subtype (i.e., mucinous, colloid, or tubular), tumor size 2 cm or smaller, negative surgical margins by at least 2 mm, and negative lymph nodes on sentinel lymph node biopsy or axillary lymph node dissection.

xviii. Assessment
- Inspect the site for erythema, drainage, ecchymosis, wound abscess, hematoma formation, bleeding, warmth, or a nonhealing surgical or catheter site.
- Assess the patient for pain at the treatment site.
- Examine the skin for late effects such as scarring and thickening of the skin.

xix. Collaborative management for APBI
- Treat pain with over-the-counter or prescription pain medication.
- Prescribe antibiotics for wound abscess or catheter site infection.
- Refer to surgery to consider excision of nonhealing sinus tract.
- Obtain new baseline mammogram six months after completion of RT, then annually.

xx. Patient and family education
- Educate the patient and family on the procedure and possible acute and late side effects.

- Instruct the patient and family on site care and dressing change.
- Report symptoms of infection such as fever, redness, swelling, warmth, or drainage.
- After removal of the catheter, keep the catheter site clean and apply antibiotic cream.
- Cover with a clean adhesive bandage or dressing until there is no drainage and the site has closed.
- Arrange home health services if the patient or caregiver is unable to perform dressing changes.

3. Acute side effects—Skin
   a) Acute radiation dermatitis (see section IV.C—Skin reactions)
   b) Transient erythema can occur after the first fraction as a result of an inflammatory response, which leads to dilation of capillaries, increased vascular permeability, and edema and may subside within 24–48 hours (Lawenda & Johnstone, 2011; McQuestion, 2011).
   c) Erythema results from dilation of the blood vessels, expansion of the papillae from edema in the upper dermis, swollen endothelial cells, arteriole obstruction with fibrin thrombi, lymphocytic infiltration, and small foci of hemorrhage in the upper dermis. Erythema becomes more evident by the third and fourth week of therapy and is localized to the treatment field (Lawenda & Johnstone, 2011; McQuestion, 2006, 2011).
   d) Inflammation results from the invasion of neutrophils within the first week of therapy and is followed by the migration of eosinophils, lymphocytes, macrophages, mast cells, and plasma cells into the dermis resulting in an inflammatory exudate (Lawenda & Johnstone, 2011).
   e) Pruritus, scaling, and hyperpigmentation occurs during the fourth to fifth week of therapy. Hyperpigmentation results from increased melanin production in the basal layer as well as flattening of dermal papillae and thinning of the epidermis (Lawenda & Johnstone, 2011; McQuestion, 2006).
   f) Moist desquamation tends to occur in areas of increased friction, such as the axilla or the inframammary fold, and also may occur on the chest wall at doses greater than 40 Gy. Moist desquamation results from eradication of all stem cells from the basal layer with exposure of the dermis. Bullae form in the suprabasal and subepidermal layers and shed. A fibrinous layer then covers the denuded surface. Both dermal and subepidermal edema persists with development of an epidermal inflammatory infiltrate and stromal fibrin formation. The treatment field is tender, moist, and red with leaking of serous fluid and may be associated with discomfort or pain (Lawenda & Johnstone, 2011; McQuestion, 2006).
   g) Reepithelialization usually occurs within 10 days of the development of moist desquamation (Lawenda & Johnstone, 2011).
   h) Reepithelialization is complete by the sixth to eighth week after completion of therapy (Lawenda & Johnstone, 2011).
   i) Risk factors: The severity of skin changes, both during and after RT, is influenced by both patient-related and treatment-related factors.
      (1) Patient-related factors (McQuestion, 2011)
         (a) Older age
         (b) Breast size
         (c) Smoking history
         (d) Malnutrition
         (e) Chronic sun exposure
         (f) Comorbidities (e.g., diabetes, renal failure)
         (g) Seroma drainage prior to and during treatment
         (h) Dehiscence or infection of the surgical wound
      (2) Treatment-related factors (McQuestion, 2011)
         (a) Cumulative dose delivered
         (b) Location of treatment field
         (c) Fraction size and schedule
         (d) Techniques employed
         (e) Larger treatment field
         (f) Duration of treatment
         (g) Use of bolus material
   j) Assessment
      (1) Prior to the initiation of RT, assess the skin to ensure that surgical incisions have healed and are without evidence of infection.
      (2) Evaluate the skin weekly, as needed, and at routine follow-up.
      (3) Assess fatigue, pain, range of motion, and lymphedema at each appointment.

k) Documentation
  (1) Radiation dermatitis (NCI CTEP, 2010)
      (a) 1—Faint erythema or dry desquamation
      (b) 2—Moderate to brisk erythema; patchy moist desquamation, mostly confined to skin folds and creases; moderate edema
      (c) 3—Moist desquamation other than skin folds and creases; bleeding induced by minor trauma or abrasion
      (d) 4—Skin necrosis or ulceration of full-thickness dermis; spontaneous bleeding from involved site; skin graft indicated; life-threatening consequences
      (e) 5—Death
  (2) Fatigue (NCI CTEP, 2010)
      (a) 1—Fatigue relieved by rest
      (b) 2—Fatigue not relieved by rest; limiting instrumental ADL
      (c) 3—Fatigue not relieved by rest; limiting self-care ADL
  (3) Pain (NCI CTEP, 2010)
      (a) 1—Mild pain
      (b) 2—Moderate pain; limiting instrumental ADL
      (c) 3—Severe pain; limiting self-care ADL
l) Collaborative management for acute skin reactions
  (1) Prevention
      (a) Delay RT until all surgical sites are healed.
      (b) Identify factors that may increase the risk for skin reaction and take measures to decrease the risk for each factor, such as poor nutritional status, other comorbidities, medications, and smoking.
      (c) Use immobilization devices to reduce appositional skin folds, such as arm-positioning boards, breast boards, wingboards, positioning molds, and breast-immobilization devices (Alpha Cradle, n.d.; Bionix Radition Therapy, n.d.). Review previous treatment records in patients who have had previous RT in the same treatment field when considering reirradiation.
      (d) Caution or avoidance should be taken in patients with collagen vascular disease.
  (2) Intervention
      (a) Dry desquamation
          i. Use products likely to be effective in reducing the intensity of radiation dermatitis (McQuestion, 2011; ONS, 2010)
             • Hyaluronic acid
             • Calendula cream
          ii. Products are often used for skin reactions although are not evidence based (McQuestion, 2011; ONS, 2010).
          iii. Use a moisturizing cream that is unscented, lanolin free, and water based to maintain moisture at the skin surface and to maintain skin pliability (McQuestion, 2011).
          iv. Avoid lotions that contain alcohol, perfume, and other irritants.
          v. Use caution when using products that contain metal salts, such as antiperspirants and talcum powder (Graham & Graham, 2009; McQuestion, 2011; ONS, 2010; Théberge, Harel, & Dagnault, 2009).
      (b) Pruritus
          i. Aloe vera gel can soothe and cool the skin but will not moisturize the skin.
          ii. An oral or topical antihistamine may be helpful with pruritus.
          iii. Hydrophilic, hydrogel, and hydrocolloid dressings also may be soothing but do not expedite the healing process (MacMillan et al., 2007; McQuestion, 2011).
          iv. Colloidal oatmeal soaps and lotions can relieve pruritus.
      (c) Moist desquamation
          i. Apply a protective atraumatic dressing. Mepilex® Lite and

Mepilex Transfer (Mölnlycke Health Care) soft silicone foam dressings minimize maceration, maintain a moist environment, and do not stick to the wound (MacBride et al., 2008; Mölnlycke Health Care, n.d.).

ii. Manage pain with either over-the-counter or prescription medications.

iii. Treat infection but avoid the prophylactic use of antimicrobials to prevent resistance with overuse (McQuestion, 2006).

- Silver sulfadiazine has a lower toxicity and hypersensitivity profile and a lower incidence of resistance (McQuestion, 2006).
- Nystatin cream or powder can be used for *Candida* infections. Powder is not recommended with moist desquamation.

m) Patient and family education

(1) Discuss possible side effects associated with RT for breast cancer and which symptoms to report.

(2) Teach the patient the following self-care considerations.

(a) Avoid tight-fitting clothes, underwire bras, and heavy breast prostheses, which can cause additional skin irritation.

(b) Use a mild, unscented, nonalkaline soap to prevent further drying of the skin in the radiation treatment field (Bolderston et al., 2006; McQuestion, 2011).

(c) Use a washcloth or the tips of fingers to clean the breast or chest wall. Pat the skin dry or allow to air dry.

(d) Avoid extreme temperature changes, such as heating pads and ice packs, to prevent thermal injury.

(e) Avoid talcum powder and cornstarch in moist areas, such as skin folds and the axilla, which can create an environment for bacterial and fungal infections.

(f) Avoid scratching the skin, which can cause additional trauma to the skin.

(g) Avoid shaving under the arm to help minimize friction.

(h) Avoid adhesive tapes in the treatment field to prevent skin tears.

(i) Avoid sun exposure to the treatment fields.

(j) Avoid chlorinated pools and hot tubs, which can cause additional drying of the skin.

(k) Avoid lakes and rivers until the skin has healed to prevent infection.

4. Late side effects—Skin

a) Late skin reactions result from injury to the dermis (see section IV.C—Skin reactions).

b) Atrophy results from a decreased population of the dermal fibroblasts and reabsorption of collagen fibers (Harper, Franklin, Jenrette, & Aguero, 2010).

c) Remaining atypical fibroblasts are stimulated by growth factors that are produced in response to injury. As a response to the growth factors, the proliferation of the atypical fibroblasts results in deposition of dense fibrous tissue resulting in fibrosis. Radiation-induced fibrosis is characterized by edema formation, progressive induration, and thickening of the dermis (Harper et al., 2010).

d) Pigmentation changes can manifest as either hyperpigmentation or hypopigmentation. Some patients may experience hyperpigmentation, whereas other patients with darker-pigmented skin may actually develop hypopigmentation as a result of complete eradication of all melanocytes (Harper et al., 2010).

e) Telangiectasias are dilated blood vessels that result from injury of the reticular dermis and are visible through an atrophied dermal layer (Harper et al., 2010).

f) Assessment

(1) Assess for atrophy, fibrosis, pigmentation changes, and telangiectasias.

(2) Assess for skin breakdown, nonhealing wounds, tissue necrosis, and evidence of local recurrence.

g) Prevention: Patients should be taught to

(1) Avoid sun exposure, including tanning beds and booths, because the treatment area will be more sensitive to the sun.

(2) Use sunscreen with SPF 30 or greater.

(3) Avoid products that contain alcohol, perfume, or other harsh chemicals that irritate the skin.

h) Intervention

(1) Apply moisturizing lotions to the skin daily and as needed.

(2) Refer to physical therapy to increase elasticity, reduce fibrosis, and reduce scar formation, which could limit range of motion.

(3) Rule out cancer recurrence for patients presenting with nonhealing wounds, rash, or other skin changes prior to referral to a wound care specialist.

i) Patient and family education

(1) Discuss possible permanent skin changes associated with RT.

(2) Avoid sun exposure or tanning beds/booths and use sunscreen with SPF 30 or greater or keep the area covered.

(3) Moisturize the skin daily.

(4) Avoid products with alcohol, perfume, or other harsh chemicals that can irritate the skin.

5. Late side effects—Lymphedema

a) Abnormal accumulation of lymphatic fluid in interstitial spaces leads to persistent swelling (Fu, Ridner, & Armer, 2009a).

b) Lymphatic fluid is a clear liquid composed of protein, salts, water, and white blood cells (ACS, 2006; Singer, 2009).

c) The lymphatic system plays a key role in immune surveillance by transporting harmful substances within the lymphatic fluid to the lymph nodes, which subsequently present the substances to the immune system, which then elicits a response to protect the body (ACS, 2006).

d) Impaired lymphatic flow from the tissues can result in lymphedema and occurs when the amount of fluid exceeds the lymphatic system's ability to drain the fluid (ACS, 2006; Poage, Singer, Armer, Poundall, & Shellabarger, 2008).

e) Disruption of lymph nodes and vessels makes it difficult for the lymph system to drain fluid from distal areas (ACS, 2006; Poage et al., 2008).

f) If the undamaged portion of the lymphatic system is unable to remove fluid from that portion of the body, the protein-rich fluids continue to build, resulting in lymphedema (ACS, 2006; Poage et al., 2008).

(1) Primary lymphedema is a result of a genetic alteration that predisposes a patient to developing lymphedema (ACS, 2006; Fu et al., 2009a).

(2) Secondary lymphedema results from blockage or interruption in the lymphatic system and can result from surgery or RT (ACS, 2006; Fu et al., 2009a).

(a) Most common type of lymphedema

(b) Can occur months to years after completion of cancer treatment

g) Mild to moderate edema and thickening and faint pink hue of the breast can occur during the first six months after completion of RT and usually disappear by 12–18 months after completion of RT (Hunt et al., 2001).

h) Incidence and risk factors

(1) Most patients diagnosed with lymphedema have received treatment for breast cancer.

(a) An estimated 5%–60% of patients treated for breast cancer will develop lymphedema (ACS, 2006; Poage et al., 2008).

(b) Patients have developed lymphedema as late as 30 years after completion of treatment (ACS, 2006; Poage et al., 2008).

(c) With the advent of breast conservation and sentinel lymph node biopsy, the incidence of lymphedema has decreased (Hamner & Fleming, 2007).

(2) The severity of lymphedema can vary from patient to patient. Lymphostasis, impaired lymph movement, is a precursor to lymphedema. Lymphostasis does not result in visible symptoms. Lymphedema actually begins before visible changes are noted (ACS, 2006).

(3) Risk factors (Singer, 2009)

(a) Mastectomy (Sclafani & Baron, 2008; Tsai et al., 2009)

(b) Sentinel lymph node biopsy and axillary lymph node dissection (Sclafani & Baron, 2008)

(c) RT to the breast or chest wall and/or draining lymphatics: Shrinks the lymph nodes, which causes scarring of the lymphatic system and impeded flow of lymphatic fluid (ACS, 2006; Tsai et al., 2009)

(d) Axillary recurrence

(e) Multiple lymph nodes involved

(f) Postoperative infection, hematoma, or seroma

(g) BMI greater than 30

(4) Stage

(a) No consensus has been established regarding lymphedema grading or staging.

(b) The International Society of Lymphology staging system includes

four stages (ACS, 2006; Fu et al., 2009a).

   i. Stage 0—No swelling or pitting of the skin, but the patient may experience a heaviness of the affected arm caused by fluid buildup, which may be present for months to years.

   ii. Stage I—First stage with visible symptoms. When pressure is applied to the arm, an indention or pitting may be noted. This may not be evident in the early morning but progresses throughout the day and is reversible with elevation or compression of the arm.

   iii. Stage II—Increased edema is present, the skin pits, and the tissue becomes hardened and thickened. The patient has an increased risk of developing cellulitis, and swelling is not reduced with elevation of the arm.

   iv. Stage III—Affects the deeper dermal layer. The arm is large and swollen and the skin becomes inflamed, thickened, and tough, and lymph fluid may actually leak through the damaged skin. Irreversible without treatment.

(5) Assessment

  (a) Comparative circumferential measurement (ACS, 2006; Fu et al., 2009a)

   i. Uses a flexible, nonstretch tape measure to measure the affected arm and unaffected arm at several locations for comparison. Proximal to the metacarpals of the hand, the wrist, and every 4 cm from the wrist to the axilla should be measured.

   ii. A measurement of 1–2 cm more in the affected arm or 1–2 cm above baseline is often considered a sign of lymphedema.

  (b) Water displacement (ACS, 2006; Fu et al., 2009a; Singer, 2009)

   i. More accurate way of determining the circumference of the arm

   ii. Requires specialized equipment and training

   iii. The affected arm is submerged in a container of water. The displaced water flows into another container and is measured

   iv. Does not localize the location of edema or the shape of the extremity

  (c) Optoelectronic volumetry (Fu et al., 2009a)

   i. Method uses infrared light to calculate the volume and shape of the limb.

   ii. Volume changes can be calculated in seconds.

(6) Documentation of limb edema (NCI CTEP, 2010)

  (a) 1—Inter-limb difference of 5%–10% discrepancy in volume or circumference at point of greatest visible difference; swelling or obscuration of anatomic architecture on close inspection

  (b) 2—Greater than 10%–30% inter-limb discrepancy in volume or circumference at the point of greatest visible difference; readily apparent obscuration of anatomic architecture; obliteration of skin folds; readily apparent deviation from normal anatomic contour; limiting instrumental ADL

  (c) 3—Greater than 30% inter-limb discrepancy in volume; gross deviation from normal anatomic contour; limiting self care ADL

(7) Collaborative management of lymphedema

  (a) Obtain baseline measurement of both arms prior to initiation of RT and at each follow-up; document the locations of where measurements are obtained so that there is consistency with each visit.

  (b) Refer to a certified lymphedema therapist for combination therapy or complete decongestive therapy, which includes manual lymphatic drainage, compression, exercise, and skin care (ACS, 2006; National Lymphedema Network [NLN], 2010).

   i. Manual lymphatic drainage stimulates the absorption of lymphatic fluid and transportation of stagnant lymphatic fluid to areas where the lymphatic system is functioning (ACS, 2006).

ii. Compression helps reduce swelling and helps stagnant fluid in the arm to move into functioning lymphatic passageways. Pressure on the outside of the arm decreases internal pressure in the lymphatic system and maximizes the effects of the muscles pumping lymph throughout the body. Compression garments, pumps, and bandaging are used (ACS, 2006).

iii. Exercise should include flexing and curling of the hand and arm; stretching to maintain or restore range of motion, increase flexibility, improve lymphatic flow, and reduce fibrosis; aerobic activity to encourage lymphatic flow through muscular contraction; and strength training to protect muscles from fatigue, which will stimulate lymphatic fluid production (ACS, 2006).

iv. Keep the skin clean and moisturized.

(c) Monitor for signs and symptoms of lymphangitis.

   i. Rash

  ii. Blotchy, erythematous skin

 iii. Pruritus

 iv. Discoloration

  v. Increased swelling and sense of heaviness above baseline

 vi. Pain

vii. Sudden onset of chills and fever; treat with antibiotics. Penicillin is the drug of choice, but amoxicillin and cefazolin can be considered. For patients with a penicillin allergy, a cephalosporin can be prescribed (Auwaerter, 2010; NLN, 2010).

(8) Patient and family education

(a) ACS (2006) and NLN (2010) recommendations

  i. Discuss the signs and symptoms of lymphedema, as well as edema of the breast, and the importance of early recognition because lymphedema can lead to significant functional and psychological morbidity (ACS, 2006; Fu, Chen, Haber, Guth, & Axelrod, 2010; Poage et al., 2008; Smoot et al., 2010). These include decreased flexibility of the affected arm, swollen limb, visible skin changes including tightness and pitting, feeling of heaviness, tingling, fatigue, fullness, numbness, and aching.

ii. Educate the patient that edema of the breast can persist for 12–18 months after completion of RT and that compression bras can reduce edema.

iii. Wear a compression sleeve while awake.

iv. Assess the skin daily and report signs and symptoms of infection such as warmth, erythema, pain, increased swelling, fever of 100.5°F (38.1°C) or greater, chills, and heaviness of the arm.

 v. Maintain clean and supple skin by keeping the affected arm clean and moisturized. Use pH-neutral or oil-based lotions and soaps. The use of low-pH lotions can slow or prevent bacterial growth.

vi. Avoid cuts. Use an electric razor to remove underarm hair. Cut nails straight across. Avoid cutting the cuticles with scissors. Push the cuticles back with a cuticle stick. Wear a thimble when sewing to avoid pinpricks.

vii. Prevent insect bites by using an insect repellent.

viii. Avoid having blood draws, IV insertions, and injections in the affected arm.

ix. Wear protective gloves when gardening or cleaning.

 x. Clean breaks in the skin with warm water and soap, apply an over-the-counter antibacterial cream, and cover with a sterile dressing.

xi. Prevent sunburns by using sunscreen with SPF 30 or greater.

    xii. Avoid extreme temperature changes. Use the unaffected arm to test water temperature. Use caution when cooking with hot water and oils. Wear oven mitts when cooking.

   xiii. Avoid tight clothes and jewelry.

   xiv. Avoid carrying briefcases and purses on the affected shoulder.

   xv. Use the unaffected arm for blood pressure assessment.

   xvi. Treat pain with NSAIDs. If pain is unresponsive to over-the-counter medications, prescription pain medication may be indicated.

  xvii. Maintain a healthy weight.

  xviii. Drink plenty of water.

   xix. Exercise regularly but avoid straining the arm muscles and over-tiring the arm. Rest and elevate the arm as needed.

   xx. Use caution with air travel because of changes in barometric pressure. Wear a compression garment. Stretch frequently. Avoid carrying and lifting heavy luggage. Drink plenty of water or fruit juice during the flight.

(b) Trials are under way to determine whether axillary reverse mapping is safe and feasible in preventing lymphedema by enhancing lymphatic preservation (Bedrosian et al., 2010; Boneti et al., 2008; Noguchi, 2010; Thompson et al., 2007).

(c) Lymphatic venous anastomosis is being studied to determine whether microsurgery for lymphedema is beneficial in managing lymphedema when nonsurgical management has failed (Campisi et al., 2010; Damstra, Voesten, van Schelven, & van der Lei, 2009).

(d) The FDA approved low-level laser therapy (LLLT) in 2006 for the management of lymphedema in postmastectomy patients (Fu, Ridner, & Armer, 2009b; Morgan-Hazelwood & Balaicuis, 2010).

   i. LLLT affects the synthesis of fibroblasts and collagen, which influences the tissue repair process.

   ii. LLLT can be used in conjunction with manual lymphatic drainage.

   iii. Safety and effectiveness need to be determined when the laser is used beyond two three-week treatment blocks.

6. Late side effects—Secondary malignancy

  a) Secondary malignancy is a late but rare side effect of RT that can occur years after RT.

  b) A secondary malignancy is a new cancer that occurs within a previous radiation treatment field (Kaufman, Jacobson, Hershman, Desai, & Neugut, 2008).

    (1) Incidence and risk factors

      (a) RT for breast cancer treatment has been reported to increase the risk of developing squamous cell carcinoma of the upper to middle third of the esophagus as opposed to adenocarcinomas, which are primarily located in the lower third of the esophagus (Zablotska, Chak, Das, & Neugut, 2005).

      (b) Postmastectomy radiation has been found to increase the risk of developing an ipsilateral lung carcinoma because of the volume of lung tissue included in the treatment field (Deutsch et al., 2003; Kaufman et al., 2008; Zablotska & Neugut, 2003).

        i. Because smoking is a risk factor for developing lung cancer, the effects of radiation combined with the carcinogenic effects of cigarette smoking may have a synergistic effect and increase the risk for developing lung cancer (Iyer & Jhingran, 2006; Kaufman et al., 2008).

      ii. Patients who smoke are also at higher risk for developing postmastectomy radiation-induced lung cancer (Kaufman et al., 2008).

    (c) Angiosarcoma, fibrosarcoma, malignant fibrous histiocytomas, and osteosarcoma are rare radiation-associated sarcomas that have been documented in the literature (Di Tommaso & Fabbri, 2003; Fineberg & Rosen, 1994; Hildebrandt, Mittag, Gütz, Kunze, & Haustein, 2001; Orta, Suprun, Goldfarb, Bleiweiss, & Jaffer, 2006; Rudman et al., 2002).

(2) Patient and family education

    (a) Instruct the patient to report symptoms of esophageal cancer, including unintentional weight loss, difficulty swallowing, hoarseness, persistent cough, heartburn, sensation that food is getting stuck, and fatigue. Refer to gastroenterology for upper endoscopy and biopsy.

    (b) Instruct the patient to report symptoms of lung cancer, including a persistent cough, chest pain, arm and shoulder pain, hemoptysis, shortness of breath, wheezing, hoarseness, swelling of the face or neck, loss of appetite, unintentional weight loss, fatigue, and recurrent episodes of pneumonia and bronchitis. Refer to pulmonologist for chest x-ray, CT scan, and biopsy.

    (c) Instruct the patient to report skin changes, pain, swelling, and nodules in the previous radiation treatment field.

    (d) Discuss with the patient risk factors such as alcohol use, smoking, use of chewing tobacco, gastroesophageal reflux disease, obesity, and a diet high in fat and low in fruits and vegetables.

(3) Collaborative management

    (a) Follow the ACS guidelines for the early detection of cancer.

    (b) Refer for smoking cessation.

    (c) Refer to dietitian for nutrition counseling.

    (d) Encourage the patient to continue routine follow-up care with primary care physician and specialists.

7. Late side effects—Radiation pneumonitis

    a) Can occur between six weeks and six months after completion of RT and tends to be related to the volume of lung included in the radiation treatment field, the cumulative dose, and treatment technique (Hunt et al., 2001)

    b) Risk is greater in patients treated with comprehensive chest wall RT than those who received whole breast RT (Hunt et al., 2001).

    c) Radiation-induced lung changes conform to the radiation treatment portals (Iyer & Jhingran, 2006).

    d) Patient and family education: Report symptoms of radiation pneumonitis such as cough, shortness of breath, low-grade fever, and chest fullness.

    e) Collaborative management

      (1) Chest x-ray or CT imaging to confirm diagnosis of radiation pneumonitis and rule out other causes

      (2) High-dose steroids, such as prednisone, can be useful in reducing inflammation.

      (3) Radiation pneumonitis can lead to bacterial infection; treat with antibiotics.

      (4) Oxygen therapy may be indicated for chronic radiation pneumonitis.

8. Late side effects—Brachial plexopathy

    a) The brachial plexus supplies the entire nerve supply of the shoulders and upper extremities. Roots of spinal nerves C5 thru C8 and T1 form the brachial plexus. The brachial plexus extends both laterally and inferiorly on either side of the last four cervical vertebrae and first thoracic vertebrae and passes above the first rib posterior to the clavicle then enters the axilla (Tortora & Derrickson, 2006).

    b) Brachial plexopathy is a condition that results from changes in action potentials and conduction time and is accompanied by altered vascular permeability, anomalies of microtubule assembly, and neurilemmal damage. With time, extensive fibrosis can develop in connective tissue surrounding nerves, which results in decreased vascularity and direct pressure on the plexus (Gosk, Rutowski, Urban, Wiecek, & Rabczyński, 2007; Recht, 2011).

    c) Radiation toxicity to the brachial plexus is the most common radiation toxicity affecting the peripheral nervous system (Dropcho, 2010).

    d) Neuropathy after RT includes changes in electrophysiology, histochemistry, and fibrosis of the tissue surrounding the nerves (Gosk, Rutowski, Reichert, & Rabczyński, 2007).

e) Total radiation dose, fractionation dose, treatment technique, overlapping treatment fields, increased dose to the axilla and supraclavicular fossa, concurrent chemotherapy, and the premorbid state of the irradiated nerves can contribute to the development of brachial plexopathy (Gosk, Rutowski, Reichert, et al., 2007; Kamenova et al., 2009; Schierle & Winograd, 2004).

f) Brachial plexopathy can develop months to years after completion of RT (Gosk, Rutowski, Reichert, et al., 2007; Kamenova et al., 2009; Schierle & Winograd, 2004).

(1) Assessment

    (a) Assess the patient for symptoms associated with brachial plexopathy (Gosk, Rutowski, Reichert, et al., 2007; Kamenova et al., 2009; Schierle & Winograd, 2004).

        i. Pain

        ii. Numbness—Fourth and fifth digit on affected side

        iii. Paresthesia

        iv. Dysesthesia

        v. Swelling of the upper extremity

        vi. Weakness of the hand, wrist, and arm

        vii. Inability to extend or lift the wrist

        viii. Muscle atrophy

        ix. Decreased muscle stretch exercises

    (b) Obtain a CT scan or MRI of the brachial plexus to diagnose brachial plexopathy. A diffuse, ill-defined loss of tissue plane is consistent with radiation-induced injury to the brachial plexus (Bowen, Verma, Brandon, & Fiedler, 1996).

    (c) Electromyography studies can be useful in the diagnosis of brachial plexopathy. Nerve conduction velocities can differentiate brachial plexopathy from other neurologic dysfunctions but cannot differentiate between radiation-induced brachial plexopathy and metastatic brachial plexopathy. Electromyography findings may include increases in latency, re-

duction in amplitude, and slowing in conduction velocity (Gosk, Rutowski, Reichert, et al., 2007; Schierle & Winograd, 2004).

(2) Documentation

    (a) Brachial plexopathy (NCI CTEP, 2010)

        i. 1—Asymptomatic; clinical or diagnostic observations only; intervention not indicated

        ii. 2—Moderate symptoms; limiting instrumental ADL

        iii. 3—Severe symptoms; limiting self-care ADL

    (b) Peripheral motor neuropathy (NCI CTEP, 2010)

        i. 1—Asymptomatic; clinical or diagnostic observations only; intervention not indicated

        ii. 2—Moderate symptoms; limiting instrumental ADL

        iii. 3—Severe symptoms; limiting self-care ADL; assistive device indicated

        iv. 4—Life-threatening consequences; urgent intervention indicated

        v. 5—Death

    (c) Peripheral sensory neuropathy (NCI CTEP, 2010)

        i. 1—Asymptomatic; loss of deep tendon reflexes or paresthesia

        ii. 2—Moderate symptoms; limiting instrumental ADL

        iii. 3—Severe symptoms; limiting self-care ADL

        iv. 4—Life-threatening consequences; urgent intervention indicated

        v. 5—Death

(3) Collaborative management

    (a) Determine whether the plexopathy is disease related or treatment related.

    (b) Refer to physical therapist to prevent atrophy, frozen shoulder, lymphedema, and muscle spasms.

    (c) Refer to occupational therapist to maintain functional status.

    (d) Manage pain.

        i. The use of tricyclic antidepressants, dual reuptake inhibitors of both serotonin and norepinephrine antidepressants, calcium channel alpha-2-delta li-

gands, topical lidocaine, opioid analgesics, and tramadol may be useful in the treatment of neuropathic pain (Gosk, Rutowski, Reichert, et al., 2007; O'Connor & Dworkin, 2009; Schierle & Winograd, 2004).

  ii. Refer for consideration of a transcutaneous electrical nerve stimulation unit or dorsal column stimulator for intractable pain (Schierle & Winograd, 2004).

(4) Patient and family education
  (a) Instruct the patient to report symptoms of brachial plexopathy.
  (b) Educate the patient on potential injury resulting from motor and sensory changes.
  (c) Educate the patient and family on the importance of early physical therapy to prevent muscular atrophy, frozen shoulder, and lymphedema.
  (d) Educate the patient and family on the importance of early occupational therapy to help maintain the patient's functional status.

9. Late side effects—Bone toxicity and rib fracture
  a) RT doses do not typically result in profound acute injury to bony structures (Hoebers, Ferguson, & O'Sullivan, 2011).
  b) Because of the slow metabolic turnover rate of bone, there is a latent period before changes are clinically evident (Hoebers et al., 2011).
  c) Late effects of RT include damage to osteoblasts, decreased matrix formation, and osteopenia within the previous treatment field and can be seen on radiograph one year following the completion of treatment (Hoebers et al., 2011; Iyer & Jhingran, 2006).
  d) Repair follows bone atrophy with bone deposition on unresorbed trabeculae (Hoebers et al., 2011; Iyer & Jhingran, 2006).
  e) Radiographs show mottled areas of bone with osteopenia, course trabeculation, and focal areas of increased bone density, referred to as *radiation-induced osteitis* (Hoebers et al., 2011).
  f) Rib fracture increases in incidence with a higher total radiation dose, hypofractionation, low machine energy, and larger volume of rib or chest wall included in the RT fields (Hoebers et al., 2011).
  g) Rib fractures tend to be painless, identified incidentally on radiograph, and involve the anterior aspects of the third to fifth ribs (Mitchell & Logan, 1998).
  h) Patient and family education
    (1) Report symptoms of bone toxicity.
      (a) Chest pain
      (b) Pain with cough or deep inspiration
      (c) Difficulty breathing
      (d) Pain with movement
      (e) Rib swelling
      (f) Rib bruising
      (g) Chest wall deformity
    (2) Encourage the patient to cough frequently despite pain to decrease the risk for developing pneumonia.
    (3) Discuss positioning to promote comfort and reduce pain associated with rib fracture.
  i) Collaborative management
    (1) Obtain rib films to confirm rib fracture and rule out metastatic disease.
    (2) Treat pain with over-the-counter or prescription pain medication.
    (3) Assess for signs of respiratory distress.

10. Late side effects—Cardiac and vascular toxicity
  a) Radiation-induced cardiac complications result from injury to the heart as a result of radiation to adjacent tissues.
  b) Cardiac complications may result from damage to microvasculature and macrovasculature (Demirci, Nam, Hubbs, Nguyen, & Marks, 2009; Senkus-Konefka & Jassem, 2007).
  c) Damage to the microvasculature begins with injury to endothelial cells (Demirci et al., 2009; Senkus-Konefka & Jassem, 2007).
  d) Capillary swelling and progressive obstruction of the vessel lumen result in ischemia and can lead to fibrosis (Demirci et al., 2009; Senkus-Konefka & Jassem, 2007).

e) Macrovascular damage from injury to the larger vessels leads to the exacerbation of atherosclerotic lesion formation (Demirci et al., 2009; Senkus-Konefka & Jassem, 2007).

f) Damage to the pericardium can result in fibrous thickening, pericardial adhesions, and excessive pericardial fluid (Demirci et al., 2009; Senkus-Konefka & Jassem, 2007).

g) Valvular damage can result in thickening, fibrosis, and calcification of the cusp or leaflets of the valves (Demirci et al., 2009; Senkus-Konefka & Jassem, 2007).

h) For patients receiving RT, the mechanism and pathology of coronary artery disease are similar to those of the general population, but it tends to develop at a younger age and in patients with risk factors such as hypertension, obesity, and smoking (Demirci et al., 2009; Senkus-Konefka & Jassem, 2007).

i) The different features of radiation-induced cardiac change are the presence of more fibrotic changes in the media and adventitia, depletion of media smooth muscle, and predominance of coronary artery ostial stenosis (Demirci et al., 2009; Senkus-Konefka & Jassem, 2007).

j) Radiation-induced cardiac complications are a concern for patients receiving RT for left-sided breast cancer.

k) Fewer cardiac complications develop with modern treatment techniques when radiation is delivered tangentially (Demirci et al., 2009; Lenihan & Esteva, 2008).

l) Older RT techniques increased the risk of death associated with radiation-induced cardiac toxicity because of significant exposure of the coronary arteries and/or myocardium (Evans et al., 2006).

m) For patients receiving radiation following breast-conserving surgery or mastectomy, the most common affected vessel is the left anterior descending coronary artery because this artery lies close to the edge of the tangential RT fields (Buchholz, Strom, & McNeese, 2003).

n) In addition, patients receiving radiation to the supraclavicular fossa often receive a significant dose to the proximal carotid artery (Senkus-Konefka & Jassem, 2007).

o) Treatment-related risk factors (Senkus-Konefka & Jassem, 2007)
  (1) Hormonal therapy
  (2) Systemic chemotherapy

  (3) Therapeutic doses of 40–50 Gy or greater to partial volumes of the heart

p) Incidence is higher when additional cardiovascular risk factors are present (Giraud, Henni, Yassa, & Cosset, 2011).

q) Patient-related risk factors (Giraud et al., 2011)
  (1) Obesity
  (2) Menopausal status
  (3) Younger age
  (4) Smoking
  (5) Diabetes mellitus
  (6) Hypertension
  (7) Hypercholesterolemia
  (8) Physical inactivity

r) Patient and family education: Instruct the patient to report symptoms of radiation-induced cardiac toxicity.
  (1) Chest pain
  (2) Fatigue
  (3) Shortness of breath
  (4) Discomfort lying flat

s) Collaborative management
  (1) Treatment technique and the skill of the radiation oncologist are key factors in limiting radiation-induced cardiac toxicity (Bird & Swain, 2008).
  (2) Deep inspiration breath-hold technique can reduce cardiac volume in the RT field (Lee & Harris, 2009; Stranzl & Zurl, 2008).
  (3) Refer to cardiologist for further evaluation and treatment recommendations.

References

Alpha Cradle. (n.d.). Alpha Cradle®: The leader in repositioning for radiation therapy: Breast forms. Retrieved from http://www.alpha cradle.com/category/products/breast-forms

American Cancer Society. (2006). *Lymphedema: Understanding and managing lymphedema after cancer treatment.* Atlanta, GA: Author.

Anné, P.R., & Curran, W.J., Jr. (2010). Radiation therapy in breast-conserving therapy for invasive breast cancer. In H. Silberman & A.W. Silberman (Eds.), *Principles and practice of surgical oncology: Multidisciplinary approach to difficult problems* (pp. 385–396). Philadelphia, PA: Lippincott Williams & Wilkins.

Auwaerter, P. (2010). Lymphangitis. In J.G. Bartlett, P.G. Auwaerter, & P. Pham (Eds.), *Johns Hopkins ABX guide.* Retrieved from http://www.hopkinsguides.com/hopkins/ub

Bedrosian, I., Babiera, G.V., Mittendorf, E.A., Kuerer, H.M., Pantoja, L., Hunt, K.K., ... Meric-Bernstam, F. (2010). A phase I study to assess the feasibility and oncologic safety of axillary reverse mapping in breast cancer patients. *Cancer, 116,* 2543–2548. doi:10.1002/cncr.25096

Bensaleh, S., Bezak, E., & Borg, M. (2009). Review of MammoSite brachytherapy: Advantages, disadvantages and clinical outcomes. *Acta Oncologica, 48*, 487–494. doi:10.1080/02841860802537916

Bionix Radiation Therapy. (n.d.). Bionix® Radiation Therapy: Breast and lung devices. Retrieved from http://www.bionixrt.com/RT_Pages/Breast_Lung.html

Bird, B.H., & Swain, S.M. (2008). Cardiac toxicity in breast cancer survivors: Review of potential cardiac problems. *Clinical Cancer Research, 14*, 14–24. doi:10.1158/1078-0432.CCR-07-1033

Bolderston, A., Lloyd, N.S., Wong, R.K., Holden, L., Robb-Blenderman, L., & Supportive Care Guidelines Group of Cancer Care Ontario Program in Evidence-based Care. (2006). The prevention and management of acute skin reactions related to radiation therapy: A systematic review and practice guidelines. *Supportive Care in Cancer, 14*, 802–817. doi:10.1007/s00520-006-0063-4

Boneti, C., Korourian, S., Bland, K., Cox, K., Adkins, L.L., Henry-Tillman, R.S., & Klimberg, V.S. (2008). Axillary reverse mapping: Mapping and preserving arm lymphatics may be important in preventing lymphedema during sentinel lymph node biopsy. *Journal of the American College of Surgeons, 206*, 1038–1042. doi:10.1016/j.jamcollsurg.2007.12.022

Bowen, B.C., Verma, A., Brandon, A.H., & Fiedler, J.A. (1996). Radiation-induced brachial plexopathy: MR and clinical findings. *American Journal of Neuroradiology, 17*, 1932–1936.

Buchholz, T.A., & Haffty, B.G. (2008). Breast cancer: Locally advanced and recurrent disease, postmastectomy radiation, and systemic therapies. In E.C. Halperin, C.A. Perez, & L.W. Brady (Eds.), *Perez and Brady's principles and practice of radiation oncology* (5th ed., pp. 1292–1317). Philadelphia, PA: Lippincott Williams & Wilkins.

Buchholz, T.A., Strom, E.A., & McNeese, M.D. (2003). The breast. In J.D. Cox & K.K. Ang (Eds.), *Radiation oncology: Rationale, techniques, results* (pp. 333–385). St. Louis, MO: Mosby.

Campisi, C., Bellini, C., Campisi, C., Accogli, S., Bonioli, E., & Boccardo, F. (2010). Microsurgery for lymphedema: Clinical research and long-term results. *Microsurgery, 30*, 256–260. doi:10.1002/micr.20737

Chronowski, G.M., & Buchholz, T.A. (2007). Accelerated partial breast irradiation. *Current Problems in Cancer, 31*, 1–28. doi:10.1016/j.currproblcancer.2006.10.001

Contura. (n.d.). Instructions for daily Contura MLB dressing changes. Retrieved from http://www.senorx.com/products/apbi/contura/documents/MM0256A-ConturaDailyDressingChangesv5.pdf

Damstra, R.J., Voesten, H.G.J., van Schelven, W.D., & van der Lei, B. (2009). Lymphatic venous anastomosis (LVA) for treatment of secondary arm lymphedema. A prospective study of 11 LVA procedures in 10 patients with breast cancer related lymphedema and a critical review of the literature. *Breast Cancer Research and Treatment, 113*, 199–206. doi:10.1007/s10549-008-9932-5

Demirci, S., Nam, J., Hubbs, J.L., Nguyen, T., & Marks, L.B. (2009). Radiation-induced cardiac toxicity after therapy for breast cancer: Interaction between treatment era and follow-up duration. *International Journal of Radiation Oncology, Biology, Physics, 73*, 980–987. doi:10.1016/j.ijrobp.2008.11.016

Deutsch, M., Land, S.R., Begovic, M., Wieand, H.S., Wolmark, N., & Fisher, B. (2003). The incidence of lung carcinoma after surgery for breast carcinoma with and without postoperative radiotherapy. *Cancer, 98*, 1362–1368. doi:10.1002/cncr.11655

Di Tommaso, L., & Fabbri, A. (2003). Cutaneous angiosarcoma arising after radiotherapy treatment of a breast carcinoma. Description of a case and review of the literature [Abstract]. *Pathologica, 95*, 196–202.

Dropcho, E.J. (2010). Neurotoxicity of radiation therapy. *Neurologic Clinics, 28*, 217–234. doi:10.1016/j.ncl.2009.09.008

Evans, E.S., Prosnitz, R.G., Yu, X., Zhou, S.M., Hollis, D.R., Wong, T.Z., ... Marks, L.B. (2006). Impact of patient-specific factors, irradiated left ventricular volume, and treatment set-up errors on the development of myocardial perfusion defects after radiation therapy for left-sided breast cancer. *International Journal of Radiation Oncology, Biology, Physics, 66*, 1125–1134.

Fineberg, S., & Rosen, P.P. (1994). Cutaneous angiosarcoma and atypical vascular lesions of the skin and breast after radiation therapy for breast carcinoma. *American Journal of Clinical Pathology, 102*, 757–763.

Fu, M.R., Chen, C.M., Haber, J., Guth, A.A., & Axelrod, D. (2010). The effects of providing information about lymphedema on the cognitive and symptom outcomes of breast cancer survivors. *Annals of Surgical Oncology, 17*, 1847–1853. doi:10.1245/s10434-010-0941-3

Fu, M.R., Ridner, S.H., & Armer, J. (2009a). Post-breast cancer lymphedema: Part 1. *American Journal of Nursing, 109*(7), 48–54.

Fu, M.R., Ridner, S.H., & Armer, J. (2009b). Post-breast cancer lymphedema: Part 2. *American Journal of Nursing, 109*(8), 34–41.

Giraud, P., Henni, M., Yassa, M., & Cosset, J.-M. (2011). Heart. In D.C. Shrieve & J.S. Loeffler (Eds.), *Human radiation injury* (pp. 316–322). Philadelphia, PA: Lippincott Williams & Wilkins.

Gosk, J., Rutowski, R., Reichert, P., & Rabczyński, J. (2007). Radiation-induced brachial plexus neuropathy—Aetiopathogenesis, risk factors, differential diagnostics, symptoms and treatment. *Folia Neuropathologica, 45*, 26–30.

Gosk, J., Rutowski, R., Urban, M., Wiecek, R., & Rabczyński, J. (2007). Brachial plexus injuries after radiotherapy—Analysis of 6 cases. *Folia Neuropathologica, 45*, 31–35.

Graham, P.H., & Graham, J.L. (2009). Use of deodorants during adjuvant breast radiotherapy: A survey of compliance with standard advice, impact on patients and a literature review on safety. *Journal of Medical Imaging and Radiation Oncology, 53*, 569–573. doi:10.1111/j.1754-9485.2009.02125.x

Haffty, B.G., Buchholz, T.A., & Perez, C.A. (2008). Early stage breast cancer. In E.C. Halperin, C.A. Perez, & L.W. Brady (Eds.), *Perez and Brady's principles and practice of radiation oncology* (5th ed., pp. 1175–1291). Philadelphia, PA: Lippincott Williams & Wilkins.

Hamner, J.B., & Fleming, M.D. (2007). Lymphedema therapy reduces the volume of edema and pain in patients with breast cancer. *Annals of Surgical Oncology, 14*, 1904–1908. doi:10.1245/s10434-006-9332-1

Harper, J.L., Franklin, L.E., Jenrette, J.M., & Aguero, E.G. (2010, July 24). Skin toxicity during breast irradiation: Pathophysiology and sequence of radiation-induced skin changes. Retrieved from http://www.medscape.com/viewarticle/493434_3

Hildebrandt, G., Mittag, M., Gütz, U., Kunze, M.L., & Haustein, U.F. (2001). Cutaneous breast angiosarcoma after conserving treatment of breast cancer. *European Journal of Dermatology, 11*, 580–583.

Hoebers, F.J.P., Ferguson, P.C., & O'Sullivan, B. (2011). Bone. In D.C. Shrieve & J.S. Loeffler (Eds.), *Human radiation injury* (pp. 481–498). Philadelphia, PA: Lippincott Williams & Wilkins.

Hologic. (2010, July 20). Am I a candidate for MammoSite 5-day targeted radiation therapy? Retrieved from http://www.mammosite.com/breast-mastectomy/mammosite-right-me.cfm

Hopwood, P., Haviland, J.S., Sumo, G., Mills, J., Bliss, J.M., & START Trial Management Group. (2010). Comparison of patient-reported breast, arm, and shoulder symptoms and body image after radiotherapy for early breast cancer: 5 year follow-up in the randomized standardisation of breast radiotherapy (START) trials. *Lancet Oncology, 11*, 231–240. doi:10.1016/s1470-2045-09-70382-1

Hunt, K.K., Robb, J.L., Strom, E.A., & Ueno, N.T. (Eds.). (2001). *M.D. Anderson cancer care series: Breast cancer.* New York, NY: Springer.

Iyer, R., & Jhingran, A. (2006). Radiation injury: Imaging findings in the chest, abdomen and pelvis after therapeutic radiation. *Cancer Imaging, 6*(Spec. No. A), S131–S139. doi:10.1102/1470-7330.2006.9095

Kamenova, B., Braverman, A.A., Schwartz, M., Sohn, C., Lange, C., Efiom-Ekaha, D., … Yoon, H. (2009). Effective treatment of the brachial plexus syndrome in breast cancer patients by early detection and control of loco-regional metastases with radiation or systemic therapy. *International Journal of Clinical Oncology, 14*, 219–224. doi:10.1007/s10147-008-0838-3

Kaufman, E.L., Jacobson, J.S., Hershman, D.L., Desai, M., & Neugut, A.I. (2008). Effect of breast cancer radiotherapy and cigarette smoking on risk of second primary lung cancer. *Journal of Clinical Oncology, 26*, 392–398. doi:10.1200/JCO.2007.13.3033

Lawenda, B.D., & Johnstone, P.A.S. (2011). Skin. In D.C. Shrieve & J.S. Loeffler (Eds.), *Human radiation injury* (pp. 499–515). Philadelphia, PA: Lippincott Williams & Wilkins.

Lee, L.J., & Harris, J.R. (2009). Innovations in radiation therapy (RT) for breast cancer. *Breast, 18*(Suppl. 3), S103–S111. doi:10.1016/S0960-9776-09-70284-x

Lehman, M., & Hickey, B. (2010). The less than whole breast radiotherapy approach. *Breast, 19*, 180–187. doi:10.1016/j.breast.2010.03.005

Lenihan, D.J., & Esteva, F.J. (2008). Multidisciplinary strategy for managing cardiovascular risks when treating patients with early breast cancer. *Oncologist, 13*, 1224–1234. doi:10.1634/theoncologist.2008-0112

MacBride, S.K., Wells, M.E., Hornsby, C., Sharp, L., Finnila, K., & Downie, L. (2008). A case study to evaluate a new soft silicone dressing, Mepilex Lite, for patients with radiation skin reactions. *Cancer Nursing, 31*(1), E8–E14. doi:10.1097/01.NCC.0000305680.06143.39

MacMillan, M.S., Wells, M., MacBride, S., Raab, G.M., Munro, A., & MacDougall, H. (2007). Randomized comparison of dry dressings versus hydrogel in management of radiation-induced moist desquamation. *International Journal of Radiation Oncology, Biology, Physics, 68*, 864–872. doi:10.1016/j.ijrobp.2006.12.049

McBride, W.H., & Withers, H.R. (2008). Biologic basis of radiation therapy. In E.C. Halperin, C.A. Perez, & L.W. Brady (Eds.), *Perez and Brady's principles and practice of radiation oncology* (5th ed., pp. 76–108). Philadelphia, PA: Lippincott Williams & Wilkins.

McQuestion, M. (2006). Evidence-based skin management in radiation therapy. *Seminars in Oncology Nursing, 22*, 163–173. doi:10.1016/j.soncn.2006.04.004

McQuestion, M. (2011). Evidence-based skin care management in radiation therapy: Clinical update. *Seminars in Oncology Nursing, 27*(2), e1–e17. doi:10.1016/j.soncn.2011.02.009

Mitchell, M.J., & Logan, P.M. (1998). Radiation-induced changes in bone. *Radiographics, 18*, 1125–1136.

Mölnlycke Health Care. (n.d.). Wound care: Mepilex® Lite. Retrieved from http://www.molnlycke.com/com/Wound-Care-Products/Product-selector---Wound-division/Tabs/Products/Mepilex-Lite/?activeTab=2

Morgan-Hazelwood, W., & Balaicuis, J. (2010). A new advance in lymphedema therapy. *Oncology Nurse-APN/PA, 3*(4), 32–34.

National Cancer Institute Cancer Therapy Evaluation Program. (2010). *Common terminology criteria for adverse events* [v.4.03]. Retrieved from http://evs.nci.nih.gov/ftp1/CTCAE/CTCAE_4.03_2010-06-14_QuickReference_8.5x11.pdf

National Lymphedema Network. (2010). Treatments for lymphedema. Retrieved from http://www.lymphnet.org/lymphedemaFAQs/overview.htm

Noguchi, M. (2010). Axillary reverse mapping for breast cancer. *Breast Cancer Research and Treatment, 119*, 529–535. doi:10.1007/s10549-009-0578-8

O'Connor, A.B., & Dworkin, R.H. (2009). Treatment for neuropathic pain: An overview of recent guidelines. *American Journal of Medicine, 122*(Suppl. 10), S22–S32. doi:10.1016/j.amjmed.2009.04.007

Oncology Nursing Society. (2010). ONS putting evidence into practice: Radiodermatitis: Evidence table. Retrieved from http://www.ons.org/Research/PEP/media/ons/docs/research/outcomes/radiodermatitis/evidencetable.pdf

Orta, L., Suprun, U., Goldfarb, A., Bleiweiss, I., & Jaffer, S. (2006). Radiation-associated extraskeletal osteosarcoma of the chest wall. *Archives of Pathology and Laboratory Medicine, 130*, 198–200.

Poage, E., Singer, M., Armer, J., Poundall, M., & Shellabarger, M.J. (2008). Demystifying lymphedema: Development of the lymphedema Putting Evidence Into Practice® card. *Clinical Journal of Oncology Nursing, 12*, 951–964. doi:10.1188/08.CJON.951-964

Pollock, J. (2007). Partial breast irradiation: A community hospital approach. *Community Oncology, 4*(1), 37–42.

Recht, A. (2011). Brachial plexus. In D.C. Shrieve & J.S. Loeffler (Eds.), *Human radiation injury* (pp. 246–253). Philadelphia, PA: Lippincott Williams & Wilkins.

Rudman, F., Jr., Stanec, S., Stanec, M., Stanec, Z., Margaritoni, M., Žic, R., Šeparović, V. (2002). Rare complication of breast cancer irradiation: Postirradiation osteosarcoma. *Annals of Plastic Surgery, 48*, 318–322.

Sanders, M.E., Scroggins, T., Ampil, F.L., & Li, B.D. (2007). Accelerated partial breast irradiation in early-stage breast cancer. *Journal of Clinical Oncology, 25*, 996–1002. doi:10.1200/JCO.2006.09.7436

Schierle, C., & Winograd, J.M. (2004). Radiation-induced brachial plexopathy: Review. Complications without a cure. *Journal of Reconstructive Microsurgery, 20*, 149–152. doi:10.1055/s-2004-820771

Sclafani, L.M., & Baron, R.H. (2008). Sentinel lymph node biopsy and axillary dissection: Added morbidity of the arm, shoulder and chest wall after mastectomy and reconstruction. *Cancer Journal, 14*, 216–222. doi:10.1097/PPO.0b013e31817fbe5e

Senkus-Konefka, E., & Jassem, J. (2007). Cardiovascular effects of breast cancer radiotherapy. *Cancer Treatment Reviews, 33*, 578–593. doi:10.1016/j.ctrv.2007.07.011

Singer, M. (2009). Lymphedema in breast cancer: Dilemmas and challenges. *Clinical Journal of Oncology Nursing, 13*, 350–352. doi:10.1188/09.CJON.350-352

Smoot, B., Wong, J., Cooper, B., Wanek, L., Topp, K., Byl, N., & Dodd, M. (2010). Upper extremity impairments in women with or without lymphedema following breast cancer treatment. *Journal of Cancer Survivorship, 4,* 167–178. doi:10.1007/s11764-010-0118-x

Stranzl, H., & Zurl, B. (2008). Postoperative irradiation of left-sided breast cancer patients and cardiac toxicity. Does deep inspiration breast-hold (DIBH) technique protect the heart? *Strahlentherapie und Onkologie, 184,* 354–358. doi:10.1007/s00066-008-1852-0

Théberge, V., Harel, F., & Dagnault, A. (2009). Use of axillary deodorant and effect on acute skin toxicity during radiotherapy for breast cancer: A prospective randomized noninferiority trial. *International Journal of Radiation Oncology, Biology, Physics, 75,* 1048–1052. doi:10.1016/j.ijrobp.2008.12.046

Thompson, M., Korourian, S., Henry-Tillman, R., Adkins, L., Mumford, S., Westbrook, K.C., & Klimberg, V.S. (2007). Axillary reverse mapping (ARM): A new concept to identify and enhance lymphatic preservation. *Annals of Surgical Oncology, 14,* 1890–1895. doi:10.1245/s10434-007-9412-x

Tortora, G.J., & Derrickson, B. (2006). The spinal cord and spinal nerves. In G.J. Tortora & B. Derrickson (Eds.), *Principles of anatomy and physiology* (11th ed., pp. 439–472). Hoboken, NJ: Wiley.

Tsai, R.J., Dennis, L.K., Lynch, C.F., Snetselaar, L.G., Zamba, G.K., & Scott-Conner, C. (2009). The risk of developing arm lymphedema among breast cancer survivors: A meta-analysis of treatment factors. *Annals of Surgical Oncology, 16,* 1959–1972. doi:10.1245/s10434-009-0452-2

Wazer, D.E., & Arthur, D.W. (2008). Breast: Stage Tis. In E.C. Halperin, C.A. Perez, & L.W. Brady (Eds.), *Perez and Brady's principles and practice of radiation oncology* (5th ed., pp. 1162–1174). Philadelphia, PA: Lippincott Williams & Wilkins.

Whelan, T.J., Pignol, J.P., Levine, M.N., Julian, J.A., MacKenzie, R., Parpia, S., … Freeman, C. (2010). Long-term results of hypofractionated radiation therapy for breast cancer. *New England Journal of Medicine, 362,* 513–520.

Zablotska, L.B., Chak, A., Das, A., & Neugut, A.I. (2005). Increased risk of squamous cell esophageal cancer after adjuvant radiation therapy for primary breast cancer. *American Journal of Epidemiology, 161,* 330–337. doi:10.1093/aje/kwi050

Zablotska, L.B., & Neugut, A.I. (2003). Lung carcinoma after radiation therapy in women treated with lumpectomy or mastectomy for primary breast carcinoma. *Cancer, 97,* 1404–1411. doi:10.1002/cncr.11214

Zeiss. (2010, July 20). Intrabeam® radiotherapy system. Retrieved from http://meditec.zeiss.com/intrabeam

D. Thoracic
  1. Indications
    a) Non-small cell lung cancer (NSCLC)
      (1) Most common type of lung cancer, accounting for about 80% of all lung cancer cases (Aupérin et al., 2010)
      (2) The TNM staging system provides common language to describe extent of disease and define prognosis. In 2009, the International Association for the Study of Lung Cancer (IASLC) revised the classification of the TNM system (Thomas & Gould, 2010).
      (3) Surgery remains the standard of care for stage I and II NSCLC; however, approximately 40% of patients present at a locally advanced stage (Schrump, Giaccone, Kelsey, & Marks, 2008).
      (4) The PORT Meta-Analysis Trialists Group (2005) concluded that postoperative radiation is not indicated for completely resected stage I or II NSCLC.
      (5) Inoperable patients with stage I or II disease can be treated with standard EBRT or stereotactic body radiation therapy (SBRT) depending on the size and location of tumor. Standard RT is delivered in 1.8–2 Gy daily fractions whereas SBRT dosing can range between 10 and 20 Gy per daily fraction (Timmerman, Solberg, Kavanagh, & Lo, 2010).
      (6) Patients with unresectable stage III disease may receive chemoradiation or RT alone if unable to tolerate chemotherapy. Radiation total dose of 60–70 Gy can be delivered in 1.8–2 Gy daily fractions (Schild, Ramalingam, & Vallièresl, 2010).
      (7) Concomitant chemoradiation shows improved patient survival over sequential chemoradiation (Aupérin et al., 2010).
      (8) RT remains the standard of care for nonsurgical candidates and patients with locally advanced disease (Rosenzweig et al., 2008).
      (9) RT is effective for palliation of symptoms in stage IV disease. RT may be used to manage pain, airway obstruction, hemoptysis, and superior vena cava syndrome.
    b) Small cell lung cancer (SCLC)
      (1) Classified as either limited stage, when disease is confined to one radiation port field, or extensive stage, which cannot be included in one RT port.
      (2) According to the IASLC system, limited stage is consistent with TNM stages I to IIIB, whereas extensive stage defines patients with distant metastases. TNM staging can be important for SCLC, particularly in the clinical trial setting (NCI, 2011).
      (3) RT plays an important role in preventing local recurrence in limited-stage SCLC. Clinical trials offering concurrent chemoradiation have proven sur-

vival benefits for patients with limited-stage SCLC (Baldini, 2010).

(4) Accelerated hyperfractionation is a recommended radiation delivery schedule for limited-stage SCLC. The total dose of 45 Gy is delivered in divided 1.5 Gy fractions twice daily for three weeks (Baldini, 2010).

(5) Decreased length of time from first day of chemotherapy to the last day of radiation has shown improved survival in patients with limited-stage SCLC (De Ruysscher et al., 2006).

(6) Prophylactic cranial irradiation may be given to patients who have had a good response to chemotherapy. Some studies have shown a 5% improved survival in patients who received prophylactic cranial irradiation (Edelman & Gandora, 2009).

c) Esophageal cancer

(1) Common subtypes are squamous cell carcinoma and adenocarcinoma.

(2) Forty percent of esophageal cancers are squamous cell carcinoma, and 60% of those cases arise in the middle third of the esophagus within the thorax (Hershock, 2005).

(3) Treatment usually consists of multiple modalities, most commonly chemoradiation (cisplatin/5-fluorouracil [5-FU]) with or without surgical resection. Preoperative chemoradiation has shown an increase in the three-year survival rates and prolonged median disease-free survival compared to surgery alone in several randomized studies (Alberts & Goldberg, 2009).

(4) In the preoperative setting, a total dose of 45–50.4 Gy may be administered in daily 1.8 Gy fractions. In the curative setting, nonsurgical patients may receive a total dose of 60–66.6 Gy administered in 1.8–2 Gy daily fractions, often given with concurrent chemotherapy (Alberts & Goldberg, 2009).

d) Metastatic cancer

(1) Lungs are the most common site for distant metastases for many malignant tumors, with the exception of GI cancers (Prommer & Casciato, 2009).

(2) Metastatic tumors to the lung can be treated with conventional RT or SBRT. Studies have shown that patients with metastatic tumors to the lung tolerate SBRT with less severe toxicities than patients with primary lung cancers.

Generally, these patients have peripherally based tumors and stronger lung function than patients with primary lung cancer (Heinzerling & Timmerman, 2010).

e) Thymoma

(1) Rare tumor that arises in the anterior mediastinum

(2) RT field normally includes the entire mediastinum and adjacent lung (Loehrer, Henley, & Kesler, 2010).

(3) RT is not indicated in completely resected stage I disease; however, studies have shown a role for radiation in other stages. For subtotal resections, recommended total dose is 60 Gy given in less than 2 Gy daily fractions (Loehrer et al., 2010).

f) Malignant mesothelioma

(1) Rare but aggressive malignancy of the pleura commonly associated with asbestos exposure

(2) RT is primarily administered in the postoperative setting but may be primary treatment for nonsurgical candidates.

(3) Challenges exist because of the large GTV, which can lead to serious side effects, including fatal pneumonitis (Robinson, Baas, & Kindler, 2010).

2. Techniques

a) 3DCRT: 3DCRT is the standard radiation technique used to treat lung cancer. This technique can precisely target tumors in the thoracic area while avoiding critical organs (Keall, Belderbos, & Kong, 2010).

b) IMRT

(1) IMRT adjusts beam intensity within the target volume to decrease normal surrounding tissues' exposure to radiation. This can be beneficial in treating node-positive lung cancers to help decrease the risk of esophagitis (Keall et al., 2010).

(2) This approach may help reduce the percentage of lung volume receiving

more than 20 Gy, which may help decrease the risk of pneumonitis (Keall et al., 2010).

- c) IGRT
  - (1) IGRT uses x-ray imaging during treatments to locate and focus dosing beams more precisely on tumors. The tumor is able to be visualized almost simultaneously during treatment delivery.
  - (2) Tumors in the thoracic area can move because of patient respirations or weight loss over time. Daily imaging can be used to verify tumor position prior to treatment delivery (Haas, 2008).
- d) SBRT
  - (1) SBRT consists of hypofractionated delivery of high radiation doses to visible lung tumors up to 5–7 cm. Dose generally ranges between 10 and 20 Gy per fraction (Zimmermann et al., 2006).
  - (2) This is a definitive treatment option for patients with early-stage NSCLC who are not surgical candidates or who decline surgery (Zimmermann et al., 2006).
  - (3) Clinical trials have demonstrated local control rates of 88% with SBRT for inoperable early-stage NSCLC (Senan & Lagerwaard, 2010).
  - (4) Hypofractionated dosing can provide local control for metastatic lung tumors. Studies have shown a two-year local control rate of 80% when SBRT was used to treat metastatic lung tumors. Less than 5% of patients developed severe toxicities (Bogart, 2010).
  - (5) The high dose per fraction can increase the risk of toxicities. Fistula development, pneumonitis, and hemopytsis can occur when treating centrally located tumors. Peripheral lesions treated with SBRT can lead to increased skin toxicities, rib fractures, and brachial plexopathy (Bogart, 2010).
  - (6) With hypofractionated treatment, the patient's treatment course is shorter, which can limit nursing and patient interaction. This may present nursing challenges regarding patient education and symptom management (Smink & Schneider, 2008).
- e) Brachytherapy
  - (1) Endobronchial HDR
    - (a) Can be used for local control and symptom management in advanced NSCLC. Not enough evidence exists to support using endobronchial HDR in place of EBRT for symptom relief (Zorilla, Reveiz, Ospina, & Yepes, 2008).
    - (b) HDR has been used for palliation of symptoms including hemoptysis, postobstructive pneumonia, dyspnea, and pain. Studies have shown 50%–100% of patients reporting relief of their symptoms (Moore-Higgs, 2003).
  - (2) Esophageal HDR
    - (a) May be used as a boost after the completion of EBRT
    - (b) May be used as treatment with curative intent for patients without evidence of metastases and tumors smaller than 10 cm. Total dose is usually 10 Gy, delivered in two 5 Gy fractions (Posner, Minsky, & Ilson, 2008).
    - (c) Effective modality for palliation of dysphagia
  - (3) LDR brachytherapy
    - (a) LDR brachytherapy can be used with surgical resection for NSCLC.
    - (b) Approximately 40–60 ^{125}I seeds are sutured in mesh, which is then placed along the staple line after lung resection.
    - (c) The total delivered radiation dose to the local tissues (staple line) is usually around 10 Gy at a 1 cm distance from the staple line, which essentially expands the surgical margin by another centimeter (Haji-Momenian, Santos, Fernando, & Dupuy, 2010).
- f) Proton therapy
  - (1) EBRT that delivers proton beams to the tumor site while limiting radiation dose to surrounding critical structures
  - (2) Widesott, Amichetti, and Schwarz (2008) conducted a review that showed limited data to support the application of proton therapy for the treatment of NSCLC.
  - (3) Promising studies have been done using proton therapy; however, more evidence is needed to justify it as standard of care in the treatment of lung cancer (Pijls-Johannesma, Grutters, Verhaegen, Lambin, & De Ruysscher, 2010).
  - (4) It is not considered standard treatment for thoracic malignancies at this time.

3. Acute side effects
   a) Cough
      (1) Pathophysiology
         (a) Decreased function of cilia and mucus-secreting glands causes bronchial mucosa irritation, edema, and hypervascularity (Knopp, 1997).
         (b) Cough may initially become more productive during radiation as a result of airways opening up (Haas, 2004).
         (c) Respiratory mucosa continues to become drier during RT, possibly leading to a nonproductive cough (Haas, 2004).
      (2) Incidence and risk factors
         (a) Many patients present with a cough prior to initiation of treatment. Estfan and LeGrand (2004) reported that 60% of patients with advanced lung cancer have a cough.
         (b) Continued smoking increases cough.
      (3) Assessment
         (a) Determine whether cough is productive or nonproductive; note sputum color and consistency.
         (b) Perform auscultation of breath sounds.
         (c) Monitor oxygen saturation level.
         (d) Determine hydration and nutritional status.
         (e) Check for fever, chills, and diaphoresis.
      (4) Documentation (NCI CTEP, 2010)
         (a) 1—Mild symptoms; nonprescription intervention indicated
         (b) 2—Moderate symptoms; medical intervention indicated; limiting instrumental ADL
         (c) 3—Severe symptoms; limiting self-care ADL
      (5) Collaborative management
         (a) Antitussives: Hydrocodone has fewer GI and CNS toxicities compared with codeine (Estfan & LeGrand, 2004).
         (b) Expectorants
         (c) Bronchodilators (i.e., inhalers, nebulizers)
         (d) Supplemental oxygen as needed
         (e) Chest x-ray if indicated
      (6) Patient and family education
         (a) Advise patient to increase fluids when cough becomes produc-

tive, if not contraindicated (Haas, 2004).
         (b) Instruct patient to avoid smoke-filled areas.
         (c) Instruct on use of medications, including suppressants, expectorants, and bronchodilators.
         (d) Instruct on use of home humidification and/or home oxygen if needed.
         (e) Instruct the patient to report any signs or symptoms of infection, including fevers or change in color of secretions, shortness of breath, or dyspnea.
   b) Esophagitis
      (1) Pathophysiology
         (a) Irritation and inflammation of the lining of the esophagus within the RT field
         (b) The epithelium is very radiosensitive, and irritation usually occurs two to three weeks from the beginning of treatment.
      (2) Incidence and risk factors
         (a) Esophagitis is a common dose-limiting complication for thoracic radiation. Primary radiation-related toxicity leads to distress, weight loss, and hospitalizations (Duffy & Krishnasamy, 2009).
         (b) Concurrent chemoradiation can increase esophageal toxicity versus sequential treatment (Aupérin et al., 2010).
      (3) Assessment
         (a) Assess for dysphagia and odynophagia.
         (b) Assess for swallowing impairment.
         (c) Nutritional status impairment can result; thus, close monitoring of patient weight is a necessity.
         (d) Assess for candidiasis (thrush).
      (4) Documentation
         (a) Pharynx and esophagus (NCI CTEP, 2010)
            i. 1—Symptomatic, able to eat regular diet
            ii. 2—Symptomatic and altered eating and swallowing
            iii. 3—Severely altered eating/swallowing; tube feeding or TPN or hospitalization indicated
            iv. 4—Life-threatening consequences; urgent intervention indicated
            v. 5—Death

(b) Pain location and intensity

(c) Effectiveness of pain intervention (Catlin-Huth, Haas, & Pollock, 2002)

   i. 0—No relief

   ii. 1—Pain relieved 25%

   iii. 2—Pain relieved 50%

   iv. 3—Pain relieved 75%

   v. 4—Pain relieved 100%

(5) Collaborative management

(a) Duffy and Krishnasamy (2009) reported that minimal evidence exists regarding the optimal way to manage acute radiation esophagitis.

(b) Consult dietitian at onset of treatment.

(c) Use of swish-and-swallow solutions that contain a topical anesthetic prior to meals and as needed may be helpful.

(d) Pain medications, including over-the-counter medications and/or narcotics (oral, liquid, or transdermal). Consult for pain management if needed.

(e) Administer antifungals if candidiasis is present or suspected.

(f) Use of amifostine during radiation has shown to decrease the incidence of esophagitis (Vujaskovic et al., 2002) (see section X.A—Radioprotectors).

(g) Although controversial, consider a feeding tube in cases of declining nutritional status.

(6) Patient and family education

(a) Increase caloric intake with supplements, and decrease spicy foods.

(b) Encourage small, frequent meals.

(c) Take pain medication prior to eating.

(d) Report any sudden increase in pain or change in ability to swallow.

(e) Educate that acute side effects may last at least three to four weeks after completion of treatment.

c) Dyspnea

(1) Pathophysiology

(a) Dyspnea is a subjective finding of breathlessness reported by many patients with lung cancer who receive thoracic RT.

(b) Dyspnea can increase a patient's level of anxiety and fatigue (Haas, 2004).

(2) Incidence and risk factors

(a) Occurs in 15%–55% of patients at initial cancer diagnosis (Eaton, 2009)

(b) Can be exacerbated by various factors including asthma, anemia, pulmonary embolism, anxiety, and smoking

(3) Assessment

(a) Heart and lung breath sounds, use of accessory muscles

(b) Painful breathing

(c) Skin color

(d) Breathing pattern and rate

(e) Oxygen saturation level

(f) Signs of infection including cough, fever, or increased white blood cell count

(g) Anxiety, fear, or depression (Eaton, 2009)

(4) Documentation (NCI CTEP, 2010)

(a) 1—Shortness of breath with moderate exertion

(b) 2—Shortness of breath with minimal exertion; limiting instrumental ADL

(c) 3—Shortness of breath at rest; limiting self-care ADL

(d) 4—Life-threatening consequences; urgent intervention indicated

(e) 5—Death

(5) Collaborative management

(a) Supplemental oxygen as needed

(b) Chest x-ray, if infection is suspected

(c) Bronchodilators to relieve airway constriction

(d) Corticosteroids to decrease lung irritation

(e) Anxiolytics to decrease anxiety

(f) Psychosocial management

(6) Patient and family education

(a) Instruct on medications including bronchodilators, steroids, pain management, and anxiolytics.

(b) Teach the patient alternative breathing techniques (e.g., pursed-lip breathing).

(c) Provide ideas to help conserve energy.

(d) Provide emotional support.

(e) Encourage smoking cessation if indicated.

  d) Skin reactions may occur in patients receiving thoracic radiation. SBRT to peripheral tumors can increase radiation skin dose (see section IV.C—Skin reactions).

  e) Patients with lung cancer frequently experienced fatigue (see section IV.B—Fatigue).

4. Late or delayed side effects

  a) Radiation pneumonitis

    (1) Pathophysiology

      (a) Interstitial pulmonary inflammation—Several cell populations of the lung, including alveolar macrophages, type II cells, fibroblasts, and endothelial cells, are involved in a network of interactions leading to inflammation and pulmonary fibrosis (Abratt & Morgan, 2002).

      (b) Damage to the pneumocytes and endothelial cells and to the interstitium leads to a release of surfactant and exudate into the alveoli and to interstitial edema. This occurs over the first month and is referred to as the early phase of the latent period (Abratt & Morgan, 2002).

      (c) Inflammatory response continues with capillary obstruction and increase in leukocytes, plasma cells, macrophages, fibroblasts, and collagen fibers. Alveolar septa become thickened, and the alveolar space becomes smaller. This phase lasts from one to several months and is termed the intermediate or acute pneumonitis phase (Abratt & Morgan, 2002).

    (2) Incidence and risk factors

      (a) Symptomatic pneumonitis occurs in 5%–15% of patients irradiated for mediastinal lymphoma, lung cancer, and breast cancer (Knopp, 1997).

      (b) Advanced technology, including IMRT, IGRT, and proton therapy, has helped reduce the incidence and severity of radiation pneumonitis (Liao, Travis, & Komaki, 2010).

      (c) The volume of lung receiving 20 Gy has been a standard parameter to assess the predictability of lung toxicity in NSCLC. In SCLC, the rate of radiation pneumonitis is decreased if less than 25% of the total lung receives more than 20 Gy (Krug, Kris, Rosenzweig, & Travis, 2008).

      (d) Occurs three to six months after a fractionated course of irradiation. Symptoms usually resolve in six to eight weeks without any long-term effects (Liao et al., 2010).

      (e) High-risk factors for developing radiation pneumonitis include low performance status, decreased pretreatment pulmonary function, chronic obstructive pulmonary disease, lower lobe tumor location, once-daily RT dose fractionation, RT combined with chemotherapy, and larger radiation doses (greater than 2.67 Gy) per fraction (Liao et al., 2010). Additional studies are needed to determine the role of the independent variables.

      (f) Clinically significant radiation pneumonitis occurs in an estimated 13%–37% of patients treated for lung cancer with combination chemotherapy and irradiation (Rodrigues, Lock, D'Souza, Yu, & Van Dyk, 2004).

      (g) The development of risk models and increased knowledge about molecular events related to developing radiation pneumonitis may be two important strategies to help understand and predict radiation-induced lung injury (Liao et al., 2010).

    (3) Assessment

      (a) Symptoms may include dyspnea, nonproductive cough, low-grade fever, tachycardia, and pleuritic chest pain.

      (b) Chest x-ray may reveal diffuse infiltrate corresponding to the RT field, but this is not always evident (Liao et al., 2010).

      (c) CT scan can reveal evidence of increased lung density and discrete and solid consolidation in corresponding RT field (McDonald, Rubin, Phillips, & Marks, 1995).

    (4) Documentation

      (a) Cough (NCI CTEP, 2010)—As listed previously

(b) Hemoptysis (Catlin-Huth et al., 2002)
  i. 0—None
  ii. 1—Specks of blood in mucus
  iii. 2—Pink-tinged mucus
  iv. 3—Small clots of blood in mucus
  v. 4—Frank blood in mucus
(c) Mucus color (Catlin-Huth et al., 2002)
  i. 0—Clear
  ii. 1—White
  iii. 2—Yellow
  iv. 3—Green
  v. 4—Brown
  vi. 5—Red (hemoptysis)
(d) Dyspnea (NCI CTEP, 2010)—As listed previously
(e) Oxygen saturation level

(5) Collaborative management
  (a) The use of cytoprotective agents during radiation treatment such as amifostine may reduce radiation-induced lung toxicity (Schild et al., 2010) (see section X.A—Radioprotectors).
  (b) Corticosteroids remain the treatment of choice for radiation pneumonitis, providing symptomatic relief, but do not reverse or prevent fibrosis and may be contraindicated.
  (c) Bronchodilators
  (d) Expectorants, humidifier, increased hydration, and antitussives
  (e) Supplemental oxygen
  (f) Fatigue management (see section IV.B—Fatigue)
  (g) Share information about symptom management (e.g., home health, medical oncology, hospice) with all nurses caring for the patient.

(6) Patient and family education
  (a) Inform the patient and family about interventions to manage cough and shortness of breath.
  (b) Teach the patient and family the signs and symptoms of radiation pneumonitis.
  (c) Instruct the patient to alternate rest and activity.
  (d) Advise the patient to avoid irritants (e.g., tobacco, pollutants).
  (e) Teach the patient and family the signs and symptoms (e.g., fever, cough, dyspnea) to report to the healthcare team.

  (f) Provide written steroid taper instructions for the patient to follow when appropriate.

b) Radiation fibrosis
  (1) Pathophysiology
    (a) Fibrosis develops together with loss of capillaries, increase in the thickness of the alveolar septa, and obliteration of the alveolar space as a result of radiation.
    (b) Fibrosis occurs six months or longer after completion of RT (Abratt & Morgan, 2002).
  (2) Incidence and risk factors
    (a) Almost 70% of patients with lung cancer treated with radiation will have radiographic evidence of pulmonary fibrosis (Madani et al., 2007).
    (b) Fibrosis is almost always evident after a patient develops pneumonitis. However, it can occur in patients without prior pneumonitis (Knopp, 1997).
    (c) Fibrosis usually is asymptomatic if it is limited to less than 50% of one lung (McDonald et al., 1995).
    (d) Fibrosis usually stabilizes in one to two years (Liao et al., 2010).
  (3) Assessment
    (a) If symptoms present, they usually include dyspnea associated with progressive chronic cor pulmonale.
    (b) Symptoms are proportional to the extent of lung parenchyma involved and the preexisting pulmonary reserve.
    (c) Retraction of the involved lung with elevation of the hemidiaphragm is the predominant finding (Nicolaou, 2003).
    (d) CT imaging is the preferred diagnostic study.
    (e) Pulmonary function studies are the most objective evaluation of the functional late effects of radiation lung toxicity. Studies may show mild deterioration as fibrosis develops.
  (4) Collaborative management
    (a) Delanian, Porcher, Balla-Mekias, and Lefaix (2003) suggested that six months of pentoxifylline and tocopherol (vitamin E) may stimulate the regression of superficial radiation-induced fibrosis.

(b) Currently, no effective treatment for radiation fibrosis exists.

(5) Patient and family education

(a) Teach the patient and family the signs and symptoms of fibrosis.

(b) Teach methods to avoid further respiratory compromise, including pulmonary rehabilitation.

c) Radiation myelopathy

(1) Pathophysiology: Spinal cord changes in radiation myelopathy may include white matter lesions, vasculopathies, and glial reactions (Schultheiss, Kun, Ang, & Stephens, 1995).

(2) Incidence and risk factors

(a) Radiation myelopathy is a rare, well-described, serious complication of spinal cord irradiation. Recovery from radiation-induced motor sequelae is rare, whereas the regeneration of sensory losses is relatively frequent (Esik et al., 2003).

(b) Risk of radiation myelopathy sometimes limits delivery of the dose necessary for tumor control or for reirradiation.

(c) When RT is given in a conventional fractionation schedule of 1.8–2 Gy per day, the incidence of radiation myelopathy is less than 1% for total doses of 50–55 Gy and less than 10% for total doses of 61 Gy (Kirkpatrick, van der Kogel, & Schultheiss, 2010).

(d) The dose per fraction, total dose, and absolute length of cord irradiated play an important role in determining whether radiation damage to the spinal cord occurs.

(3) Assessment

(a) Assess for Lhermitte sign, which is most frequently characterized by a sensation similar to an electric shock passing down the spine in the cervico-caudal direction. The pain may be felt in the upper or lower limbs (Esik et al., 2003).

(b) Symptoms may develop after a latent period from six months and on (Schultheiss et al., 1995). Severity of symptoms is often progressive.

(c) Symptoms can include paresthesia or sensory deficits (either unilateral or bilateral), leg weakness, clumsiness, diminished proprio-ception, paralysis, and bladder or anal dysfunction/incontinence.

(d) Examination

i. Complete neurologic examination

ii. Pain assessment

iii. Hyperreflexia and Babinski reflex often are present.

iv. MRI may show cord swelling with decreased intensity of T1-weighted images and increased intensity on T2-weighted images (Wang, Shen, & Jan, 1992).

v. Myelogram may be normal or may show slight widening of the spinal cord (Schultheiss et al., 1995).

(4) Documentation (NCI CTEP, 2010)

(a) Peripheral motor neuropathy

i. 1—Asymptomatic: clinical or diagnostic observations only; intervention not indicated

ii. 2—Moderate symptoms; limiting instrumental ADL

iii. 3—Severe symptoms; limiting self-care ADL; assistive device indicated

iv. 4—Life-threatening consequences; urgent intervention indicated

v. 5—Death

(b) Ataxia

i. 1—Asymptomatic: clinical or diagnostic observations only; intervention not indicated

ii. 2—Moderate symptoms; corticosteroids indicated

iii. 3—Severe symptoms; limiting self-care ADL; mechanical assistance indicated

(c) Urinary incontinence

i. 1—Occasional (e.g., with coughing, sneezing, etc.), pads not indicated

ii. 2—Spontaneous; pads indicated; limiting instrumental ADL

iii. 3—Intervention indicated (e.g., clamp, collagen injections); operative intervention indicated; limiting self-care ADL

(d) Fecal incontinence

i. 1—Occasional use of pads

ii. 2—Daily use of pads required

iii. 3—Severe symptoms; elective operative intervention indicated

(5) Collaborative management

    (a) Careful dose calculation and administration of RT

    (b) Interventions

        i. Evaluate for other etiologies, including tumor progression, infection, or trauma.

        ii. Administer corticosteroid as needed.

        iii. Provide a referral to rehabilitation to maximize function.

(6) Patient and family education

    (a) Educate on neurologic symptoms to report.

    (b) Instruct regarding injury prevention secondary to neurologic and sensory deficits, including fall prevention.

    (c) Instruct on corticosteroid administration, tapering, and potential side effects.

    (d) Progression of symptoms depends upon the degree to which the lesion transects the spinal cord and the level of injury.

d) Cardiac injury

  (1) Pathophysiology

    (a) Acute inflammation and progressive fibrosis of the pericardial, myocardial, and endocardial (valvular and arterial) tissues (Veinot & Edwards, 1996)

    (b) Certain cytokines and growth factors, such as tumor growth factor-beta1 and interleukin-1 beta, may stimulate radiation-induced endothelial proliferation, fibroblast proliferation, collagen deposition, and fibrosis leading to advanced lesions of atherosclerosis (Basavaraju & Easterly, 2002).

    (c) Other late complications include myocardial fibrosis and cardiomyopathy, accelerated coronary artery disease, conduction abnormalities, and valvular dysfunction (Lund et al., 1996).

  (2) Incidence and risk factors

    (a) Risk of cardiac damage correlates with radiation dose volume and fractionation.

    (b) Pericardial disease was considered the most common side effect of radiation to the heart; however, with modern radiation techniques, incidence has greatly decreased (Yahalom & Portluck, 2008).

    (c) Risk of radiation-induced cardiac injury may be further increased by the concomitant use of anthracycline-based chemotherapy, especially when larger cumulative doses of doxorubicin (greater than 450 mg/m^2) are used, when radiation and chemotherapy are given concurrently, and when high dose volumes of cardiac radiation are administered (Shapiro et al., 1998).

    (d) A significantly higher risk of death from ischemic heart disease has been reported for patients treated with radiation for Hodgkin lymphoma and breast cancer (Basavaraju & Easterly, 2002).

    (e) Little is known about the prevalence of heart disease that is present before initiation of RT.

  (3) Assessment

    (a) Clinical manifestations

        i. Shortness of breath

        ii. Chest pain

        iii. Fatigue

        iv. Lower extremity swelling

        v. Syncope

    (b) Physical examination

        i. Arrhythmias

        ii. Altered respiratory status

        iii. Lower extremity edema

    (c) Cardiac function studies

        i. Electrocardiogram

        ii. Resting echocardiograph and exercise echocardiography

        iii. CT or MRI

  (4) Documentation

    (a) Fatigue (NCI CTEP, 2010)

        i. 1—Fatigue relieved by rest

        ii. 2—Fatigue not relieved by rest; limiting instrumental ADL

        iii. 3—Fatigue not relieved by rest; limiting self-care ADL

    (b) Dyspnea

    (c) Chest pain

  (5) Collaborative management

    (a) Prevention

        i. Use treatment strategies that use lower total radiation doses and minimize cardiac exposure.

        ii. Avoid concurrent cardiotoxic chemotherapeutic agents when possible.

        iii. If the patient has a pacemaker, have it checked weekly if pacemaker dose might exceed 2 Gy (Yahalom & Portluck, 2008).

    (b) Early detection

        i. Refer to cardiology for evaluation and recommendations to reduce the degree of initial cardiac injury and slow the progression of vascular, myocardial, and valvular fibrosis.

        ii. Regular electrocardiogram and echocardiograms if indicated

        iii. Aggressive treatment of cardiac risk factors, especially hyperlipidemia, both at the time of cardiac therapy and during follow-up

  (6) Patient and family education

    (a) Importance of routine follow-up with cardiologist and cardiac rehabilitation if indicated

    (b) Compliance with recommendations for cardiac health, including following a healthy diet, maintaining an ideal weight, and engaging in regular exercise

    (c) Signs and symptoms of heart disease to report

e) Esophageal injury

  (1) Pathophysiology

    (a) Each abnormality is directly related to the tissue injury that occurs with high-dose radiation and the subsequent healing process.

    (b) Abnormalities include impaired motility with and without mucosal edema, stricture, ulceration and pseudodiverticulum, and fistula.

  (2) Incidence and risk factors

    (a) Radiation-induced esophageal injury is more frequent when RT and chemotherapy are combined than it is with RT alone.

    (b) Abnormal motility occurred 4–12 weeks following RT alone and as early as one week if concurrent chemoradiation had been given (Lepke & Libshitz, 1983).

    (c) Strictures may develop four to eight months following completion of RT. Ulceration, pseudodiverticulum, and fistula formation do not develop in a uniform time frame (Lepke & Libshitz, 1983).

    (d) Although rare complications occur, the exact incidence of these abnormalities is not well documented in the literature.

  (3) Assessment

    (a) Clinical manifestations

        i. Dysphagia

        ii. Hemoptysis with ulceration

        iii. Weight loss

        iv. Chest pain

    (b) Physical examination

        i. Weight loss

        ii. Difficulty swallowing solid foods

    (c) Additional studies: Upper endoscopy

  (4) Documentation: Nutritional alteration (NCI CTEP, 2010)

    (a) Anorexia

        i. 1—Loss of appetite without alteration in eating habits

        ii. 2—Oral intake altered without significant weight loss or malnutrition; oral nutritional supplements indicated

        iii. 3—Associated with significant weight loss or malnutrition (e.g., inadequate oral caloric and fluid intake); tube feeding or TPN indicated

        iv. 4—Life-threatening consequences; urgent intervention indicated

        v. 5—Death

    (b) Nausea

        i. 1—Loss of appetite without alteration in eating habits

        ii. 2—Oral intake decreased without significant weight loss, dehydration, or malnutrition

        iii. 3—Inadequate oral caloric or fluid intake; tube feeding, TPN, or hospitalization indicated

    (c) Dyspepsia

        i. 1—Mild symptoms; intervention not indicated

ii. 2—Moderate symptoms; medical intervention indicated

iii. 3—Severe symptoms; surgical intervention indicated

(5) Collaborative management for esophageal injury

(a) Management depends on the specific injury.

(b) Refer to gastroenterologist for evaluation for potential interventions, which may include esophageal dilation, cauterization of bleeding, or placement of a stent.

(c) Obtain nutritional consult.

(6) Patient and family education

(a) Provide information on dietary suggestions and restrictions.

(b) Teach the signs and symptoms to report, including increased pain or difficulty swallowing.

(c) Provide emotional support.

References

Abratt, R.P., & Morgan, G.W. (2002). Lung toxicity following chest irradiation in patients with lung cancer. *Lung Cancer, 35,* 103–109. doi:10.1016/S0169-5002(01)00334-8

Alberts, S.R., & Goldberg, R.M. (2009). Gastrointestinal tract cancers. In D.A. Casciato (Ed.), *Manual of clinical oncology* (6th ed., pp. 188–192). Philadelphia, PA: Lippincott Williams & Wilkins.

Aupérin, A., Le Péchoux, C., Rolland, E., Curran, W.J., Furuse, K., Fournel, P., … Pignon, J.P. (2010). Meta-analysis of concomitant versus sequential radiochemotherapy in locally advanced non-small cell lung cancer. *Journal of Clinical Oncology, 28,* 2181–2190. doi:10.1200/JCO.2009.26.2543

Baldini, E.H. (2010). Thoracic radiotherapy in the treatment of limited stage small cell lung cancer. Retrieved from http://www.uptodateonline.com

Basavaraju, S.R., & Easterly, C.E. (2002). Pathophysiological effects of radiation on atherosclerosis development and progression, and the incidence of cardiovascular complications. *Medical Physics, 29,* 2391–2403.

Bogart, J.A. (2010). Stereotactic body radiation therapy for early-stage lung cancer: Are we "all in." *Journal of Thoracic Oncology, 5,* 927–929. doi:10.1097/JTO.0b013e3181e3a319

Catlin-Huth, C., Haas, M., & Pollock, V. (Eds.). (2002). *Radiation therapy patient care record: A tool for documenting nursing care.* Pittsburgh, PA: Oncology Nursing Society.

Delanian, S., Porcher, R., Balla-Mekias, S., & Lefaix, J.L. (2003). Randomized, placebo-controlled trial of combined pentoxifylline and tocopherol for regression of superficial radiation-induced fibrosis. *Journal of Clinical Oncology, 21,* 2545–2550. doi:10.1200/JCO.2003.06.064

De Ruysscher, D., Pijls-Johannesma, M., Bentzen, S.M., Minken, A., Wanders, R., Lutgens, L., … Lambin, P. (2006). Time between the first day of chemotherapy and the last day of chest radiation is the most important predictor of survival in limited-disease small-cell lung cancer. *Journal of Clinical Oncology, 24,* 1057–1063. doi:10.1200/JCO.2005.02.9793

Duffy, M., & Krishnasamy, M. (2009). A review of evidence to inform the pharmacological management of pain associated with radiation-induced oesophagitis in patients diagnosed with primary lung cancer. *Australian Journal of Cancer Nursing, 10,* 19–22.

Eaton, L.H. (2009). Dyspnea. In L.H. Eaton & J.M. Tipton (Eds.), *Putting evidence into practice: Improving oncology patient outcomes* (pp. 135–140). Pittsburgh, PA: Oncology Nursing Society.

Edelman, M., & Gandora, D.R. (2009). Lung cancer. In D.A. Casciato (Ed.), *Manual of clinical oncology* (6th ed., pp. 169–187). Philadelphia, PA: Lippincott Williams & Wilkins.

Esik, O., Csere, T., Stefanits, K., Lengyel, Z., Sáfrány, G., Vönöczky, K., … Trón, L. (2003). A review on radiogenic Lhermitte's sign. *Pathology Oncology Research, 9,* 115–120.

Estfan, B., & LeGrand, S. (2004). Management of cough in advanced cancer. *Journal of Supportive Oncology, 2,* 523–526.

Haas, M.L. (2004). *Pocket guide to lung cancer.* Sudbury, MA: Jones and Bartlett.

Haas, M.L. (2008). Advances in radiation therapy for lung cancer. *Seminars in Oncology Nursing, 24,* 34–40. doi:10.1016/j.soncn.2007.11.010

Haji-Momenian, S., Santos, R.S., Fernando, H.C., & Dupuy, D.E. (2010). Percutaneous therapeutic technologies for medically inoperable lung cancer. In H.I. Pass, D.P. Carbone, D.H. Johnson, J.D. Minna, G.V. Scagliotti, & A.T. Turrisi III (Eds.), *Principles and practice of lung cancer: The official reference text of the IASCL* (4th ed., pp. 510–515). Philadelphia, PA: Lippincott Williams & Wilkins.

Heinzerling, J.H., & Timmerman, R.D. (2010). Stereotactic body radiation therapy for primary and metastatic lung tumors. Retrieved from http://www.uptodateonline.com

Hershock, D. (2005). Approach to chemotherapy and radiation for gastric and esophageal cancer. In M.L. Kochman (Ed.), *The clinician's guide to gastrointestinal oncology* (pp. 23–52). Thorofare, NJ: SLACK Inc.

Keall, P., Belderbos, J., & Kong, F.M. (2010). Physical basis of modern radiotherapy: Dose and volume. In H.I. Pass, D.P. Carbone, D.H. Johnson, J.D. Minna, G.V. Scagliotti, & A.T. Turrisi III (Eds.), *Principles and practice of lung cancer: The official reference text of the IASCL* (4th ed., pp. 549–564). Philadelphia, PA: Lippincott Williams & Wilkins.

Kirkpatrick, J.P., van der Kogel, A.J., & Schultheiss, T.E. (2010). Radiation dose-volume effects in the spinal cord. *International Journal of Radiation Oncology, Biology, Physics, 7*(Suppl. 3), S42–S49. doi:10.1016/j.ijrobp.2009.04.095

Knopp, J.M. (1997). Lung cancer. In K.H. Dow, J.D. Bucholtz, R. Iwamoto, V. Fieler, & L. Hilderley (Eds.), *Nursing care in radiation oncology* (2nd ed., pp. 293–315). Philadelphia, PA: Saunders.

Krug, L.M., Kris, M.G., Rosenzweig, K., & Travis, W.D. (2008). Small cell and other neuroendocrine tumors of the lung. In V.T. DeVita Jr., T.S. Lawrence, & S.A. Rosenberg (Eds.), *Cancer: Principles and practice of oncology* (8th ed., pp. 946–971). Philadelphia, PA: Lippincott Williams & Wilkins.

Lepke, R.A., & Libshitz, H.I. (1983). Radiation-induced injury of the esophagus. *Radiology, 148,* 375–378.

Liao, Z., Travis, E.L., & Komaki, R. (2010). Radiation treatment-related lung damage. In H.I. Pass, D.P. Carbone, D.H. Johnson, J.D. Minna, G.V. Scagliotti, & A.T. Turrisi III (Eds.), *Principles and practice of lung cancer: The official reference text of the IASCL* (4th ed., pp. 601–634). Philadelphia, PA: Lippincott Williams & Wilkins.

Loehrer, P.J., Henley, J., & Kesler, K. (2010). Thymoma and thymic carcinoma. In H.I. Pass, D.P. Carbone, D.H. Johnson, J.D. Minna, G.V. Scagliotti, & A.T. Turrisi III (Eds.), *Principles and practice of lung cancer: The official reference text of the IAS-CL* (4th ed., pp. 929–942). Philadelphia, PA: Lippincott Williams & Wilkins.

Lund, M.B., Ihlen, H., Voss, B.M., Abrahamsen, A.F., Nome, O., Kongerud, J., ... Forfang, K. (1996). Increased risk of heart valve regurgitation after mediastinal radiation for Hodgkin's disease: An echocardiographic study. *Heart, 75,* 591–595. doi:10.1136/hrt.75.6.591

Madani, I., De Ruyck, K., Goeminne, H., De Neve, W., Thierens, H., & Van Meerbeeck, J. (2007). Predicting the risk of radiation-induced lung injury. *Journal of Thoracic Oncology, 2,* 864–874. doi:10.1097/JTO.0b013e318145b2c6

McDonald, S., Rubin, P., Phillips, T.L., & Marks, L.B. (1995). Injury to the lung from cancer therapy: Clinical syndromes, measurable endpoints and potential scoring systems. *International Journal of Radiation Oncology, Biology, Physics, 31,* 1187–1203. doi:10.1016/0360-3016(94)00429-O

Moore-Higgs, G.J. (2003). New advances in radiotherapy for lung cancer. In M. Haas (Ed.), *Contemporary issues in lung cancer: A nursing perspective* (pp. 83–91). Sudbury, MA: Jones and Bartlett.

National Cancer Institute. (2011, February). Small cell lung cancer treatment (PDQ®). Retrieved from http://www.cancer.gov/cancertopics/pdq/treatment/small-cell-lung/healthprofessional

National Cancer Institute Cancer Therapy Evaluation Program. (2010). *Common terminology criteria for adverse events* [v.4.03]. Retrieved from http://evs.nci.nih.gov/ftp1/CTCAE/CTCAE_4.03_2010-06-14_QuickReference_5x7.pdf

Nicolaou, N. (2003). Prevention and management of radiation toxicity. In R. Pazdur, L.R. Coia, W.J. Hoskins, & L.D. Wagman (Eds.), *Cancer management: A multidisciplinary approach* (7th ed., pp. 909–939). New York, NY: Oncology Group.

Pijls-Johannesma, M., Grutters, J.P., Verhaegen, F., Lambin, P., & De Ruysscher, D. (2010). Do we have enough evidence to implement particle therapy as standard treatment in lung cancer? A systematic literature review. *Oncologist, 15,* 93–103. doi:10.1634/theoncologist.2009-0116

PORT Meta-Analysis Trialists Group. (2005). Postoperative radiotherapy for non-small cell lung cancer. *Cochrane Database of Systemic Reviews* 2005, Issue 2. Art. No.: CD002142. doi:10.1002/14651858.CD002142.pub2

Posner, M.C., Minsky, B.D., & Ilson, D.H. (2008). Cancer of the esophagus. In V.T. DeVita Jr., T.S. Lawrence, & S.A. Rosenberg (Eds.), *Cancer: Principles and practice of oncology* (8th ed., pp. 994–1043). Philadelphia, PA: Lippincott Williams & Wilkins.

Prommer, E.E., & Casciato, D.A. (2009). Thoracic complications. In D.A. Casciato (Ed.), *Manual of clinical oncology* (6th ed., pp. 595–610). Philadelphia, PA: Lippincott Williams & Wilkins.

Robinson, B.W., Baas, P., & Kindler, H.L. (2010). Malignant mesothelioma. In H.I. Pass, D.P. Carbone, D.H. Johnson, J.D. Minna, G.V. Scagliotti, & A.T. Turrisi III (Eds.), *Principles and practice of lung cancer: The official reference text of the IAS-CL* (4th ed., pp. 945–960). Philadelphia, PA: Lippincott Williams & Wilkins.

Rodrigues, G., Lock, M., D'Souza, D., Yu, E., & Van Dyk, J. (2004). Prediction of radiation pneumonitis by dose-volume histogram parameters in lung cancer—A systematic review. *Radiotherapy and Oncology, 71,* 127–138. doi:10.1016/j.radonc.2004.02.015

Rosenzweig, K.E., Movsas, B., Bradley, J., Gewanter, R.M., Gopal, R.S., Komaki, R.U., ... Langer, C.J. (2008). *ACR Appropriateness Criteria® nonsurgical treatment for non-small-cell lung cancer: Poor performance status or palliative intent.* Reston, VA: American College of Radiology.

Schild, S.E., Ramalingam, S.S., & Vallièresl, E. (2010). Management of stage III non-small cell lung cancer. Retrieved from http://www.uptodate.com/contents/management-of-stage-iii-non-small-cell-lung-cancer

Schrump, D.S., Giaccone, G., Kelsey, C.R., & Marks, L.B. (2008). Non–small-cell lung cancer. In V.T. DeVita Jr., T.S. Lawrence, & S.A. Rosenberg (Eds.), *Cancer: Principles and practice of oncology* (8th ed., pp. 897–938). Philadelphia, PA: Lippincott Williams & Wilkins.

Schultheiss, T.E., Kun, L.E., Ang, K.K., & Stephens, L.C. (1995). Radiation response of the central nervous system. *International Journal of Radiation Oncology, Biology, Physics, 31,* 1093–1112. doi:10.1016/0360-3016(94)00655-5

Senan, S., & Lagerwaard, F. (2010). Stereotactic radiotherapy for stage I lung cancer: Current results and new developments. *Cancer/Radiothérapie, 14,* 115–118. doi:10.1016/j.canrad.2009.11.003

Shapiro, C.L., Hardenbergh, P.H., Gelman, R., Blanks, D., Hauptman, P., Recht, A., ... Henderson, I.C. (1998). Cardiac effects of adjuvant doxorubicin and radiation therapy in breast cancer patients. *Journal of Clinical Oncology, 16,* 3493–3501.

Smink, K.A., & Schneider, S.M. (2008). Overview of stereotactic body radiotherapy and the nursing role. *Clinical Journal of Oncology, 12,* 889–893. doi:10.1188/08.CJON.889-893

Thomas, K.W., & Gould, M.K. (2009). Tumor node metastasis (TNM) staging system for non-small cell lung cancer. Retrieved from http://www.uptodate.com/contents/tumor-node-metastasis-tnm-staging-system-for-non-small-cell-lung-cancer

Timmerman, R.D., Solberg, T.D., Kavanagh, B.D., & Lo, S. (2010). Stereotactic techniques for lung cancer treatment. In H.I. Pass, D.P. Carbone, D.H. Johnson, J.D. Minna, G.V. Scagliotti, & A.T. Turrisi III (Eds.), *Principles and practice of lung cancer: The official reference text of the IASCL* (4th ed., pp. 589–597). Philadelphia, PA: Lippincott Williams & Wilkins.

Veinot, J.P., & Edwards, W.D. (1996). Pathology of radiation-induced heart disease: A surgical and autopsy study of 27 cases. *Human Pathology, 27,* 766–773.

Vujaskovic, Z., Feng, Q.F., Rabbani, Z.N., Samulski, T.V., Anscher, M.S., & Brizel, D.M. (2002). Assessment of the protective effect of amifostine on radiation-induced pulmonary toxicity. *Experimental Lung Research, 28,* 577–590. doi:10.1080/01902140290096791

Wang, P.Y., Shen, W.C., & Jan, J.S. (1992). MR imaging in radiation myelopathy. *American Journal of Neuroradiology, 13,* 1049–1058.

Widesott, L., Amichetti, M., & Schwarz, M. (2008). Proton therapy in lung cancer: Clinical outcomes and technical issues. A systematic review. *Radiotherapy and Oncology, 86,* 154–164. doi:10.1016/j.radonc.2008.01.003

Yahalom, J., & Portluck, C.S. (2008). Cardiac toxicity. In V.T. DeVita Jr., T.S. Lawrence, & S.A. Rosenberg (Eds.), *Cancer: Principles and practice of oncology* (8th ed., pp. 2683–2687). Philadelphia, PA: Lippincott Williams & Wilkins.

Zimmermann, F.B., Geinitz, H., Schill, S., Thamm, R., Nieder, C., Schratzenstaller, U., & Molls, M. (2006). Stereotactic hypofractionated radiotherapy in stage I (T1-2 N0 M0) non-small-cell lung cancer (NSCLC). *Acta Oncologica, 45,* 796–801. doi:10.1080/02841860600913210

Zorilla, A.F.C., Reveiz, L., Ospina, E.G., & Yepes, A. (2008). Palliative endobronchial brachytherapy for non-small cell lung cancer. *Cochrane Database of Systematic Reviews* 2008, Issue 2. Art. No.: CD004284. DOI: 10.1002/14651858.CD004284.pub2

E. Gastrointestinal/abdomen
1. Radiation to abdominal structures may be used for treatment of certain malignancies of the GI tract (e.g., distal esophageal/GI junction or gastric tumors, pancreatic or biliary tract cancers, liver cancer, or obstructive colon/colorectal tumors) or other tumors that may develop in the abdominal cavity (such as desmoid tumors or sarcomas) (see Table 13).
   a) Incidental irradiation of stomach or small bowel may occur during treatment for lower thoracic cancers (esophageal, lung) or pelvic malignancies (cervical, prostate, rectal) or with para-aortic RT for testicular cancers or treatment to the thoracic or lumbar spine (Kavanagh et al., 2010).
   b) Side effects of radiation exposure to the stomach or small bowel may be either acute or chronic and are mediated by the total radiation dose, exposure volume, treatment factors (chemotherapy), and other patient factors.
      (1) Major dose-limiting structures in the abdomen include the small intestine, stomach, liver, kidneys, and spinal cord.
      (2) For some clinical situations, advanced treatment planning techniques (such as IMRT) have demonstrated benefit in minimizing toxicity by more effectively limiting doses to sensitive GI structures (Zelefsky et al., 2006).

2. Anorexia
   a) Pathophysiology
      (1) Anorexia may occur as a manifestation of the primary cancer diagnosis or may develop or be exacerbated by treatment effects.
      (2) Radiation to the abdomen produces alterations in GI function (enteritis/colitis) related to denudement/atrophy of small bowel villi and flattening of the large bowel epithelial surface (Holland, 2007).
      (3) Anorexia is associated with early satiety, taste and smell alterations, meat aversions, and nausea and vomiting (Adams, Shepard, et al., 2009; Tipton, 2009a).
      (4) Anorexia is associated with increased morbidity and mortality (Adams, Shepard, et al., 2009).
   b) Incidence
      (1) Approximately half of all patients with cancer, and up to 70% of patients with advanced disease (Yavuzsen, Davis, Walsh, LeGrand, & Lagman, 2005), will experience anorexia (Adams, Shepard, et al., 2009). Prevalence of weight loss is highest among patients with pancreatic or gastric cancer (von Meyenfeldt, 2005).
      (2) Patients with poor nutritional status or who experience significant weight loss

Table 13. General Radiation Treatment Principles for Gastrointestinal Cancers

Tumor Type	Incidence*	General Radiation Treatment Principles
Colon cancer	101,340	45–50 Gy in 25–28 fractions; boost to the tumor bed may be considered for close or positive margins; often given with 5-fluorouracil (5-FU) as a radiosensitizer.
Pancreatic cancer	44,030	Neoadjuvant/adjuvant therapy: 45–54 Gy (1.8–2 Gy/day); definitive treatment (unresectable): 50–60 Gy (1.8–2 Gy/day); often given in combination with 5-FU–based chemotherapy.
Rectal cancer	39,870	May be considered preoperatively or postoperatively; 45–50 Gy in 25–28 fractions with 5.4–9 Gy boost (54 Gy for unresectable tumors); often given in combination with 5-FU–based chemotherapy.
Liver and intrahepatic bile duct cancer	26,190	Radiation to the liver is limited by the radiosensitivity of the organ and ability to reliably localize the target volume. Recommended dose limit of 35 Gy for treatment of the whole liver, 52 Gy for half of the liver, and 70 Gy for 30% of the liver (Cheng & Huang, 2004). Radiofrequency ablation may be considered for patients with small tumors (smaller than 3 cm) that are not a candidate for curative therapy (i.e., resection).
Gastric cancer	21,520	Curative or palliative treatment for unresectable disease, or adjuvant therapy if incomplete resection or positive surgical margins present. Dose of 45–50.4 Gy in 25–28 fractions; prophylactic antiemetics should be offered with antacids and antidiarrheal agents on an as-needed basis.
Gallbladder/biliary cancer	9,250	Limited data exist to define standard radiation therapy parameters or benefit for biliary tract cancers. Doses of 45–50 Gy in 25–28 fractions may be considered (generally in combination with 5-FU–based chemotherapy) in unresectable or adjuvant treatment settings.

*Estimated new cases in 2011 from American Cancer Society, 2011

during treatment are at greater risk for adverse clinical outcomes, including decreased response to or tolerance of chemotherapy and RT (Cunningham & Bell, 2000; Jatoi & Loprinzi, 2001; Tipton, 2009a), prolonged disease or treatment-related symptoms, reduced functional status, or diminished quality of life (Adams, Shepard, et al., 2009).

(3) Treatment side effects such as mucositis, dysphagia, nausea, vomiting, and diarrhea contribute to anorexia and weight loss.

c) Assessment

(1) Factors that contribute to anorexia and weight loss are age, nicotine use, medical conditions (e.g., severe chronic obstructive pulmonary disease, diseases affecting metabolism), malignant symptoms, and socioeconomic conditions, such as living alone and low income (Brown, 2002). Other symptoms associated with weight loss are depression, infection, dyspnea, pain, fatigue, and the cumulative effect of several symptoms (McMahon & Brown, 2000).

(2) Weight change: Compare usual weight with present weight, time interval in which weight loss occurred, and weight at each visit. Weight loss of 5% in one month or 1%–2% per week is an indicator of malnutrition (Beaver, Matheny, Roberts, & Myers, 2001).

(3) Nutritional screening tools are available, such as the Patient-Generated Subjective Global Assessment, the Mini Nutritional Assessment, and the Malnutrition Screening Tool (Makhija & Baker, 2008; Tipton, 2009a). Screening assists in identifying patients who are malnourished or at risk, prompting more detailed nutritional assessment and dietitian consult for vulnerable patients (Davies, 2005).

(4) Dietary intake: Three-day food diary, including one weekend day (Brown, 2002)

(5) Functional status, such as decreased ability to care for self and maintain nutritional status, as measured by the Karnofsky Performance Status and Eastern Cooperative Oncology Group performance status (McMahon & Brown, 2000)

(6) Physical examination findings to evaluate for signs of malnutrition, such as weakness, loss of body fat, loss of muscle mass, and fluid status (McMahon & Brown, 2000)

(7) Laboratory findings such as serum albumin, prealbumin, iron levels, and electrolytes may be helpful in assessing nutritional or hydration status (Davies, 2005).

(8) Symptoms affecting nutrition, such as pain, mucositis, infection, fatigue, and depression

d) Collaborative management of anorexia

(1) Nonpharmacologic management

(a) The aim of nutritional intervention should be to maintain or improve functional status (von Meyenfeldt, 2005).

(b) Weight loss of 10% body weight over six months or 5% over one month is associated with worse clinical outcome (Nitenberg & Raynard, 2000). Goal is weight loss of less than 5% during treatment (Beaver et al., 2001).

i. Identify and correct underlying contributors to anorexia (e.g., mucositis, constipation) (Dy et al., 2008).

ii. Nutritional counseling: Implement an individualized nutritional teaching program (Adams, Cunningham, Caruso, Norling, & Shepard, 2009). Nutritional counseling had a favorable impact on weight maintenance and quality of life among patients with GI malignancies undergoing treatment (Isenring, Capra, & Bauer, 2004; Ravasco, Monteiro-Grillo, Vidal, & Camilo, 2005).

iii. Encourage oral liquid nutritional supplements (Garg, Yoo, & Winquist, 2010).

iv. Enhance calorie intake (small, frequent meals and calorie-dense foods); limit beverage intake around mealtime; take advantage of the time of day when the patient has best appetite.

v. Avoid extremes in taste or smell, and encourage pleasant eating environment and presentation of food (Laviano, Meguid, Inui, Muscaritoli, & Rossi-Fanelli, 2005).

vi. Manage symptoms (nausea, vomiting, pain, constipation, depression).

vii. Exercise may improve physical functioning, body composition, and muscle strength (Brown, 2002).

(2) Pharmacologic management

(a) Progestins—Recommended

i. Megestrol acetate dose range 160–1,600 mg/day, although there is insufficient evidence to recommend an exact dose (Adams, Cunningham, et al., 2009). In a randomized trial, the addition of olanzapine to megestrol acetate resulted in improved appetite, weight gain, and increased quality of life in patients with advanced GI and lung cancers compared to megestrol acetate alone (Navari & Brenner, 2010).

ii. Medroxyprogesterone acetate 300–1,000 mg/day (Brown, 2002)

iii. Potential dose-related adverse effects of progestinal agents include thromboembolic events, breakthrough bleeding, peripheral edema, hyperglycemia, hypertension, and renal suppression (Adams, Cunningham, et al., 2009). Dose low and titrate to decrease occurrence of adverse events (Adams, Cunningham, et al., 2009).

(b) Corticosteroids—Recommended

i. Dexamethasone, methylprednisolone, and prednisolone (Adams, Cunningham, et al., 2009)

ii. Improve treatment-related nausea and vomiting, appetite, food intake, performance status, and quality of life (Inoue et al., 2003; Yavuzsen et al., 2005)

(c) Metoclopramide

i. Decreases nausea and early satiety; does not stimulate appetite directly (Yavuzsen et al., 2005)

ii. Dose of 5–10 mg prior to meals enhances gastric motility and is useful for managing early satiety, delayed gastric emptying, and nausea/vomiting, but not anorexia specifically (Adams, Cunningham, et al., 2009).

(d) Other drugs that have been investigated in patients with cancer experiencing anorexia or weight loss, but as yet lack compelling evidence of benefit, include cyproheptadine, pentoxifylline, erythropoietin, eicosapentaenoic acid, androgenic steroids, ghrelin, interferon, NSAIDs, and thalidomide (Adams, Cunningham, et al., 2009; Yavuzsen et al., 2005). Drugs not likely to be effective include hydrazine sulfate, melatonin, and cannabinoids (Adams, Cunningham, et al., 2009).

e) Documentation (NCI CTEP, 2010)

(1) 1—Loss of appetite without alteration in eating habits

(2) 2—Oral intake altered without significant weight loss or malnutrition; oral nutritional supplements indicated

(3) 3—Associated with significant weight loss or malnutrition (e.g., inadequate oral caloric and/or fluid intake); tube feeding or TPN indicated

(4) 4—Life-threatening consequences; urgent intervention indicated

(5) 5—Death

f) Patient and family education (Cunningham & Bell, 2000)

(1) Educate the patient and family on the fundamentals of good nutrition.

(2) Give examples of sources of nutritious calories and protein.

(3) Teach the patient how to complete a food diary.

(4) Instruct the patient and family on symptoms to report that affect food intake.

(5) Encourage patient and family participation in development and implementation of the plan for nutrition.

(6) Related Web sites

    (a) Cancer*Care*: www.cancercare.org

    (b) CancerSymptoms.org: www.cancersymptoms.org/anorexia-from-cancer-treatment

    (c) Caring4Cancer: www.caring4cancer.com/go/cancer/effects/lesscommon/weight-loss-and-anorexia.htm

    (d) NCI: www.cancer.gov/cancertopics/pdq/supportivecare/nutrition/Patient

3. Nausea and vomiting

  a) Pathophysiology

    (1) Acute effects—Physiologic causes of nausea

      (a) Mechanisms of radiation-induced nausea are likely multifactorial and are related to the treatment field, dose, and fractionation schedule (Schnell, 2003).

      (b) The chemoreceptor trigger zone (CTZ) is located within the area postrema in the brain (Urba, 2007).

      (c) Vomiting center and vagal nuclei are stimulated by radiation or chemical mediators (Wickham, 2004).

      (d) Activation of neurotransmitter receptors—serotonin, substance P, dopamine, NK1, and other receptors that stimulate the CTZ in the area postrema in the brain (Holland, 2007; Wickham, 2004)

      (e) Rapidly dividing cells within the GI tract (specifically the small intestine) are particularly sensitive to radiation damage (Urba, 2007). Stimulation of enterochromaffin cells by abdominal radiation liberates serotonin (5-HT) that binds to 5-HT_3 receptors on vagal terminals, which activates the CTZ (Horiot, 2004).

      (f) Radiation to the brain can directly affect the CTZ (Hogan & Grant, 1997).

        i. Nausea is mediated by the CNS, cerebral cortex, and autonomic nervous system (Wickham, 2004).

        ii. The stomach relaxes, and gastric acid secretion is inhibited. A contraction of the small intestine causes the alkaline contents of the small bowel to be propelled into the stomach (Murphy-Ende, 2006).

      (g) Vomiting is mediated through the vomiting center and activated by several inputs, including the CTZ, cerebral cortex, limbic region, and afferent vagal and visceral nerves (Wickham, 2004).

    (2) Late effects (gastric): Result from a combination of vascular damage, progressive fibrosis, and loss of mucosal/epithelial cells (Czito & Willett, 2011)

      (a) Chronic gastritis—Ulceration and mucosal atrophy with evidence of antral stenosis

      (b) Dyspepsia—Persistent, vague gastric symptoms developing months after treatment completion

      (c) Risk of late gastric ulceration or perforation limits radiation doses to 50 Gy when the treatment field includes a large portion of the stomach (Kavanagh et al., 2010).

  b) Incidence

    (1) Acute effects

      (a) Treatment field is considered the most important factor, but others include treatment volume, dose, fractionation, and technique (Urba, 2007).

      (b) Overall incidence of nausea and vomiting in patients undergoing RT (all sites) has been reported between 28% and 39% (Enblom, Axelsson, Steineck, Hammar, & Börjeson, 2009; Maranzano et al., 2010).

      (c) Onset may occur within the first 24 hours of treatment and within 10–15 minutes following TBI and hemibody radiation (Feyer et al., 2011).

      (d) Approximately 50% of people who receive conventionally fractionated radiation to the abdomen have onset of symptoms within 40–90 minutes, and nausea may persist for up to 24 hours after exposure (Urba, 2007).

      (e) High risk (greater than 90%) with TBI and total nodal irradiation (Feyer et al., 2011; Multinational Association of Supportive Care in Cancer [MASCC], 2010)

(f) Moderate risk (60%–90%) with hemibody, upper abdomen, and upper body RT (Feyer et al., 2011; MASCC, 2010)

(g) Low risk (30%–60%) for head and neck, cranium, craniospinal, pelvis, and lower thorax RT alone (Feyer et al., 2011; MASCC, 2010); risk increases with concomitant chemotherapy.

(h) Minimal risk (less than 30%) for RT to other sites, including breast and extremities (Feyer et al., 2011; MASCC, 2010); risk increases with concomitant chemotherapy.

(2) Chronic effects

(a) Gastric atrophy and ulceration may occur after doses of 45 Gy or more (Engelking, 2004; Holland, 2007; Kavanagh et al., 2010).

(b) Symptoms may present months to years after cessation of treatment (Holland, 2007).

c) Assessment

(1) Risk factors

(a) Incidence and severity of past nausea and vomiting, precipitating factors

(b) Age—More likely in patients at younger age (Holland, 2007).

(c) Sex—More likely in menstruating women (Wickham, 2004).

(d) Susceptibility to motion sickness (Hickok, Roscoe, & Morrow, 2001)

(e) Unsuccessful past treatment of nausea and vomiting (Holland, 2007)

(f) Patients with anxiety (Holland, 2007)

(g) Other possible causes—Concurrent chemotherapy, emetic potential of chemotherapy, other drugs (e.g., opioids), infection, constipation, intestinal obstruction, hypercalcemia, electrolyte abnormalities, and increased intracranial pressure (Holland, 2007; Wickham, 2004)

(2) Symptom assessment

(a) Occurrence, frequency, intensity, onset, and duration of nausea and vomiting. Use patient report such as diaries, journals, and logs (Holland, 2007).

(b) Review of medications

(c) Signs and symptoms of dehydration (e.g., poor skin turgor, electrolyte imbalance, light-headedness or dizziness with postural changes, nausea, increased weakness or fatigue, concentrated urine, orthostatic hypotension, oral cavity moisture)

(d) Physical examination

i. Height and weight

ii. Vital signs (including orthostatic blood pressure and pulse)

• Decrease in systolic blood pressure greater than 20 mm Hg, diastolic blood pressure greater than 10 mm Hg

• Compensatory increase in heart rate

iii. Mental status, skin turgor, oral cavity, bowel sounds, abdominal tenderness or distension, neurologic examination

iv. Complete blood count to rule out associated infection and dehydration

v. Electrolytes: Rule out dehydration—check chloride and potassium levels because of loss in emesis, blood urea nitrogen, creatinine ratio, and CO_2 (Wickham, 2004). Check calcium level to rule out hypercalcemia (Murphy-Ende, 2006).

vi. Oral intake over last 24-hour period

d) Collaborative management of nausea and vomiting

(1) Pharmacologic

(a) 5-HT$_3$ receptor antagonists block the stimulation of 5-HT$_3$ receptors at various points in the body and are useful to prevent radiation-induced emesis (Spratto & Woods, 2008).

i. Management of constipation if present

ii. Headache, light-headedness, and sedation are other common side effects.

iii. Ondansetron, granisetron, and dolasetron have similar efficacy (Gralla et al., 1999).

iv. Some patients have successful control with a second 5-HT$_3$ antagonist despite inadequate control with a first (de Wit et al., 2001).

(b) Dopamine receptor antagonists bind to dopamine-2 and other receptors to vomiting impulses.

    i. Children and young adults are at risk for extrapyramidal symptoms.

    ii. Prophylactic diphenhydramine may be used.

    iii. Dopamine-2 receptor antagonists include phenothiazines, the most commonly used being prochlorperazine, butyrophenone, haloperidol, and substituted benzamides (metoclopramide) (Wickham, 2004).

(c) Controlled-release metoclopramide, 20–80 mg every 12 hours for a maximum period of 12 weeks, has demonstrated a 40%–60% decrease in the severity of nausea over the first two weeks of treatment and an approximate 50% reduction in the severity of vomiting over the first four weeks of treatment (Wilson et al., 2002).

(d) Corticosteroids (e.g., dexamethasone, prednisone, prednisolone)—Inhibition of prostaglandin synthesis. May cause insomnia, anxiety, or euphoria (Spratto & Woods, 2008). A trend toward better emetic control in patients receiving ondansetron combined with dexamethasone on days 1–5 in comparison to ondansetron alone in patients receiving upper abdominal RT has been reported (Wong et al., 2006).

(e) Benzodiazepines—Anxiolytics and amnesiacs, such as alprazolam and lorazepam, may be useful for the treatment of anticipatory nausea and vomiting (Friend et al., 2009).

(f) NK1 antagonists block the NK1 receptors in the brain. The NK1 receptor antagonist is more effective in the prevention of delayed emesis. When NK1 antagonists were given with other antiemetics, acute emesis also decreased. Aprepitant is approved for prevention of acute and delayed emesis with highly emetogenic chemotherapy (Spratto & Woods, 2008).

(g) High risk for radiation-induced nausea and vomiting: TBI or total nodal irradiation

    i. 5-HT$_3$ antagonists give complete control rates of 50%–90% (Gralla et al., 1999; Spitzer, Friedman, Bushnell, Frankel, & Raschko, 2000).

    ii. Addition of corticosteroids may be beneficial.

    iii. Use a serotonin receptor antagonist with or without a corticosteroid before each fraction and for at least 24 hours afterward (Feyer, Stewart, & Titlbach, 1998; Gralla et al., 1999; Maranzano et al., 2005).

    iv. Patients receiving concurrent chemotherapy should be given an antiemetic agent based on the level of emetogenicity of chemotherapy and risk factors associated with radiation-induced emesis (MASCC, 2010).

(h) Moderate risk for radiation-induced nausea and vomiting: Upper abdomen, hemibody irradiation or upper-body irradiation, lower thoracic spine

    i. Use a serotonin receptor antagonist before each fraction for the entire duration of treatment (Maranzano et al., 2005).

    ii. Serotonin receptor antagonists are more effective than metoclopramide, phenothiazines, or placebo in this setting (Lanciano et al., 2001). Efficacy may decrease after the first week.

    iii. An optional short course of dexamethasone in addition to a serotonin receptor antagonist may be considered (MASCC, 2010).

(i) Low risk for radiation-induced nausea and vomiting: Radiation to lower thorax, pelvis, head and neck, or cranium and craniospinal RT. Prophylactic or rescue treatment with a serotonin receptor antagonist is recommended (Maranzano et al., 2005; MASCC, 2010).

(j) Minimal risk for radiation-induced nausea and vomiting: Radiation to extremities and breast. Treatment with a dopamine or serotonin receptor antagonist on an as-needed basis (Maranzano et al., 2005; MASCC, 2010)

(2) Nonpharmacologic management

    (a) Use in combination with prescribed antiemetic therapy.

    (b) May be effective by producing physiologic relaxation, which may decrease nausea and vomiting, serve as a distraction, and enhance control (Lotfi-Jam et al., 2008; Tipton et al., 2007)

      i. Systematic desensitization

      ii. Exercise

      iii. Hypnosis

      iv. Music therapy

      v. Relaxation/progressive muscle relaxation

      vi. Imagery: Mentally take self away by focusing on images of a relaxing place (Friend et al., 2009).

e) Documentation (NCI CTEP, 2010)

(1) Nausea

    (a) 1—Loss of appetite without alteration in eating habits

    (b) 2—Oral intake decreased without significant weight loss, dehydration, or malnutrition

    (c) 3—Inadequate oral caloric or fluid intake; tube feeding, TPN, or hospitalization indicated

(2) Vomiting

    (a) 1—One to two episodes (separated by 5 minutes) in 24 hours

    (b) 2—Three to five episodes (separated by 5 minutes) in 24 hours

    (c) 3—Six or more episodes (separated by 5 minutes) in 24 hours; tube feeding, TPN, or hospitalization indicated

    (d) 4—Life-threatening consequences; urgent intervention indicated

    (e) 5—Death

f) Patient and family education

(1) Teach patients who are at high or intermediate risk to self-administer antiemetics before treatment on a daily basis.

(2) Instruct the patient to record nausea and vomiting in a diary.

(3) If the patient is vomiting, the patient should check weight daily.

(4) Teach symptoms of dehydration, such as excessive thirst, dizziness, palpitations, and fever.

(5) Practice dietary modifications such as eating small, frequent meals, eating foods that are cold or at room temperature, avoiding favorite foods to prevent food aversions, and avoiding fatty, spicy, salty, and sweet foods that may aggravate nausea (Wickham, 2004).

(6) Prepare meals when not feeling nauseated; share task of cooking with family members.

(7) Instruct the patient on nonpharmacologic methods to alleviate nausea.

(8) Use self-care guidelines for radiation-induced nausea and vomiting (Wickham, 2004).

(9) Related Web sites

    (a) ACS: www.cancer.org

    (b) ASCO's patient site: www.cancer.net

    (c) NCCN: www.nccn.org

    (d) NCI: www.cancer.gov

4. Diarrhea/proctitis

  a) Pathophysiology

    (1) Acute effects

      (a) Radiation affects the rapidly dividing cells of the small and large bowel.

        i. Crypt stem cells responsible for cellular replacement are affected, resulting in denudement and atrophy of villi in the small bowel and flattening of the epithelial surface in the large bowel (Engelking, 2004).

        ii. Loss of epithelial absorptive function results in loss of water, electrolytes, protein, and blood. Conjugated bile salts are not absorbed, enter the colon, and are deconjugated by bacterial flora, resulting in water retention and diarrhea (Engelking, 2004).

        iii. Decreased lactase production in the small bowel causes accumulation of lactose (Engelking, 2004).

      (b) Diarrhea occurs as a result of hypermotility of bowels, loss of absorptive surface with decreased absorption of nutrients and bile salts, and decreased or absent lactase resulting in lactose intolerance (Engelking, 2004).

(c) Symptoms may include nausea, vomiting, abdominal cramping or pain, watery diarrhea, flatus, bleeding, and anemia. Symptoms of proctitis include mucoid rectal discharge, rectal pain, and rectal bleeding (Saclarides, 1997).

(d) Diarrhea can significantly affect quality of life with physical and psychosocial consequences (Engelking, 2004).

(e) Symptoms usually develop during treatment (or shortly thereafter) and resolve within two to six weeks of completing therapy.

(2) Chronic effects (small/large bowel)

(a) Median onset of 8–12 months, but can develop up to 15 years after RT. Result of vascular insufficiency caused by damaged cells in blood vessels and connective tissue in the bowel wall (Engelking, 2004; Saclarides, 1997).

(b) Mucosal ulcerations may result in perforation, fistula, or abscess formation, and fibrotic tissue from healing can cause stenosis or adhesion formation leading to strictures or obstruction (Crane & Janjan, 2003). Possible symptoms include nausea and vomiting, as well as abdominal cramping, bloating, chronic diarrhea, malabsorption with weight loss, and chronic blood loss.

(c) The volume of small bowel in the field affects the incidence and type of complications seen (Saclarides, 1997).

(d) The small intestine is sensitive to late effects and is a dose-limiting structure in the treatment of the abdomen and pelvis.

(e) The large bowel is less radiosensitive, but radiation injury may result in colitis.

b) Incidence and risk factors

(1) Acute

(a) Most patients receiving radiation to the abdomen, pelvis, or rectum will show signs of acute enteritis (Saclarides, 1997).

(b) Incidence increases with higher dose fraction, larger treatment volume, concomitant chemotherapy, prior abdominal or pelvic surgery, and history of colitis, ileitis, or irritable bowel syndrome (Engelking & Sauerland, 2001; Holland, 2007).

(c) Usually begins to occur at 10–30 Gy (Engelking, 2004)

(2) Chronic effects: Occur in 5%–15% of patients treated with lower abdominal or pelvic irradiation (Engelking & Sauerland, 2001)

c) Assessment

(1) Individual risk factors

(a) Prior abdominal surgery

(b) History of pelvic inflammatory disease or colitis

(c) History of lactose intolerance (Holland, 2007)

(d) History of cardiovascular disease, hypertension, or diabetes (Holland, 2007)

(2) Usual pattern of elimination

(3) Change in bowel pattern: Onset, frequency, amount, and character of stools, blood in stool

(4) Presence of other symptoms such as flatus, pain or cramping, nausea, abdominal distension, fecal incontinence or urgency, timing of onset of symptoms (Tipton, 2009b)

(5) Nutritional status: Weight and height, change in eating habits, amount of residue in diet

(6) Signs of dehydration: Poor skin turgor for age, serum electrolyte imbalance, increased weakness, orthostatic hypotension, and weight loss

(7) Level of stress, coping patterns, and impact of symptoms on usual lifestyle

(8) Abdominal and rectal examination for bowel sounds, inflamed hemorrhoids (Tipton, 2009b)

(9) Elevated temperature

(10) Comorbid conditions that can exaggerate side effects (diabetes, lactose intolerance, baseline chronic GI abnormalities) (Engelking, 2004)

(11) Assessment of medication use, including over-the-counter medications; recent antibiotic history

(12) Imaging (abdominal CT, upper GI series) and endoscopy often are required to establish the diagnosis.

d) Collaborative management of acute and chronic diarrhea

(1) Dietary modification

(a) Include low-residue foods such as baked, broiled, or steamed meat, fish, and poultry; refined grains; cooked vegetables; canned fruit and applesauce; bananas; and juices and nectars (McCallum & Polisena, 2000).

(b) Include potassium-rich foods.

(c) Avoid fried and fatty foods, lactose products, foods high in fiber, strong spices and herbs, caffeine, alcohol, and tobacco.

(d) Avoid foods that are too hot or cold. Evaluate on a case-by-case basis (Engelking, 2004).

(2) Drink adequate fluids (2,000–3,000 ml/day). Some fluids should contain some salt and sugar, such as clear broth, gelatin desserts, and sports drinks or soft drinks with some carbonation removed (Saltz, 2003).

(3) Pharmacologic management: Goals are inhibition of intestinal motility, reduction in intestinal secretions, and promotion of absorption. Few studies specifically addressing radiation-induced diarrhea have reached the level of evidence necessary for practice recommendations (Muehlbauer et al., 2009).

(a) Loperamide hydrochloride—Recommended: Loperamide slows GI peristalsis, which increases GI transit time and promotes water reabsorption. Start with 4 mg at the first episode of diarrhea, followed by 2 mg after each unformed stool, with a maximum of 12–16 mg in 24 hours (Wilkes, Ingwersen, & Barton-Burke, 2002). This agent should be avoided in patients with suspected bowel obstruction.

(b) Diphenoxylate/atropine—Recommended: Diphenoxylate slows GI transit time. It appears to have similar efficacy to loperamide in mild to moderate diarrhea (Saltz, 2003). It is associated with more CNS side effects, including dizziness, nausea, vomiting, and blurred vision (Engelking, 2004). Dose is one to two tablets every four hours as needed, not to exceed eight tablets in 24 hours.

(c) Certain probiotic preparations, such as *Lactobacillus casei* DN-114 001 and VSL #3, may reduce the incidence and severity of diarrhea associated with radiation enteritis; however, evidence is insufficient to recommend its routine use for enteritis prevention during abdominal or pelvic RT (Visich & Yeo, 2010).

(d) Bulk-forming agents—Psyllium fiber, methylcellulose, and pectin absorb water and enhance stool bulk but may cause abdominal discomfort and bloating in some people (Engelking, 2004; Singh, 2007).

(e) Paregoric or tincture of opium may be used, alternating with loperamide.

(f) Cholestyramine is a bile salt sequestering agent (Engelking, Wickham, & Sauerland, 2007). Dose is one package after each meal and at bedtime.

(g) Steroid foam may be given rectally for proctitis.

(h) Narcotics may be needed for relief of abdominal pain.

e) Documentation (NCI CTEP, 2010)

(1) Diarrhea

(a) 1—Increase of less than four stools per day over baseline; mild increase in ostomy output compared to baseline

(b) 2—Increase of four to six stools per day over baseline; moderate increase in ostomy output compared to baseline

(c) 3—Increase of seven or more stools per day over baseline; incontinence; hospitalization indicated; severe increase in ostomy output compared to baseline; limiting self-care ADL

(d) 4—Life-threatening consequences; urgent intervention indicated

(e) 5—Death

f) Patient and family education

(1) Educate the patient and family about expected side effects prior to therapy.

(2) Teach diarrhea management.

    (a) Record the number and consistency of daily bowel movements and when to seek medical attention (e.g., rectal spasms, excessive cramping, watery or bloody stools, continued diarrhea not relieved by treatment) (Engelking, 2004).

    (b) Teach signs and symptoms of dehydration, such as excessive thirst, fever, dizziness or light-headedness, and palpitations.

    (c) Teach dietary modifications as described previously.

    (d) Give specific instructions on how to take antidiarrheal medications.

    (e) Provide recommendations for proper skin care: Sitz baths and moisture barrier creams and ointments.

    (f) Instruct the patient to report symptoms such as change in stools, rectal bleeding, or pain in follow-up.

    (g) Related Web sites

        i. ASCO patient Web site: www.cancer.net

        ii. NCI: www.cancer.gov

        iii. OncoLink, sponsored by Abramson Cancer Center of the University of Pennsylvania: www.oncolink.upenn.edu

References

Adams, L.A., Cunningham, R.S., Caruso, R.A., Norling, M.J., & Shepard, N. (2009). ONS PEP resource: Anorexia. In L.H. Eaton & J.M. Tipton (Eds.), *Putting evidence into practice: Improving oncology patient outcomes* (pp. 31–36). Pittsburgh, PA: Oncology Nursing Society.

Adams, L.A., Shepard, N., Caruso, R.A., Norling, M.J., Belansky, H., & Cunningham, R.S. (2009). Putting evidence into practice®: Evidence-based interventions to prevent and manage anorexia. *Clinical Journal of Oncology Nursing, 13,* 95–102. doi:10.1188/09.CJON.95-102

American Cancer Society. (2011). Cancer facts and figures 2011. Retrieved from http://www.cancer.org/Research/CancerFactsFigures/CancerFactsFigures/cancer-facts-figures-2011

Beaver, M.E., Matheny, K.E, Roberts, D.B., & Myers, J.N. (2001). Predictors of weight loss during radiation therapy. *Otolaryngology—Head and Neck Surgery, 125,* 645–648. doi:10.1067/mhn.2001.120428

Brown, J.K. (2002). A systematic review of the evidence on symptom management of cancer-related anorexia and cachexia. *Oncology Nursing Forum, 29,* 517–532. doi:10.1188/02.ONF.517-532

Catlin-Huth, C., Haas, M., & Pollock, V. (Eds.). (2002). *Radiation therapy patient care record: A tool for documenting nursing care.* Pittsburgh, PA: Oncology Nursing Society.

Cheng, S.H., & Huang, A.T. (2004). Liver and hepatobiliary tract. In C.A. Perez, E.C. Halperin, L.W. Brady, & R.K. Schmidt-Ullrich (Eds.), *Principles and practice of radiation oncology* (4th ed., pp. 1589–1606). Philadelphia, PA: Lippincott Williams & Wilkins.

Crane, C.H., & Janjan, N.A. (2003). The stomach and small intestine. In J.D. Cox & K.K. Ang (Eds.), *Radiation oncology: Rationale, technique, results* (8th ed., pp. 444–464). St. Louis, MO: Elsevier Mosby.

Cunningham, R.S., & Bell, R. (2000). Nutrition in cancer: An overview. *Seminars in Oncology Nursing, 16,* 90–98. doi:10.1053/on.2000.7141

Czito, B.G., & Willett, C.G. (2011). Stomach. In D.C. Shrieve, & J.S. Loeffler (Eds.), *Human radiation injury* (pp. 444–452). Philadelphia, PA: Lippincott Williams & Wilkins.

Davies, M. (2005). Nutritional screening and assessment in cancer-associated malnutrition. *European Journal of Oncology Nursing, 9*(Suppl. 2), S64–S73. doi:10.1016/j.ejon.2005.09.005

de Wit, R., de Boer, A.C., Linden, G.H.M., Stoter, G., Sparreboom, A., & Verweij, J. (2001). Effective cross-over to granisetron after failure to ondansetron, a randomized double blind study in patients failing ondansetron plus dexamethasone during the first 24 hours following highly emetogenic chemotherapy. *British Journal of Cancer, 85,* 1099–1101. doi:10.1054/bjoc.2001.2045

Dy, S.M., Lorenz, K.A., Naeim, A., Sanati, H., Walling, A., & Asch, S.M. (2008). Evidence-based recommendations for cancer fatigue, anorexia, depression, and dyspnea. *Journal of Clinical Oncology, 26,* 3886–3895. doi:10.1200/JCO.2007.15.9525

Enblom, A., Axelsson, B.B., Steineck, G., Hammar, M., & Börjeson, S. (2009). One third of patients with radiotherapy-induced nausea consider their antiemetic treatment insufficient. *Supportive Care in Cancer, 17,* 23–32. doi:10.1007/s00520-008-0445-x

Engelking, C. (2004). Diarrhea. In C.H. Yarbro, M.H. Frogge, & M. Goodman (Eds.), *Cancer symptom management* (3rd ed., pp. 528–550). Sudbury, MA: Jones and Bartlett.

Engelking, C., & Sauerland, C. (2001). Maintenance of normal elimination. In D. Watkins-Bruner, G. Moore-Higgs, & M. Haas (Eds.), *Outcomes in radiation therapy: Multidisciplinary management* (pp. 530–562). Sudbury, MA: Jones and Bartlett.

Engelking, C., Wickham, R.J., & Sauerland, C. (2007). Radiation-induced nausea, vomiting, and diarrhea. In M.L. Haas, W.P. Hogle, G.J. Moore-Higgs, & T.K. Gosselin-Acomb (Eds.), *Radiation therapy: A guide to patient care* (pp. 589–608). St. Louis, MO: Mosby Elsevier.

Feyer, P.C., Maranzano, E., Molassiotis, A., Roila, F., Clark-Snow, R.A., & Jordan, K. (2011). Radiotherapy-induced nausea and vomiting (RINV): MASCC/ESMO guideline for antiemetics in radiotherapy: Update 2009. *Supportive Care in Cancer, 19*(Suppl. 1), 5–14. doi:10.1007/s00520-010-0950-6

Feyer, P.C., Stewart, A.L., & Titlbach, O.J. (1998). Aetiology and prevention of emesis induced by radiotherapy. *Supportive Care in Cancer, 6,* 253–260. doi:10.1007/s005200050163

Friend, P.J., Johnston, M.P., Tipton, J.M., McDaniel, R.W., Barbour, L.A., Starr, P., ... Ripple, M.L. (2009). ONS PEP resource: Chemotherapy-induced nausea and vomiting. In L.H. Eaton & J.M. Tipton (Eds.), *Putting evidence into practice: Improving oncology patient outcomes* (pp. 71–83). Pittsburgh, PA: Oncology Nursing Society.

Garg, S., Yoo, J., & Winquist, E. (2010). Nutritional support for head and neck cancer patients receiving radiotherapy: A systematic review. *Supportive Care in Cancer, 18,* 667–677. doi:10.1007/s00520-009-0686-3

Gralla, R.J., Osoba, D., Kris, M.G., Kirkbride, P., Hesketh, P.J., Chinnery, L.W., ... Pfister, D.G. (1999). Recommendations for the use of antiemetics: Evidence-based, clinical practice guidelines. *Journal of Clinical Oncology, 17,* 2971–2994.

Hickok, J.T., Roscoe, J.A., & Morrow, G.R. (2001). The role of patients' expectations in the development of anticipatory nausea related to chemotherapy for cancer. *Journal of Pain and Symptom Management, 22*, 843–850. doi:10.1016/S0885-3924(01)00317-7

Hogan, C.M., & Grant, M. (1997). Physiologic mechanisms of nausea and vomiting in patients with cancer. *Oncology Nursing Forum, 24*(Suppl. 7), 8–12.

Holland, J.C. (2007). Gastrointestinal cancers. In M.L. Haas, W.P. Hogle, G.J. Moore-Higgs, & T.K. Gosselin-Acomb (Eds.), *Radiation therapy: A guide to patient care* (pp. 166–194). St. Louis, MO: Elsevier Mosby.

Horiot, J.C. (2004). Prophylaxis versus treatment: Is there a better way to manage radiotherapy-induced nausea and vomiting? *International Journal of Radiation Oncology, Biology, Physics, 60*, 1018–1025. doi:10.1016/j.ijrobp.2004.07.722

Inoue, A., Yamada, Y., Matsumura, Y., Shimada, Y., Muro, K., Gotoh, M., … Shirao, K. (2003). Randomized study of dexamethasone treatment for delayed emesis, anorexia and fatigue induced by irinotecan. *Supportive Care in Cancer, 11*, 528–532. doi:10.1007/s00520-003-0488-y

Isenring, E.A., Capra, S., & Bauer, J.D. (2004). Nutrition intervention is beneficial in oncology outpatients receiving radiotherapy to the gastrointestinal or head and neck area. *British Journal of Cancer, 91*, 447–452. doi:10.1038/sj.bjc.6601962

Jatoi, A., Jr., & Loprinzi, C.L. (2001). Current management of cancer-associated anorexia and weight loss. *Oncology, 15*, 497–502, 508.

Kavanagh, B.D., Pan, C.C., Dawson, L.A., Das, S.K., Li, X.A., Ten Haken, R.K., & Miften, M. (2010). Radiation dose-volume effects in the stomach and small bowel. *International Journal of Radiation Oncology, Biology, Physics, 76*, S101–S107. doi:10.1016/j.ijrobp.2009.05.071

Lanciano, R., Sherman, D.M., Michalski, J., Preston, A.J., Yocom, K., & Friedman, C. (2001). The efficacy and safety of once-daily Kytril (granisetron hydrochloride) tablets in the prophylaxis of nausea and emesis following fractionated upper abdominal radiotherapy. *Cancer Investigation, 19*, 763–772.

Laviano, A., Meguid, M.M., Inui, A., Muscaritoli, M., & Rossi-Fanelli, F. (2005). Therapy insight: Cancer anorexia-cachexia syndrome—When all you can eat is yourself. *Nature Clinical Practice Oncology, 2*, 158–165. doi:10.1038/ncponc0112

Lotfi-Jam, K., Carey, M., Jefford, M., Schofield, P., Charleson, C., & Aranda, S. (2008). Nonpharmacologic strategies for managing common chemotherapy adverse effects: A systematic review. *Journal of Clinical Oncology, 26*, 5618–5629. doi:10.1200/JCO.2007.15.9053

Makhija, S., & Baker, J. (2008). The Subjective Global Assessment: A review of its use in clinical practice. *Nutrition in Clinical Practice, 23*, 405–409. doi:10.1177/0884533608321214

Maranzano, E., De Angelis, V., Pergolizzi, S., Lupattelli, M., Frata, P., Spagnesi, S., … Di Gennaro, D. (2010). A prospective observational trial on emesis in radiotherapy: Analysis of 1020 patients recruited in 45 Italian radiation oncology centres. *Radiotherapy and Oncology, 94*, 36–41. doi:10.1016/j.radonc.2009.11.001

Maranzano, E., Feyer, P.C., Molassiotis, A., Rossi, R., Clark-Snow, R.A., Olver, I., … Roila, F. (2005). Evidence-based recommendations for the use of antiemetics in radiotherapy. *Radiotherapy and Oncology, 76*, 227–233. doi:10.1016/j.radonc.2005.07.002

McCallum, P.O., & Polisena, C.G. (2000). *The clinical guide to oncology nutrition.* Chicago, IL: American Dietetic Association.

McMahon, K., & Brown, J.K. (2000). Nutritional screening and assessment. *Seminars in Oncology Nursing, 16*, 106–112. doi:10.1053/on.2000.5549

Muehlbauer, P.M., Thorpe, D., Davis, A., Drabot, R., Rawlings, B.L., & Kiker, E. (2009). Putting evidence into practice: Evidence-based interventions to prevent, manage, and treat chemotherapy- and radiotherapy-induced diarrhea. *Clinical Journal of Oncology Nursing, 13*, 336–341. doi:10.1188/09.CJON.336-341

Multinational Association of Supportive Care in Cancer. (2010). *MASCC antiemetic guidelines.* Retrieved from http://www.mascc.org/mc/page.do?sitePageId=88041

Murphy-Ende, K. (2006). Nausea and vomiting. In D. Camp-Sorrell & R.A. Hawkins (Eds.), *Clinical manual for the oncology advanced practice nurse* (2nd ed., pp. 465–471). Pittsburgh, PA: Oncology Nursing Society.

National Cancer Institute Cancer Therapy Evaluation Program. (2010). *Common terminology criteria for adverse events* [v.4.03]. Retrieved from http://evs.nci.nih.gov/ftp1/CTCAE/CTCAE_4.03_2010-06-14_QuickReference_5x7.pdf

Navari, R.M., & Brenner, M.C. (2010). Treatment of cancer-related anorexia with olanzapine and megestrol acetate: A randomized trial. *Supportive Care in Cancer, 18*, 951–956. doi:10.1007/s00520-009-0739-7

Nitenberg, G., & Raynard, B. (2000). Nutritional support of the cancer patient: Issues and dilemmas. *Critical Reviews in Oncology/Hematology, 34*, 137–168. doi:10.1016/S1040-8428(00)00048-2

Ravasco, P., Monteiro-Grillo, I., Vidal, P.M., & Camilo, M.E. (2005). Dietary counseling improves patient outcomes: A prospective, randomized, controlled trial in colorectal cancer patients undergoing radiotherapy. *Journal of Clinical Oncology, 23*, 1431–1438. doi:10.1200/JCO.2005.02.054

Saclarides, T.J. (1997). Radiation injuries of the gastrointestinal tract. *Surgical Clinics of North America, 77*, 261–268.

Saltz, L.B. (2003). Understanding and managing chemotherapy-induced diarrhea. *Journal of Supportive Oncology, 1*, 35–46.

Schnell, F.M. (2003). Chemotherapy-induced nausea and vomiting: The importance of acute antiemetic control. *Oncologist, 8*, 187–198. doi:10.1634/theoncologist.8-2-18

Singh, B. (2007). Psyllium as therapeutic and drug delivery agent. *International Journal of Pharmaceutics, 334*, 1–14. doi:10.1016/j.ijpharm.2007.01.028

Spitzer, T.R., Friedman, C.J., Bushnell, W., Frankel, S.R., & Raschko, J. (2000). Double-blind, randomized, parallel-group study on the efficacy and safety of oral granisetron and oral ondansetron in the prophylaxis of nausea and vomiting in patients receiving hyperfractionated total body irradiation. *Bone Marrow Transplantation, 26*, 203–210. doi:10.1038/sj.bmt.1702479

Spratto, G.R., & Woods, A.L. (2008). *PDR nurse's drug handbook.* Montvale, NJ: Thomson Delmar Learning.

Tipton, J.M. (2009a). Anorexia. In L.H. Eaton & J.M. Tipton (Eds.), *Putting evidence into practice: Improving oncology patient outcomes* (pp. 25–29). Pittsburgh, PA: Oncology Nursing Society.

Tipton, J.M. (2009b). Diarrhea. In L.H. Eaton & J.M. Tipton (Eds.), *Putting evidence into practice: Improving oncology patient outcomes* (pp. 119–124). Pittsburgh, PA: Oncology Nursing Society.

Tipton, J.M., McDaniel, R.W., Barbour, L., Johnston, M.P., Kayne, M., LeRoy, P., & Ripple, M.L. (2007). Putting evidence into practice: Evidence-based interventions to prevent, manage, and treat chemotherapy-induced nausea and vomiting. *Clinical Journal of Oncology Nursing, 11*, 69–78. doi:10.1188/07.CJON.69-78

Urba, S. (2007). Radiation-induced nausea and vomiting. *Journal of the National Comprehensive Cancer Network, 5*, 60–65.

Visich, K.L., & Yeo, T.P. (2010). The prophylactic use of probiotics in the prevention of radiation therapy-induced diarrhea. *Clinical Journal of Oncology Nursing, 14*, 467–473. doi:10.1188/10.CJON.467-473 von Meyenfeldt, M. (2005). Cancer-associated malnutrition: An introduction. *European Journal of Oncology Nursing, 9*(Suppl. 2), S35–S38. doi:10.1016/j.ejon.2005.09.001

Wickham, R. (2004). Nausea and vomiting. In C.H. Yarbro, M.H. Frogge, & M. Goodman (Eds.), *Cancer symptom management* (3rd ed., pp. 187–207). Sudbury, MA: Jones and Bartlett.

Wilkes, G.M., Ingwersen, K., & Barton-Burke, M. (2002). *2002 oncology nursing drug handbook.* Sudbury, MA: Jones and Bartlett.

Wilson, J., Plourde, J.-Y., Marshall, D., Yoshida, S., Chow, W., Harsanyi, Z., … Darke, A. (2002). Long-term safety and clinical effectiveness of controlled-release metoclopramide in cancer-associated dyspepsia syndrome: A multicentre evaluation. *Journal of Palliative Care, 18,* 84–91.

Wong, R.K.S., Paul, N., Ding, K., Whitehead, M., Brundage, M., Fyles, A., … Pater, J. (2006). 5-hydroxytryptamine-3 receptor antagonist with or without short-course dexamethasone in the prophylaxis of radiation induced emesis: A placebo-controlled randomized trial of the National Cancer Institute of Canada Clinical Trials Group (SC19). *Journal of Clinical Oncology, 24,* 3458–3464. doi:10.1200/JCO.2005.04.4685

Yavuzsen, T., Davis, M.P., Walsh, D., LeGrand, S., & Lagman, R. (2005). Systematic review of the treatment of cancer-associated anorexia and weight loss. *Journal of Clinical Oncology, 23,* 8500–8511. doi:10.1200/JCO.2005.01.8010

Zelefsky, M.J., Chan, H., Hunt, M., Yamada, Y., Shippy, A.M., & Amols, H. (2006). Long-term outcome of high dose intensity modulated radiation therapy for patients with clinically localized prostate cancer. *Journal of Urology, 176,* 1415–1419. doi:10.1016/j.juro.2006.06.002

F. Bladder
1. Incidence and risk factors: Bladder cancer is the fourth most common cancer in men and the eighth most common cancer in women (Sharma, Ksheersagar, & Sharma, 2009). It is most common in older, White men. Cigarette smoking increases the risk of developing bladder cancer as much as 50% in men and 30% in women (Sharma et al., 2009).
2. Staging
   a) Bladder cancer is classified as noninvasive, muscle-invasive, or metastatic disease.
   b) Noninvasive tumors, according to the American Joint Committee on Cancer (AJCC) TNM staging system, include stage I tumors that are Ta, Tis, or T1. Invasive tumors are classified as stage II–IV and include T2–T4 tumors (Edge et al., 2010).
   c) More than 80% of patients with bladder cancer present with noninvasive disease. Noninvasive tumors respond well to local therapy but tend to recur in 30%–70% of patients and can progress to invasive cancer (Hegarty & Kamat, 2008). Eighty-two percent of patients with no residual disease may have up to 10-year survival compared to 57% survival for those who have residual disease (Hegarty & Kamat, 2008).
   d) Twenty percent of the patients who present with muscle-invasive disease will die from their disease within two years of their diagnosis without treatment (Langsenlehner et al., 2010).
   e) Depending on the stage and grade of disease or recurrence, bladder cancer may be treated with surgery, intravesical immunotherapy or chemotherapy, IV chemotherapy, RT, or a combination of these. It is important for nurses to understand the various treatment options and the side effects that can occur from RT to the bladder.
3. Treatment
   a) Treatment for noninvasive tumors is transurethral resection of the bladder tumor (TURBT) for low-grade tumors. The purpose of TURBT is to remove all visible tumors, send specimens to pathology for diagnosis, and determine the grade and type of tumor (Overstreet, Zhao, Sims, & Cash, 2009).
   b) Intravesical therapy is used to prevent post-TURBT implantation of tumor cells, treat any residual disease, prevent recurrence, and postpone or decrease tumor progression (Urdaneta, Solsona, & Palou, 2008). Intravesical therapy may be recommended if recurrences persist, the disease progresses to a higher grade, or muscle-invasive disease is present (Sharma et al., 2009).
      (1) According to NCCN (2011) guidelines, the treatment of choice for intermediate or high-risk noninvasive bladder cancer can be TURBT and intravesical therapy using alkylating agents or antitumor antibiotics such as thiotepa, docetaxel, mitomycin C, valrubicin, doxorubicin, and epirubicin or immunotherapy with bacillus Calmette-Guérin (BCG) (Urdaneta et al., 2008). Conflicting evidence exists as to whether BCG or intravesical chemotherapy is better in controlling disease recurrences when compared to chemotherapy (Shelley, Wilt, Barber, & Mason, 2004). Optimal maintenance schedules for administering the therapies are part of the debate concerning progression or recurrence (Urdaneta et al., 2008).
      (2) Other agents, such as gemcitabine and BCG with interferon alpha, are currently under study (NCCN, 2011).
      (3) Tumors tend to recur at the original site and are multifocal (Milosevic et al., 2007). Failure to respond to TURBT

and intravesical therapy may indicate the need for cystectomy.

c) RT for the management of bladder cancer

(1) Single-modality RT with curative intent was used from the 1950s through the 1980s (Troiano et al., 2009).

  (a) Comparison trials on candidates for cystectomy versus RT as definitive treatment were difficult to compare because cystectomy patients had less-advanced tumors at diagnosis, were younger in age, and had fewer comorbidities. Five-year survival rates were not significantly different in the RT-alone group.

  (b) Retrospective studies from various institutions showed little uniformity in imaging, field size, dose and fractionation, and patient fluid intake restriction. Although a 50% response rate was found, only 30%–50% maintained a complete tumor regression without recurrence, and 50% of the patients developed distant metastasis (Choueiri & Raghavan, 2008; Milosevic et al., 2007).

  (c) Strong evidence has demonstrated that a substantial proportion of patients who have small tumors at presentation are cured with RT and are able to maintain normal bladder function (Milosevic et al., 2007).

  (d) Definitive EBRT produces complete regression of muscle-invasive bladder cancer in about 70% of patients (Milosevic et al., 2007).

(2) RT can be used as part of multimodality treatment for invasive bladder cancer.

  (a) Treatment can include TURBT, chemotherapy, and RT.

  (b) Chemotherapy can be used in the neoadjuvant or adjuvant setting with surgery and RT (Choueiri & Raghavan, 2008).

d) Surgery

(1) For muscle-invasive bladder cancers, radical cystectomy with urinary diversion and pelvic lymph node dissection provides a local control rate of 90%, but five-year overall survival is about 50% because of distant metastatic disease (Fernando & Sandler, 2007).

  (a) Although less-invasive surgical techniques such as robotic-assisted cystectomy have emerged over the past few years, bladder preservation options may be considered for patients who are not candidates for surgery or for those who choose not to have a cystectomy (Langsenlehner et al., 2010; Overstreet et al., 2009).

  (b) Response rates are better with combination chemotherapy and cystectomy (Troiano et al., 2009). In the past, single-agent chemotherapy treatment produced response rates of only 15%–25% (Raghavan, 2003).

e) Chemotherapy

(1) Increasing data support the use of neoadjuvant chemotherapy for T2 and T3 muscle-invasive disease. A survival benefit was found in two randomized trials after three cycles of methotrexate, vinblastine, doxorubicin, and cisplatin (MVAC) before cystectomy (Grossman et al., 2003; Sherif et al., 2004). Chemotherapy with cisplatin-based combinations has shown strong evidence of significant benefit in overall survival irrespective of type of surgery or radiation treatment (Choueiri & Raghavan, 2008).

(2) Currently, data support adjuvant chemotherapy to delay recurrences for patients with high risk of relapse. Three cycles of MVAC has shown to be effective, although gemcitabine and cisplatin have been found to be less toxic and better tolerated by patients (Lorusso et al., 2000; Roberts et al., 2006). Patients with extensive disease commonly receive adjuvant chemotherapy because RT alone rarely cures pelvic wall recurrences (Zietman & Shipley, 2007).

(3) Chemotherapy drugs such as 5-FU, cisplatin, gemcitabine, and paclitaxel act

as radiosensitizers, making normal and malignant cells more sensitive to radiation (Choueiri & Raghavan, 2008).

(a) Concurrent cisplatin and RT is the most common and most studied multimodality treatment used to treat muscle-invasive bladder cancer. Strong evidence shows that up to 70% of patients are tumor free within the bladder when examined at the initial post-treatment cystoscopy (Shipley et al., 2002). Persistent or recurrent muscle-invasive tumors require salvage cystectomy with urinary diversion when multimodality chemoradiation fails (Perdonà et al., 2008).

(b) Patients who present with metastatic or unresectable disease usually are treated with chemotherapy and/or RT. In patients with locally advanced or metastatic bladder cancer, the combination of gemcitabine and cisplatin had a similar survival advantage when compared with MVAC in a 2005 phase III multicenter study by von der Maase et al.

f) Targeted therapy remains investigational at this time with EGFRs, monoclonal antibodies, and vascular endothelial growth factor inhibitors being tested in phase II trials (Yafi, Cury, & Kassouf, 2009).

g) Preoperative RT

(1) A randomized trial evaluated 338 patients with T2–T4 disease who received planned preoperative RT followed in four weeks by cystectomy (von der Maase et al., 2005). The study found 65% downstaging, with no tumor found in the surgical specimen of 42% of patients, and a 44% overall survival at five years (Choueiri & Raghavan, 2008). Pelvic and distant metastasis recurrence rates were 16% and 43%, respectively (Pollack, Zagars, Dinney, Swanson, & von Eschenbach, 1994).

(2) Prior to 1983, all patients received 50 Gy preoperative RT followed in four weeks by cystectomy with pelvic disease control rate of 91% (Zietman & Shipley, 2007).

(3) More recently, the pelvic disease control rate was 73%, despite improved surgical techniques, staging, and use of systemic chemotherapy (Zietman & Shipley, 2007).

(4) Contradictory evidence has been reported that cystectomy alone had lower rates of pelvic recurrence (Skinner & Lieskovsky, 1984).

(5) Low-dose RT of 8.5–20 Gy is occasionally used in the United States prior to partial cystectomy to prevent autotransplantation of tumors (Zietman & Shipley, 2007).

h) Postoperative RT

(1) The main advantage of postoperative RT is the ability to perform pathologic staging after cystectomy.

(2) Postoperative RT is most commonly used with extravesical disease, positive resection margins, or involved pelvic lymph nodes with doses of 40–50 Gy given by external beam.

(3) Late GI complications can occur because of the large volume of small bowel in the pelvis following cystectomy (Troiano et al., 2009).

4. RT techniques for bladder cancer

a) Hyperfractionated RT has been used with 1 Gy three times daily to a total dose of 84 Gy with significant improved survival (Edsmyr, Andersson, Esposti, Littbrand, & Nilsson, 1985).

(1) Failure to achieve a complete response decreases with increasing T stage (Stuschke & Thames, 1997).

(2) Moderate evidence shows that hyperfractionated RT provides a survival benefit at 5 and 10 years and an increased local control rate compared with conventional fractionation (Milosevic et al., 2007).

(3) More evidence is needed for hyperfractionated RT to be routinely used in clinical practice.

b) Some evidence suggests that palliative hypofractionated RT, three fractions in one week, provides the same relief of symptoms as 10 fractions in two weeks. This therapy can be considered for palliation of bladder symptoms in incurable bladder cancer but should be used cautiously because of possible adverse effects (Milosevic et al., 2007).

c) IMRT uses beams with varying intensities across the fields to improve and individualize RT dose distributions to match the tumor shape.

(1) Normal tissue sparing is limited to the bowel and the rectum. Image guided strategies are used to reduce treatment margins. The bladder is treated when

empty. Previously, three-field box technique was the standard with greater toxicity to the bowel and the bladder (Søndergaard et al., 2009).

(2) Modern bladder-sparing approaches such as TURBT and combined chemotherapy and RT are able to show results equal to surgery in survival and disease control (Sandhu & Mundt, 2009). When used with partial bladder irradiation and image-guided localization, these techniques may preserve bladder function and quality of life (Sandhu & Mundt, 2009).

d) Treatment volumes for RT need to be tailored for differences in bladder and tumor position on a daily basis because variation can occur in bladder and rectal filling (Milosevic et al., 2007).

(1) Radiation treatment volumes for muscle-invasive bladder cancer should include the primary bladder tumor and pelvic lymph nodes.

(2) According to Milosevic et al. (2007), a radiation dose of 50–70 Gy should be given in 1.8–2.5 Gy fractions over four to seven weeks to the primary tumor and 40–50 Gy in 1.8–2 Gy fractions over four to five weeks to the lymph nodes.

(3) NCCN (2011) guidelines recommend a radiation dose of 45 Gy given in 1.8 Gy fractions over five weeks and 20 Gy given in 1.8 Gy fractions to the boost sites of disease in the bladder.

e) Interstitial RT delivers a high dose of radiation to a small area of the bladder using ^{192}Ir, sparing the surrounding normal tissues.

(1) The largest patient population was studied in France by Rozan et al. (1992). Partial cystectomy was performed in 58% of the patients; 17% had local recurrence, and long-term overall survival was 67%.

(2) Level 3 evidence shows that interstitial RT can be an effective alternative to EBRT in selected patients who have unifocal and small tumors. Interstitial RT involves the placement of radioactive seeds into or near tumors that lie within the bladder to focally treat the disease (Milosevic et al., 2007).

(3) Interstitial RT is not used widely in the United States because of the development of refined EBRT, the lengthy hospital stays required for radiation precautions related to brachytherapy, and increased morbidity from urinary leakage (Zietman & Shipley, 2007).

f) Strong evidence of multiple meta-analyses supports treatment of patients with noninvasive bladder cancer with TURBT followed by intravesical BCG or other intravesical chemotherapy (Milosevic et al., 2007; Urdaneta et al., 2008).

(1) Data support better local control of muscle-invasive disease using combination systemic chemotherapy and RT versus single-modality therapy (Choueiri & Raghavan, 2008). Quality-of-life issues come into play with cystectomy versus bladder preservation. Although survival is important, quality of life after cystectomy needs to be considered (Porter, Wei, & Penson, 2005).

(2) Moderate evidence shows that palliative RT for invasive bladder carcinoma can rapidly provide tumor-related symptom relief, particularly hematuria. Single-modality RT should be considered as a viable option for older patients who are not candidates for surgery (Sandhu & Mundt, 2009).

(3) Multimodality therapy of TURBT, chemotherapy, and RT shows encouraging results in achieving a complete response, bladder preservation, and overall survival. Total dose to the tumor and bladder should not be below 55–60 Gy (Fokdal, Høyer, & von der Maase, 2006). Moderate evidence shows that this combined therapy can be used as an alternative for patients who are not surgical candidates or who prefer not to have cystectomy.

(4) No randomized trials have compared radical cystectomy alone with RT alone (Shelley et al., 2004).

(a) Previous trials have suggested an overall benefit after cystectomy compared with definitive RT or RT alone (Bloom, Hendry, Wallace, & Skeet, 1982; Miller, 1977; Sell et al., 1991). However, the patient population was small, and most patients did not receive the designated treatment.

(b) Complications may occur after surgery (Perdonà et al., 2008). RT and surgery have improved since these trials (Fokdal et al., 2006).

(c) RT is generally well tolerated, with 82%–97% of patients completing their prescribed therapy. The benefit of bladder preservation needs to be weighed against the risk of recurrence or progression of disease (Perdonà et al., 2007).

(d) Level 3 evidence indicates that the ideal candidate for curative EBRT with or without concurrent chemotherapy is an individual with a small solitary tumor (smaller than 5 cm) with no associated carcinoma in situ, no evidence of lymph node or distant metastases, and a normally functioning bladder (Milosevic et al., 2007). The patient will require lifelong surveillance with immediate treatment of new disease (Milosevic et al., 2007).

(5) Randomized trials of planned RT before cystectomy precluded the use of chemoradiation (Choueiri & Raghavan, 2008). The intent of preoperative RT was to reduce the size of the tumor so the patient would have less-extensive surgery, to decrease local and distant recurrence, and to improve survival (Overstreet et al., 2009).

(a) Patients with locally extensive T3 or T4 disease are most likely to experience downsizing of their tumor with preoperative RT but are at risk for local recurrence or distant metastasis (Milosevic et al., 2007). Compared to cystectomy alone, preoperative RT appeared to improve pelvic disease control in this group of patients (91% versus 72%) (Cole et al., 1995).

(b) Overall survival benefit with combined preoperative RT plus radical surgery compared with radical RT plus salvage cystectomy from randomized phase III trials conducted from 1964 to 1983 remains controversial (Huncharek, Muscat, & Geschwind, 1998; Shelley et al., 2004). Major advances in RT and surgery have taken place since these trials (Shelley et al., 2004).

(c) Planned preoperative RT is not routinely used in modern practice because of the availability of effective systemic treatment (Milosevic et al., 2007).

(6) Patients need to be informed about the advantages and disadvantages of treatment options in order to make an informed decision. With newer and less-invasive surgical techniques, continuing studies on response rates and survival rates are ongoing. Multimodality chemoradiation along with the patient's overall health needs to be considered before treatment decisions are made. Conflicting evidence, as stated previously, does not provide conclusive information on the use of RT, optimal doses, or combination therapy for bladder cancer (Choueiri & Raghavan, 2008). According to Milosevic et al. (2007), large randomized trials still are needed to address biologic factors that influence radiation response and improve local tumor control and patient survival.

5. Irritative bladder symptoms (IBS)

a) Pathophysiology

(1) IBS is a group of symptoms that includes dysuria, frequency, hesitancy, nocturia, and urgency. These symptoms may occur as acute or early symptoms and can be seen during treatment and up to 12 months after treatment is completed (Marks, Carroll, Dugan, & Anscher, 1995).

(2) Because of the nature of bladder cancer, it may be difficult to differentiate whether the symptoms are from the tumor or from the RT (Sengeløv & von der Maase, 1999).

(3) Early or acute urinary symptoms are a result of injury and inflammation of the epithelial layer of the bladder mucosa caused by the ionizing radiation (Muruve, 2009).

(4) Submucosal inflammation eventually may lead to fibrosis, perineural inflammation, and surface ulceration (Muruve, 2009).

(5) Side effects and long-term complications from RT may vary because of the amount of irradiated bladder volume, field setup, beam quality, fraction size, total dose, previous surgeries, and overall condition of the patient (Muruve, 2009).

(6) Long-term effects (later than 12 months) are mainly fibrovascular and include luminal occlusion, vascular telangiectasia, and necrosis of the vessel

walls. These changes cause ischemia and fibrosis, leading to loss of muscle tone with dysfunctional voiding (Muruve, 2009).

    (7) Side effects usually are decreased when normal tissue is spared. However, when treating bladder cancer, because of the proximity of the bladder neck and exposure to the urethra to radiation, side effects are not decreased when comparing conformal beam radiation with four-box small field therapy (Muruve, 2009).

    (8) With IMRT, higher doses can be delivered to the target area. Fewer RTOG grade 2 bladder complications such as moderate urinary frequency, generalized telangiectasia, intermittent macroscopic hematuria, and intermittent urinary incontinence occur when compared with conformal radiation (Muruve, 2009).

b) Incidence

    (1) Occurrence of urinary symptoms that appear during RT can vary from 2% to 47% with reported mean of 17.8% (Muruve, 2009).

    (2) Symptoms of IBS occur in 2%–12% of patients whose whole bladder radiation doses reach 50–60 Gy. Partial treatment of the bladder using 50–75 Gy has a 5%–20% complication rate for IBS (Muruve, 2009).

    (3) Symptoms usually subside within several weeks but can still be present one year after completion of radiation (Muruve, 2009).

c) Assessment: Includes urologic voiding pattern related to frequency of urination, urgency, nocturia, dysuria, and time of day that the symptoms are better or worse. If symptoms are moderate to severe, have the patient keep a diary to record voiding patterns and symptoms (Berry, 2004).

d) Collaborative management of IBS

    (1) Acute effects

        (a) Encourage the patient to increase daily fluid intake to two to three liters (unless contraindicated for cardiac or other medical reasons). Increasing fluid intake keeps the urine more diluted and less irritating to the bladder mucosa and helps to wash out clots that can cause an obstruction of urine flow (Kelly & Miaskowski, 1996; Kuck & Ricciardi, 2005).

        (b) Encourage the patient to avoid caffeine and spicy drinks and food because they can irritate the bladder mucosa (Kuck & Ricciardi, 2005).

        (c) Obtain urinalysis, culture, and sensitivity.

        (d) Administer pharmacologic agents as prescribed to relieve symptoms (Berry, 2004).

           i. Phenazopyridine hydrochloride has analgesic and anesthetic effects on the urinary tract and can be useful for the irritative effects of RT. Warn the patient that this drug will color the urine orange. Dose is 200 mg three times a day after meals for two days.

           ii. Urimax® (Xanodyne Pharmaceuticals) (contains hyoscyamine sulfate and methylene blue) is a urinary antiseptic indicated for treatment of irritative voiding and pain of the urinary tract. This drug may discolor urine or stools a blue-green color. Dosage is usually one tablet of 200 mcg or 400 mcg four times a day with a full 8 oz. of water with each dose.

           iii. Flavoxate hydrochloride is an antispasmodic used for managing urgency, frequency, nocturia, suprapubic pain, and incontinence associated with cystitis. Dose is usually 100–200 mg three to four times a day.

    (2) Long-term effects

        (a) Long-term effects that can occur years after initial therapy include contracted bladder, ulcer formation, fistulas, and bladder dysfunction (mainly IBS) (Muruve, 2009).

        (b) For persistent symptoms of slight to moderate IBS, continue to have patient obtain prescriptions for medications.

        (c) For symptoms that cause severe IBS, refer the patient to a urologist for possible surgical intervention.

        (d) For suspected ulcer or fistula, refer the patient to a urologist for possible surgical intervention.

6. Urinary tract infection (UTI)

a) Pathophysiology

  (1) UTI or whole bladder infection can occur as an early or late side effect of radiation to the bladder. It is not a common acute side effect of RT but can occur as a secondary symptom because of the nature of bladder cancer (Muruve, 2009).

  (2) Inflammatory changes in the bladder mucosa can occur with exposure of subepithelial tissues to the caustic effects of urine.

b) Incidence: Occurrence of UTI is 9%–22%, including both early and late symptoms (Henningsohn, Wijkström, Dickman, Bergmark, & Steineck, 2002).

c) Assessment (Kelly & Miaskowski, 1996)

  (1) Obtain urinalysis, with microscopic analysis and culture and sensitivity, if indicated for symptoms. Check urine for color, clarity, and odor.

  (2) Check the patient's temperature.

  (3) Check the patient for diaphoresis or chills.

  (4) Assess for lower abdominal or flank pain.

  (5) Obtain a complete blood count to assess for an elevated white blood count, which may indicate an infection.

d) Collaborative management of UTI

  (1) Administer an antibiotic, such as sulfamethoxazole-trimethoprim, ciprofloxacin, nitrofurantoin, or levofloxacin, as guided by the urine culture and sensitivity (Berry, 2004).

  (2) Monitor the patient for signs and symptoms of allergic reaction to the antibiotic.

  (3) The patient may need to be admitted to the hospital for IV antibiotic therapy if oral antibiotics do not relieve infection in 7–14 days.

7. Hemorrhagic cystitis with irritative or hemorrhagic symptoms

a) Pathophysiology

  (1) Vascular changes can occur along with endothelial edema and thickening, with a progressive depletion of a blood supply to the irradiated tissue, or frank hematuria (Muruve, 2009).

  (2) Concurrent chemotherapy may increase the damaging effects of irradiation, as seen with cyclophosphamide and ifosfamide, which can cause hemorrhagic cystitis with gross hematuria, irritative voiding symptoms, and bladder contracture (Muruve, 2009).

b) Incidence: Slight to moderate IBS along with hematuria was reported by 19%–49% of patients and more severe IBS plus hematuria by 33%–48% of patients (Muruve, 2009).

  (1) Symptoms of acute cystitis usually subside two to eight weeks after treatment (Volpe, 2000).

  (2) The trigone of the bladder is more sensitive to radiation side effects than the dome of the bladder (Muruve, 2009).

  (3) With the use of IMRT and conformal radiation, higher doses of radiation can be delivered to the tumor, but tissue injury to nontarget organs can still occur (Smit & Heyns, 2010).

c) Assessment (Kelly & Miaskowski, 1996)

  (1) Monitor for presence of blood in the urine. Obtain a urinalysis with microscopic analysis; observe color, clarity, and odor.

  (2) Monitor for other signs of bleeding (e.g., patient complaining of dizziness, light-headedness, headache, pallor, decrease in blood pressure, weak pulse, or fatigue).

  (3) Monitor for signs of fluid volume loss (e.g., poor skin turgor).

  (4) Monitor for anemia. Obtain a complete blood count; check if hemoglobin and hematocrit are within normal limits.

  (5) Monitor the patient's intake and output (Kuck & Ricciardi, 2005; Overstreet et al., 2009).

  (6) Obtain physician order for prothrombin time and international normalized ratio to assess bleeding tendencies.

  (7) Check frequency of urination; clots may obstruct urinary flow. The patient should void every two hours.

  (8) Obtain order for type and crossmatch for a blood transfusion as needed.

d) Collaborative management

  (1) Acute effects

(a) If the patient is unable to void, notify the physician because an order to catheterize may be needed. The patient may need a physician to perform either intermittent or continuous bladder irrigations with saline (Smit & Heyns, 2010).

(b) Obtain order for blood transfusion (packed red blood cells) if hemoglobin and hematocrit are low.

(c) Conjugated estrogens have been shown to normalize the prolonged bleeding time and improve hemostasis in patients with hemorrhagic cystitis (Liu et al., 1990; Smit & Heyns, 2010).

(d) Pentoxifylline, which is useful in providing relief from radiation fibrosis, enhances blood flow and oxygenation of the tissue. Usual dose is 400 mg orally three times a day for six weeks (Muruve, 2009).

(e) Pentosan polysulfate sodium is useful in treating the pain or discomfort of interstitial cystitis. Usual dose is 100 mg orally three times a day. Alert the patient that this drug is a weak anticoagulant; it is contraindicated in patients on anticoagulant therapy (Smit & Heyns, 2010).

(f) Flavoxate hydrochloride is an antispasmodic used for managing urgency, frequency, nocturia, suprapubic pain, and incontinence associated with cystitis.

(g) If the patient is concurrently receiving chemotherapeutic agents that can cause hemorrhagic cystitis, administer sodium-2-mercaptoethane sulfonate for the prevention of hemorrhagic cystitis as prescribed. The compound is given to detoxify acrolein, the by-product of cyclophosphamide, which causes the hemorrhagic cystitis (Liu et al., 1990; Marks et al., 1995).

(2) Long-term effects

(a) Hyperbaric oxygen—The breathing of 100% oxygen is thought to increase vascular density. Stimulation of angiogenesis leads to the repair of tissue damaged from radiation (Corman, McClure, Pritchett, Kozlowski, & Hampson, 2003).

Various regimens are used, but in general 100% oxygen is given at pressures of 1.5–2.5 atm (atmospheres) for 45–120 minutes once daily for about 20–30 times (Smit & Heyns, 2010). Radiation cystitis response rate is 60%–92% with use of hyperbaric oxygen (Smit & Heyns, 2010).

(b) Alum can be instilled intravesically for the treatment of hemorrhagic cystitis. Alum controls hemorrhage by causing protein precipitation in the interstitial spaces and cell membranes, which leads to contraction of bleeding vessels (Goswami, Mahajan, Nath, & Sharma, 1993). Adequate renal function is necessary. Complete response is from 50% to 100% (Smit & Heyns, 2010).

(c) Using a transurethral catheter, intermittent or continuous bladder irrigation can be performed until the bleeding stops (Smit & Heyns, 2010).

8. Obstructive symptoms (Muruve, 2009)

a) Pathophysiology: A decrease in force or caliber of urine flow, including urinary retention, decrease in caliber of urinary stream, leakage, or dribbling

(1) Normal smooth muscle may be replaced by fibroblasts and collagen deposition, causing severe scarring known as fibrosis.

(2) Fibrosis leads to tissue hypoxia (ischemia) and necrosis. Mucosal ischemia and epithelial damage increase as these tissues develop more submucosal fibrosis with exposure to the caustic effects of urine. Clinical findings show ulcer formation, radiation neuritis, and postradiation fibrosis. The patient usually experiences suprapubic and pubic pain and discomfort (Muruve, 2009).

b) Incidence: Severe obstructive complications have been reported at 7%–36%, with patients reporting urinary incontinence, urine leakage requiring incontinence pads, and urethral stricture with use of a urinary catheter (Fokdal et al., 2006).

c) Assessment

(1) Pain, discomfort

(2) Urinary frequency and urgency due to incomplete voiding

(3) Decrease in bladder capacity

(4) Change in caliber or flow of urine, such as weak urine stream

(5) Loss of control of urine

(6) Inability to void

(7) Obtain blood for electrolytes, blood urea nitrogen, and creatinine to assess renal function.

d) Collaborative management

(1) Acute effects

  (a) Antispasmodics are indicated for neurogenic bladder problems such as retention, urinary overflow, incontinence, nocturia, urinary frequency, or urgency.

    i. Oxybutynin chloride

    ii. Tolterodine tartrate

    iii. Belladonna and opium suppositories (Overstreet et al., 2009)

  (b) Alpha-1 blocker medications are useful for obstructive urinary symptoms because they help to relax the smooth muscles in the body, which may help improve urinary flow. Additional antihypertensive medications should be cautiously used to minimize any hypotensive effect of the combination of medications (Overstreet et al., 2009).

    i. Tamsulosin hydrochloride

    ii. Terazosin hydrochloride

    iii. Doxazosin mesylate

    iv. Alfuzosin hydrochloride

  (c) Urinary antiseptics include combination products such as methylene blue, which can cause discoloration of urine, possible rash, flushing of skin, or dizziness (Overstreet et al., 2009).

(2) Long-term effects

  (a) For obstructive urinary symptoms unrelieved with medications, patients may need to have an indwelling catheter placed or be taught to perform intermittent self-catheterization.

  (b) Patients with obstructive urinary symptoms unrelieved with oral pharmacologic management may require cystectomy.

9. Assessment: Other diagnostic tests that may be useful in determining the extent of radiation side effects (Muruve, 2009)

a) Imaging studies

(1) IV pyelogram is useful in evaluating anatomic abnormalities, such as strictures, fistula formation, and renal calcifications, in the genitourinary tract.

(2) A computed axial tomography scan can be useful in diagnosing bladder fistulas and bladder wall thickening and detecting extraluminal masses. The bladder may be viewed intravesically with air or contrast dye.

(3) Renal ultrasonography, an alternative to IV pyelogram, can be used to assess for hydronephrosis, a result of scarring or calculus disease.

(4) MRI urogram may be useful to assess abnormalities of the urinary tract, such as obstruction and hematuria (Leyendecker, Barnes, & Zagoria, 2008).

b) Urodynamics may be helpful in assessing bladder volume, flow rate, decreased bladder compliance, and postvoid residual urine caused by injury to the innervation of the bladder.

c) Cystoscopy may be useful in confirming acute radiation changes seen in the bladder mucosa, such as telangiectasia, diffuse erythema, increase in submucosal vascularity, and mucosal edema (Muruve, 2009).

10. Documentation

a) Urinary frequency/urgency (NCI CTEP, 2010)

(1) 1—Present

(2) 2—Limiting instrumental ADL; medical intervention indicated

b) Dysuria (Catlin-Huth, Haas, & Pollock, 2002)

(1) 0—None

(2) 1—Mild symptoms requiring no intervention

(3) 2—Symptoms relieved with therapy

(4) 3—Symptoms not relieved despite therapy

c) Urinary retention (NCI CTEP, 2010)

(1) 1—Urinary, suprapubic or intermittent catheter placement not indicated; able to void with some residual

(2) 2—Placement of urinary, suprapubic or intermittent catheter placement indicated; medication indicated

(3) 3—Elective operative or radiologic intervention indicated; substantial loss of affected kidney function or mass

(4) 4—Life-threatening consequences; organ failure; urgent operative intervention indicated

(5) 5—Death

d) Urinary incontinence (NCI CTEP, 2010)

(1) 1—Occasional (e.g., with coughing, sneezing, etc.); pads not indicated

_____

(2) 2—Spontaneous; pads indicated; limiting instrumental ADL

(3) 3—Intervention indicated (e.g., clamp, collagen injections); operative intervention indicated; limiting self-care ADL

e) Skin sensation (Catlin-Huth et al., 2002)
(1) 0—No problem
(2) 1—Pruritus
(3) 2—Burning
(4) 3—Painful

f) Mucous membrane alteration (Catlin-Huth et al., 2002)
(1) Drainage
  (a) 0—Absent
  (b) 1—Present
(2) Drainage odor
  (a) 0—Absent
  (b) 1—Present

11. Patient and family education
a) Encourage the patient to quit smoking and to avoid tobacco products because smoking has been found to be a prognostic risk factor for bladder cancer (Sharma et al., 2009).

b) Instruct the patient about the possibility of bladder irritation from pelvic irradiation.
(1) Instruct the patient to drink two to three liters of fluid per day (if not contraindicated) to help decrease irritation to the bladder mucosa (Berry, 2004).
(2) Instruct the patient to void every two to four hours, empty bladder before sleep, and drink fluids during the night if awakened to help decrease irritation of the bladder mucosa caused by urine being in the bladder (Kelly & Miaskowski, 1996).
(3) Instruct the patient to decrease intake of caffeinated drinks such as coffee, tea, and soda, alcohol, and other bladder irritants (Kuck & Ricciardi, 2005).

c) Instruct the patient about the signs and symptoms of bladder infection, such as burning or stinging on urination, increased frequency of urination, pain in the abdomen over the bladder, low back pain, low-grade fever, foul-smelling urine, blood in urine, increased urge to urinate, and painful sexual intercourse, and to call the nurse or healthcare provider if they occur.
(1) Instruct the patient to take temperature daily and to call the physician if temperature is 100°F (37.8°C) or higher.
(2) Instruct the patient to call the physician if symptoms are unrelieved or persist even with pain medications or oral antibiotics.

d) For urinary incontinence
(1) Instruct the patient to practice pelvic floor exercises (Kegel exercises). Instruct the patient to tighten the muscles that are used to stop and release urine flow to the count of three and then release, and repeat 10 times once to twice a day. These exercises can help to strengthen muscles to regain control of urination (ACS, 2011).
(2) Instruct the patient on how to urinate on schedule until frequency and urgency decrease to manageable intervals.
(3) Instruct the patient to take medications as prescribed to relax bladder muscles and to call for a refill when 5–10 tablets are left (Berry, 2004).
(4) Instruct the patient on options to help manage these symptoms, such as the use of incontinence pads, a penile clamp, or a condom (Texas) catheter with leg bag.
(5) Instruct the patient on how to self-catheterize if instructed to do so by the physician.
(6) Instruct the patient in perineal skin care due to incontinence (Berry, 2004).
  (a) Keep skin in perineum and genital area clean with soap and water.
  (b) Use a moisture barrier on the skin, if needed, to protect the skin from excoriation.
  (c) Wear loose clothing to help prevent moisture buildup on the skin.
  (d) Wear incontinence pads to absorb moisture; change frequently to prevent skin excoriation.
  (e) Instruct the patient to call the physician if skin becomes reddened or irritated.
(7) Monitor the patient's compliance to instructions on incontinence (Kuck & Ricciardi, 2005).

(8) Monitor effectiveness of instructions given to the patient and family (Kuck & Ricciardi, 2005).

12. Related Web sites

a) ACS information on bladder cancer and side effects from RT: www.cancer.org/Cancer/BladderCancer/DetailedGuide/bladder-cancer-treating-radiation

b) ASCO's patient site: www.cancer.net/patient/Cancer+Types/Bladder+Cancer

c) Bladder Cancer Web Café—Information, resources, and support: http://blcwebcafe.org

d) Cleveland Clinic—Treatment options for bladder cancer: www.clevelandclinic.org/lp/bladder-cancer/index.html

e) eMedicineHealth: www.emedicinehealth.com/bladder_cancer/article_em.htm

f) Macmillan Cancer—Support for people with cancer: www.macmillan.org.uk/Cancerinformation/Cancertypes/Bladder/Treatingbladdercancer/Radiotherapy.aspx

g) MedicineNet: www.medicinenet.com/bladder_cancer/article.htm

h) MedlinePlus information on urinary incontinence: www.nlm.nih.gov/medlineplus/urinaryincontinence.html

i) NCI bladder cancer information: www.cancer.gov/cancertopics/types/bladder

j) Urology Channel—Information on types, incidence, and treatment for bladder cancer: www.urologychannel.com/bladdercancer/overview-of-bladder-cancer.shtml

k) WebMD information on bladder cancer health—RT for the bladder: www.webmd.com/cancer/bladder-cancer/radiation-therapy-for-bladder-cancer

References

American Cancer Society. (2011). Side effects of radiation therapy: Sexual side effects of radiation. Retrieved from http://www.cancer.org/Treatment/TreatmentsandSideEffects/PhysicalSideEffects/index

Berry, D. (2004). Bladder disturbances. In C.H. Yarbro, M.H. Frogge, & M. Goodman (Eds.), *Cancer symptom management* (3rd ed., pp. 505–511). Sudbury, MA: Jones and Bartlett.

Bloom, H.J., Hendry, W.F., Wallace, D.M., & Skeet, R.G. (1982). Treatment of T3 bladder cancer: Controlled trial of pre-operative radiotherapy and radical cystectomy versus radical radiotherapy. *British Journal of Urology, 54,* 136–151.

Catlin-Huth, C., Haas, M., & Pollock, V. (Eds.). (2002). *Radiation therapy patient care record: A tool for documenting nursing care.* Pittsburgh, PA: Oncology Nursing Society.

Choueiri, T.K., & Raghavan, D. (2008). Chemotherapy for muscle-invasive bladder cancer treated with definitive radiotherapy: Persisting uncertainties. *Nature Clinical Practice Oncology, 5,* 444–454. doi:10.1038/ncponc1159

Cole, C.J., Pollack, A., Zagars, G.K., Dinney, C.P., Swanson, D.A., & von Eschenbach, A.C. (1995). Local control of muscle invasive bladder cancer: Preoperative radiotherapy and cystectomy versus cystectomy alone. *International Journal of Radiation Oncology, Biology, Physics, 32,* 331–340. doi:10.1016/0360-3016(95)00086-E

Corman, J.M., McClure, D., Pritchett, R., Kozlowski, P., & Hampson, N.B. (2003). Treatment of radiation induced hemorrhagic cystitis with hyperbaric oxygen. *Journal of Urology, 169,* 2200–2202. doi:10.1097/01.ju.0000063640.41307.c9

Edge, S.B., Byrd, D.R., Compton, C.C., Fritz, A.G., Greene, F.L., & Trotti, A., III. (Eds.). (2010). *AJCC cancer staging manual* (7th ed.). New York, NY: Springer.

Edsmyr, F., Andersson, L., Esposti, P.L., Littbrand, B., & Nilsson, B. (1985). Irradiation therapy with multiple small fractions per day in urinary bladder cancer. *Radiotherapy and Oncology, 4,* 197–203. doi:10.1016/S0167-8140(85)80084-0

Fokdal, L., Høyer, M., & von der Maase, H. (2006). Radical radiotherapy for urinary bladder cancer: Treatment outcomes. *Expert Review of Anticancer Therapy, 6,* 269–279. doi:10.1586/14737140.6.2.269

Fernando, S.A., & Sandler, H.M. (2007). Multimodality therapy for muscle invasive bladder tumors. *Seminars in Oncology, 34,* 129–134. doi:10.1053/j.seminoncol.2006.12.009

Goswami, A.K., Mahajan, R.K., Nath, R., & Sharma, S.K. (1993). How safe is 1% alum irrigation in controlling intractable vesical hemorrhage. *Journal of Urology, 149,* 264–267.

Grossman, H.B., Natale, R.B., Tangen, C.M., Speights, V.O., Vogelzang, N.J., Trump, D.L., ... Crawford, E.D. (2003). Neoadjuvant chemotherapy plus cystectomy alone for locally advanced bladder cancer. *New England Journal of Medicine, 349,* 859–866. doi:10.1056/NEJMoa022148

Hegarty, P.K., & Kamat, A.M. (2008). Management of bladder cancer. *Minerva Urologica Nefrologica, 60,* 255–264.

Henningsohn, L., Wijkström, H., Dickman, P.W., Bergmark, K., & Steineck, G. (2002). Distressful symptoms after radical radiotherapy for urinary bladder cancer. *Radiotherapy and Oncology, 62,* 215–225. doi:10.1016/S0167-8140(01)00455-8

Huncharek, M., Muscat, J., & Geschwind, J.F. (1998). Planned preoperative radiation therapy in muscle invasive bladder cancer: Results of a meta-analysis. *Anticancer Research, 18*(3B), 1931–1934.

Kelly, L.P., & Miaskowski, C. (1996). An overview of bladder cancer: Treatment and nursing implications. *Oncology Nursing Forum, 23,* 459–469.

Kuck, A.W., & Ricciardi, E. (2005). Alterations in elimination. In J.K. Itano & K.N. Taoka (Eds.), *Core curriculum for oncology nursing* (4th ed., pp. 318–344). St. Louis, MO: Elsevier Saunders.

Langsenlehner, T., Döller, C., Quehenberger, F., Stranzl-Lawatsch, H., Langsenlehner, U., Pummer, K., & Kapp, K.S. (2010). Treatment results of radiation therapy for muscle invasive cancer. *Strahlentherapie und Onkologie, 186,* 203–209. doi:10.1007/s00066-010-2053-1

Leyendecker, J.R., Barnes, C.E., & Zagoria, R.J. (2008). MR urography: Techniques and clinical applications. *Radiographics, 28,* 23–46. doi:10.1148/rg.281075077

Liu, Y.K., Harty, J.I., Steinbock, G.S., Holt, H.A., Jr., Goldstein, D.H., & Amin, M. (1990). Treatment of radiation or cyclophosphamide induced hemorrhagic cystitis using conjugated estrogen. *Journal of Urology, 144,* 41–43.

Lorusso, V., Manzione, L., De Vita, F., Antimi, M., Selvaggi, F.P., & De Lena, M. (2000). Gemcitabine plus cisplatin for advanced transitional cell carcinoma of the urinary tract: A phase II multicenter trial. *Journal of Urology, 164,* 53–56. doi:10.1016/S0022-5347(05)67447-2

Marks, L.B., Carroll, P.R., Dugan, T.C., & Anscher, M.S. (1995). The response of the urinary bladder, urethra, and ureter to radiation and chemotherapy. *International Journal of Radiation Oncology, Biology, Physics, 31*, 1257–1280. doi:10.1016/0360-3016(94)00431-J

Miller, L.S. (1977). Bladder cancer: Superiority of preoperative irradiation and cystectomy in clinical stages B2 and C. *Cancer, 39*(Suppl. 2), 973–980. doi:10.1002/1097-0142(197702)39:2+<973::AID-CNCR2820390737>3.0.CO;2-O

Milosevic, M., Gospodarowicz, M., Zietman, A., Abbas, F., Haustermans, K., Moonen, L., ... Shipley, W. (2007). Radiotherapy for bladder cancer. *Urology, 69*(Suppl. 1), 80–92. doi:10.1016/j.urology.2006.05.060

Muruve, N.A. (2009). Radiation cystitis. Retrieved from http://emedicine.medscape.com/article/442319-overview

National Cancer Institute Cancer Therapy Evaluation Program. (2010). *Common terminology criteria for adverse events* [v.4.03]. Retrieved from http://evs.nci.nih.gov/ftp1/CTCAE/CTCAE_4.03_2010-06-14_QuickReference_5x7.pdf

National Comprehensive Cancer Network. (2011). *NCCN Clinical Practice Guidelines in Oncology: Bladder cancer* [v.2.2011]. Retrieved from http://www.nccn.org/professionals/physician_gls/pdf/bladder.pdf

Overstreet, D.L., Zhao, H., Sims, T.W., & Cash, J. (2009). Treatment of bladder cancer. In J. Held-Warmkessel (Ed.), *Site-specific cancer series: Genitourinary cancers* (pp. 53–72). Pittsburgh, PA: Oncology Nursing Society.

Perdonà, S., Autorino, R., Damiano, R., De Sio, M., Morrica, B., Gallo, L., ... Di Lorenzo, G. (2008). Bladder-sparing, combined-modality approach for muscle-invasive bladder cancer: A multi-institutional, long-term experience. *Cancer, 112*, 75–83. doi:10.1002/cncr.23137

Pollack, A., Zagars, G.K., Dinney, C.P., Swanson, D.A., & von Eschenbach, A.C. (1994). Preoperative radiotherapy for muscle-invasive bladder carcinoma: Long term follow-up and prognostic factors for 338 patients. *Cancer, 74*, 2819–2827. doi:10.1002/1097-0142(19941115)74:10<2819::AID-CNCR2820741013>3.0.CO;2-L

Porter, M.P., Wei, J.T., & Penson, D.F. (2005). Quality of life issues in bladder cancer patients following cystectomy and urinary diversion. *Urologic Clinics of North America, 32*, 207–216. doi:10.1016/j.ucl.2005.01.002

Raghavan, D. (2003). Progress in the chemotherapy of metastatic cancer of the urinary tract. *Cancer, 97*(Suppl. 8), 2050–2055. doi:10.1002/cncr.11280

Roberts, J.T., von der Maase, H., Sengeløv, L., Conte, P.F., Dogliotti, L., Oliver, T., ... Arning, M. (2006). Long-term survival results of a randomized trial comparing gemcitabine/cisplatin and methotrexate/vinblastine/doxorubicin/cisplatin in patients with locally advanced metastatic bladder cancer. *Annals of Oncology, 17*(Suppl. 5), v118–v122. doi:10.1093/annonc/mdj965

Rozan, R., Albuisson, E., Donnarieix, D., Giraud, B., Mazeron, J.J., Gerard, J.P., ... Douchez, J. (1992). Interstitial iridium-192 for bladder cancer (a multicentric survey: 205 patients). *International Journal of Radiation Oncology, Biology, Physics, 24*, 469–477. doi:10.1016/0360-3016(92)91061-Q

Sandhu, A., & Mundt, A.J. (2009). Radiation therapy for urologic malignancies in the elderly. *Urologic Oncology, 27*, 643–652. doi:10.1016/j.urolonc.2009.07.019

Sell, A., Jakobsen, A., Nerstrøm, B., Sørensen, B.L., Steven, K., & Barlebo, H. (1991). Treatment of advanced bladder cancer category T2 T3 and T4a: A randomized multicenter study of preoperative irradiation and cystectomy versus radical irradiation and early salvage cystectomy for residual tumor. DAVECA protocol 8201. Danish Vesical Cancer Group. *Scandinavian Journal of Urology and Nephrology: Supplementum, 138*, 193–201.

Sengeløv, L., & von der Maase, H. (1999). Radiotherapy in bladder cancer. *Radiotherapy and Oncology, 52*, 1–14. doi:10.1016/S0167-8140(99)00090-0

Sharma, S., Ksheersagar, P., & Sharma, P. (2009). Diagnosis and treatment of bladder cancer. *American Family Physician, 80*, 717–723.

Shelley, M.D., Wilt, T.J., Barber, J., & Mason, M.D. (2004). A meta-analysis of randomised trials suggests a survival benefit for combined radiotherapy and radical cystectomy compared with radical radiotherapy for invasive bladder cancer: Are these data relevant to practice? *Clinical Oncology, 16*, 166–171.

Sherif, A., Holmberg, L., Rintala, E., Mestad, O., Nilsson, J., Nilsson, S., & Malmström, P.U. (2004). Neoadjuvant cisplatinum based combination chemotherapy in patients with invasive bladder cancer: A combined analysis of two Nordic studies. *European Urology, 45*, 297–303. doi:10.1016/j.eururo.2003.09.019

Shipley, W.U., Kaufman, D.S., Zehr, E., Heney, N.M., Lane, S.C., Thakral, H.K., ... Zietman, A.L. (2002). Selective bladder preservation by combined modality protocol treatment: long term outcomes of 190 patients with invasive bladder cancer. *Urology, 60*, 62–67. doi:10.1016/S0090-4295(02)01650-3

Skinner, D.G., & Lieskovsky, G. (1984). Contemporary cystectomy with pelvic node dissection compared to preoperative radiation therapy plus cystectomy in management of invasive bladder cancer. *Journal of Urology, 131*, 1069–1072.

Smit, S.G., & Heyns, C.F. (2010). Management of radiation cystitis. *Nature Reviews Urology, 7*, 206–214. doi:10.1038/nrurol.2010.23

Søndergaard, J., Høyer, M., Petersen, J.B., Wright, P., Grau, C., & Muren, L.P. (2009). The normal tissue sparing obtained with simultaneous treatment of the pelvic lymph nodes and bladder using intensity-modulated radiotherapy. *Acta Oncologica, 48*, 238–244. doi:10.1080/02841860802251575

Stuschke, M., & Thames, H.D. (1997). Hyperfractionated radiotherapy of human tumors: Overview of the randomized clinical trials. *International Journal of Radiation Oncology, Biology, Physics, 37*, 259–267. doi:10.1016/S0360-3016(96)00511-1

Troiano, M., Corsa, P., Raguso, A., Cossa, S., Piombino, M., Guglielmi, G., & Parisi, S. (2009). Radiation therapy in urinary cancer: state of the art and perspective. *Radiologica Medica, 114*, 70–82. doi:10.1007/s11547-008-0347-5

Urdaneta, G., Solsona, E., & Palou, J. (2008). Intravesical chemotherapy and BCG for the treatment of bladder cancer: evidence and opinion. *European Urology Supplements, 7*, 542–547. doi:10.1016/j.eursup.2008.04.006

Volpe, H.M. (2000). Radiation therapy. In J. Held-Warmkessel (Ed.), *Contemporary issues in prostate cancer: A nursing perspective* (pp. 150–157). Sudbury, MA: Jones and Bartlett.

von der Maase, H., Sengelov, L., Roberts, J.T., Ricci, S., Dogliotti, L., Oliver, T., ... Arning, M. (2005). Long-term survival results of randomized trial comparing gemcitabine plus cisplatin, with methotrexate, vinblastine, doxorubicin, plus cisplatin in patients with bladder cancer. *Journal of Clinical Oncology, 23*, 4602–4608. doi:10.1200/JCO.2005.07.757

Yafi, F.A., Cury, F.L., & Kassouf, W. (2009). Organ-sparing strategies in the management of invasive bladder cancer. *Expert Review of Anticancer Therapy, 9*, 1765–1775. doi:10.1586/era.09.151

Zietman, A.L., & Shipley, W.U. (2007). Bladder cancer. In L.L. Gunderson & J.E. Tepper (Eds.), *Clinical radiation oncology* (2nd ed., pp. 1237–1260). Philadelphia, PA: Elsevier Churchill Livingstone.

G. Male pelvis/prostate
1. Urinary dysfunction side effects include frequency, urgency, hesitancy, retention, dysuria, nocturia, and cystitis. Use of conformal techniques such as IMRT or 3DCRT can reduce effects.
   a) Pathophysiology
      (1) Acute—Urinary frequency/urgency results from changes in the urinary bladder and prostate gland. Acute or early reactions are characterized primarily by changes occurring rapidly within hours, such as increased endothelial cell swelling, vascular permeability, and edema, as well as lymphocyte adhesion and infiltration. Ionizing radiation causes irritation and inflammation of the bladder, resulting in urinary symptoms of frequency/urgency dysuria and cystitis. Radiation-induced cell kill has been proposed to have a role as a triggering event; it is now clear that an orchestrated, active biologic response is brought about by the early release of cytokines (Bentzen, 2006). This response is mediated by various cell types, including inflammatory, stromal, endothelial, and parenchymal cells actively responding through the release or activation of downstream cytokines, growth factors, or chemokines (Bentzen, 2006).
         (a) Normal function depends upon the successful interaction of the bladder wall mucosa, muscle layers, and supporting neurovascular structures. Smooth muscle edema occurring early in RT can contribute to early changes in reservoir function (Delanian, Porcher, Rudant, & Lefaix, 2005), thus causing an increase in urinary frequency, urgency, nocturia, and dysuria. Moderate to severe acute genitourinary effects are caused by irritation of the bladder detrusor or urothelial inflammation (cystitis, urethritis, or both) resulting in urgency, frequency, or dysuria. Prostatic inflammation may result in prolonged or incomplete voiding, especially in the setting of coincident benign hypertrophy (Pisansky, 2006).
         (b) Radiation to the prostate can contribute to the described associated urinary morbidity. Moderate to severe urinary symptoms can occur in up to one-third of patients treated with EBRT (Pisansky, 2006).
      (2) Late—Interstitial fibrosis occurs in irradiated tissue, which can be accompanied by obliterative endarteritis and telangiectasia. Apoptosis of endothelial cells is an important feature in radiation-induced acute alterations in the vascular system of irradiated organs (Rodemann & Blaese, 2007). Thin-walled dilated vessels may rupture, resulting in painless hematuria.
   b) Incidence
      (1) Late genitourinary symptoms include urinary frequency, urgency, hematuria, and incontinence; 29% of the patients experienced grade 2 or higher late genitourinary morbidity (Karlsdóttir, Muren, Wentzel-Larsen, & Dahl, 2008).
      (2) Males with obstructive symptoms (increased frequency, urgency, weak urinary flow) that may be caused by an enlarged prostate should be assessed before initiation of RT and during therapy (Pisansky, 2006). Androgen deprivation therapy (ADT) has been found to decrease prostate volume by 30%–50% (Karlsdóttir et al., 2008). The reduction of the prostate volume thereby decreases the amount of bladder tissue irradiated, which has been shown to reduce the severity of urinary and rectal toxicities. ADT may be continued for several months after RT because of a possible benefit from synergy between ADT and RT (Karlsdóttir et al., 2008).
      (3) Incidence rates are dependent upon specific treatment planning and modality. Even when escalated radiation doses of 81 Gy are used, rectal toxicity is significantly lower related to the enhanced conformity of IMRT (Zelefsky et al., 2008). UTIs are not common during EBRT.
         (a) Zelefsky et al. (2008) reported the toxicity results of 1,571 patients treated with 3DCRT or IMRT after a medial follow-up of 10 years. They concluded that serious late toxicities were unusual despite high doses of radiation. The higher doses of radiation were associated with increased GI and genitourinary grade 2 toxicities, but the risk of proctitis was significantly

reduced with IMRT. Acute symptoms were a precursor of late toxicities in these patients.

(b) IMRT to the prostate resulted in less rectal toxicity. For acute toxicity and late GI and genitourinary toxicity, incidence was lower after simultaneously integrated boost IMRT as compared to 3DCRT, but these differences were not statistically significant (Al-Mamgani, Heemsbergen, Peeters, & Lebesque, 2009).

c) Assessment
(1) Presence of urinary urgency, frequency, hesitancy, dysuria, hematuria, and nocturia
(2) Reports of weakened urinary stream, obstructive symptoms, or urge or stress incontinence
(3) Elevated temperature greater than 99.5°F (37.5°C)
(4) Discolored or cloudy urine
(5) Bladder spasms
(6) Physical examination
(a) Palpate and percuss abdomen and suprapubic area to assess for bladder distension or tenderness.
(b) Allow symptoms (fever, pain, cloudy urine, or hematuria) to indicate what testing should be performed (e.g., a urinalysis or urine culture to detect the presence of bacteria and red and white blood cells).

d) Documentation (NCI CTEP, 2010)
(1) Urinary frequency
(a) 1—Present
(b) 2—Limiting instrumental ADL; medical management indicated
(2) Urinary incontinence
(a) 1— Occasional (e.g., with coughing or sneezing); pads not indicated
(b) 2—Spontaneous; pads indicated; limiting instrumental ADL
(c) 3—Intervention indicated (e.g., clamp, collagen injections); operative intervention indicated; limiting self-care ADL
(3) Urinary retention
(a) 1—Urinary, suprapubic, or intermittent catheter placement not indicated; able to void with some residual
(b) 2—Urinary, suprapubic, or intermittent catheter placement indicated; medication indicated

(c) 3—Elective operative or radiologic intervention indicated; substantial loss of affected kidney function or mass
(d) 4—Life-threatening consequences; organ failure; urgent operative intervention indicated
(e) 5—Death
(4) Pain (with urination)
(a) 1—Mild pain
(b) 2—Moderate pain; limiting instrumental ADL
(c) 3—Severe pain; limiting self-care ADL

e) Collaborative management
(1) Acute effects of urinary symptoms (Iwamoto & Maher, 2001)
(a) Maintain hydration throughout daytime while decreasing fluid intake in the evening to reduce the incidence of nocturia.
(b) Instruct the patient to avoid caffeinated products.
(c) Administer appropriate medication as prescribed.
i. Ibuprofen 400–800 mg three to four times daily orally. Relieves pain by inhibiting cyclooxygenase and lipoxygenase and reduces prostaglandin synthesis (Epocrates Rx, 2010). May be contraindicated if hematuria is present.
ii. Oxybutynin chloride 5 mg two to three times daily orally, not to exceed 5 mg daily or 10–15 mg daily as extra large tablets. Inhibits the action of acetylcholine and has antispasmodic action on smooth muscle. Inform the patient that this medication may cause drowsiness or blurred vision (Epocrates Rx, 2010).
iii. Phenazopyridine 200 mg up to three times daily orally. Acts on urinary mucosa to produce an analgesic effect. Caution the patient that urine will turn a reddish-orange color (Epocrates Rx, 2010).
iv. Tamsulosin hydrochloride 0.4 mg once daily orally; can be increased to 0.8 mg daily if ineffective. To be taken 30 minutes after dinner. Decreases contractions of smooth mus-

cle within the prostatic capsule by binding to alpha-1 receptors (Epocrates Rx, 2010).

    v. Terazosin hydrochloride 1 mg orally; may be increased to 5–10 mg daily (at bedtime). Usual maintenance dose is 5–10 mg once daily. Decreases contractions of smooth muscle within the prostatic capsule by binding to alpha-1 receptors (Epocrates Rx, 2010).

    vi. Doxazosin mesylate 1–8 mg daily orally with gradual dose escalation. Decreases contractions of smooth muscle within the prostatic capsule by binding to alpha-1 receptors (Epocrates Rx, 2010).

    (d) Consider temporary suspension of RT.

    (e) Refer the patient to a urologist for evaluation and possible cystoscopy if symptoms persist (Gomez, Alektiar, & Zelefsky, 2009).

(2) Long-term effects of urinary symptoms

    (a) Late effects generally are managed by long-term administration of urinary analgesics, antispasmodics, or alpha-1 receptor–blocking agents mentioned under acute effects.

    (b) If long-term effects are a result of decreased bladder capacity or urethral strictures, surgical or endoscopic evaluation may be necessary (Pisansky, 2006).

f) Patient and family education

(1) Inform the patient and family of the potential for urinary side effects from pelvic irradiation including the signs and symptoms of UTI and radiation-induced cystitis.

(2) Instruct the patient in dietary interventions, and promote adequate hydration.

(3) Reassure the patient as to the availability of medications should symptoms become problematic. Thoroughly review side effect profiles and possible drug interactions with the patient as appropriate.

2. Proctitis/diarrhea

  a) Pathophysiology: See section V.E—Gastrointestinal/abdomen.

  b) Incidence of lower GI side effects: Rates are dependent on treatment planning and

technique. Radiation proctitis, which may occur in severe and persistent form, may require colostomy in a small number of patients (Muehlbauer et al., 2009; Zelefsky et al., 2008). Acute rectal morbidity includes rectal discomfort, tenesmus, and diarrhea. Urinary morbidity includes frequency, nocturia, and dysuria in varying degrees.

(1) With 3DCRT

    (a) Acute—Moderate to severe adverse effects including proctitis or (when pelvic nodal treatment is given) enteritis develop in 40% of patients treated with high-dose (greater than 74 Gy) RT (Pisansky, 2006).

    (b) Chronic—Zelefsky et al. (2008) reported the incidence of late treatment-related toxicity after 3DCRT in 1,100 patients, finding that 99 patients (6%) developed greater than grade 2 late toxicity. The median time was 17 months.

(2) With IMRT

    (a) Acute—A Dutch dose escalation trial showed a significant decrease in grade 2 or greater GI toxicity with IMRT versus 3DCRT, 20% and 61%, respectively, $p = 0.001$ (Al-Mamgani et al., 2009; Budiharto, Haustermans, & Kovacs, 2010).

    (b) Late—Zelefsky et al. (2008) found that IMRT was associated with significantly reduced risk of GI toxicities compared with conventional 3DCRT (13% to 5%, $p < 0.001$).

c) Assessment of symptoms: See section V.E—Gastrointestinal/abdomen.

d) Documentation

(1) Elimination alteration (NCI CTEP, 2010)

    (a) Diarrhea (patients without colostomy): See section V.E—Gastrointestinal/abdomen.

(b) Diarrhea (patients with colostomy): See section V.E—Gastrointestinal/abdomen.

(c) Proctitis (NCI CTEP, 2010)

    i. 1—Rectal discomfort, intervention not indicated

    ii. 2—Symptoms (e.g., rectal discomfort, passing blood or mucus); medical intervention indicated; limiting instrumental ADL

    iii. 3—Severe symptoms; fecal urgency or stool incontinence; limiting self-care ADL

    iv. 4—Life-threatening consequences; urgent intervention indicated

    v. 5—Death

(d) Other factors

    i. Weight change

    ii. Compliance with dietary recommendations and fluid intake

    iii. May be helpful to use a daily documentation of dietary intake and bowel pattern sheet

(2) Skin sensation: See section IV.C—Skin reactions.

e) Collaborative management

(1) Acute effects of diarrhea (see section V.E—Gastrointestinal/abdomen)

(a) Dietary management: Goal is to minimize diarrhea and abdominal cramping and to initiate dietary interventions at start of treatment (Muehlbauer et al., 2009).

    i. Consult a dietitian at the onset of diarrhea or at start of treatment for diarrhea prevention interventions.

    ii. Use of ONS Putting Evidence Into Practice resource for diarrhea (Muehlbauer et al., 2009) to help teach patients how to make appropriate food choices, including

      • Restrict milk products. Low lactose to handle lactase deficiency.

      • Avoid greasy and fatty foods.

      • May consider adding psyllium and other soluble fiber (pectin, applesauce), and avoid whole grains, nuts, and legumes.

      • Avoid or limit caffeine to less than three servings daily.

      • Use high-potency probiotics (pills or powders) daily from first day of RT until the end of scheduled treatment.

    iii. If severe diarrhea continues, a treatment break may be required.

(b) Fluid and nutrient balance: Goal is intake of adequate amounts of fluid and nutrients to prevent dehydration, electrolyte imbalance, and weight loss.

    i. Clear juices, broth, and decaffeinated tea

    ii. Juices high in electrolytes (e.g., Gatorade®)

    iii. Lactose-free liquid supplements

(c) Skin alteration from diarrhea (see sections IV.C—Skin reactions; V.E—Gastrointestinal/abdomen)

    i. If appropriate, suggest the use of sanitary pads or adult incontinence briefs for rectal discharge or stool incontinence.

    ii. Instruct the patient to maintain good personal hygiene using mild soap and tepid water to gently wash skin.

    iii. Use plain, unscented, lanolin-free, hydrophilic cream if skin is intact.

    iv. Use over-the-counter medications (Preparation H® [Pfizer Consumer Healthcare], Tucks® wipes [McNeil-PPC, Inc.]) as instructed by the patient's healthcare provider.

(d) Medications/pharmacologic interventions: After three or more watery bowel movements a day, initiation of medication should begin.

    i. Initial treatment: Anticholinergic medications (see section V.E—Gastrointestinal/abdomen)

    ii. If experiencing proctitis, consider administering appropriate medication as prescribed.

      • Hydrocortisone preparations (cream, ointment, suppository, or foam) can be used up to four times daily (Gomez et al., 2009).

- Send stool for testing for *Clostridium difficile* toxin if early into treatment or not responding to pharmaceuticals (can be caused by chemotherapy, RT, prolonged hospitalization, and high doses of antibiotics). Initiate appropriate antibiotic therapy as prescribed by the patient's healthcare provider.

iii. If no response to pharmacologic interventions
  - Consult proctologist or gastroenterologist if diarrhea or rectal bleeding is unresolved by pharmacologic interventions. Colonoscopy, more invasive treatments, or surgery may be needed in severe cases (Wong et al., 2010).
  - Treatment breaks may be considered during therapy.

(2) Long-term effects of diarrhea

  (a) Maintain low-fiber diet to decrease stool bulk.

  (b) Maintain good anal and personal hygiene.

  (c) Continue the use of sanitary pads or adult incontinence briefs as needed.

  (d) Continue long-term use of medications for both urinary morbidity (as described previously) and antidiarrheal/proctitis medications also as described with the possible addition of hydrocortisone enemas (Pisansky, 2006).

  (e) Close follow-up with proctologist/gastroenterologist if indicated
  i. Argon plasma coagulation, a noncontact coagulation technique where a tube expressing argon is inserted into the rectum via endoscope. Argon plasma coagulation ameliorates rectal bleeding associated with hemorrhagic radiation proctitis in 80%–90% of cases. It improves diarrhea and tenesmus in 60%–70% of cases, usually achieved in one or two treatment sessions (Postgate, Saunders, Tjandra, & Vargo, 2007).

  ii. Laser treatment to cauterize bleeding vessels within the rectum (Wong et al., 2010). Use with precaution, as laser treatments may sometimes cause ulceration because of poor wound healing after RT.

  iii. Formalin instillation or topical application for chronic hemorrhagic proctitis (Wong et al., 2010). In three prospective studies using 4% formalin applied to the rectum, 80 patients achieved a 67%–89% response rate over a period of 20 months (Garg et al., 2006).

  iv. Hyperbaric oxygen treatments (Wong et al., 2010): Hyperbaric oxygen uses increased oxygen pressure to telangietatic vessels and reverses the ischemic component of chronic radiation proctopathy and promotes angiogenesis with healing of rectal mucosa. Analysis of several small studies for a total of 83 patients showed an improvement in up to 65% of patients, but it may require 40–90 sessions to be effective (Garg et al., 2006).

f) Patient and family education (see section V.E—Gastrointestinal/abdomen)

  (1) Inform the patient that diarrhea is an expected side effect of radiation to the pelvis.

  (2) Teach dietary modifications.

  (3) Instruct the patient and family in comfort measures (sitz baths, tepid water cotton cloth soaks).

  (4) Explain protocol for perianal hygiene (use mild soap, do not rub, pat dry).

  (5) Instruct the patient and family regarding signs and symptoms of dehydration.

  (6) Instruct the patient to keep a log of the number and consistency of bowel movements per day.

  (7) Inform the patient and family of medications available to alleviate treatment-related side effects. Thoroughly review side effect profiles and possible drug interactions. Instruct the patient regarding appropriate use of suppositories, foams, ointments, or enemas if prescribed.

(8) Post-treatment late effects: Instruct the patient on reporting symptoms, including changes in stools and rectal bleeding or pain, and those to report at follow-up visits and when to call physician.

(9) Use teaching tools to enhance understanding.

3. Sexual dysfunction (see section IV.F—Sexual dysfunction)

a) Pathophysiology—Radiation can result in erectile dysfunction by accelerating microvascular angiopathy in the arteriolar system supplying the corporal muscles causing cavernosal fibrosis or stenosis of the pelvic arteries, thereby leading to impotence. Zelefsky et al. (2008) concluded that the predominant etiology of radiation-induced impotence was vascular disruption as opposed to radiation damage of the nerve bundles. High doses of radiation to the corpus spongiosum significantly increase the risk of erectile dysfunction; the dose to this region is addressed during RT planning (Pisansky, 2006).

b) Incidence

(1) Sexual dysfunction and quality of life are interrelated (Katz, 2007). The term *sexual dysfunction* can pertain not only to impotence but also to erectile dysfunction, lack of sexual enjoyment, inability to satisfy a partner, and orgasmic dysfunction. Quality of life has been described as "present when the hopes of an individual are matched and fulfilled by experience. The opposite is also true: A poor quality of life occurs when the hopes do not meet with the experience" (Calman, 1984, pp. 124–125).

(2) The exact incidence of erectile dysfunction as a treatment-related side effect is difficult to determine because of the absence of a uniform definition and because older men experience erectile dysfunction as a result of concomitant medical conditions (diabetes, hypertension) and commonly prescribed pharmacologic agents (beta-blockers) (O'Rourke, 2007).

(3) Prior studies have documented the dependence of long-term sexual function outcomes on patients' baseline functional status. Compromised pretreatment function may make patients more vulnerable to additional treatment-related dysfunction, whereas very advanced dysfunction (e.g., severe erectile dysfunction) may leave little residual for additional treatment-related worsening (Chen, Clark, & Talcott, 2009).

(4) Phan, Syed, Puthawala, Sharma, and Khan (2007) treated 309 patients with prostate cancer with EBRT and HDR brachytherapy. They reported that overall, 62% of the patients maintained baseline (sexual) ability, while 38% reported a decrease in erectile function. In the latter group, 10%, 18%, and 10% of the patients had mild, moderate, and complete impotence, respectively.

(5) Chen et al. (2009) reported that half of the patients with normal baseline function who underwent EBRT and four-fifths of patients with normal baseline function who had brachytherapy retained some useful function. For those with intermediate baseline function, 29% preserved an ability to have sexual intercourse after EBRT, and 38% preserved that ability after brachytherapy. Patients with poor baseline function fared dismally after all treatments.

c) Assessment

(1) Baseline dysfunction prior to initiation of treatment

(2) Baseline sexual activity level

(3) Baseline satisfaction/dissatisfaction with intercourse

(4) Medications and comorbid conditions (hypertension, diabetes, peripheral vascular disease, and neuropathy)

(5) Decreased ability to achieve erection

(6) Decreased sensation during intercourse

(7) Decreased ability to achieve orgasm

d) Documentation (in addition to baseline and existing symptoms): See section IV.F—Sexual dysfunction.

e) Collaborative management

(1) Acute effects of sexual dysfunction (see section IV.F—Sexual dysfunc-

tion) (Galbraith & Crighton, 2008; O'Rourke, 2007)

   (a) Factors such as stress and impaired coping may contribute to acute onset of impotence.

   (b) Interventions for acute onset of impotence would not significantly differ from those for long-term effects (refer to interventions later).

(2) Long-term effects of sexual dysfunction (see section IV.F—Sexual dysfunction)

   (a) The patient and spouse may need to be referred for professional counseling regarding the physical and psychological effects of sexual dysfunction.

   (b) Referral to urology for other alternative treatments

   i. Other nonsurgical approaches include urethral suppositories, intracavernous injections, and vacuum devices.

   ii. Penile prostheses may be used after proper education of the patient and partner.

f) Patient and family education

(1) Sexual issues must be incorporated into the general discussion of side effects of treatment, rather than being raised as a separate issue, to reduce embarrassment and provide permission for the men to raise sexual issues in future discussions. Maliski, Heilemann, and McCorkle (2001) demonstrated that a weekly homecare intervention over eight weeks focusing on assisting couples with immediate postoperative care, intimacy, communication, and psychosocial support helped the couples to obtain, evaluate, and manage information, thus leading them to regain mastery over their lives (O'Rourke, 2007).

(2) The patient should verbalize understanding of importance of communication between both partners regarding concerns or issues of sexual dysfunction.

(3) The patient should verbalize understanding of side effects of RT as it relates to sexual dysfunction.

(4) Instruct the patient and significant other about alternative medical and surgical interventions that may be available to them.

(5) Inform the patient of the availability of medications to treat some forms of sexual dysfunction. Thoroughly review side effect profiles and drug interactions of prescribed medications.

(6) The patient and partner are informed about resuming intercourse and sexual activity after therapy.

(7) The patient and partner should inform nurse or physician of continued sexual dysfunction.

(8) Teaching tools for specific site

4. Prostate brachytherapy

   a) Procedure description: Radioactive sources are placed directly into the prostate tissue for the purpose of eradicating malignant cells from within the prostate gland. They may be permanent (i.e., left in the prostate, such as radioactive seeds) or temporary (removed after treatment) sources. It has the advantage of delivering higher doses to the tumor with reduced toxicity to normal tissues. Brachytherapy, also referred to as interstitial implantation, is commonly used to treat patients with low- or intermediate-risk prostate cancer.

   b) Contraindications: Gomez et al. (2009) established absolute and relative contraindications for prostate brachytherapy.

   (1) Absolute contraindications are history of severe urinary symptoms including recurrent urethral strictures/transurethral resection of the prostate (TURP) procedures, international prostate symptom score (IPSS, used to assess the severity of urinary symptoms) of 16 or higher, medically poor surgical candidate, or overt seminal vesicle invasion.

   (2) Relative contraindications are prior history of TURP or transurethral needle ablation of the prostate, IPSS less than 15, and patient requires continuous use of alpha-blockers or prostate gland larger than 60 ml (ADT may be given for volume reduction).

   c) Indications: LDR and HDR implants can be used as monotherapy or as a boost in combination with EBRT and/or androgen ablation (Gomez et al., 2009; Mohler et al., 2010; Potters et al., 2005).

   (1) Candidates for LDR prostate brachytherapy include patients whose cancer is clinically confined to the prostate (T1c or T2, Gleason score 2–6, prostate-specific antigen [PSA] less than 10 ng/ml) and who have a life

expectancy of greater than five years (Mohler et al., 2010; NCCN, 2011).

   (a) Patients with more aggressive disease are treated with combination of brachytherapy and EBRT with or without ADT. The most common criteria are clinical stage T2c or higher, Gleason score 4+3 or higher, PSA greater than 10, and/or 50% or more of biopsy cores involved (Gomez et al., 2009). The addition of EBRT increases the rate and severity of side effects. Combination therapy including the addition of EBRT or ADT remains unconfirmed until randomized trials are completed (Potters et al., 2005).

   (b) ^{103}Pd and ^{125}I are the most common isotopes in use and the most extensively studied, but the use of ^{131}Cs for LDR has increased because of its shorter half-life (Sahgal et al., 2008). Despite differences in the half-lives and energies of these two isotopes, no differences have been established in survival outcomes. However, proper placement of the isotopes within the prostate is associated with improved biochemical outcomes (Zelefsky et al., 2007).

(2) Candidates for HDR prostate brachytherapy include patients with both favorable (stage less than T2a) and unfavorable (stage T2b or higher) disease. HDR prostate brachytherapy allows the radiation oncologist to modulate the intensity of the radiation by varying the time the source spends at each dwell position within the implant (Demanes, Rodriguez, Schour, Brandt, & Altieri, 2005). HDR brachytherapy has been shown to have decreased rates of acute dysuria, urinary frequency/urgency, and rectal pain as compared to LDR brachytherapy (Gomez et al., 2009).

d) Treatment: The practice of prescribing LDR versus HDR brachytherapy for prostate malignancies is based on the patient's clinical stage including not just TNM stage but also Gleason score and PSA level.

  (1) LDR: Consists of inserting needles directly into the prostate gland using a transperineal approach under the guidance of transrectal ultrasound. This is an operative procedure during which the patient can undergo either general or epidural anesthesia (Buyyounouski, Horowitz, & Pollack, 2009; Gomez et al., 2009). Small radioactive seeds then are placed into the gland through the needles.

   (a) Sources most commonly used include the following radioactive isotopes (Gomez et al., 2009).

     i. ^{125}I, with a 59.6-day half-life

     ii. ^{103}Pd, with a 17-day half-life

   (b) The number of needles used depends on the size of the prostate gland. Multiple needles are inserted and immediately removed following the procedure. A typical prostate will receive 70–100 seeds.

  (2) HDR

   (a) HDR brachytherapy is administered in an operative procedure during which a template is secured to the perineum, and, under the guidance of transrectal ultrasound, needles are inserted through the holes in the template and into the prostate gland. As the needles are removed, plastic catheters are left in place and secured by way of the template.

   (b) After radiation planning is complete, the catheters are secured to an HDR afterloader, and the radiation source is directed into and out of each catheter. Iridium dwell time varies according to source strength and radiation plan.

   (c) Typically, treatments are given in three to four fractions ranging from 5.5 to 7 Gy/fraction (Gomez et al., 2009).

   (d) This procedure requires overnight inpatient hospitalization and interstitial catheter care to be administered by either radiation oncology nurses or inpatient staff nurses (Gomez et al., 2009).

   (e) The most commonly used isotopes are ^{125}I and ^{103}Pd (Buyyounouski et al., 2009).

e) Side effects: Acute and late side effects from prostate brachytherapy can be influenced by a number of different factors that include prostate size greater than 60 g, history of TURP, higher pretreatment American Urology Association scores or IPSS score (both scores are used to determine the severity of urinary symptoms), and addition of EBRT. Comorbid disease such as diabetes and hypertension can have an adverse effect on erectile function (Pisansky, 2006).

(1) Acute side effects

    (a) Side effects during the acute phase are caused by procedural trauma, and later effects are a result of urethral obstruction, incontinence, and bleeding from radiation exposure (Chen, D'Amico, Neville, & Earle, 2006; Pisansky, 2006).

    (b) Urinary frequency/urgency is a result of changes in both the prostate and the urinary bladder. This can cause an increase in urinary frequency, urgency, nocturia, and dysuria.

    (c) Changes can occur to the bladder causing urinary urgency, frequency, retention/distended bladder, dysuria, nocturia, hematuria, weakened stream/obstructive symptoms, urge incontinence, stress incontinence, and discolored or cloudy urine (Gomez et al., 2009; Pisansky, 2006).

    (d) Changes can occur to the bowels, including softer, more frequent stools, nighttime bowel frequency, diarrhea, abdominal cramping, bloating, flatulence, bowel urgency, feeling of incomplete bowel evacuation, incontinence of stools, rectal irritation/ulceration (proctitis), rectal bleeding, rectal discharge, and tenesmus (Chen et al., 2006; Pisansky, 2006).

    (e) Inflamed hemorrhoids

    (f) Skin ulceration in the gluteal folds

(2) Late side effects

    (a) Previous studies have shown that the use of TURP, prostate size, and poor preimplantation urinary function are associated with higher rates of urinary toxicity (Chen et al., 2006).

    (b) Interstitial fibrosis occurs in radiated tissue, which can be accompanied by obliterative endarteritis and telangiectasia. Late reactions occurring months to years after radiation exposure are primarily the result of radiation-dependent depletion of tissue-specific stem cells or progenitor cells, leading to fibrosis, organ dysfunc-

tion, and necrosis (Rodemann & Blaese, 2007).

    (c) Urinary symptoms vary significantly and can persist for several years after implant. Keys et al. (2009) reported on 712 patients who underwent brachytherapy for localized prostate cancer. Of these patients, 6% experienced severe urinary toxicity at five years after brachytherapy. Statistics vary as to how many men will develop long-term cystitis from RT.

    (d) Changes can continue with bladder symptoms: 1%–2% with urethral stricture; incontinence in 1% or less (Gomez et al., 2009).

    (e) Demanes et al. (2005) reported on 209 patients, 67% of whom were able to preserve some level of sexual function. Grade 1 and 2 late GI toxicities were noted in 2% of the patients, and grade 1 morbidity consisted of self-limited rectal bleeding.

    (f) The exact incidence of erectile dysfunction as a treatment-related side effect is difficult to determine because of the absence of a uniform definition and because older men may experience erectile dysfunction as a result of medical conditions or medications (O'Rourke, 2007).

f) Collaborative management for LDR brachytherapy: Predominantly outpatient procedure

(1) Acute effects

    (a) Educate the patient about the differences between palladium and iodine implant (half-life, exposure precautions).

    (b) Inform the patient and family of acute and late effects.

    (c) An indwelling catheter may be required until acute postoperative swelling of smooth muscle decreases and urinary obstructive symptoms subside.

    (d) If a displaced seed is found, use tongs or a long-handled instrument to place it in a container with water and contact the radiation safety officer and the oncology department as soon as possible.

    (e) Educate the patient and family about exposure precautions as in-

dicated by institutional policy (see Patient and family education).

(f) Educate about the side effects of medications prescribed to alleviate urinary or bowel morbidity.

(g) Urinary-specific management: See section V.G—Site-specific management.

(h) Bowel management: See section V.G—Site-specific management.

(i) Proctitis: See section V.G—Site-specific management.

(2) Late effects

(a) The patient and partner may need to be referred for professional counseling regarding the physical and psychological effects of sexual dysfunction.

   i. Encourage communication regarding fears or concerns of sexual dysfunction (O'Rourke, 2007).

   ii. Identify resources that may be helpful in managing the effects of sexual dysfunction. Nurses need to be aware of the importance of quality of life for these men and their partners and how the disease and treatment can affect quality of life (O'Rourke, 2007).

(b) Administer appropriate medication as prescribed.

   i. Sildenafil 25–100 mg orally 30 minutes to 4 hours before sexual activity. Gomez et al. (2009) reported success rates of 70%–80% with sildenafil treatment among patients who have received RT to the prostate.

   ii. Other PDE5 inhibitors, such as tadalafil or vardenafil hydrochloride, may be useful in treating impotence. However, no studies have examined the effectiveness of tadalafil or vardenafil among patients treated with RT.

(c) Refer the patient to urology for other alternative treatments. Other nonsurgical approaches include urethral suppositories, intracavernous injections, and vacuum devices.

g) Collaborative management for HDR prostate brachytherapy (brachytherapy catheter care)

(1) Keep area open to air as much as possible and monitor for signs and symptoms of infection.

(2) Keep perineal template as clean as possible.

(3) Some discharge may occur while catheters are in place; frequent pad changes may be necessary to maintain patient hygiene and comfort. Monitor for bleeding and maintain catheter placement.

(4) Decrease bowel movements while catheters or template is in place.

(a) Loperamide hydrochloride as instructed by physician or healthcare provider to promote mild constipation, thereby decreasing the need for bowel movements and accidental displacement or movement of brachytherapy catheters.

(b) Low-fiber diet to decrease stool bulk

(5) Minimize patient activity to avoid brachytherapy catheter displacement and maintain patency of indwelling urinary catheter.

(6) Collect and monitor urinary output for the first 24 hours after implantation.

(7) Inpatient staff nurses need to be aware that patients receiving HDR prostate brachytherapy in the radiation oncology department via remote afterloader are not radioactive when they return to the floor because the radioactive source remains in the afterloader machine in radiation oncology. When patients are treated in this manner, special precautions are unnecessary on the inpatient unit. If a radioisotope is housed in the patient while the patient is on the inpatient unit, then precautions must be taken, including personal dosimeters or radiation badges. Nurses and staff must minimize exposure to the radioactive source (see section III—Radiation protection and safety).

(8) Administer pain medications as needed for postoperative discomfort and acute and late urinary and bowel morbidity, as well as for late effect potency issues.

h) Patient and family education

(1) For brachytherapy

(a) Instruct the patient on the brachytherapy procedure and precautions as advised by the radiation oncologist.

(b) Teach the patient and family about the side effects from prostate brachytherapy. The side effects are similar to EBRT and include diarrhea, dysuria, rectal bleeding, cystitis, and urinary retention but may differ in time to onset and severity.

(c) Teach the patient and family about dietary modifications: Maintaining hydration throughout the daytime while decreasing fluid intake in the evening to reduce the incidence of nocturia, avoiding caffeinated products and following a low-fiber/low-residue diet (Iwamoto & Maher, 2001). Consider the addition of bulk agents to absorb excess fluid if loose stools are present.

(d) Teach the patient and family about the need for NSAIDs, antispasmodics, or alpha-1 receptor blocking agents for urinary symptoms. If the patient is experiencing diarrhea, teach about antidiarrheal medications. If the patient is experiencing proctitis or impotence, teach about appropriate medications.

(e) Instruct the patient and partner to always use a condom during sexual intercourse and during any act in which ejaculation may occur. Seed migration and loss is not limited to the venous system but also can occur through other mechanisms such as through the urinary tract, ejaculation, or distal displacement because of the action of the perineal muscles (Saibishkumar et al., 2009). Loss (of radioactive seeds) most frequently occurred within the first month after implant (Sommerkamp, Rupprecht, & Wannenmacher, 1988).

(f) Much controversy exists over the recommendation that patients minimize their exposure to children and pregnant women. Kono, Miyamoto, Oohashi, and Fukushi (2011) suggested that based on anterior skin surface exposure rates, patients with permanent prostate brachytherapy implants do not need to be concerned about being a radiation risk to the public following the procedure. Exposure

information usually is dictated by institutional policy.

(g) Patients should be advised to notify the radiation oncologist and radiation safety officer where they received their implant if they discover a seed that may have been passed through their ejaculate or urine.

(2) For urinary side effects (Chen et al., 2009; Demanes et al., 2005)

(a) Instruct the patient on expected urinary side effects and possible long-term complications of prostate brachytherapy.

(b) Instruct the patient to report treatment-related sequelae promptly as well as any changes from baseline urinary function, including signs and symptoms of urinary infection.

(c) Instruct the patient in dietary interventions as appropriate.

(d) Reassure the patient as to the availability of medications if symptoms become problematic. Thoroughly review side effect profiles and possible drug interactions with patient.

(e) Inform the patient that a referral to urology for alternative treatments for urinary dysfunction is an option.

(3) For lower GI side effects

(a) Inform the patient of lower GI–related side effects and possible complications associated with prostate brachytherapy.

(b) Encourage the patient to report any side effects or changes from baseline bowel function promptly.

(c) Instruct the patient in dietary interventions as appropriate.

(d) Teach the patient the signs and symptoms of dehydration.

(e) Instruct the patient to monitor frequency, consistency, and presence of blood in bowel movements.

(f) Instruct the patient in appropriate hygiene techniques.

(g) Instruct the patient in appropriate use of sitz baths.

(h) Inform the patient and family of medications available to alleviate treatment-related side effects. Thoroughly review side effect profiles and possible drug interactions. Instruct in appropriate use of any suppositories, foams, ointments, or enemas if prescribed.

(4) For erectile dysfunction (Galbraith & Crighton, 2008)

(a) Instruct the patient about the importance of communication between both partners regarding concerns and issues of sexual dysfunction.

(b) Explain side effects as they relate to sexual dysfunction resulting from RT.

(c) Instruct the patient and significant other about medical and surgical interventions that may be available.

(d) Inform the patient of the availability of medication to treat some forms of sexual dysfunction. Thoroughly review side effect profiles and drug interactions of prescribed medications.

(e) Inform the patient and significant other that a referral for professional counseling regarding the physical and psychological effects of sexual dysfunction is available.

References

Al-Mamgani, A., Heemsbergen, W.D., Peeters, S.T., & Lebesque, J.V. (2009). Role of intensity-modulated radiotherapy in reducing toxicity in dose escalation for localized prostate cancer. *International Journal of Radiation Oncology, Biology, Physics, 73,* 685–691. doi:10.1016/j.ijrobp.2008.04.063

Bentzen, S.M. (2006). Preventing or reducing late side effects of radiation therapy: Radiobiology meets molecular pathology. *Nature Reviews Cancer, 6,* 702–713. doi:10.1038/nrc1950

Budiharto, T., Haustermans, K., & Kovacs, G. (2010). External beam radiotherapy for prostate cancer. *Journal of Endourology, 24,* 781–789. doi:10.1089/end.2009.0436

Buyyounouski, M.K., Horwitz, E.M., & Pollack, A. (2009). Prostate cancer. In B.G. Haffty & L.D. Wilson (Eds.), *Handbook of radiation oncology: Basic principles and clinical protocols* (pp. 565–582). Sudbury, MA: Jones and Bartlett.

Calman, K.C. (1984). Quality of life in cancer patients—An hypothesis. *Journal of Medical Ethics, 10,* 124–127.

Chen, A.B., D'Amico, A.V., Neville, B.A., & Earle, C.C. (2006). Patient and treatment factors associated with complications after prostate brachytherapy. *Journal of Clinical Oncology, 24,* 5298–5304. doi:10.1200/JCO.2006.07.9954

Chen, R.C., Clark, J.A., & Talcott, J.A. (2009). Individualizing quality-of-life outcomes reporting: How localized prostate cancer treatments affect patients with different levels of baseline urinary, bowel, and sexual dysfunction. *Journal of Clinical Oncology, 27,* 3916–3922. doi:10.1200/JCO.2008.18.6486

Delanian, S., Porcher, R., Rudant, J., & Lefaix, J.L. (2005). Kinetics of response to long-term treatment combining pentoxifylline and tocopherol in patients with superficial radiation-induced fibrosis. *Journal of Clinical Oncology, 23,* 8570–8579. doi:10.1200/JCO.2005.02.4729

Demanes, D.J., Rodriguez, R.R., Schour, L., Brandt, D., & Altieri, G. (2005). High-dose-rate intensity-modulated brachytherapy with external beam radiotherapy for prostate cancer: California endocurietherapy's 10-year results. *International Journal of Radiation Oncology, Biology, Physics, 61,* 1306–1316. doi:10.1016/j.ijrobp.2004.08.014

Epocrates Rx® [version 3.15]. (2010). Retrieved from http://epocrates.com

Galbraith, M.E., & Crighton, F. (2008). Alterations of sexual function in men with cancer. *Seminars in Oncology Nursing, 24,* 102–114. doi:10.1016/j.soncn.2008.02.010

Garg, A., Mai, W., McGary, J.E., Grant, W.H., Butler, B., & Teh, B.S. (2006). Radiation proctopathy in the treatment of prostate cancer. *International Journal of Radiation Oncology, Biology, Physics, 66,* 1294–1305.

Gomez, D.R., Alektiar, K.M., & Zelefsky, M.J. (2009). Brachytherapy. In B.G. Haffty & L.D. Wilson (Eds.), *Handbook of radiation oncology: Basic principles and clinical protocols* (pp. 111–139). Sudbury, MA: Jones and Bartlett.

Iwamoto, R.R., & Maher, K.E. (2001). Radiation therapy for prostate cancer. *Seminars in Oncology Nursing, 17,* 90–100. doi:10.1053/sonu.2000.23071

Karlsdóttir, A., Muren, L.P., Wentzel-Larsen, T., & Dahl, O. (2008). Late gastrointestinal morbidity after three-dimensional conformal radiation therapy for prostate cancer fades with time in contrast to genitourinary morbidity. *International Journal of Radiation Oncology, Biology, Physics, 70,* 1478–1486. doi:10.1016/j.ijrobp.2007.08.076

Katz, A. (2007). Quality of life for men with prostate cancer. *Cancer Nursing, 30,* 302–308. doi:10.1097/01.NCC.0000281726.87490.f2

Keys, M., Miller, S., Moravan, V., Pickles, T., McKenzie, M., Pai, H., … Morris, W.J. (2009). Predictive factors of acute and late urinary toxicity after permanent prostate brachytherapy: Long-term outcome in 712 consecutive patients. *International Journal of Radiation Oncology, Biology, Physics, 73,* 1023–1032. doi:10.1016/j.ijrobp.2008.05.022

Kono, Y., Miyamoto, Y., Oohashi, S., & Fukushi, M. (2011). Radiation exposure to general public after permanent brachytherapy for prostate cancer. *Radiation Protection Dosimetry, 146,* 229–230. doi: 10.1093/rpd/ncr156

Maliski, S.L., Heilemann, M.S.V., & McCorkle, R. (2001). Mastery of postprostatectomy incontinence and impotence: His work, her work, our work. *Oncology Nursing Forum, 28,* 985–992.

Mohler, J., Bahnson, R.R., Boston, B., Busby, J.A., D'Amico, A., Eastman, J.A., … Walsh, P.C. (2010). NCCN clinical practice guidelines in oncology: Prostate cancer. *Journal of the National Comprehensive Cancer Network, 8,* 162–200.

Muehlbauer, P.M., Thorpe, D., Davis, A., Drabot, R., Rawlings, B.L., & Kiker, E. (2009). Putting evidence into practice: Evidence-based interventions to prevent, manage, and treat chemotherapy- and radiotherapy-induced diarrhea. *Clinical Journal of Oncology Nursing, 13,* 336–341. doi:10.1188/09.CJON.336-341

National Cancer Institute Cancer Therapy Evaluation Program. (2010). *Common terminology criteria for adverse events* [v.4.03]. Retrieved from http://ctep.cancer.gov/protocolDevelopment/electronic _applications/ctc.htm

National Comprehensive Cancer Network. (2011). *NCCN Clinical Practice Guidelines in Oncology: Prostate cancer* [v.4.2011]. Retrieved from http://www.nccn.org/professionals/physician_ gls/pdf/prostate.pdf

O'Rourke, M.E. (2007). Choose wisely: Therapeutic decisions and quality of life in patients with prostate cancer. *Clinical Journal of Oncology Nursing, 11,* 401–408. doi:10.1188/07.CJON.401-408

Phan, T.P., Syed, A.M., Puthawala, A., Sharma, A., & Khan, F. (2007). High dose rate brachytherapy as a boost for the treatment of localized prostate cancer. *Journal of Urology, 177,* 123–127. doi:10.1016/j.juro.2006.08.109

Pisansky, T.M. (2006). External beam radiotherapy for localized prostate cancer. *New England Journal of Medicine, 355,* 1583–1591. doi:10.1056/NEJMct055263

Postgate, A., Saunders, B., Tjandra, J., & Vargo, J. (2007). Argon plasma coagulation in chronic radiation proctitis. *Endoscopy, 39,* 361–365. doi:10.1055/s-2007-966284

Potters, L., Morgenstern, C., Calugaru, E., Fearn, P., Jassal, A., Presser, J., & Mullen, E. (2005). 12-year outcomes following permanent prostate brachytherapy in patients with clinically localized prostate cancer. *Journal of Urology, 173,* 1562–1566. doi:10.1097/01. ju.0000154633.73092.8e

Rodemann, H.P., & Blaese, M.A. (2007). Responses of normal cells to ionizing radiation. *Seminars in Radiation Oncology, 17,* 81–88. doi:10.1016/j.semradonc.2006.11.005

Sahgal, A., Jabbari, S., Chen, J., Pickett, B., Roach, M., III, Weinberg, V., ... Pouliot, J. (2008). Comparison of dosimetric and biologic effective dose parameters for prostate and urethra using ^{131}Cs and ^{125}I for prostate permanent implant brachytherapy. *International Journal of Radiation Oncology, Biology, Physics, 72,* 247–254. doi:10.1016/j.ijrobp.2008.05.013

Saibishkumar, E.P., Borg, J., Yeung, I., Cummins-Holder, C., Landon, A., & Crook, J. (2009). Sequential comparison of seed loss and prostate dosimetry of stranded seeds with loose seeds in ^{125}I permanent implant for low-risk prostate cancer. *International Journal of Radiation Oncology, Biology, Physics, 73,* 61–68. doi:10.1016/j.ijrobp.2008.04.009

Sommerkamp, H., Rupprecht, M., & Wannenmacher, M.A. (1988). Seed loss in interstitial radiotherapy of prostatic carcinoma with I-125. *International Journal of Radiation Oncology, Biology, Physics, 14,* 389–392. doi:10.1016/0360-3016(88)90448-8

Wong, M.T.C., Lim, J.F., Ho, K.S., Ooi, B.S., Tang, C.L., & Eu, K.W. (2010). Radiation proctitis: A decade's experience. *Singapore Medical Journal, 51,* 315–319.

Zelefsky, M.J., Kuban, D., Levy, L.B., Potters, L., Beyer, D.C., Blasko, J.C., ... Horwitz, E.M. (2007). Multi-institutional analysis of long-term outcome for stages T1–T2 prostate cancer treated with permanent seed implantation. *International Journal of Radiation Oncology, Biology, Physics, 67,* 327–333. doi:10.1016/j. ijrobp.2006.08.056

Zelefsky, M.J., Levin, E.J., Hunt, M., Yamada, Y., Shippy, A.M., Jackson, A., & Amols, H. (2008). Incidence of late rectal and urinary toxicities after three-dimensional conformal radiotherapy and intensity-modulated radiotherapy for localized prostate cancer. *International Journal of Radiation Oncology, Biology, Physics, 70,* 1124–1129. doi:10.1016/j.ijrobp.2007.11.044

H. Female pelvis
1. Introduction
   a) Pelvic RT is used to treat gynecologic cancers (cervical, endometrial, ovarian, vaginal, and vulvar), bladder cancer, and colon cancer.
   b) Gynecologic cancer incidence: In 2010, an estimated 83,750 new cases for female genital cancers were diagnosed, with an estimated 27,710 deaths (ACS, 2011).
   c) Typical daily dose of external radiation to pelvic fields is 18–20 Gy.
   d) Intracavitary radiation (see section VIII.B— LDR and HDR brachytherapy), also known as brachytherapy, may consist of intracavitary applicators such as the following.
      (1) HDR vaginal cylinder
      (2) Syed template
      (3) Tandem and ovoids
         (a) Fletcher-Suit-Delclos
         (b) Henschke applicator
         (c) Manchester
      (4) Tandem and colpostat
2. Skin changes
   a) Pathophysiology
      (1) Acute effects
         (a) Hyperpigmentation occurs after two to four weeks of treatment. With cumulative dose reaching 20 Gy, the patient may experience dryness, pruritus, or flaking of the skin or dry desquamation in the genital area. This is a result of the decreased ability of the basal layer to replace surface layers, shedding of the epidermis, and decreased functioning of the sweat and sebaceous glands (McQuestion, 2011).
         (b) At doses of 30–40 Gy, extracapillary cell damage occurs with increased capillary blood flow, hyperemia, and edema. If severe, epilation results, leading to moist desquamation that can occur at doses of 45–60 Gy (McQuestion, 2011). See section IV.C—Skin reactions.
      (2) Late effects
         (a) Typically defined as effects having an onset at least three months after treatment. Symptoms can be slight to severe and can worsen over time (Azria, Betz, Bourgier, Sozzi, & Ozsahin, 2010).
         (b) May include fibrosis, atrophy, ulceration, pigmentation changes,

friability, and telangiectasias (Azria et al., 2010; Chopra & Bogart, 2010).

b) Evaluation before and during treatment
  (1) Risk factors
    (a) Skin folds in perineum within the treatment field
    (b) Concomitant use of chemotherapy or radiosensitizing agents before, during, or after radiation may increase late effects (Vale et al., 2010).
    (c) Prior to treatment, confirm drug/dose of adjuvant chemotherapy to avoid treatment with drugs that may cause a radiation recall effect.
    (d) Autoimmune diseases or other comorbid conditions
    (e) Medications—Use of steroids may lead to thinning of skin, thereby increasing skin reaction to EBRT (Mayo Clinic, 2010).
  (2) Clinical manifestations
    (a) Pruritus is often associated with early signs of dry desquamation and is a commonly reported symptom in the first two to three weeks (Sparks, 2007).
    (b) Discomfort/pain is associated with moist desquamation.
  (3) Physical examination (see section IV.C—Skin reactions)
  (4) Documentation (see sections IV.B—Fatigue; IV.C—Skin reactions; and IV.D—Pain)
    (a) Use the ONS *Radiation Therapy Patient Care Record* assessment tool for pelvis, female (Catlin-Huth, Haas, & Pollock, 2002).
    (b) Document any changes in vaginal discharge (i.e., amount, color, odor).

c) Collaborative management
  (1) Acute effects (see section IV.C—Skin reactions)
  (2) Late effects (see section IV.C—Skin reactions)

d) Patient and family education (Moore-Higgs, 2007)
  (1) Perform nutritional evaluation and education to ensure proper diet to enhance tissue healing; maintain adequate nutritional and fluid intake.
  (2) Instruct on the signs and symptoms of infection and enforce the need to report them (e.g., fever, chills, drainage, odor).
  (3) Instruct on use of pain medications and antipruritic medications.
  (4) General recommendations for the patient (ONS, 2010)
    (a) Use only mild soap and pat dry with a soft towel.
    (b) May use unscented, lanolin-free, water-based lubricant or moisturizing cream.
    (c) Avoid use of cosmetic or perfumed products on irradiated skin.
    (d) Do not use cornstarch or baby powder, especially in the area with skin folds.
    (e) Wear loose clothing made from soft fabric or cotton.
    (f) Avoid the use of tapes and other adhesives within the treatment field to avoid mechanical skin injury.
    (g) Do not use ice or heating pads on the skin in the area being treated.
    (h) Avoid swimming in lakes or chlorinated pools and using hot tubs or saunas.
    (i) Avoid sun exposure following radiation treatment for lifetime. Use sunscreen with an SPF of at least 30 at all times.
  (5) Recommendations for management of moist desquamation
    (a) Consider use of specialized dressings for moist desquamation, bleeding, exudates, or drainage.
    (b) When selecting a dressing, consider the principles of wound healing, patient comfort, need for frequency of dressing changes, product evaluation, and cost.
    (c) Do not use irritants (e.g., soaps, oils, perfumes, powders).

3. Urinary frequency/dysuria/cystitis
  a) Pathophysiology
    (1) Acute effects

(a) Acute cystitis usually becomes symptomatic after 10–14 days of treatment and results in dysuria, increased frequency, urgency, hesitancy, and increased nocturia (Moore-Higgs, 2007).

(b) The symptoms usually resolve within one month of completing treatment (Moore-Higgs, 2007).

(c) The normal tissue tolerance to therapeutic irradiation to the bladder is 65–80 Gy (Chopra & Bogart, 2010).

(2) Late effects

(a) Adverse effects usually are secondary to chronic fibrosis and progressive endarteritis in poorly oxygenated submucosal and muscular tissues, with eventual tissue scarring. This is expressed by radiation cystitis, defunctionalized bladder due to scarring, hemorrhagic cystitis due to breakdown of mucosa secondary to loss of supporting submucosal blood supply, ureteral and urethral strictures, and fistulas (Elliott & Malaeb, 2011).

(b) Ureteral stricture and radiation cystitis are the most common urinary complications after RT for cervical cancer (Elliott & Malaeb, 2011).

b) Incidence

(1) Incidence depends on factors related to radiation timing, dose, and volume. Acute symptoms subside within several weeks following RT (Nicolaou, 2003).

(2) Acute symptoms can vary from 23% to 80% among patients receiving pelvic irradiation for a variety of tumors (Maduro, Pras, Willemse, & de Vries, 2003).

(3) Because of the various sites of treatment, doses, and fractionation schedules, late effects to the bladder differ for each patient.

(4) Severe effects include hemorrhagic cystitis, incontinence, fistula, and conditions requiring surgery (Maduro et al., 2003).

(5) Hemorrhagic cystitis occurs in 1%–2% of patients after pelvic radiation.

(6) The risk of cystitis increases as a function of the bladder dose, ranging from 3% for patients receiving 50 Gy or less to 12% in patients receiving at least 80 Gy to the bladder (Moore-Higgs, 2007).

(7) Cervical cancer: Minor grade 1 or 2 urinary tract complications occurred most often during the first three years after treatment. Acute cystitis toxicity (grade 1 and grade 2) was reported in 28% of patients (Ferrero, Martínez, & Maciá, 2009).

(8) Endometrial cancer: Low-grade adverse effects were reported in 11%–16% of the patients. The majority tended to be grade 1. The lower rate of urinary adverse effects after uterine RT compared to cervical RT may be related to differences in follow-up, in anatomic position relative to the ureters, or the lower dose EBRT delivered as adjuvant therapy after hysterectomy rather than high dose of brachytherapy and EBRT used as sole therapy in cervical cancer (Elliott & Malaeb, 2011).

c) Assessment of symptoms (Bickley & Szilagyi, 2009)

(1) Clinical

(a) Symptoms indicative of bladder irritation (i.e., changes from baseline including urinary frequency, dysuria, urgency, nocturia, and hematuria)

(b) Urge incontinence (occurs at the time of sensation of bladder fullness associated with the immediate desire to urinate)

(c) Stress incontinence associated with activity

(d) Obstructive symptoms (e.g., decrease in flow or force of flow, hesitancy)

(2) Physical examination (Bickley & Szilagyi, 2009)

(a) Palpate and percuss abdomen and suprapubic area to assess for bladder distension or tenderness.

(b) As indicated by symptoms (fever, pain, cloudy urine, or hematuria), obtain a urinalysis and urine culture to detect the presence of bacteria and red and white blood cells.

(c) Consider postvoid residual ultrasound of bladder to identify incomplete voiding.

d) Documentation: Elimination alteration (Catlin-Huth et al., 2002)

(1) Urinary frequency/urgency

(a) 0—Normal

(b) 1—Increase in frequency or nocturia up to two times the normal

(c) 2—Increase more than two times the normal but less than hourly

(d) 3—Hourly or more with urgency, requiring catheter

(2) Urinary incontinence
　(a) 0—Absent
　(b) 1—Present

(3) Urinary retention
　(a) 0—Absent
　(b) 1—Present

(4) Dysuria
　(a) 0—None
　(b) 1—Mild symptoms requiring no intervention
　(c) 2—Symptoms relieved with therapy
　(d) 3—Symptoms not relieved despite therapy

(5) Drainage: Rectovaginal fistula
　(a) 0—Absent
　(b) 1—Present

(6) Type of drainage
　(a) Fecal
　(b) Urinary

e) Collaborative management
(1) Acute effects of urinary frequency/dysuria: Interventions for acute effects of urinary symptoms
　(a) Adequate hydration: Instruct the patient to drink one to three liters of fluids per day while decreasing fluid intake in the evening to reduce the incidence of nocturia (Ramphal, 2004).
　(b) Encourage the patient to avoid acidic, alcoholic, or carbonated beverages, spicy foods, caffeine products (e.g., coffee, tea, cola), and chocolates (Moore-Higgs, 2007; Ramphal, 2004).
　(c) Send urine specimen for urinalysis and cultures to rule out infectious processes that may be contributing to symptoms.
　(d) Administer appropriate medication as prescribed.
　　i. Ibuprofen 400–800 mg orally three to four times daily; relieves pain by inhibiting prostaglandin synthesis (Spratto & Woods, 2008)
　　ii. Urinary tract analgesics, such as phenazopyridine hydrochloride, are helpful to control discomfort.
　　iii. Antispasmodics, such as hyoscyamine sulfate or oxybu-

tynin chloride, provide relief from symptoms of dysuria (Moore-Higgs, 2007).
　(e) As a last resort, treatment break may be considered.

(2) Late genitourinary complications
　(a) Persistent irritative voiding symptoms
　(b) Severe late radiation cystitis and hematuria may occur in 3%–5% of patients (Chopra & Bogart, 2010).
　(c) Urethral stricture and bladder neck contracture occur in less than 5% of patients, but the risk increases in patients treated with combined surgery and RT. Treatment with outpatient dilation is generally successful in alleviating symptoms, although repeat dilation may be necessary (Chopra & Bogart, 2010).
　(d) Hyperbaric oxygen therapy has emerged as a potential primary option for the management of hemorrhagic cystitis (Yoshida et al., 2008).

f) Patient and family education (Moore-Higgs, 2007)
(1) Inform the patient and family of the potential for urinary side effects from pelvic irradiation.
(2) Educate the patient and family on the signs and symptoms of UTI and radiation-induced cystitis and instruct to report first sign of symptoms.
(3) Instruct the patient in dietary interventions and promote adequate hydration (Moore-Higgs, 2007).
(4) Reassure the patient as to the availability of medications should symptoms become problematic. Thoroughly review side effect profiles and possible drug interactions with the patient as appropriate.

4. Diarrhea/proctitis (ONS, 2009)
a) Definition of diarrhea: An abnormal increase in the liquidity and frequency of stools
b) Pathophysiology (see section V.E—Gastrointestinal/abdomen)
c) Incidence
(1) Cervical cancer: The small bowel is incidentally irradiated during radiation to the pelvis. Radiation-induced small-bowel mucositis can be expressed as cramping and diarrhea from interference with nutrient absorption, typically

developing one to two weeks after the start of RT. Weight loss can be a secondary consequence (Kavanagh et al., 2010).

(2) Concurrent chemotherapy adds to radiation-induced acute bowel toxicity. In a Gynecological Oncology Group study, patients with cervical cancer who received 45 Gy pelvic RT alone experienced a 5% (9/186) rate of grade 3–4 GI toxicity versus 14% (26/183) with RT plus weekly cisplatin (40 mg/m²) (Kavanagh et al., 2010).

d) Late effects of RT

(1) Effects to the GI tract, including stricture and ulceration, can occur secondary to radiation endarteritis and chronic ischemia (Chopra & Bogart, 2010).

(2) Chronic or late radiation proctitis generally occurs one to two years after undergoing RT and is due to epithelial atrophy and fibrosis associated with the obliterative "endarteritis" seen in other late radiation toxicity syndromes (Chopra & Bogart, 2010).

(3) Changes to the mucosa can include pallor with friability and telangiectasias (Chopra & Bogart, 2010).

e) Assessment of symptoms (see section V.E—Gastrointestinal/abdomen)

f) Documentation

(1) Diarrhea (patient without colostomy) (see section V.E—Gastrointestinal/abdomen)

(2) Diarrhea (patients with colostomy) (see section V.E—Gastrointestinal/abdomen)

(3) Lower GI including pelvis: RTOG Acute Radiation Morbidity Scoring Criteria (RTOG, 2011)

(a) 0—None

(b) 1—Increased frequency or change in quality of bowel habits not requiring medication; rectal discomfort not requiring analgesics

(c) 2—Diarrhea requiring parasympatholytic drugs (e.g., Lomotil); mucous discharge not necessitating sanitary pads; rectal or abdominal pain requiring analgesics

(d) 3—Diarrhea requiring parenteral support; severe mucous or blood discharge necessitating sanitary pads; abdominal distension (flat plate radiograph demonstrates distended bowel loops)

(e) 4—Acute or subacute obstruction, fistula, or perforation; GI bleeding requiring transfusion; abdominal pain or tenesmus requiring tube decompression or bowel diversion

(f) Other factors

i. Documentation of daily weight

ii. Compliance with dietary recommendations and fluid intake: May be helpful to use a daily documentation sheet for dietary intake and bowel pattern such as the Weekly Bowel Pattern Recording Sheet (see Engelking, 2004, p. 551).

(4) Skin sensation (see section IV.C—Skin reactions)

g) Collaborative management (ONS, 2009)

(1) Acute effects of diarrhea (see section V.E—Gastrointestinal/abdomen)

(a) Consultation with dietitian

(b) Dietary guidelines recommended by expert opinion (Muehlbauer, Thorpe, Davis, Drabot, Kiker, et al., 2009)

i. Choose low-fiber, low-residue foods (rice, noodles, Cream of Wheat®, well-cooked eggs, bananas, white toast, canned or cooked fruit without the skin, skinned turkey or chicken, fish, and mashed potatoes).

ii. Avoid insoluble fiber (raw fruit, vegetables, whole-grain bread, nuts, popcorn, skins, seeds, and legumes).

iii. Avoid spicy, greasy, fatty, or fried foods.

iv. Avoid milk products.

v. Avoid alcohol.

vi. Drink plenty of fluids, such as water, diluted cranberry juice, broth, and decaffeinated tea or coffee.

vii. Eat small, frequent meals.

viii. Drink liquids at room temperature.

ix. Increase intake of foods high in sodium and potassium, such as bananas and potatoes.

(c) Medications/pharmacologic interventions

i. Likely to be effective for prevention of radiation-induced diarrhea (Muehlbauer,

Thorpe, Davis, Drabot, Kiker, et al., 2009)
- Psyllium fiber supplements
- Probiotic supplements
  - *Lactobacillus acidophilus*
  - *Lactobacillus rhamnosus*

ii. Initial treatment is anticholinergic medications (see section V.E—Gastrointestinal/abdomen). Oral opiates such as loperamide and diphenoxylate are evidence-based recommendations for practice (Muehlbauer, Thorpe, Davis, Drabot, Kiker, et al., 2009).

iii. Octreotide 100 mcg subcutaneously three times daily is likely to be effective (Muehlbauer, Thorpe, Davis, Drabot, Kiker, et al., 2009).

iv. The value of a registered dietitian on the team cannot be overstated. A registered dietitian can make recommendations that could help alleviate diarrhea, decrease dehydration, and maintain nutritional status (Muehlbauer, Thorpe, Davis, Drabot, Rawlings, et al., 2009).

v. Other interventions
- Eliminating sorbitol-containing substances, such as sugar-free gums and sugar-free candies, may help to diminish diarrhea.
- Encouraging intake of oral rehydration solutions, such as sports drinks, also assists with rehydration and electrolyte repletion (Muehlbauer, Thorpe, Davis, Drabot, Rawlings, et al., 2009).

vi. Note what is unlikely to be of benefit and what not to use based on evidence from Muehlbauer, Thorpe, Davis, Drabot, Kiker, et al. (2009).

(2) Frequency and surgical management of chronic complications related to pelvic radiation: Twenty-five patients had received RT for colorectal carcinoma, 10 for prostate cancer, 7 for carcinoma of the cervix, and 6 other tumors. Patients presented with one or more complications, including radiation

enteritis (60%), strictures (53%), fistulae (17%), nonhealing wounds (15%), and de novo cancers in the irradiated fields (10%). Low anastomotic strictures (10%) were initially treated with dilation under sedation. Six patients (12%) ultimately required permanent diversion. All radiation-induced fistulae required an operation (Turina, Mulhall, Mahid, Yashar, & Galandiuk, 2008).

h) Patient and family education (see section V.E—Gastrointestinal/abdomen) (ONS, 2009)

(1) Inform the patient that diarrhea is an expected side effect of radiation to the pelvis and usually occurs after 2.5–3 weeks of treatment.

(2) Teach dietary modifications.

(3) Instruct the patient and family in comfort measures (e.g., sitz bath, tepid water cotton cloth soaks).

(4) Explain the protocol for perianal hygiene (mild soap, do not rub, pat dry).

(5) Describe the signs and symptoms of dehydration.

(6) Instruct the patient to keep a log of the number and consistency of bowel movements per day.

(7) Inform the patient and family of medications available to alleviate treatment-related side effects. Thoroughly review side effect profiles and possible drug interactions. Instruct in the appropriate use of any suppositories, foams, ointments, or enemas if prescribed.

(8) Post-treatment late effects: Instruct the patient on reporting symptoms, including changes in stools, rectal bleeding, or pain, at follow-up visits and when to call the physician.

5. Sexual dysfunction (see section IV.F—Sexual dysfunction): Sexuality is an integral part of normal life for most people and is an important aspect of quality of life (Katz, 2005).

a) Pathophysiology

(1) Acute effects

(a) Altered sexual functioning is the most compromised quality-of-life issue after treatment of gynecologic cancers, affecting 40%–100% of patients (Audette & Waterman, 2010).

(b) As the abdominal dose escalates above 1.5 Gy, amenorrhea can occur with ensuing premature menopause (Shell, 2007).

(c) Depletion of estrogens and androgens will cause young women to experience what their older counterparts have already been through, including troublesome hot flashes, mood swings, vaginal thinning, and decreased vaginal lubrication. As a result, dyspareunia often follows, which may influence a decrease in sexual arousal, and intercourse will no longer be pleasurable (Shell, 2007).

(d) As long as a woman is not bleeding heavily from a tumor in her bladder, rectum, uterus, cervix, or vagina, she can usually have sex during pelvic RT. The outer genitals and vagina are just as sensitive as before. Unless intercourse or touching is painful, a woman should still be able to reach orgasm (ACS, 2011).

(2) Late effects

(a) Up to 88% of women treated with pelvic radiation for cervical cancer develop vaginal stenosis as a consequence of therapy (Wolf, 2006).

(b) The only prognostic factor associated with increased risk of stenosis was age greater than 50 years (odds ratio of 2.26). Vaginal stenosis is a common complication of pelvic and vaginal RT, occurring in 38% of patients. Stenosis occurs most often in the first year after treatment (Brand, Bull, & Cakir, 2006).

(c) The vaginal epithelium is affected in a similar manner as the bladder epithelium. The radiation causes thinning and pale atrophic changes over time and may be traumatized by intercourse or masturbation.

(d) Women treated with abdominal pelvic irradiation have an increased rate of uterine dysfunction lending to miscarriage, preterm labor, low-birth-weight infants, and placental abnormalities (Wo & Viswanathan, 2009).

(e) Early menopause results from low-dose ovarian radiation. Ovarian transposition may decrease the rates of ovarian dysfunction (Wo & Viswanathan, 2009).

b) Incidence

(1) The prevention or treatment of sexual morbidity may improve psychological adjustment and quality of life in patients with gynecologic cancer receiving treatment with hysterectomy, chemotherapy, or RT (Levin et al., 2010).

(2) Women report a wide variety of symptoms after treatment for cervical cancer. One-third of women report severe symptoms related to the vagina, including it feeling narrow, tighter, shorter, or smaller; decreased sexual desire; feeling less feminine or desirable; less frequent intercourse; loss of vaginal lubrication with intercourse; and inability to achieve orgasm (Tornatta, Carpenter, Schilder, & Cardenes, 2009).

(3) Cervical cancer: Vaginal stenosis is a common complication of pelvic and vaginal RT, occurring in 38% of patients. Stenosis occurs most often in the first year after treatment, with patients older than age 50 being most at risk (Brand et al., 2006).

(4) A study of the patterns of long-term survival suggested that nurses play a key role in responding to cervical cancer survivors' unique experiences with illness and recovery. Clinicians must use a variety of interview probes and evidence-based psychosocial and educational approaches to assist patients in their journey (Clemmens, Knafl, Lev, & McCorkle, 2008).

(a) Clinicians need to use direct questions regarding vaginal symptoms. Most patients may not initiate conversation related to this sensitive topic (Tornatta et al., 2009).

(b) The PLISSIT (**P**ermission, **L**imited **I**nformation, **S**pecific **S**uggestions, and **I**ntensive **T**herapy) model provides nurses and other healthcare providers with a framework for intervention to address

patients' psychosexual concerns (Smith, 2010).

(c) The BETTER model was developed to assist healthcare providers to include sexuality assessment in the care of patients with cancer. It is similar to the PLISSIT model in that the first level of intervention involves bringing up the topic (B). The second level involves explaining (E) that sexuality is part of quality of life, and patients should be aware that they can talk about this with the care team. Care providers should then tell (T) the patient that appropriate resources will be found to address their concerns, and that although the timing (T) may not be appropriate now, they can ask for information at any time. Patients should be educated (E) about the sexual side effects of their treatment, and finally, a record (R) should be made in the patient's medical record to report that this topic has been discussed (Katz, 2005).

(d) Show genuine interest and concern by looking at the patient and avoiding facial or verbal expressions despite what the patient tells you. Maintain a nonjudgmental attitude (Hughes, 2009).

(e) Ask open-ended questions such as: "How have things been going sexually?" and "What sexual changes have you noticed?"(Hughes, 2009).

(5) Endometrial cancer: The incidence of grade 2–3 or symptomatic vaginal toxicity was 14% in a retrospective chart review of patients with histologically confirmed endometrial cancer who underwent hysterectomy and bilateral salpingo-oophorectomy with or without lymph node dissection and adjuvant intravaginal brachytherapy between 1995 and 2009 at the Hospital of the University of Pennsylvania (Bahng, Dagan, Brunner, & Lin, 2011).

c) Assessment of symptoms

(1) Risk factors

(a) Sexual dysfunction needs to be assessed prior to the start of radiation because it may lead to a greater risk for sexual problems after therapy.

(b) Preradiation surgical interventions influence the risk of sexual dysfunction.

(2) Clinical examination

(a) Questionnaires can be used to assess topics such as sexual behavior or sexual arousal. The following areas can be briefly surveyed during a discussion with a patient: Marital status and availability of current sexual partner(s); frequency of sexual activity; presence of female sexual dysfunction (e.g., lack of desire, orgasmic difficulties); and presence of sexual dysfunction in the partner (e.g., premature ejaculation, erectile difficulties) (Women's Health and Education Center, 2009).

(b) Survivorship initiatives are now a critical focus for many cancer institutions and governmental organizations. These programs formulate comprehensive treatment plans for cancer survivors and promote research in this area. Posttreatment resources and sexual health programs are integral parts of these survivorship initiatives (Women's Health and Education Center, 2009).

(c) Sexual history is very important. Never make assumptions that patients are too old or too young to be sexually active. Create a climate that is conducive to confidentiality and trust. Maintain a nonjudgmental attitude (Hughes, 2009).

(3) Physical examination

(a) Check external genitalia and perineum for skin changes over vulva and around anus for lesions, inflammation, or skin breakdown.

(b) Examine the patient for vaginal stenosis.

(c) Check for vaginal discharge or vaginal bleeding.

(4) Psychological examination

(a) History of sexual abuse

(b) Body image: Radiation will cause either temporary or permanent gonadal failure as well as changes in body image. Scars from surgery and weight loss during chemotherapy and RT affect body image. It is common for women to avoid appearing naked in front of a partner, which can lead to distance between them (Katz, 2009).

d) Collaborative management (Hughes, 2009; Katz, 2005, 2009; Sadovsky et al., 2010)

(1) Acute effects (see section IV.F—Sexual dysfunction)

   (a) Prepare the patient for the acute effects that RT will cause to sexual function.

     i. Support the patient on concerns of sexual dysfunction.

     ii. Encourage open communication between the patient and partner. The most difficult aspect of discussing sexuality with patients is getting started. A simple question such as "How are things going sexually?" can be all it takes to initiate a conversation that can be a very positive influence on the patient's postdiagnosis sexual relationships (Hughes, 2009).

     iii. Refer patients with history of sexual abuse or marital problems to a social worker, family counselor, or sex therapist (Hughes, 2009; Sadovsky et al., 2010).

   (b) Educate the patient in the use of pain medication prior to sexual activity to help manage symptoms (e.g., pain) before engaging in activity. Teach proper positioning for continued sexual activity to prevent discomfort, depending on therapy or problem (Audette & Waterman, 2010).

   (c) RT can cause vaginal dryness and vaginal stenosis. The use of vaginal dilators and lubricants can improve these symptoms (Katz, 2009).

(2) Long-term effects (see section IV.F—Sexual dysfunction)

   (a) Vaginal stenosis: To maintain patency of the vagina, women are recommended to perform regular vaginal dilation. The patient should be taught the use of vaginal dilator to be used three times per week because it will be necessary to have continued cancer surveillance vaginal examinations (Audette & Waterman, 2010).

   (b) Lack of vaginal lubrication: Educate the patient on the use of vaginal lubricants. Two kinds of lubricants are water based and silicone based. Oil-based products are not recommended.

     i. Water-based lubricants are easiest to find, usually in drug stores or supermarkets. They tend to dry out more quickly and need to be reapplied or reactivated with the addition of water. Many contain glycerin and may predispose patients to vaginal yeast infections (Katz, 2009).

       • K-Y® Jelly (Johnson & Johnson)

       • Astroglide® (Biofilm, Inc.), which has the ability to remain slick for an extended period of time

       • Replens® (Lil' Drug Store Products, Inc.)

     ii. Silicone-based lubricants are available through online retailers or in sex stores. These are not absorbed into the tissue and sit on top of the mucous membranes and therefore remain slick for a long time. Any excess must be removed with soap and water.

e) Documentation (Catlin-Huth et al., 2002)

(1) Sexuality alteration (see section IV.F—Sexual dysfunction)

(2) Mucous membrane alteration

   (a) Drainage

     i. 0—Absent

     ii. 1—Present

   (b) Drainage odor

     i. 0—Absent

     ii. 1—Present

   (c) Vaginal bleeding

     i. 0—None

     ii. 1—Spotting requiring two pads per day

     iii. 2—Requiring two or more pads every day but not requiring transfusion

     iv. 3—Requiring transfusion

     v. 4—Catastrophic bleeding, requiring major nonelective intervention

f) Patient and family education (Audette & Waterman, 2010; Hughes, 2009; Katz, 2009)

(1) Sexual issues must be incorporated into the general discussion of side effects of treatment, rather than being raised as a separate issue, to reduce any embar-

rassment while providing permission for the women to raise sexual issues in future discussions (Hughes, 2009; Katz, 2005, 2009).

(2) The patient and partner should be able to verbalize a good understanding of the potential impact of pelvic irradiation on sexual function.

(3) The patient and partner should be made aware of alternative techniques for sexual intercourse to minimize sexual discomfort or dysfunction.

(4) The patient and partner are informed about resuming intercourse and masturbation after therapy.

(5) The patient and partner should inform the nurse or physician of continued sexual dysfunction.

g) Related Web sites

(1) ACS, "Preventing Pain During Sex": www.cancer.org/Treatment/Treatments andSideEffects/PhysicalSideEffects/ SexualSideEffectsinWomen/Sexuality fortheWoman/sexuality-for-women -with-cancer-preventing-pain

(2) ACS, "Sexuality for the Woman With Cancer": www.cancer.org/Treatment/ TreatmentsandSideEffects/Physical SideEffects/SexualSideEffectsin Women/SexualityfortheWoman/index

(3) OncoLink, "Vaginal Dilators for Radiation Therapy": www.oncolink .org/coping/article.cfm?c=4&s=46&ss =95&id=993

References

American Cancer Society. (2011). Cancer facts and figures 2011. Retrieved from http://www.cancer.org/Research/CancerFactsFigures/CancerFactsFigures/cancer-facts-figures-2011

American Cancer Society. (2011). Sex and pelvic radiation. Retrieved from http://www.cancer.org/Treatment/TreatmentsandSideEffects/PhysicalSideEffects/SexualSideEffectsinWomen/SexualityfortheWoman/sexuality-for-women-with-cancer-pelvic-rad

Audette, C., & Waterman, J. (2010). The sexual health of women after gynecologic malignancy. *Journal of Midwifery and Women's Health, 55,* 357–362. doi:10.1016/j.jmwh.2009.10.016

Azria, D., Betz, M., Bourgier, C., Sozzi, W.J., & Ozsahin, M. (2010). Identifying patients at risk for late radiation-induced toxicity. *Critical Reviews in Oncology/Hematology.* Advance online publication. doi:10.1016/j.critrevonc.2010.08.003

Bahng, A.Y., Dagan, A., Bruner, D.W., & Lin, L.L. (2011). Determination of prognostic factors for vaginal mucosal toxicity associated with intravaginal high-dose rate brachytherapy in patients with endometrial cancer. *International Journal of Radiation Oncology, Biology, Physics.* Advance online publication. doi:10.1016/j.ijrobp.2010.10.071

Bickley, L.S., & Szilagyi, P.G. (2009). *Guide to physical examination and history taking* (10th ed., pp. 427–428). Philadelphia, PA: Lippincott Williams & Wilkins.

Brand, A.H., Bull, C.A., & Cakir, B. (2006). Vaginal stenosis in patients treated with radiotherapy for carcinoma of the cervix. *International Journal of Gynecological Cancer, 16,* 288–293. doi:10.1111/j.1525-1438.2006.00348.x

Catlin-Huth, C., Haas, M., & Pollock, V. (Eds.). (2002). *Radiation therapy patient care record: A tool for documenting nursing care.* Pittsburgh, PA: Oncology Nursing Society.

Chopra, R.R., & Bogart, J.A. (2010). Radiation therapy-related toxicity (including pneumonitis and fibrosis). *Hematology/Oncology Clinics of North America, 24,* 625–642. doi:10.1016/j.hoc.2010.03.009

Clemmens, D.A., Knafl, K., Lev, E.L., & McCorkle, R. (2008). Cervical cancer: Patterns of long-term survival. *Oncology Nursing Forum, 30,* 897–903. doi:10.1188/08.ONF.897-903

Elliott, S.P., & Maleab, B.S. (2011). Long-term urinary adverse effects of pelvic radiotherapy. *World Journal of Urology, 29,* 35–41. doi:10.1007/s00345-010-0603-x

Engelking, C. (2004). Diarrhea. In C.H. Yarbro, M.H. Frogge, & M. Goodman (Eds.), *Cancer symptom management* (3rd ed., pp. 528–558). Sudbury, MA: Jones and Bartlett.

Ferrero, V.T, Martínez, F.J.A., & Maciá, R.C. (2009). Evaluation of toxicity of surgery and/or chemoirradiation treatment of uterine cervix cancer. *Clinical and Translational Oncology, 11,* 109–113.

Hughes, M.K. (2009). Sexuality and cancer: The final frontier for nurses [Online exclusive]. *Oncology Nursing Forum, 36,* E241–E246. doi:10.1188/09.ONF.E241-E246

Katz, A. (2005). The sounds of silence: Sexuality information for cancer patients. *Journal of Clinical Oncology, 23,* 238–241. doi:10.1200/JCO.2005.05.101

Katz, A. (2009). *Woman cancer sex.* Pittsburgh, PA: Oncology Nursing Society.

Kavanagh, B.D., Pan, C.C., Dawson, L.A., Das, S.K., Li, X.A., Ten Haken, R.K., & Miften, M. (2010). Radiation dose-volume effects in the stomach and small bowel. *International Journal of Radiation Oncology, Biology, Physics, 76*(Suppl. 3), S101–S107. doi:10.1016/j.ijrobp.2009.05.071

Levin, A.O., Carpenter, K.M., Fowler, J.M., Brothers, B.M., Andersen, B.L., & Maxwell, G.L. (2010). Sexual morbidity associated with poorer psychological adjustment among gynecological cancer survivors. *International Journal of Gynecological Cancer, 20,* 461–470. doi:10.1111/IGC.0b013e3181d24ce0

Maduro, J.H., Pras, E., Willemse, P.H.B., & de Vries, E.G.E. (2003). Acute and long-term toxicity following radiotherapy alone or in combination with chemotherapy for locally advanced cervical cancer. *Cancer Treatment Reviews, 29,* 471–488. doi:10.1016/S0305-7372(03)00117-8

Mayo Clinic. (2010). Prednisone and other corticosteroids: Balance the risk and benefits. Retrieved from http://www.mayoclinic.com/health/steroids/HQ01431

McQuestion, M. (2011). Evidence-based skin care management in radiation therapy: Clinical update. *Seminars in Oncology Nursing, 27*(2), e1–e17. doi:10.1016/j.soncn.2011.02.009

Moore-Higgs, G. (2007). Gynecologic cancers. In M.L. Haas, W.P. Hogle, G.J. Moore-Higgs, & T.K. Gosselin-Acomb (Eds.), *Radiation therapy: A guide to patient care* (pp. 207–233). St. Louis, MO: Mosby.

Muehlbauer, P.M., Thorpe, D., Davis, A.B., Drabot, R.C., Kiker, E.S., & Rawlings, B.L. (2009). ONS PEP resource: Diarrhea. In L.H. Eaton & J.M. Tipton (Eds.), *Putting evidence into practice: Improving oncology patient outcomes* (pp. 125–134). Pittsburgh, PA: Oncology Nursing Society.

Muehlbauer, P.M., Thorpe, D., Davis, A.B., Drabot, R.C., Rawlings, B.L., & Kiker, E.S. (2009). Putting evidence into practice:

Evidence-based interventions to prevent, manage, and treat che-motherapy- and radiotherapy-induced diarrhea. *Clinical Journal of Oncology Nursing, 13,* 336–341. doi:10.1188/09.CJON.336-341

Nicolaou, N. (2003). Prevention and management of radiation toxicity. In R. Pazdur, L. Coia, W. Hoskins, & L. Wagman (Eds.), *Cancer management: A multidisciplinary approach* (7th ed., pp. 909–939). New York, NY: Oncology Group.

Oncology Nursing Society. (2009). ONS PEP: Diarrhea. Retrieved from http://www.ons.org/Research/PEP/Diarrhea

Oncology Nursing Society. (2010). ONS PEP: Radiodermatitis expert opinion table. Retrieved from http://www.ons.org/Research/PEP/media/ons/docs/research/outcomes/radiodermatitis/expert opiniontable.pdf

Radiation Therapy Oncology Group. (2011). Acute radiation morbidity scoring criteria. Retrieved from http://www.rtog.org/Research Associates/AdverseEventReporting/AcuteRadiationMorbidity ScoringCriteria.aspx

Ramphal, S.R. (2004). A clinical approach to dysuria in women. *Continuing Medical Education, 22,* 66–70.

Sadovsky, R., Basson, R., Krychman, M., Morales, A.M., Schover, L., Wang, R., & Incrocci, L. (2010). Cancer and sexual problems. *Journal of Sexual Medicine, 7,* 349–373. doi:10.1111/j.1743 -6109.2009.01620.x

Shell, J. (2007). Sexuality and sexual dysfunction. In M.L. Haas, W.P. Hogle, G.J. Moore-Higgs, & T.K. Gosselin-Acomb (Eds.), *Radiation therapy: A guide to patient care* (pp. 609–626). St. Louis, MO: Mosby.

Smith, L.E. (2010). Sexual function of the gynecologic cancer survivor. *Oncology, 24*(Suppl. 10), 41–44.

Sparks, S. (2007). Radiodermatitis. In M.L. Haas, W.P. Hogle, G.J. Moore-Higgs, & T.K. Gosselin-Acomb (Eds.), *Radiation therapy: A guide to patient care* (pp. 511–522). St. Louis, MO: Mosby.

Spratto, G.R., & Woods, A.L. (2008). *PDR nurse's drug handbook.* Montvale, NJ: Thomson Reuters.

Tornatta, J.M., Carpenter, J.S., Schilder, J., & Cardenes, H.R. (2009). Representations of vaginal symptoms in cervical cancer survivors. *Cancer Nursing, 32,* 378–384. doi:10.1097/ NCC.0b013e3181a54c39

Turina, M., Mulhall, A.M., Mahid, S.S., Yashar, C., & Galandiuk, S. (2008). Frequency and surgical management of chronic complications related to pelvic radiation. *Archives of Surgery, 143,* 46–52. doi:0.1001/archsurg.2007.7

Vale, C., Nightingale, A., Spera, N., Whelan, A., Hanley, B., & Tierney, J.F. (2010). Late complications from chemoradiotherapy for cervical cancer: Reflections from cervical cancer survivors 10 years after the National Cancer Institute alert. *Clinical Oncology, 22,* 588–589. doi:10.1016/j.clon.2010.05.017

Wo, J.Y., & Viswanathan, A.N. (2009). The impact of radiotherapy on fertility, pregnancy, and neonatal outcomes of female cancer patients. *International Journal of Radiation Oncology, Biology, Physics, 73,* 1304–1312. doi:10.1016/j.ijrobp.2008.12.016

Wolf, J.K. (2006). Prevention and treatment of vaginal stenosis resulting from pelvic radiation therapy. *Community Oncology, 3,* 665–668.

Women's Health and Education Center. (2009). Cancer, sexual health and intimacy. Retrieved from http://www.womenshealthsection. com/content/gyno/gyno014.php3

Yoshida, T., Kawashima, A., Ujike, T., Uemura, M., Nishimura, K., & Miyoshi, S. (2008) Hyperbaric oxygen therapy for radiation-induced hemorrhagic cystitis. *International Journal of Urology, 15,* 639–641. doi:10.1111/j.1442-2042.2008.02053.x

I. Bone metastases
1. Introduction: The management of bone metastases has changed considerably in the past decade, resulting in improved longevity for patients with cancer (Biermann, Holt, Lewis, Schwartz, & Yaszemski, 2009).
   a) Bone metastases may occur by three main mechanisms.
      (1) Direct extension
      (2) Retrograde venous flow: Retrograde venous embolism is believed to be the major mechanism by which intra-abdominal cancers spread to the vertebrae. Intra-abdominal pressure increases, causing blood to be diverted from the systemic caval system to the valveless vertebral plexus of Batson, allowing the caudal and cranial flow of blood (Galasko, 1981).
      (3) Seeding with tumor emboli via the blood circulation (Coleman, 2006). Bone marrow is the initial site of seeding.
   b) When a metastatic lesion grows in the medullary cavity, the surrounding bone is remodeled by either osteoclastic or osteoblastic processes (Clines & Guise, 2008).
      (1) The extent of the resulting bone resorption or deposition is highly variable and depends on the type and location of the tumor.
      (2) Osteoclastic and osteoblastic remodeling processes determine whether a predominantly lytic, sclerotic, or mixed pattern results (Clines & Guise, 2008).
   c) Nearly any primary cancer in the body can metastasize to bone; cancers commonly associated with bone metastases are breast, lung, and prostate (Lutz et al., 2011).
2. RT is a major tool in the management of metastatic cancer to the bone (Lutz et al., 2011).
   a) Radiation typically is delivered in 1–10 daily fractions (Saarto, Janes, Tenhunen, & Kouri, 2002).
   b) The location of the metastasis will determine the dose and overall treatment time.
      (1) When a metastatic lesion is close to very radiosensitive tissue, such as the small bowel, small daily doses in multiple fractions are used. This exploits the key weakness of tumor cells because they cannot repair radiation damage as well as healthy cells (Lutz et al., 2011). In addition, using low daily radiation doses results in minimal impact on normal tissues but lethal impact on cancer cells.

(2) Conversely, when the metastasis is within an area containing radioresistant normal tissues, such as muscle, then a large single dose of radiation may be given (Roodman, 2004).

   (a) Little evidence exists of clinical superiority between a single fraction of 8 Gy and multiple daily fractions to a total dose of up to 30 Gy (McKee, 2005).

   (b) However, a meta-analysis of 11 trials cautioned that although single- and multiple-fraction courses had similar rates of pain relief in patients with metastatic bone lesions, both the incidence of subsequent fracturing and the need to re-treat were higher in patients receiving a single treatment (Sze, Shelley, Held, & Mason, 2008).

3. Indications

  a) Pain and spinal cord compression are the most common reasons for referral for palliative RT (Fairchild et al., 2009).

    (1) Appropriate diagnostic imaging is important to determine the treatment strategy. Imaging can include plain films, CT scans, and MRI (Abrahm, 2004). This is particularly important in spinal lesions where the status of the spinal cord may need to be evaluated.

    (2) The Revised Evaluation System for the Prognosis of Metastatic Spine Tumors, a scoring system to determine the prognosis of tumors that have spread to the spine, can be calculated for the patient with spinal metastasis causing cord compression by evaluating the tumor type, interval between tumor diagnosis and spinal cord compression, other bone or visceral metastases, ambulatory status, and duration of motor deficits (Biermann et al., 2009; Tokuhashi, Matsuzaki, Oda, Oshima,

& Ryu, 2005). Those with higher scores have a longer survival and improved spinal cord function after surgical intervention.

    (3) Patients may be initially referred for spinal surgery rather than RT (Putz, Wiedenhöfer, Gerner, & Fürstenberg, 2008). When cord effacement or compression is noted on MRI or CT, patients have better outcomes if initially managed with surgical decompression and fixation followed by RT (Bilsky, Laufer, & Burch, 2009).

  b) Prevention of fracture

    (1) Skeletal metastases are predominantly lytic or blastic (sclerotic). In some patients, especially those with prostate cancer, these tend to be predominantly blastic (sclerotic) (Schuettpelz & Link, 2011).

    (2) Lytic lesions generally are associated with increased morbidity and reduction in survival (Coleman, 2006).

    (3) Pain, hypercalcemia, pathologic fractures, spinal cord compression, and bone marrow suppression can result (Coleman, 2006).

    (4) Metastases within weight-bearing sites, such as the vertebrae and the hip joints, and in areas susceptible to fracture, such as the proximal or mid-humerus and mid-femur, often are treated with RT without the presence of symptoms such as pain.

    (5) These lesions typically are identified through imaging such as bone scans. A multidisciplinary approach is advantageous with the expertise of an orthopedic or neurosurgeon.

    (6) Some patients with impending fracture, or those deemed to be at high risk for a fracture, may be managed by surgical fixation or use of a novel approach such as vertebroplasty, a surgical procedure that provides stability to an unstable spine, relieving pain and delaying spinal cord compression (Tancioni et al., 2011).

    (7) Some RT centers have "virtual consultation" services available and an immediate opinion can be obtained from a colleague at another location (Grabarz et al., 2006). The potential benefits to the patient can include rapid referrals and intervention.

  c) Pathologic fractures—prefixation/postfixation

(1) Certain sites are at significant risk for fracture caused by local bone destruction exacerbated by weight bearing.

(2) Patients may be asymptomatic prior to the actual break or collapse.

(3) Clinical loss of function may be major; however, local symptoms are sometimes muted and a history of significant trauma is absent.

(4) The diagnosis of impending pathologic fracture is made following an evaluation on the basis of a high index of suspicion by the clinical staff.

(5) The fractures are managed surgically in an effort to improve medium-term quality of life and independence.

(6) In the majority of cases, internal fixation is preferred where technically feasible (Shiue et al., 2010). Following internal fixation, the patient often is referred for postoperative RT.

(7) RT is started in approximately four to five weeks, or as soon as the sutures are removed and the wound has healed.

(8) Postoperative radiation dosages are similar to the dosages used for patients who do not undergo internal fixation of the fracture (a single fraction of 8 Gy or a short course of 10 daily fractions totaling 30 Gy).

4. Documentation
   a) During the initial clinical assessment, the clinician must document careful evaluation of pain (location, intensity, character, analgesic use) and loss of function (motor, sensory, ambulation).
   b) The American Spinal Injury Association developed a classification for spinal cord injuries, adapted from the Frankel scale, to standardize the classification of spinal cord injuries (Abrahm, 2004; American Spinal Injury Association, 2011). Patients are segregated into five categories: A, B, C, D, and E (see Figure 20).
   c) The Edmonton Symptom Assessment System is a tool for screening multiple symptoms such as pain, fatigue, and anxiety and is used initially at consultation and following any intervention (Bruera, Kuehn, Miller, Selmser, & Macmillan, 1991).
   d) Post-treatment documentation of outcomes allows healthcare providers to determine outcomes and improve patient care.

5. RT techniques
   a) EBRT is the mainstay of treatment.
   b) Many RT centers provide rapid response programs where the patient can be assessed, undergo simulation and planning, and begin RT on the same day.
   c) Treatments in the past tended to use relatively simple beam arrangement with little attempt to shape the beams in order to better conform to the shape of the target volume other than by using lead blocks.
      (1) Modern conformal delivery methods employ very sophisticated collimation methods to shape each individual beam used in treatment. This results in a much more accurate dose delivery and sparing of the dose-limiting surrounding normal tissues (Jin, Wen, Ren, Glide-Hurst, & Chetty, 2011).
      (2) The need to maximize dose and tissue sparing has resulted in an increased use of sophisticated radiation techniques such as IMRT with or without cone beam guidance (Jin et al., 2011).

Figure 20. American Spinal Injury Association Impairment Scale (AIS) for Classification of Spinal Injuries

A = Complete. No sensory or motor function is preserved in the sacral segments S4–S5.

B = Sensory Incomplete. Sensory but not motor function is preserved below the neurological level and includes the sacral segments S4–S5 (light touch, pin prick at S4–S5: or deep anal pressure [DAP]), AND no motor function is preserved more than three levels below the motor level on either side of the body.

C = Motor Incomplete. Motor function is preserved below the neurological level**, and more than half of key muscle functions below the single neurological level of injury (NLI) have a muscle grade less than 3 (Grades 0–2).

D = Motor Incomplete. Motor function is preserved below the neurological level**, and at least half (half or more) of key muscle functions below the NLI have a muscle grade greater than 3.

E = Normal. If sensation and motor function as tested with the ISNCSCI are graded as normal in all segments, and the patient had prior deficits, then the AIS grade is E. Someone without an initial SCI does not receive an AIS grade.

** For individuals to receive a grade of C or D (i.e., motor incomplete status), they must have either (1) voluntary anal sphincter contraction or (2) sacral sensory sparing with sparing of motor function more than three levels below the motor level for that side of the body. The Standards at this time allow even non-key muscle function more than three levels below the motor level to be used in determining motor incomplete status (AIS B versus C).

Note: When assessing the extent of motor sparing below the level for distinguishing between AIS B and C, the *motor level* on each side is used; whereas to differentiate between AIS C and D (based on proportion of key muscle functions with strength grade 3 or greater), the *single neurological level* is used.

ISNCSCI—International Standards for the Neurological Classification of Spinal Cord Injury

Note. From "International Standards for Neurological Classification of Spinal Cord Injury," by American Spinal Injury Association, 2011. Retrieved from http://www.asia-spinalinjury.org/publications/59544_sc_Exam_Sheet_r4.pdf. Copyright 2011 by American Spinal Injury Association. Reprinted with permission.

d) Stereotactic RT may be used and involves the use of high doses of radiation typically given in one to three fractions. The dose is precisely delivered with minimal scatter to surrounding normal tissue, such as the spinal cord if a vertebral metastasis is being targeted (Haley & Gerszten, 2009; Sahgal et al., 2009; Sahgal, Larson, & Chang, 2008).

e) Patients may be referred for possible repeat treatments if symptoms return or radiologic evidence suggests recurrence (Jeremic, Shibamoto, & Igrutinovic, 2002).

f) Fractionation: A course of treatment may range from 800 cGy (8 Gy) in 1 fraction to 3,000 cGy (30 Gy) in 10 daily fractions. Little evidence supports the use of the different treatment schedules (Fairchild et al., 2009).

g) Hemibody irradiation and radiopharmaceuticals

(1) For multiple bone metastases, hemibody radiation or injected radioisotopes or radiopharmaceuticals may be used.

(2) Hemibody RT is usually prescribed for the lower body (pelvis and femora) employing a single fraction of 8 Gy. A phase II trial from Denmark reported significant pain reduction in 76% of 37 patients, almost all of whom had widespread metastatic prostate cancer (Berg et al., 2009). One-third of patients experienced grade 1–2 diarrhea peaking about two weeks after treatment.

(3) ^{89}Sr, rhenium-186, and ^{153}Sm are radiopharmaceuticals used to treat widespread bone metastases. Their indications and use, either alone or in combination with bisphosphonates, have been reported as likely to be effective (Aiello-Laws, Ameringer, Delzer, Peterson, & Reynolds, 2009; Paes & Serafini, 2010). Patients need to continue taking analgesics, as it may take two to three weeks for a response (Aiello-Laws et al., 2009). Adverse effects such as leukocytopenia and thrombocytopenia may occur (Aiello-Laws et al., 2009). Paes and Serafini (2010) argued that with the inception of the newer isotopes such as ^{186}Re and its reduced side effect profile, systemic radiopharmaceuticals should be the preferred adjunctive therapy for pain palliation in patients with extensive osseous metastases.

h) Outcomes: Although a number of reports have suggested symptom benefits for patients receiving palliative RT, few address or claim a survival benefit (McKee, 2005). A large, single-institution study involving 350 patients identified several patient factors associated with longer-term survival: Single or few metastases, the absence of prior chemotherapy, good performance status (Eastern Cooperative Oncology Group score lower than 3), the absence of visceral or cerebral metastases, and the site of origin (Katagiri et al., 2005).

6. Bisphosphonates

a) Many patients, particularly those with lytic bone metastases from prostate and breast primaries, may already be taking bisphosphonates.

b) These drugs are known to be potent inhibitors of osteoclast-mediated bone resorption with clinical utility in the treatment of osteolytic bone metastases (Vallet, Smith, & Raje, 2010).

c) They exhibit direct antitumor activity in vitro and can reduce the skeletal tumor burden in vivo. However, their precise mode of activity remains unclear (Vallet et al., 2010).

7. Side effects

a) Early RT side effects occur during treatment or approximately a week after treatment ends (e.g., mucositis, bone pain flare). Early effects are uncomfortable but reversible.

b) Late RT side effects typically occur three to six months or later after treatment and can include spinal cord demyelinization, stricture formation, and scarring. Late effects are potentially permanent and may require intervention (Berg et al., 2009).

c) The low doses associated with palliative RT tend to have some early and few late normal tissue effects.

d) Extremity (appendicular skeleton) metastases rarely involve the distal appendicular skeleton (beyond the elbow or knee) (Leeson, Makley, & Carter, 1986).

(1) Assessments include pain related to bone pain flare (pain worsens initially from patient's baseline and improves after a few days), erythema, or tenderness or dryness of skin.

(2) Documentation: Pain score (improved or worsened), palliating factors, condition of skin, and education provided to patient and family

(3) Collaborative management: Use of analgesics including NSAIDs, opiates,

and dexamethasone for bone pain flare (Hird et al., 2009). If opiates are used for pain management, a bowel program is likely to be effective (Bisanz et al., 2009).

(4) Patient and family education: Pain management, bowel program, skin care

e) Spine (axial skeleton): Many patients will have multiple sites of involvement within the axial skeleton; not all cause pain.

(1) Cervical spine: Laryngitis or pharyngitis

(a) Assessment: Pain and itchiness in throat, sensation of lump in throat or that throat is closing, oral and pharyngeal assessment for stomatitis and infection, erythema or tenderness of skin, and nutritional status

(b) Documentation
   i. Symptom assessment and use of and efficacy of interventions
   ii. Interventions and patient education provided regarding appropriate foods such as those that are soft and easy to chew and swallow
   iii. Pain management, bowel program, and nutritional status

(c) Collaborative management: Patients on long-acting opiates should continue on usual dosing (baseline) but may increase breakthrough doses as necessary to control pain and prevent opiate toxicity. Dexamethasone may be used for bone flare pain. Analgesics (liquid form if available or crushed if allowed) can facilitate swallowing, and lozenges and anesthetic medications can soothe the throat. Consult with dietitian for nutritional assessment and management. Manage oral or pharyngeal infections.

(d) Patient and family education
   i. Pain management, nutrition, and skin care
   ii. Instruct the patient that if new or worsening back pain occurs, especially when lying down, coughing, sneezing, or moving, to notify the medical team immediately or report to nearest emergency department.

(2) Thoracic spine: Cough, esophagitis, or nausea

(a) Assessment: Pain, presence of erythema or itchiness of skin, and cough, which may be related to irritation of the lungs from RT. Evaluate for infection, pneumonia, esophagitis, difficulty swallowing, sensation of lump in throat, and nausea and vomiting. Assess nutritional status.

(b) Documentation: Presence of any radiation-related side effects and education provided. Include the interventions used and their efficacy.

(c) Collaborative management: Patients on long-acting opiates should continue on usual dosing (baseline) but may increase breakthrough doses as necessary to control pain and prevent opiate toxicity. Dexamethasone may be used for bone flare pain. Analgesic mouthwashes are helpful for esophagitis or mucositis. Consume soft foods, and avoid extremes in temperature in foods and fluids. Obtain dietary consult for nutritional management. Use expectorants as needed. Treat infections and pneumonia. Antiemetics such as prochlorperazine, granisetron, or ondansetron may be used to promote comfort.

(d) Patient and family education
   i. Management of pain, esophagitis, cough, and nausea
   ii. Nutritional care
   iii. If new or worsening back pain occurs, especially when lying down, coughing, sneezing, or moving, notify the medical team immediately or report to nearest emergency department.

(3) Lumbar spine: Nausea, vomiting, or diarrhea

(a) Assessment: Bone pain flare, nausea, vomiting, diarrhea, and skin reaction

(b) Documentation: Pain assessment; presence and severity of nausea, vomiting, and diarrhea; condition of skin; education provided regarding skin care; and appropriate use of analgesics, antiemetics, and antidiarrheal medications

(c) Collaborative management

    i. Pain management: Patients on long-acting opiates should continue on usual dosing (baseline) but may increase breakthrough doses as necessary to control pain and prevent opiate toxicity. Dexamethasone may be used for bone flare pain and also may be used as an antiemetic.

    ii. Antiemetics such as prochlorperazine, granisetron, or ondansetron may be used to promote comfort.

    iii. For diarrhea, rule out a bowel infection. If no infection is present, antidiarrheal medications such as loperamide (Imodium® A-D, McNeil-PPC, Inc.) (or its equivalent) may be used if diarrhea persists. In this population, diarrhea is rarely an issue because of constipation from opiate usage.

(d) Patient and family education

    i. Management of pain, nausea and vomiting, and diarrhea

    ii. Nutritional care

    iii. Instruct the patient that if new or worsening back pain occurs, especially when lying down, coughing, sneezing, or moving, to notify the medical team immediately or report to nearest emergency department.

8. Psychosocial support in this population is important. Patients and families have concerns about progression of disease, fear of impending death, and fear that their pain cannot be adequately controlled. It is imperative to address their concerns in a caring manner.

References

Abrahm, J.L. (2004). Assessment and treatment of patients with malignant spinal cord compression. *Journal of Supportive Oncology, 2,* 377–388, 391.

Aiello-Laws, L.B., Ameringer, S.W., Delzer, N.A., Peterson, M.E., & Reynolds, J.K. (2009). ONS PEP resource: Pain. In L.H. Eaton & J.M. Tipton (Eds.), *Putting evidence into practice: Improving oncology patient outcomes* (pp. 223–234). Pittsburgh, PA: Oncology Nursing Society.

American Spinal Injury Association. (2011). International standards for neurological classification of spinal cord injury. Retrieved from http://www.asia-spinalinjury.org/publications/59544_sc_Exam_Sheet_r4.pdf

Berg, R.S., Yilmaz, M.K., Høyer, M., Keldsen, N., Nielsen, O.S., & Ewertz, M. (2009). Half body irradiation of patients with multiple bone metastases: A phase II trial. *Acta Oncologica, 48,* 556–561. doi:10.1080/02841860802488128

Biermann, J.S., Holt, G.E., Lewis, V.O., Schwartz, H.S., & Yaszemski, M.J. (2009). Metastatic bone disease: Diagnosis, evaluation, and treatment. *Journal of Bone and Joint Surgery, 91,* 1518–1530.

Bilsky, M.H., Laufer, I., & Burch, S. (2009). Shifting paradigms in the treatment of metastatic spine disease. *Spine, 34*(Suppl. 22), S101–S107. doi:10.1097/BRS.0b013e3181bac4b2

Bisanz, A.K., Woolery, M.J., Lyons, H.F., Gaido, L., Yenulevich, M., & Fulton, S. (2009). ONS PEP resource: Constipation. In L.H. Eaton & J.M. Tipton (Eds.), *Putting evidence into practice: Improving oncology patient outcomes* (pp. 93–104). Pittsburgh, PA: Oncology Nursing Society.

Bruera, E., Kuehn, N., Miller, M.J., Selmser, P., & Macmillan, K. (1991). The Edmonton Symptom Assessment System (ESAS): A simple method for the assessment of palliative care patients. *Journal of Palliative Care, 7*(2), 6–9.

Clines, G.A., & Guise, T.A. (2008). Molecular mechanisms and treatment of bone metastasis. *Expert Reviews in Molecular Medicine, 10,* e7. doi:10.1017/S1462399408000616

Coleman, R.E. (2006). Clinical features of metastatic bone disease and risk of skeletal morbidity. *Clinical Cancer Research, 12,* 6243s–6249s. doi:10.1158/1078-0432.CCR-06-0931

Fairchild, A., Barnes, E., Ghosh, S., Ben-Josef, E., Roos, D., Hartsell, W., … Chow, E. (2009). International patterns of practice in palliative radiotherapy for painful bone metastases: Evidence-based practice? *International Journal of Radiation Oncology, Biology, Physics, 75,* 1501–1510. doi:10.1016/j.ijrobp.2008.12.084

Galasko, C.S.B. (1981). The anatomy and pathways of skeletal metastases. In L. Weiss & H.A. Gilbert (Eds.), *Bone metastasis* (pp. 49–63). Boston, MA: Hall Medical Publishers.

Grabarz, D., Rampersaud, R., Fehlings, M.G., Chung, A.D., Burrows, K., Bezjak, A., & Wong, R.K.S. (2006, October). *The virtual consultation project—Enhancing multidisciplinary care for patients with malignant spinal cord compression (SCC).* Paper presented at the 11th World Congress on Internet in Medicine, Toronto, Ontario, Canada. Retrieved from http://www.mednetcongress.org/fullpapers/MEDNET-54_GrabarzDanielA_e.pdf

Haley, M., & Gerszten, P.C. (2009). Stereotactic radiosurgery in the management of cancer pain. *Current Pain and Headache Reports, 13,* 277–281. doi:10.1007/s11916-009-0044-7

Hird, A., Zhang, L., Holt, T., Fairchild, A., DeAngelis, C., Loblaw, A., … Chow, E. (2009). Dexamethasone for the prophylaxis of radiation-induced pain flare after palliative radiotherapy for symptomatic bone metastases: A phase II study. *Clinical Oncology, 21,* 329–335. doi:10.1016/j.clon.2008.12.010

Jeremic, B., Shibamoto, Y., & Igrutinovic, I. (2002). Second single 4 Gy reirradiation for painful bone metastasis. *Journal of Pain and Symptom Management, 23,* 26–30. doi:10.1016/S0885-3924(01)00366-9

Jin, J.-Y., Wen, N., Ren, L., Glide-Hurst, C., & Chetty, I.J. (2011). Advances in treatment techniques: Arc-based and other intensity modulated therapies. *Cancer Journal, 3,* 166–176. doi:10.1097/PPO.0b013e31821f8318

Katagiri, H., Takahashi, M., Wakai, K., Sugiura, H., Kataoka, T., & Nakanishi, K. (2005). Prognostic factors and a scoring system for patients with skeletal metastasis. *Journal of Bone and Joint Surgery–British Volume, 87-B,* 698–703. doi:10.1302/0301-620X.87B5.15185

Leeson, M.C., Makley, J.T., & Carter, J.R. (1986). Metastatic skeletal disease distal to the elbow and knee. *Clinical Orthopaedics and Related Research, 206,* 94–99.

Lutz, S., Berk, L., Chang, E., Chow, E., Hahn, C., Hoskin, P., … Hartsell, W. (2011). Palliative radiation therapy for bone metastasis: An ASTRO evidence-based guideline. *International Journal of Radiation Oncology, Biology, Physics, 79,* 965–976. doi:10.1016/j.ijrobp.2010.11.026

McKee, L. (2005). Palliative radiotherapy for painful bone metastases, single versus multiple fraction treatment: A literature review. *Canadian Journal of Medical Radiation Technology, 36*(3), 7–16. doi:10.1016/S0820-5930(09)60173-0

Paes, F.M., & Serafini, A.M. (2010). Systemic metabolic radio-pharmaceutical therapy in the treatment of metastatic bone pain. *Seminars in Nuclear Medicine, 40,* 89–104. doi:10.1053/j.semnuclmed.2009.10.003

Putz, C., Wiedenhöfer, B., Gerner, H.J., & Fürstenberg, C.H. (2008). Tokuhashi prognosis score: An important tool in prediction of the neurological outcome in metastatic spinal cord compression: A retrospective clinical study. *Spine, 33,* 2669–2674. doi:10.1097/BRS.0b013e318188b98f

Roodman, G.D. (2004). Mechanisms of bone metastasis. *New England Journal of Medicine, 350,* 1655–1664. doi:10.1056/NEJMra030831

Saarto, T., Janes, R., Tenhunen, M., & Kouri, M. (2002). [Palliative radiotherapy for bone metastases—Single-dose radiotherapy is effective]. *Duodecim, 118,* 1889–1894.

Sahgal, A., Ames, C., Chou, D., Ma, L., Huang, K., Xu, W., … Larson, D.A. (2009). Stereotactic body radiotherapy is effective salvage therapy for patients with prior radiation of spinal metastases. *International Journal of Radiation Oncology, Biology, Physics, 74,* 723–731. doi:10.1016/j.ijrobp.2008.09.020

Sahgal, A., Larson, D.A., & Chang, E.L. (2008). Stereotactic body radiosurgery for spinal metastases: A critical review. *International Journal of Radiation Oncology, Biology, Physics, 71,* 652–665. doi:10.1016/j.ijrobp.2008.02.060

Schuettpelz, L.G., & Link, D.C. (2011). Niche competition and cancer metastasis to bone. *Journal of Clinical Investigation, 121,* 1253–1255. doi:10.1172/JCI57229

Shiue, K., Sahgal, A., Chow, E., Lutz, S.T., Chang, E.L., Mayr, N.A., … Lo, S.S. (2010). Management of metastatic spinal cord compression. *Expert Review of Anticancer Therapy, 10,* 697–708. doi:10.1586/era.10.47

Sze, W.M., Shelley, M., Held, I., & Mason, M. (2008). Palliation of metastatic bone pain: Single fraction versus multifraction radiotherapy. *Cochrane Database of Systematic Reviews* 2002, Issue 1. Art. No.: CD004721. doi:10.1002/14651858.CD004721

Tancioni, F., Lorenzetti, M.A., Navarria, P., Pessina, F., Draghi, R., Pedrazzoli, P., … Rodriguez y Baena, R. (2011). Percutaneous vertebral augmentation in metastatic disease: State of the art. *Journal of Supportive Oncology, 9,* 4–10.

Tokuhashi, Y., Matsuzaki, H., Oda, H., Oshima, M., & Ryu, J. (2005). A revised scoring system for preoperative evaluation of metastatic spine tumor prognosis. *Spine, 30,* 2186–2191.

Vallet, S., Smith, M.R., & Raje, N. (2010). Novel bone-targeted strategies in oncology. *Clinical Cancer Research, 16,* 4084–4093. doi:10.1158/1078-0432.CCR-10-0600

VI. Disease-specific management

A. Sarcomas
1. Introduction and overview of disease: Sarcomas are named for the tissue of origin and categorized as arising from soft tissues or bone.
   a) Soft tissue sarcomas are malignant tumors that arise from soft tissues such as fibrous connective tissue, fat, smooth or striated muscle, vascular tissue, peripheral neural tissue, and visceral tissue (Edge et al., 2010). They primarily arise from connective tissue (Goldberg, 2007). The most common sites are the extremities, trunk/retroperitoneum, and areas of the head and neck. Treatment approaches for soft tissue sarcomas are based on the histologic type, grade, size, depth, and location of the mass (Edge et al., 2010). Examples of tumor types include rhabdomyosarcoma, malignant fibrous histiocytoma, liposarcoma, synovial sarcoma, leiomyosarcoma, and malignant peripheral sheath tumors (Edge et al., 2010; Goldberg, 2007). Visceral sarcomas arising from within the stroma of connective tissue can be found in all organs and are extremely rare. Treatment of visceral sarcomas is based on the organ of origin (Graham, 2001).
   b) Primary malignant bone tumors (bone sarcomas) arise from the skeletal system and are extremely rare. The most common subtypes are osteosarcoma (35%), Ewing sarcoma (16%), and chondrosarcoma (30%) (Edge et al., 2010; Skubitz & D'Adamo, 2007). Treatment approaches are based on grade and size of the tumor and the presence and location of metastasis (Edge et al., 2010).
2. Histology and staging: Staging is most commonly performed using AJCC's TNM system.
   a) Histologic grade is an important prognostic indicator and often is determined using either the NCI or the French Federation of Cancer Centers Sarcoma Group systems (Kenney, Cheney, Stull, & Kraybill, 2009). Histologic subtype, degree of differentiation, mitotic activity, and necrosis are used to determine grade.
   b) Prognostic factors for soft tissue sarcomas (Edge et al., 2010)
      (1) Stage: Patients with stage I disease have a low risk for dying from their disease; patients with stage II or III disease have a progressively greater risk.
      (2) Histopathology (low grade has a better prognosis than high grade)
      (3) Molecular markers and genetic abnormalities are currently being evaluated.
      (4) Studies are needed to determine whether neurovascular and bone invasion are prognostic markers, as was previously thought.
   c) Prognostic factors for primary malignant bone tumors (Edge et al., 2010)
      (1) Tumor size (T1 has a better prognosis than T2; Ewing sarcoma tumors 8 cm or less and osteosarcoma tumors 9 cm or less have a better prognosis than larger tumors)
      (2) Histopathology (low grade is better than high grade)
      (3) Location (resectable is better than nonresectable; spine and pelvic tumors have a poorer prognosis)
      (4) Absence of spread (localized is better than metastatic)
      (5) Metastatic site (bony and hepatic metastases are worse than lung metastasis; a solitary lung metastasis is better than multiple lung lesions)
      (6) Molecular abnormalities, including gene translocations, expression of multidrug resistance genes, expression of growth factor receptors, and cell cycle regulators are being evaluated.
3. Incidence and risk factors
   a) An estimated 10,980 new cases and 3,920 deaths from soft tissue sarcomas will occur in 2011 (Siegel, Ward, Brawley, & Jemal, 2011).
      (1) Men are affected more often than women, and African Americans are at higher risk than Caucasians.
      (2) Risk factors include predisposing genetic mutations such as Li-Fraumeni syndrome and history of hereditary retinoblastoma.
      (3) Histories of ionizing radiation, chemical exposure, and chronic soft tissue

injury or lymphedema are noted risk factors for development of soft tissue sarcoma (Ray & McGinn, 2008).

b) Sarcomas of bone constitute only 0.2% of all new cancers in the United States (Edge et al., 2010). Chondrosarcoma is the most common primary bone tumor seen in adults, accounting for more than 40% of cases (ACS, 2011). Osteosarcoma is the most common malignant bone tumor in children and young adults. Etiology of bone sarcomas is often unknown. However, some correlation exists with growth spurts in teenagers. Risk factors include prior RT, history of hereditary retinoblastoma, and diagnosis of Li-Fraumeni syndrome (Larrier, 2008).

4. Radiation treatment

a) Treatment usually is directed with curative intent. Patients should be treated at a center that has expertise in the management of sarcomas and access to orthopedic surgeons, radiation oncologists, medical oncologists, and experienced pathologists.

b) Radiation has a limited role in the treatment of osteosarcoma. It is primarily used in patients who decline surgery, those with positive margins after surgery, and in cases where surgery and reconstruction are not possible (Larrier, 2008).

  (1) Radiation can be used for palliation (Larrier, 2008).

  (2) Although Ewing sarcoma often is responsive to radiation, surgical resection has been shown to provide superior control and thus is the primary choice of treatment (Skubitz & D'Adamo, 2007).

c) Management of soft tissue sarcoma of the extremity has changed dramatically from the days when amputation was the rule. Curative treatment in extremity sarcomas now emphasizes limb-sparing surgery and function-sparing RT (Goldberg, 2007).

  (1) Radiation is indicated for all moderate- and high-grade soft tissue sarcoma. Reexcision rather than adjuvant radiation is preferred for low-grade soft tissue sarcoma (Sheplan & Juliano, 2010).

  (2) The treatment plan may or may not include chemotherapy.

  (3) Use of intraoperative RT in the treatment of retroperitoneal sarcomas may improve outcomes in this difficult setting. EBRT may be given before or after surgery as well (Kaushal & Citrin, 2008).

(4) Head and neck sarcomas present unique challenges because of the heterogeneity of tumor types and presentations. However, surgical resection with as wide a margin as possible often is preferable. Radiation and/or chemotherapy may be used (Singh et al., 2008).

d) Palliative RT may be given when a sarcoma causes significant pain or is unresectable (Forscher & Casciato, 2009).

e) EBRT is the primary means of delivering radiation. Sequencing of preoperative versus postoperative RT varies. No consensus exists at this time (Kaushal & Citrin, 2008). Several aspects need to be considered when deciding between preoperative and postoperative RT, including the type of surgical procedure, planned type of wound closure, amount of expected wound tension, probable extent of operative bed, likelihood of margin-negative resection, and histologic grade of sarcoma.

  (1) Preoperative RT may allow for a smaller treatment field and a lower dose of radiation to be given.

    (a) It may make surgery easier by decreasing tumor size (Skubitz & D'Adamo, 2007).

    (b) However, irradiated tissue may make pathologic study more difficult (Cormier & Pollock, 2004).

    (c) A landmark study by O'Sullivan et al. (2002) revealed that preoperative RT was associated with a statistically higher rate of wound complications in patients with soft tissue sarcoma of the limbs than postoperative RT (35% versus 17%, respectively).

  (2) Postoperative RT has the disadvantage of treating an often large and lesser-defined postoperative volume with high radiation doses to overcome the hypoxic effect of disrupted vasculature (Swallow & Catton, 2007). The main advantage of postoperative radiation over preoperative radiation is the lower risk of wound healing complications (Swallow & Catton, 2007). Radiopaque surgical clips can be placed at the time of surgery to help delineate the tumor bed and area at high risk for disease (Kaushal & Citrin, 2008).

  (3) A retrospective study comparing preoperative RT with postoperative RT in patients with lower extremity soft tis-

sue sarcoma validated that treatment outcomes (overall survival, local control) were essentially the same, but the use of preoperative RT was associated with an elevated rate of acute wound complications for tumors larger than 5 cm. However, when radiation was used postoperatively, an increase in chronic radiation side effects (including edema and fibrosis) was noted in patients who had developed acute surgical wound complications (Cannon et al., 2006). Preoperative radiation may be favored to provide better long-term functional outcomes (Steen & Stephenson, 2008).

f) IMRT allows higher doses of radiation to be delivered to selected volumes. The dose can be shaped around normal tissue (DeLaney, Trofimov, Engelsman, & Suit, 2005), thus allowing for less toxicity. A retrospective, single-institution study at Memorial Sloan-Kettering Cancer Center showed that IMRT for soft tissue sarcoma provided a 94% control rate at five years for those with negative margins as well as those with positive/close margins. However, because of the study's modest sample size (N = 41), more studies are needed in this area (Alektiar, Brennan, Healey, & Singer, 2008).

g) Brachytherapy can be used alone or in conjunction with EBRT following surgery. This usually involves placement of afterloading catheters into the tumor bed following surgical excision of the tumor.

(1) Brachytherapy has most commonly been used for soft tissue sarcoma but more recently has also been applied to the dura and paraspinal tissues for tumors at those sites (DeLaney et al., 2005).

(2) Brachytherapy usually is performed after postoperative day 5 to minimize wound complications. A landmark prospective, randomized trial comparing resection alone with resection followed by adjuvant brachytherapy for soft tissue sarcoma revealed five-year local control rates of 82% and 69%, respectively. Local control rates were higher for high-grade sarcomas, 89% (brachytherapy arm) and 66% (no brachytherapy arm), respectively (Pisters et al., 1996).

(3) The major benefit of brachytherapy is that more normal tissue can be spared than with EBRT. Brachytherapy appears to be most effective for high-grade sarcomas (Hueman, Thornton, Herman, & Ahuja, 2008; Pisters et al., 1996).

(4) Another study revealed a five-year local control rate of 84% with an overall survival rate of 70% at one institution's nearly 15-year experience with brachytherapy alone following surgical excision for high-grade primary soft tissue sarcoma (Alektiar, Leung, Zelefsky, Healey, & Brennan, 2002). Poorer outcomes occurred with sarcomas in the shoulder and upper extremities and in cases with positive surgical margins.

(5) HDR or LDR seeds may be used when delivering brachytherapy (Ray & McGinn, 2008). For more detail on brachytherapy, see section VIII.B.

5. Intraoperative RT: Intraoperative RT uses electrons or HDR brachytherapy during surgery and provides focused radiation to the bed of resected tumors, such as retroperitoneal, pelvic, spinal, and paraspinal tumors. This delivery method focuses intense radiation to the surgical bed or area at risk while minimizing radiation injury to normal tissues (DeLaney et al., 2005).

a) Following recovery from surgery, the patient may receive additional radiation or chemotherapy (Willett, Czito, & Tyler, 2007).

b) Intraoperative RT has been used in the treatment of soft tissue sarcoma of the extremities. A retrospective study at the University of California, San Francisco demonstrated that patients receiving intraoperative RT as a boost received excellent local control with limited acute toxicities (Tran et al., 2006).

c) The combination of EBRT and intraoperative RT provides tumorcidal doses with acceptable morbidity (Hu & Harrison, 2000; Mackenzie, Reid, Barrett, & O'Dwyer, 2003; Moore-Higgs, 2007) (see section VIII.C—Intraoperative RT).

6. Acute effects

a) Acute reactions include skin reactions, pain, difficulty in coping, changes in sexuality, fatigue, nausea, diarrhea, and bone marrow suppression. (The assessment and management of all but bone marrow suppression are discussed in other sections of this manual.)

b) Bone marrow suppression is an acute effect of RT whenever significant bone mar-

row is in the field of treatment, as it is in treatment of extremity sarcoma. Mild neutropenia can occur but usually is self-limiting and does not require colony-stimulating support. As in any bone marrow suppression, patients must be given detailed neutropenia precautions. Weekly complete blood counts should be assessed as well (Shelton, 2003).

c) Abdominal RT may cause nausea, anorexia, or diarrhea (Ritari, 2007).

  (1) NCCN (2011a) guidelines for radiation-induced nausea and vomiting recommend that patients undergoing treatment to the upper abdomen receive either granisetron or ondansetron with or without dexamethasone.

  (2) Weight should be monitored weekly and dietary interventions initiated if weight loss of 10% or greater from baseline occurs (Ritari, 2007). Corticosteroids (short-term use), progestins, and individual nutrition counseling may be considered (Adams, Cunningham, Caruso, Norling, & Shepard, 2009).

  (3) Patients who experience diarrhea should be monitored closely for dehydration and educated in the use of antidiarrheal medications and dietary modifications (Ritari, 2007). Loperamide and diphenoxylate are standard therapy for patients experiencing radiation-related diarrhea. Octreotide is likely to be effective as well. In regard to prevention of diarrhea in these patients, probiotics (VSL#3® [VSL Pharmaceuticals, Inc.], *Lactobacillus acidophilus, Lactobacillus rhamnosus*) or psyllium fiber supplementation may be helpful (Muehlbauer et al., 2009).

7. Late effects

  a) Lymphedema may be present following surgery and exacerbated by RT. However, radiation-related lymphedema is more commonly seen in the weeks to months following completion of treatment.

  (1) It is more likely to occur when a large area of an extremity is irradiated with treatment fields larger than 35 cm. Efforts are made during treatment planning to spare at least 33% of the circumference of the extremity from direct radiation, thereby minimizing the risk of impaired lymph and vascular flow after treatment (Stinson et al., 1991).

  (2) Edema is more common for patients with tumors in the lower extremities versus upper extremities (Cormier & Pollock, 2004).

  b) Fibrosis can cause discomfort and permanently limit range of motion in an extremity. The patient should initiate a stretching program during treatment with the help of a physical therapist (Ritari, 2007).

  c) Joints are spared from direct radiation whenever possible. A retrospective review (Stinson et al., 1991) of 145 patients, performed by the Radiation Oncology branch of NCI, found that if 50% or more of a joint was irradiated, contracture was much more common. Physical therapy is encouraged throughout treatment to maximize flexibility and function of limbs.

  d) When the growth plate of an extremity or epiphysis is irradiated, the possibility exists for impaired growth of that extremity with resultant deformity or dysfunction (Stinson et al., 1991). Every effort is made during treatment planning to avoid direct radiation to this area, but occasionally it is unavoidable. In such cases, a thorough discussion during consultation is crucial to ensure patient and caregiver understanding of possible treatment sequelae. This is of particular importance when treating a child (Stinson et al., 1991).

  e) The incidence of bone fracture with combined-modality treatment of soft tissue sarcoma is quite low. The need for prophylactic bone fixation is rare (Cannon et al., 2006).

8. Patient and family education

  a) Assess patient and caregiver understanding of the disease process, their understanding of the treatment proposed, and their ability and readiness to learn.

  b) Assess the need for support groups, financial assistance, and resources for spiritual coping.

  c) Review the RT treatment procedures to be used, such as intraoperative RT, brachytherapy, or EBRT. Explain that an immobilization device may be fabricated for consistent positioning.

d) Review the treatment schedule, and give the patient a treatment calendar if he or she is undergoing several types of treatments (e.g., intraoperative RT plus EBRT for retroperitoneal sarcoma).

e) Review expected acute side effects and their management. This may include skin reaction, pain, difficulty in coping, changes in sexuality, fatigue, and bone marrow suppression. When a sarcoma of an extremity is being treated, teach the patient and caregiver to elevate the extremity if swelling or edema occurs.

f) Near completion of treatment, review follow-up care and appointment schedules with the patient and caregiver. Review the possible late effects and the importance of timely follow-up care.

g) Document all of the preceding in the patient's record.

9. Follow-up

a) Perform a thorough history and complete physical at each follow-up visit, typically every three to six months for two to three years following treatment, extending to every six months for two years, and then annually. Evaluate the site of disease periodically based on the estimate of locoregional recurrence using CT, MRI, or ultrasound (NCCN, 2011b). Assess the patient for distress or difficulty coping at each visit.

b) An annual chest radiograph is standard. Any abnormalities found are evaluated by chest CT or PET scan.

c) Most soft tissue sarcomas that recur do so within the first two years after completion of therapy (Goldberg, 2007). Whenever possible, surgical resection is performed. Radiation is primarily afforded to sites of disease causing adverse symptoms (Larrier, 2008).

References

Adams, L.A., Cunningham, R.S., Caruso, R.A., Norling, M.J., & Shepard, N. (2009). ONS PEP resource: Anorexia. In L.H. Eaton & J.M. Tipton (Eds.), *Putting evidence into practice: Improving oncology patient outcomes* (pp. 31–36). Pittsburgh, PA: Oncology Nursing Society.

Alektiar, K.M., Brennan, M.F., Healey, J.H., & Singer, S. (2008). Impact of intensity-modulated radiation therapy on local control in primary soft-tissue sarcomas of the extremity. *Journal of Clinical Oncology, 26,* 3440–3444. doi:10.1200/JCO.2008.16.6249

Alektiar, K.M., Leung, D., Zelefsky, M.J., Healey, J.H., & Brennan, M.F. (2002). Adjuvant brachytherapy for primary high-grade soft tissue sarcoma of the extremity. *Annals of Surgical Oncology, 9,* 48–56. doi:10.1245/aso.2002.9.1.48

American Cancer Society. (2011). Cancer facts and figures 2011. Retrieved from http://www.cancer.org/Research/CancerFactsFigures/CancerFactsFigures/cancer-facts-figures-2011

Cannon, C.P., Ballo, M.T., Zagars, G.K., Mirza, A.N., Lin, P.P., Lewis, V.O., … Pisters, P.W.T. (2006). Complications of combined modality treatment of primary lower extremity soft-tissue sarcomas. *Cancer, 107,* 2455–2461. doi:10.1002/cncr.22298

Cormier, J.N., & Pollock, R.E. (2004). Soft tissue sarcomas. *CA: A Cancer Journal for Clinicians, 54,* 94–109. doi:10.3322/canjclin.54.2.94

DeLaney, T.F., Trofimov, A.V., Engelsman, M., & Suit, H.D. (2005). Advanced-technology radiation therapy in the management of bone and soft tissue sarcomas. *Cancer Control, 12,* 27–37.

Edge, S.B., Byrd, D.R., Compton, C.C., Fritz, A.G., Greene, F.L., & Trotti, A., III. (Eds.). (2010). *AJCC cancer staging manual* (7th ed.). New York, NY: Springer.

Forscher, C.A., & Casciato, D.A. (2009). Sarcomas. In D.A. Casciato & M.C. Territo (Eds.), *Manual of clinical oncology* (6th ed., pp. 384–396). Philadelphia, PA: Lippincott Williams & Wilkins.

Goldberg, B.R. (2007). Soft tissue sarcoma: An overview. *Orthopaedic Nursing, 26,* 4–11.

Graham, D. (2001). Management of soft tissue sarcoma. *Nursing Clinics of North America, 36,* 553–565.

Hu, K.S., & Harrison, L.C. (2000). Adjuvant RT of retroperitoneal sarcoma: The role of intraoperative radiotherapy (IORT). *Sarcoma, 4,* 11–16. doi:10.1155/S1357714X00000037

Hueman, M.T., Thornton, K., Herman, J.M., & Ahuja, N. (2008). Management of extremity soft tissue sarcomas. *Surgical Clinics of North America, 88,* 539–557. doi:10.1016/j.suc.2008.04.003

Kaushal, A., & Citrin, D. (2008). The role of radiation therapy in the management of sarcomas. *Surgical Clinics of North America, 88,* 629–646. doi:10.1016/j.suc.2008.03.005

Kenney, R.J., Cheney, R., Stull, M.A., & Kraybill, W. (2009). Soft tissue sarcomas: Current management and future directions. *Surgical Clinics of North America, 89,* 235–247. doi:10.1016/j.suc.2008.09.020

Larrier, N.A. (2008). Osteosarcoma. In D.E. Wazer, G. Freeman, & L.R. Prosnitz (Eds.), *Perez and Brady's principles and practice of radiation oncology* (5th ed., pp. 1801–1807). Philadelphia, PA: Lippincott Williams & Wilkins.

Mackenzie, S., Reid, R., Barrett, A., & O'Dwyer, P.J. (2003). Management of soft tissue sarcomas of the abdomen and pelvis. *Colorectal Disease, 5,* 129–132. doi:10.1046/j.1463-1318.2003.00380.x

Moore-Higgs, G.J. (2007). Basic principles of radiation therapy. In M.L. Haas, W.P. Hogle, G.J. Moore-Higgs, & T.K. Gosselin-Acomb (Eds.), *Radiation therapy: A guide to patient care* (pp. 8–24). St. Louis, MO: Elsevier Mosby.

Muehlbauer, P., Thorpe, D., Davis, A.B., Drabot, R.C., Kiker, E.S., & Rawlings, B.L. (2009). Diarrhea. In L.H. Eaton & J.M. Tipton (Eds.), *Putting evidence into practice: Improving oncology patient outcomes* (pp. 125–134). Pittsburgh, PA: Oncology Nursing Society.

National Comprehensive Cancer Network. (2011a). *NCCN Clinical Practice Guidelines in Oncology: Antiemesis* [v.3.2011]. Retrieved from http://www.nccn.org/professionals/physician_gls/pdf/antiemesis.pdf

National Comprehensive Cancer Network. (2011b). *NCCN Clinical Practice Guidelines in Oncology: Soft tissue sarcomas* [v.1.2011]. Retrieved from http://www.nccn.org/professionals/physician_gls/PDF/sarcoma.pdf

O'Sullivan, B., Davis, A.M., Turcotte, R., Bell, R., Catton, C., Chabot, P., ... Zee, B. (2002). Preoperative versus postoperative radiotherapy in soft-tissue sarcoma of the limbs: A randomized trial. *Lancet, 359*, 2235–2241. doi:10.1016/S0140-6736(02)09292-9

Pisters, P.W.T., Harrison, L.B., Leung, D.H., Woodruff, J.M., Casper, E.S., & Brennan, M.F. (1996). Long-term results of a prospective randomized trial of adjuvant brachytherapy in soft tissue sarcoma. *Journal of Clinical Oncology, 14*, 859–868.

Ray, M.E., & McGinn, C.J. (2008). Soft tissue sarcomas (excluding retroperitoneum). In E.C. Halperin, C.A. Perez, & L.W. Brady (Eds.), *Perez and Brady's principles and practice of radiation oncology* (5th ed., pp. 1808–1821). Philadelphia, PA: Lippincott Williams & Wilkins.

Ritari, K. (2007). Soft tissue sarcomas. In M.L. Haas, W.P. Hogle, G.J. Moore-Higgs, & T.K. Gosselin-Acomb (Eds.), *Radiation therapy: A guide to patient care* (pp. 308–318). St. Louis, MO: Elsevier Mosby.

Shelton, B.K. (2003). Evidence-based care for the neutropenic patient with leukemia. *Seminars in Oncology Nursing, 19*, 133–141. doi:10.1016/S0749-2081(03)00026-3

Sheplan, L.J., & Juliano, J.J. (2010). Use of radiation therapy with soft tissue and bone sarcomas. *Cleveland Clinic Journal of Medicine, 77*(Suppl. 1), S27–S29. doi:10.3949/ccjm.77.s1.06

Siegel, R., Ward, E., Brawley, O., & Jemal, A. (2011). Cancer statistics, 2011. *CA: A Cancer Journal for Clinicians, 61*, 212–236. doi:10.3322/caac.20121

Singh, R.P., Grimer, R.J., Bhujel, N., Carter, S.R., Tillman, R.M., & Abudu, A. (2008). Adult head and neck soft tissue sarcomas: Treatment and outcome. *Sarcoma, 2008*, Article ID 654987. doi:10.1155/2008/654987

Skubitz, K.M., & D'Adamo, D.R. (2007). Sarcoma. *Mayo Clinic Proceedings, 82*, 1409–1432. doi:10.4065/82.11.1409

Steen, S., & Stephenson, G. (2008). Current treatment of soft tissue sarcoma. *Baylor University Medical Center Proceedings, 21*, 392–396.

Stinson, S.F., Delaney, T.F., Greenberg, J., Yang, J.C., Lampert, M.H., Hicks, J.E., ... Glatstein, E.J. (1991). Acute and long-term effects on limb function of combined modality limb sparing therapy for extremity soft tissue sarcoma. *International Journal of Radiation Oncology, Biology, Physics, 21*, 1493–1499. doi:10.1016/0360-3016(91)90324-W

Swallow, C.J., & Catton, C.N. (2007). Local management of adult soft tissue sarcomas. *Seminars in Oncology, 34*, 256–269. doi:10.1053/j.seminoncol.2007.03.008

Tran, Q.N.H., Kim, A.C., Gottschalk, A.R., Wara, W.M., Phillips, T.L., O'Donnell, R.J., ... Haas-Kogan, D.A. (2006). Clinical outcomes of intraoperative radiation therapy for extremity sarcomas. *Sarcoma, 2006*, Article ID 91671. doi:10.1155/SRCM/2006/91671

Willett, C.G., Czito, B.G., & Tyler, D.S. (2007). Intraoperative radiation therapy. *Journal of Clinical Oncology, 25*, 971–977. doi:10.1200/JCO.2006.10.0255

B. Lymphoma
    1. Introduction and overview of disease
        a) Lymphoma is a diverse group of neoplasms arising from uncontrolled growth of lymphocytes in lymph nodes and lymphoid tissues (Manson & Porter, 2011). The lymph system is made up of thin tubes that branch, like blood vessels, into all parts of the body. Lymph nodes are groups of small, bean-shaped organs that make and store infection-fighting cells such as T lymphocytes, B lymphocytes, and natural killer cells. Clusters of lymph nodes are found in the underarms, pelvis, neck, and abdomen. The spleen, thymus, and tonsils are part of the lymph system.
        b) The appearance of the cancer cells and the pattern in which they grow within the lymph node or bone marrow are critical for the correct diagnosis. Therefore, the initial diagnosis can only be made by biopsy. Needle aspirations or needle biopsies are inadequate because the architecture of the lymph node is extremely important for an accurate diagnosis and histologic subclassification (Ansell & Armitage, 2006). Reed-Sternberg or Reed-Sternberg–like cells help distinguish Hodgkin lymphoma (HL) from non-Hodgkin lymphoma (NHL) (Manson & Porter, 2011).
        c) HL accounts for only 0.58% of all cancers diagnosed (Hoppe, 2008). Patients usually present with painless lymphadenopathy. One-third of patients with HL present with one of the three B symptoms: fever, night sweats, and weight loss. Patients who have both weight loss and fevers have a particularly poor prognosis (Ansell & Armitage, 2006). HL generally spreads from one lymph node group to an immediately adjacent lymph node group. More than 80% of the patients with HL present with cervical lymph node involvement, and more than 50% have mediastinal disease (Hoppe, 2008).
        d) Each histologic subtype has its own unique clinical features.
            (1) Nodular sclerosis, the most common subtype, tends to affect adolescents and young adults more commonly and usually presents as localized disease that involves cervical, supraclavicular, and mediastinal regions (Ansell & Armitage, 2006).
            (2) Mixed cellularity HL is more prevalent in the pediatric and older adult groups and commonly is associated with a more advanced stage of disease and poor prognosis (Ansell & Armitage, 2006).
            (3) Lymphocyte-depletion HL (reclassified as NHL) occurs mainly in older patients. These patients present with extensive symptomatic disease without peripheral lymphadenopathy. It is most often associated with AIDS (Ansell & Armitage, 2006).
        e) NHL is diagnosed 6 times as often as HL, and its death rate is 14 times greater (Siegel, Ward, Brawley, & Jemal, 2011). It is the sixth most common malignancy in the

United States and accounts for 4% of all cancers (Siegel et al., 2011). NHL is characterized by the type of malignant cell that is involved, the histologic and immunophenotypic appearance, and how fast the cells divide and the tumor progresses (Armitage, Bierman, Bociek, & Vose, 2006; Leukemia and Lymphoma Society, 2010a). NHL has a propensity for skipping to noncontiguous lymph node groups and has a marked increase in the incidence of bone marrow involvement. The histopathologic classification of NHL has been a challenge for decades to both pathologists and clinicians (Prosnitz & Ng, 2008).

2. Incidence and risk factors
   a) Sex: Overall incidence of lymphoma is slightly higher in men than women (Leukemia and Lymphoma Society, 2010b).
   b) Age
      (1) HL has a bimodal peak. The early peak is from 25 to 30 years of age, and the second peak is from ages 75 to 80 (Manson & Porter, 2011).
      (2) The incidence of NHL rises steadily with age starting in the fourth or fifth decade.
      (3) Lymphoma is the third most common cancer in children (HL 7.2% and NHL 6.6%) (Leukemia and Lymphoma Society, 2010b).
   c) Race: More prevalent in Caucasians than in African Americans and Asian Americans (Molina, 2001).
   d) Socioeconomic status: More common in middle-class families than in lower-class families and in developed countries compared to underdeveloped countries (Molina, 2001).
   e) Environmental factors (Molina, 2001)
      (1) Occupations: Farmers, pesticide applicators, grain (flour) millers, meat workers, wood and forestry workers, chemists, painters, mechanics, machinists, and printers
      (2) Chemicals: Pesticides, herbicides, solvents, wood preservatives, and dusts
      (3) Radiation
         (a) Survivors of atomic bombs and nuclear reactor accidents
         (b) People who have received prior RT and chemotherapy
   f) Viruses and bacteria
      (1) Epstein-Barr virus is associated with Burkitt lymphoma.
      (2) Human T-cell lymphotropic virus type 1 (HTLV-1) is associated with adult T-cell leukemia and lymphoma. It is common in some parts of southern Japan, the Caribbean, South America, and Africa (Leukemia and Lymphoma Society, 2010b). It is spread through sexual intercourse and from mother to child at birth or in breast milk.
      (3) Human herpes virus 8
      (4) Hepatitis C virus
      (5) *Helicobacter pylori* bacteria are linked with mucosa-associated lymphoid tissue lymphomas of the stomach (Leukemia and Lymphoma Society, 2010b).
   g) Immunodeficiency (Prosnitz & Ng, 2008)
      (1) HIV infection: NHL is the second most common malignancy in patients with AIDS. The use of antiretroviral drugs has resulted in a decline in incidence and an improvement in treatment outcome.
      (2) Iatrogenic immunosuppression (transplant recipients)
      (3) Collagen vascular and autoimmune diseases

3. Staging and prognostic factors
   a) The staging for HL is based on the number of involved sites, whether the involved lymph nodes are on one or both sides of the diaphragm, whether the sites of involvement are bulky, whether there is contiguous extranodal involvement or disseminated extranodal disease, and whether typical systemic symptoms (B symptoms) are present (Ansell & Armitage, 2006).
   b) Prognostic factors: Used to identify if patients are at low or high risk of recurrence. Both the German Hodgkin Study Group and the European Organization for the Research and Treatment of Cancer have developed prognostic factors for early-stage HL. These include presence of a large mediastinal mass, extranodal disease, high erythrocyte sedimentation rate, and three or more lymph node areas with involvement of disease (Ansell & Armitage, 2006).

4. Radiation treatment
   a) At one time, radiation was the primary treatment for HL. It was used alone or in combination with adjuvant chemotherapy. Bulky sites were covered with large RT fields, and patients with favorable disease received total lymphoid irradiation (Yahalom, 2009). As a result of the better understanding of prognostic factors and the awareness of the long-term side effects from large treatment fields, treatment for early-stage HL includes a combination of chemotherapy agents and involved-field RT (Diehl, Thomas, & Re, 2004) (see Table 14).
      (1) The mantle field includes all of the major lymph node regions above the diaphragm. The field extends from the inferior portion of the mandible almost to the level of the insertion of the diaphragm. An individually contoured lung block is designed to conform to the patient's anatomy and tumor distribution (Hoppe, 2008).
      (2) The subdiaphragmatic field for HL is the inverted Y, which includes the retroperitoneal and pelvic lymph nodes and the spleen. With current management programs, a full inverted Y field is rarely used. Instead, portions of the Y field are treated, such as the patient's spleen with or without the para-aortic nodes. Unilateral or bilateral pelvic fields are treated in the context of combined-modality therapy (Hoppe, 2008).
      (3) *Total lymphoid irradiation* refers to sequential treatment to the mantle plus the inverted Y field. When the subdiaphragmatic field does not include the pelvis, the term used is *subtotal lymphoid irradiation* (Hoppe, 2008).
      (4) Involved-field RT is now used with combined-modality therapy. The radiation is limited to the involved site and often is tailored to include only the reduced postchemotherapy volume. It is estimated that the average involved-field RT regimen will reduce the irradiated volume by more than 80% compared to total lymphoid irradiation, thus decreasing the radiation dose to

Table 14. Treatment Options for Hodgkin Lymphoma

Disease Stage	Presentation	Treatment	Note
Early-stage favorable disease	No bulky disease or B symptoms (stages I–IIA)	Combined therapy consisting of two to four cycles of chemotherapy (typically doxorubicin, bleomycin, vinblastine, and dacarbazine [ABVD]) and involved-field radiation therapy to 20–30 Gy	–
Early-stage unfavorable disease	Involvement of two or more lymph node regions on the same side of the diaphragm, localized contiguous involvement of only one extranodal organ or site, and lymph node region(s) on the same side of the diaphragm (stages I–II)	Four to six cycles of effective chemotherapy (ABVD) followed by 20–30 Gy involved-field radiation therapy	–
Advanced-stage Hodgkin lymphoma	Involvement of lymph node regions on both sides of the diaphragm and diffuse or disseminated involvement of one or more extranodal organs or tissues	Six to eight cycles of chemotherapy (ABVD or other regimens) with or without consolidative radiation therapy	The role of radiation therapy is controversial. Radiation therapy is often added in patients who present with bulky disease or remain in uncertain complete response (i.e., unable to ascertain on radiographic films whether it is disease or scar tissue) after chemotherapy.
Progressive or relapsing disease	–	Depends on previous treatment, but options include radiation therapy, high-dose chemotherapy, and autologous stem cell transplantation.	–

Note. Based on information from Diehl et al., 2004.

the breast, heart, and lungs (Yahalom, 2009).

    (5) Total skin irradiation of cutaneous T-cell lymphoma (see section VIII.H—Total skin irradiation).

5. Side effects from RT depend on the radiation dose and the treatment field.

  a) Acute effects (Leukemia and Lymphoma Society, 2010b)

    (1) Fatigue

    (2) Hair loss

    (3) Skin reactions—Result from the depletion of actively proliferating cells in a renewing cell population (see section IV.C—Skin reactions).

    (4) Changes in taste or loss of appetite (see section V.B—Head and neck)

      (a) The taste buds are radiosensitive, and the changes may include blunting or increased sensitivity to certain tastes. Normal taste may return months after treatment is completed, but taste alterations could be permanent.

      (b) Instruct the patient to perform oral care before eating.

      (c) Instruct the patient to add spices and seasoning to food if the mantle field is not being treated.

      (d) Instruct the patient to experiment with different foods.

    (5) Mucositis (see section V.B—Head and neck)

    (6) Xerostomia (see section V.B—Head and neck)

      (a) Occurs when the salivary glands are treated with radiation. The saliva becomes thick and ropy. It occurs at 10 Gy and is permanent at 40 Gy (Bruce, 2004).

      (b) Perform frequent prophylactic dental care.

      (c) Administer fluoride treatment.

    (7) Dysphagia and esophagitis (see sections V.B—Head and neck and V.D—Thoracic)

      (a) Caused by irritation of the membranes lining the throat and esophagus. Effects usually develop after the second or third week of treatment and may continue for months after treatment.

      (b) Instruct the patient to

        i. Eat soft, bland foods such as puddings, custards, and yogurt.

        ii. Take dietary supplements.

        iii. Avoid irritants such as citrus and alcohol.

      (c) Medicate with viscous lidocaine, liquid antacids, or narcotics.

    (8) Nausea and vomiting

      (a) Administer antiemetic prior to treatment and as needed.

      (b) Schedule treatment for the end of the day to allow the patient to eat during the day.

      (c) Instruct the patient to avoid eating large meals just prior to treatment but to have a light snack so that the stomach is not completely empty.

    (9) Decreased blood counts: Check complete blood count weekly during treatment and hold treatment as needed.

  b) Long-term effects

    (1) Thyroid dysfunction

      (a) Subclinical hypothyroidism develops in approximately 50% of patients with HL (Hoppe, 2008). It is manifested by an elevation of the thyroid-stimulating hormone even with a normal thyroxine level (Hoppe, 2008).

      (b) Obtain thyroid profile (blood work) with follow-up visits.

      (c) Treat with thyroid hormone replacement as needed.

    (2) Radiation pneumonitis

      (a) May develop within 6–12 weeks after completing treatment (Hoppe, 2008). Associated with lung inflammation that is characterized by a mild, nonproductive cough, low-grade fever, and difficult breathing on exertion. Occurs in 1% or less of patients receiving mantle field irradiation. The risk may increase if the chemotherapy drug bleomycin was used in combination with RT (Hoppe, 2008).

      (b) Fewer than 5% of patients develop symptomatic pneumonitis, which is manifested by cough, fever, pleuritic chest pain, and infiltrate on chest radiograph that often conforms to the treatment fields. Symptomatic management usually is sufficient; however, a small proportion of patients require treatment with corticosteroids (Hoppe, 2008).

    (3) Cardiovascular disease

      (a) Mediastinal radiation predisposes patients to premature coronary artery disease and pericardial and

myocardial fibrosis, but modification to treatment techniques has decreased the dose of radiation to the heart (von der Weid, 2008).

(b) Refer the patient to a cardiologist if symptomatic.

(4) Radiation pericarditis (Hoppe, 2008)

(a) Occurs in less than 5% of patients. It presents as an acute febrile syndrome with chest pain and friction rub; it usually clears within a few weeks.

(b) Perform routine echocardiogram.

(c) Administer analgesics and NSAIDs.

(d) Refer the patient to a cardiologist if symptomatic.

(e) Tamponade or constrictive pericarditis is more serious. It develops in less than 1% of patients and may require surgical correction (Hoppe, 2008).

(5) Infection

(a) Herpes zoster can occur during treatment or within the first two years after treatment in 10%–15% of patients. If cutaneous eruptions are identified within 72 hours of onset, initiate acyclovir (Hoppe, 2008).

(b) Postsplenectomy sepsis is uncommon but nonetheless a potentially serious complication following splenectomy or splenic irradiation. The most serious infections occur with gram-positive organisms, including *Streptococcus pneumonia*, meningococci, and *Haemophilus* strains (Hoppe, 2008).

i. This can be minimized by establishing a regular immunization schedule against these organisms.

• Pneumococcal vaccine every five years

• Influenza vaccine every year

ii. Initiate prompt treatment of febrile disease.

(6) Lhermitte sign

(a) Definition: Paresthesias extending into the arm and legs on neck flexion and is related to the demyelination of the spinal cord (Hoppe, 2008)

(b) Develops in approximately 10%–15% of patients (Hoppe, 2008)

(c) Occurs one to two months after treatment and spontaneously resolves after two to six months (Hoppe, 2008)

(7) Secondary malignancies

(a) The mean 15-year actuarial risk for any secondary malignant neoplasm in survivors of HL or NHL is 17.6% compared with 2.6% in the general population (Fernsler & Fanuele, 1998).

(b) The following are the most common secondary malignancies in HD or NHL.

i. Leukemia: May develop after treatment with chemotherapy regimens that include alkylating agents or procarbazine (Hoppe, 2008)

ii. Breast cancer: This risk is related to the age at which women receive mantle RT and the dose. Women should begin mammographic screening as soon as five to seven years after completion of mantle RT (Hoppe, 2008). This would include MRIs of the breast along with mammograms.

iii. Thyroid cancer: Peaks at 15–19 years after RT (Fernsler & Fanuele, 1998)

iv. Lung cancer: The risk is dose related. The risk is higher among those who smoked at the time of diagnosis and who continued smoking after treatment (Hoppe, 2008).

(8) Sterility

(a) Radiation to the para-aortic and iliac lymph nodes can affect gonadal function both in men and women. Concomitant chemotherapy with alkylating agents such as cyclophosphamide and especially procarbazine has synergistic action and can lead to premature menopause and infertility (von der Weid, 2008).

(b) Suggest sperm banking prior to starting RT for men who wish to have children.

(c) Surgically move the ovaries out of the RT field (oophoropexy).

(d) Suggest freezing of embryos prior to RT.

(9) Psychosocial and economic effects: These are the most challenging effects to both survivors and healthcare providers. The severity of the problems is related to the developmental stage of the survivor (Fernsler & Fanuele, 1998).

(a) Anxiety/fear of recurrence (see section IV.E—Distress/coping)

(b) Denial of insurance

(c) Denial of job offers or rejection by the military

(d) Body image

6. Patient and family education

a) Teach the patient and family about the required treatment and the length of treatment depending upon the treatment site.

b) Teach the patient and family about the acute and late effects of treatment that the patient may experience depending upon the individual treatment site.

c) Teach the patient and family about medications that may be used to minimize side effects of treatment.

d) Teach the patient and family about appropriate healthcare risks associated with treatment and lifestyle modifications.

(1) Healthy diet

(2) Regular exercise

(3) Not smoking

(4) Limited sun exposure

(5) Breast self-examinations

e) Teach the patient and family about the need for long-term follow-up.

7. Follow-up management

a) Long-term or chronic side effects may become apparent months or years after treatment has ended. Therefore, follow-up visits should be with oncologists or practitioners who are familiar with not only the treatment course but also the potential long-term side effects. Appropriate diagnostic tests should include, but are not limited to, chest x-ray, thyroid panel, and complete blood count.

b) Patients should receive appropriate vaccinations as necessary.

8. Special circumstances

a) Older adult patients with HL: Older age is an adverse prognostic factor for survival. The poorer outcome is associated with increased treatment-related toxic effects and an increased incidence of early disease relapse often associated with suboptimal therapy (Ansell & Armitage, 2006).

b) Pregnant patients: If clinically appropriate, delay therapy until the end of the first trimester, the delivery of the neonate, or disease progression. Involved-field radiation to the neck or axilla can be safely given, and chemotherapy at full doses can be safely administered even during the first trimester if necessary (Ansell & Armitage, 2006).

References

Ansell, S.M., & Armitage, J.O. (2006). Management of Hodgkin lymphoma. *Mayo Clinic Proceedings, 81,* 419–426. doi:10.4065/81.3.419

Armitage, J.O., Bierman, P.J., Bociek, R.G., & Vose, J.M. (2006). Lymphoma 2006: Classification and treatment. *Oncology, 20,* 231–239.

Bruce, S.D. (2004). Radiation-induced xerostomia: How dry is your patient? *Clinical Journal of Oncology Nursing, 8,* 61–67. doi:10.1188/04.CJON.61-67

Diehl, V., Thomas, R.K., & Re, D. (2004). Part II: Hodgkin's lymphoma—Diagnosis and treatment. *Lancet Oncology, 5,* 19–26. doi:10.1016/S1470-2045(03)01320-2

Fernsler, J., & Fanuele, J.S. (1998). Lymphomas: Long-term sequelae and survivorship issues. *Seminars in Oncology Nursing, 14,* 321–328.

Hoppe, R.T. (2008). Hodgkin lymphoma. In E.C. Halperin, C.A. Perez, & L.W. Brady (Eds.), *Perez and Brady's principles and practice of radiation oncology* (5th ed., pp. 1721–1738). Philadelphia, PA: Lippincott Williams & Wilkins.

Leukemia and Lymphoma Society. (2010a). Disease information and support. Non-Hodgkin lymphoma. Retrieved from http://www.lls.org/#/diseaseinformation/lymphoma/nonhodgkinlymphoma/

Leukemia and Lymphoma Society. (2010b). Lymphoma. Retrieved from http://www.leukemia-lymphoma.org/all_page?item_id=7030

Manson, S., & Porter, C. (2011). Lymphomas. In C.H. Yarbro, D. Wujcik, & B.H. Gobel (Eds.), *Cancer nursing: Principles and practice* (7th ed., pp. 1458–1503). Sudbury, MA: Jones and Bartlett.

Molina, A. (2001). Non-Hodgkin's lymphoma. In R. Pazdur, L. Coia, W. Hoskins, & L. Wagman (Eds.), *Cancer management: A multidisciplinary approach* (5th ed., pp. 585–622). Melville, NY: PRR Inc.

Prosnitz, L.R., & Ng, A. (2008). Non-Hodgkin's lymphoma. In E.C. Halperin, C.A. Perez, & L.W. Brady (Eds.), *Perez and Brady's principles and practice of radiation oncology* (5th ed., pp. 1739–1765). Philadelphia, PA: Lippincott Williams & Wilkins.

Siegel, R., Ward, E., Brawley, O., & Jemal, A. (2011). Cancer statistics, 2011. *CA: A Cancer Journal for Clinicians, 61,* 212–236. doi:10.3322/caac.20121

von der Weid, N.X. (2008). Adult life after surviving lymphoma in childhood. *Supportive Care in Cancer, 16,* 339–345. doi:10.1007/s00520-007-0369-x

Yahalom, J. (2009). Does radiotherapy still have a place in Hodgkin lymphoma? *Current Hematologic Malignancy Reports, 4,* 117–124. doi:10.1007/s11899-009-0017-2

C. Benign conditions
  1. Overview/guidelines
    a) RT is primarily used as a cancer treatment modality. However, the clinical application of RT to treat benign diseases otherwise unresponsive to medical interventions is sometimes indicated. The goal for RT treatment delivery is focused on the treatment of patients with malignant tumors. Long-standing clinical experience has recognized the utility of RT to treat a complement of benign disorders. It is vital that clinicians take into account the potential for serious acute and long-term implications of RT, such as skin injury, carcinogenesis, and genetic damage from ionizing radiation, before offering RT regimens to individuals with a benign disease diagnosis (Tripuraneni, 2009).
    b) Technical considerations and guidelines (Tripuraneni, 2009)
      (1) Quality of radiation, total dose, shielding, depth of dose
      (2) Targeted skin region for a benign disorder must avoid treatment to underlying organs
      (3) Long-term risk/benefit assessment of all potential patients
      (4) Assessment of treatment consequences and natural history of benign disease
      (5) Risks and benefits of other available treatment modalities
      (6) Informed consent specific to clinical implications and outcomes
  2. Indications (Tripuraneni, 2009)
    a) Acute and chronic inflammatory diseases: Antibiotic-refractory infections, such as ankylosing spondylitis
    b) Acute and chronic painful degenerative diseases: Joint-related disease, such as heterotopic ossification
    c) Soft tissue proliferative disorders: Desmoids tumors, gynecomastia
    d) Functional disorders: Ocular diseases such as Graves ophthalmopathy, arteriovenous malformations (AVMs)
    e) Skin conditions: Keloids
    f) Other conditions: Vascular restenosis
  3. Clinical application of RT for benign conditions
    a) Ocular indications
      (1) Pterygium (definition: wing) is a triangular wedge of conjunctival tissue that extends into the cornea. Pterygia can block the visual axis, thus reducing visual acuity and hastening astig-matism. The eye appears red and irritated and the patient may have difficulty with wearing contact lenses. Pterygia occur most frequently in sunny regions; sunglass protection diminishes the occurrence (Jürgenliemk-Schulz et al., 2004).
        (a) Diagnosis is made by ophthalmologic assessment revealing a wedged-shaped growth on the cornea. Surgery is the primary therapy for pterygia; however, the recurrence rates are high and range from 20% to 30% (Luthra, Nemesure, Wu, Xie, & Leske, 2001).
        (b) Treatment: Immediate postoperative RT within eight hours to decrease recurrence. Typical application of RT is with a beta-emitting applicator and has reduced recurrence rates to 20% or less when compared to surgery alone (Tripuraneni, 2009).
        (c) Treatment dose: Varies from one single fraction of 20 Gy to multiple-fraction regimens of 8–10 Gy given immediately postoperatively followed by two more treatments at seven-day intervals. Local control was best when RT was given immediately after surgery (Pajic & Greiner, 2005).
        (d) Acute side effects include ocular irritation, scleral atrophy, and neovascularization. No late side effects have been reported (Pajic & Greiner, 2005).
        (e) Alternative methods for preventing recurrence include intraoperative or postoperative mitomycin C, postoperative thiotepa, or postoperative 5-FU (Bekibele, Baiyeroju, & Ajayi, 2004).
        (f) Pterygium may be prevented by protecting the eyes from sunlight. Nurses may facilitate prevention in their community by educating the public to wear sunglasses when spending significant time outdoors.
      (2) Graves ophthalmopathy is an inflammatory autoimmune disease characterized by inflammation and edema of the orbital tissues and the extraocular muscles (Wakelkamp et al., 2004). Graves ophthalmopathy commonly occurs in females between the ages of

40–44 and 60–64. Graves disease often is associated with hyperthyroidism; however, it can occur in euthyroid or hypothyroid patients (Bartalena, Marcocci, & Pinchera, 2002; Kaprealian, Mishra, Wang-Chesebro, & Quivey, 2010).

(a) Histologic features: The complex histologic features of Graves disease include interstitial edema, T-cell predominant lymphocytic infiltration of orbital tissues, and glycosaminoglycans in periorbital fat and extraocular muscles. The inflammatory reaction associated with Graves disease leads to venous engorgement, diminished drainage of interstitial fluid, periorbital edema, proptosis, and, uncommonly, compression of the optic nerve. This compression can cause irreversible neuronal death and diminished nerve function, which could lead to decreased visual acuity and papillary dysfunction, as well as constriction of the visual fields (Bahn, 2003; Kaprealian et al., 2010).

(b) Clinical management: Multidisciplinary approach includes medicine, surgery (orbital decompression, eye muscle or lid surgery), and radiology. First-line treatment is high-dose systemic glucocorticoids. If the patient is resistant to steroid therapy, then orbital decompression to relieve proptosis and optic neuropathy may be initiated. RT is effective either alone or in combination with other therapies (Bartalena, Tanda, Piantanida, Lai, & Pinchera, 2004). Underlying thyroid disorder, if present, must be treated systemically in addition to local-regional treatment with EBRT (Kaprealian et al., 2010).

(c) RT should be reserved for patients who are symptomatic and have not responded to high-dose steroids or for patients in whom steroids are contraindicated (Bartalena, Marcocci, Gorman, Wiersinga, & Pinchera, 2003). The risk of enhancing retinopathy with RT precludes it in patients with Graves disease who have diabetes mellitus.

(d) The most common dose of radiation is 20 Gy in 10 fractions administered using small, opposed lateral fields with a split beam or five-degree posterior angulation to avoid dose to lens with megavoltage. This treatment course can yield a 50%–80% response rate (Bradley et al., 2008). Immobilization, CT treatment planning, and beam shaping are necessary to minimize radiation beyond the retro-orbital region. Radiation treatment will take several weeks to take effect and may cause a flare of inflammation in the post-treatment phase. Because of this, patients may be maintained on steroids during the first few weeks of treatment (Alpert et al., 2003).

(e) Potential side effects associated with treatment include cataracts, radiation retinopathy, and radiation optic neuropathy, which may manifest either acutely (within days to weeks following RT) or as a late effect (six months after RT to years later) (Wakelkamp et al., 2005). When RT is precisely fractionated and planned, these side effects should not occur.

(3) Orbital pseudotumor is a benign idiopathic orbital inflammation that can simulate exophthalmos in Graves disease. It is part of the spectrum of lymphoid diseases of the orbit and may be either unilateral or bilateral. Orbital pseudotumor causes inflammation of tissues of the orbit or surrounding the eye and can cause a palpable mass resembling a tumor. Patients may present with acute pain, edema, and diplopia (Jacobs & Galetta, 2002). Pseudotumor is self-limiting; however, it can cause compression of orbital contents leading

to optic nerve atrophy, disc edema, and visual loss (Kaprealian et al., 2010).

(a) Diagnostic workup includes CT of the orbits and sclera to differentiate pseudotumor from Graves disease. Contrast-enhanced MRI with coronal views is recommended. Biopsy may be required to define the disease process.

(b) First-line treatment is systemic corticosteroids usually yielding transient responses. Complete resolution of symptoms with steroids alone occurs in only 50% of patients (Yuen & Rubin, 2003). Low-dose RT is the treatment of choice for cases in which there is a contraindication to, a poor response to, or a recurrence after steroid treatment (Yuen & Rubin, 2003). Surgery usually is not initiated.

(c) IMRT is the treatment of choice for pseudotumor once the patient has not responded to steroids. Local control rates are high and morbidity is minimal with proper RT planning and lens shielding. High-dose isodose lines that are conformal to the tumor, sparing the globe, brain, and normal tissues, are indicated in treatment planning (Kaprealian et al., 2010).

(d) Local control rates range from 74% to 100% with dose ranges of 15–25 Gy, with 20 Gy in 10 fractions being most common (Jacobs & Galetta, 2002; Kaprealian et al., 2010).

b) Skin indications: Keloids

(1) Described as benign fibroproliferative growths caused by connective tissue proliferation in response to the following factors: surgery, burns, trauma, inflammation, foreign body reactions, and spontaneous occurrence (Eng et al., 2006). Keloids are unsightly benign masses of fibrous tissue that extend beyond wounds and do not regress spontaneously.

(2) Keloids often are described as pruritic, painful, and tender. Keloids most commonly affect areas of increased skin tension. Anatomic regions include the presternal, back, and posterior neck regions and the ears, the deltoid, and the anterior chest.

(3) The treatment course for keloid management depends on the size, location,

and depth of the lesion, as well as the age of the patient. The treatment of choice for keloids is surgery followed by adjuvant treatment to stop fibroblast proliferation (Garg et al., 2004). Adjuvant treatments include cryotherapy; intralesional injections of corticosteroids; interferon, and fluorouracil. No consensus exists on treatment for keloids (Alster & Tanzi, 2003). Greater than 80% relapse rates have been reported postoperatively without adjuvant treatment (Luis et al., 2008).

(4) RT has been shown to decrease local relapse following surgery. Brachytherapy and EBRT are both used to treat keloids. Radiation targets fibroblasts, which are well oxygenated and therefore radiosensitive (Eng et al., 2006).

(5) RT is given as soon possible (usually within the first 24 hours) following surgery. The dose ranges from 10 to 15 Gy in two to five fractions. Slightly improved control has been reported with doses of 15 Gy. The fields are conformed to the surgical excision bed with custom cutouts and low energy electrons and bolus (Tripuraneni, 2009). Local control with immediate postoperative RT ranges from 70% to 90% depending on dose (Tripuraneni, 2009).

(6) RT as monotherapy is not as successful as RT following surgery. If surgery is not indicated, then treatment courses of 4 Gy given monthly for one to five treatments have been reported to yield good clinical control (Guix, 2004).

c) CNS indications

(1) AVMs

(a) Intracranial AVMs are congenital lesions within the cerebral vasculature in which blood flows from arteries to veins without passing through a capillary system. The risk of hemorrhage is about 2%–3% per year (Altschul, Smith, & Sinson, 2009). The mortality rate for an initial bleed is about 10% and rises with each subsequent bleed (Smith et al., 2009).

(b) Treatment options for AVMs include observation, surgical resection, endovascular embolization, or SRS. Patients must be assessed for SRS including age, performance status, comorbidities, and anatomic location of the AVM. The goal of SRS is to deliver a single fraction of high-dose radiation to a stereotactically defined small volume to sclerose the AVM and prevent hemorrhage.

(c) SRS techniques used to treat AVMs include cobalt beams, proton beams, modified linear accelerators, and Gamma Knife. SRS is more effective if the AVM is smaller than 3 cm and when all feeder vessels are irradiated. Conventional fractionated RT yields inferior results compared to SRS (Seegenschmiedt, 2007). Complications associated with SRS are low and depend upon the volume treated and whether the lesion had been reirradiated. Recommended dose is 15–30 Gy in one fraction (International RadioSurgery Association, 2009).

(d) Estimated obliteration rates of AVMs treated with SRS vary from 60% to 90% within two to three years following SRS (Altschul et al., 2009). During this time, patients may be at risk for hemorrhage (Maruyama et al., 2005). Patients require long-term multidisciplinary team management including radiation oncology and neurosurgery.

(2) Trigeminal neuralgia

(a) Trigeminal neuralgia is also known as tic douloureux, prosopalgia, or "suicide disease" (Morris, 2007). It is a disorder of the fifth (trigeminal) nerve causing stabbing, electric shock–like pain in the facial areas where the branches of the nerve are distributed (lips, eyes, nose, scalp, forehead, upper jaw, and lower jaw). It is not fatal; however, it is considered to be the most painful clinical disorder. It occurs in approximately 15.5 people per 100,000 worldwide (Morris, 2007).

(b) Medications such as anticonvulsants are the primary intervention; however, they only act to lessen or block the debilitating pain (Urgosik, Liscak, Novotny, Vymazal, & Vladyka, 2005). Most patients develop medication resistance and must resort to other interventions such as surgery, alcohol ablation, and SRS.

(c) Surgical intervention also may be offered to patients who become refractory to medication. Patients treated with microvascular decompression can result in complete and long-term pain relief (Brisman, 2007).

(d) Nonsurgical alternatives such as SRS are considered only for intractable pain or when the patient becomes refractory or unable to tolerate medical therapy.

(e) Patients with trigeminal neuralgia have always been heavily pretreated with either surgery and medical therapy or both. Often they experience only transient control of the debilitating pain and compromised quality of life.

(f) SRS is successful at controlling and eliminating trigeminal neuralgia pain completely. The exact mechanism is unknown; however, it is considered to be related to an electrophysiologic block with complete destruction of the involved nerve (Brisman, 2007). Treatment is a single-fraction dose of 70–90 Gy delivered to the trigeminal nerve root. Patients must have close multidisciplinary management from both radiation oncology and neurosurgical teams (Urgosik et al., 2005).

(g) Side effects associated with SRS for trigeminal neuralgia include facial numbness, ataxia, dryness of the eyes, and radiation-induced necrosis of the temporal lobe.

(3) Acoustic neuroma

(a) Acoustic neuromas (also called vestibular schwannomas) are tumors of the myelin-forming cells of the eighth cranial nerve located in the inner ear canal. Occurrence rate is approximately 1 person per 100,000 (Chang & Timmerman, 2009). As this tumor grows, it occupies a significant portion of the cerebellopontine angle and can extend into the extracanalicular spaces (Morris, 2007). Symptoms include hearing loss, headache, tinnitus, and ataxia.

(b) Treatment includes microsurgical removal, which is curative and attempts to preserve hearing.

(c) SRS is offered for disease control. SRS treatment contours the target volume of the acoustic neuroma and adjacent normal structures, including the eyes, optic nerves, and brain stem. CT and MRI images are fused and an optimal single-fraction treatment of 12–14 Gy is delivered to the target volume. This is considered the minimum dose necessary to treat the tumor. Higher doses of 16–20 Gy may provide greater tumor control; however, morbidity of facial nerve damage has been reported (Chopra, Kondziolka, Niranjan, Lunsford, & Flickinger, 2007; Foote et al., 1995; Koh et al., 2007).

(d) The goals of SRS treatment for acoustic neuroma are both tumor control and hearing preservation. Tumor control progressively improves as time passes.

(e) Research to determine whether SRS can improve hearing in patients with acoustic neuroma (Chopra et al., 2007; Koh et al., 2007): The radiobiologic effects on surrounding structures, such as the cochlea and acoustic nerve, are still not well defined in contemporary clinical practice. It is important that research continues so that improvements in hearing with SRS become a realistic treatment goal.

(f) Close follow-up of patients with acoustic neuroma is required, as 20% of tumors continue to grow following SRS (Morris, 2007).

d) Soft tissue indications

(1) Desmoid tumors/aggressive fibromatosis

(a) Desmoid tumors are rare, benign, low-grade tumors of connective tissue that are locally invasive and nonmetastasizing. Desmoid tumors arise from tendons or scar tissue; *desmoid* refers to the appearance of these tumors as an oppressive band. There is a relationship to other fibromatosis skin conditions such as keloids (Tripuraneni, 2009).

(b) Desmoid tumors account for less than 3% of all soft tissue tumors (Micke & Seegenschmiedt, 2005). These tumors appear predominantly in women 30–40 years old. Endocrine and physical factors have been linked to their onset (Micke & Seegenschmiedt, 2005).

(c) Desmoid tumors are characterized by slow and locally aggressive growth with high potential for relapse after surgical resection. Prognosis is related to the tumor's location; extra-abdominal tumors demonstrate a higher postoperative relapse rate (Nuyttens, Rust, Thomas, & Turrisi, 2000). In contemporary clinical practice, the aforementioned characteristics of desmoid tumors still are perpetuated.

(d) The treatment of choice is complete surgical resection, although this is not always possible. Postoperative local recurrence can range from 10% to 100% depending on the extent of the surgical resection and margins (Micke & Seegenschmiedt, 2005). Because of the high probability of local recurrence following surgery, RT is used either initially in unresectable or inoperable tumors or as adjuvant therapy following surgery.

(e) The recommended dose of RT is 50–60 Gy over six to seven weeks at 1.8–2 Gy per fraction (Tripuraneni, 2009). RT fields are large and encompass the entire tumor compartment with 5–7 cm around the tumor volume.

(2) Gynecomastia

(a) Gynecomastia is a benign proliferation of the glandular and/or fatty

subareolar tissue surrounding the male breast (can be unilateral or bilateral). It is caused by an imbalance between the stimulatory effect of estrogen and the inhibitory effect of androgen (Seegenschmiedt, 2007). The most common cause is the pharmacologic use of antiandrogens for prostate cancer treatment (Seegenschmiedt, 2007).

(b) Gynecomastia can occur in up to 90% of patients taking antiandrogen therapy and in up to 15% of patients taking luteinizing hormone-releasing agonists (Seegenschmiedt, 2007).

(c) If gynecomastia is hormone induced, it usually is bilateral and painful. Low-dose RT is effective in preventing and treating gynecomastia. Radiation should be given prophylactically before the administration of antiandrogens. It can still be effective once hormonal therapy has been initiated (Dicker, 2003).

(d) Portal fields cover the entire breast region. Electrons are used because of the need for shallow-depth dose characteristics. Electrons are particles that have shallow penetration and therefore are safe to use when underlying critical anatomic structures, such as lungs, heart, and spinal cord, are within the treatment field. Doses used for prophylaxis range from 8 to 15 Gy in two fractions to 20 Gy in five fractions (Tyrrell et al., 2004).

(e) Side effects are few with only mild skin erythema as a common acute side effect. The potential risk of radiation-related skin and breast cancer developing after RT for gynecomastia is low (Eng et al., 2006).

(f) Alternatives to RT include surgery (mastectomy) or hormonal therapy with either antiestrogens or aromatase inhibitors (Eng et al., 2006).

e) Bone indications
  (1) Heterotopic bone formation/ossification
    (a) Heterotopic ossification is a complication following hip arthroplasty, trauma, fracture, or CNS injury. Heterotopic ossification can occur in a variety of joints following soft tissue trauma, medullary or brain lesions, or hip, knee, elbow, and shoulder fractures or postsurgical replacement. Heterotopic ossification is a syndrome that causes soft tissues surrounding these joints to ossify and transform into osteoblastic tissue (Tripuraneni, 2009). This tissue forms mature bone. After total hip arthroplasty, heterotopic ossification occurs around the femoral neck adjacent to the greater trochanter (Neal, Gray, MacMahon, & Dunn, 2002).

    (b) Heterotopic ossification varies widely in incidence and occurs in about 30% of patients undergoing hip arthroplasty (Tripuraneni, 2009). Incidence can rise to approximately 60% if patients have hypertrophic osteoarthritis or other high-risk skeletal diseases such as trauma or ankylosing spondylitis (Neal et al., 2002).
      i. Hip symptoms include stiffness and pain. Advanced heterotopic ossification may have signs of inflammation, including fever, erythema, swelling, warmth, and tenderness. These findings require assessment of possible wound or prosthetic joint infections (Eng et al., 2006).
      ii. Diagnosis of hip heterotopic ossification is made by an anteroposterior radiograph of the pelvis and hip. It may be visible on plain films within three to four weeks postoperatively. A bone scan will demonstrate increased uptake in the soft tissues adjacent to the hip.

    (c) Treatment of heterotopic ossification is surgical excision followed by a form of prophylaxis. Surgery has a high risk of recurrence (Tripuraneni, 2009), which is limiting. It is important to identify patients who are at high risk preoperatively. Measures used to prevent heterotopic ossification from developing following total hip arthroplasty should be initiated before the fifth postoperative day, optimally within 24–48 hours of surgery (Seegenschmiedt, Makoski, & Micke, 2001).

    i. NSAIDs and EBRT have been used successfully in preventing heterotopic ossification after total hip arthroplasty.

    ii. A prospective, randomized study showed that both RT and indomethacin were effective in the prevention of postoperative heterotopic ossification (Kienapfel et al., 1999). A single dose of 7–8 Gy given through anteroposterior and posteroanterior fields and including the soft tissue surrounding the hip joint is effective.

(d) Radiation may be given as a single dose of 7 Gy to the hip and joint capsule either preoperatively (four hours prior to surgery) or postoperatively (within 72 hours), achieving similar low failure rates. Luh, Cavanaugh, Eng, and Thomas (2004) reported no clinical evidence existed suggesting an increased risk for secondary malignancies from the single-dose regimen.

f) Vascular indications

(1) Restenosis

(a) Restenosis is the renarrowing of a coronary artery after angioplasty or stenting treatment. It is the main limitation of revascularization following angioplasty with or without stent placement. The underlying mechanism is the damage caused by the angioplasty balloon on the vessel walls. The vessel response to injury is to stimulate proliferation of smooth muscle cells, leading to vascular intimal hyperplasia (thickening) and narrowing of the vessel lumen (Luis et al., 2008).

(b) Restenosis has been reported to occur within six months of percutaneous transluminal coronary angioplasty in 30%–50% of patients (Pokrajac et al., 2005).

(c) Either external or endovascular RT following percutaneous angioplasty has proved to be bene-

ficial for the prevention of restenosis following a stent implantation (Waksman et al., 2004). RT inhibits cell proliferation and is able to delay or even prevent restenosis.

(d) The key effect of ionizing radiation is the elimination of smooth muscle cells, thereby preventing proliferation. This prolongs the time required for restenosis, favoring the normal processes of vascular endothelium repair and diminishing cell migration toward the vascular lumen. Research has shown that a single fraction of 20 Gy causes a nearly complete inhibition of restenosis (Hall, Miller, & Brenner, 1999). Leon et al. (2001) demonstrated that restenosis decreased significantly in patients receiving intra-arterial ^{192}Ir afterloading following stent placement compared to those not treated.

4. Summary/future

a) RT for the treatment of benign conditions was common in the past; however, current use has sharply declined because of potential for significant long-term side effects, including the high probability of causing radiation-induced cancer. Malignancies that arose following radiation for the treatment of a benign disorder most likely were due to nonspecific targeted treatment volumes. Recently, SRS has provided highly precise delivery of radiation, resulting in a lower probability of adverse side effects. Many nonmalignant diseases can benefit from radiation treatment if given precisely with clear objectives and goals delineated by an expert multidisciplinary team of radiation oncology professionals.

b) It was a century ago when the first benign condition, a giant hairy nevus (congenital mole), was treated with radiation (Kogelnik, 1998). This initial success and additional experimental applications spurred the clinical use of radiation for nonmalignant diseases. Many of these early treatment applications resulted in devastating long-term side effects (such as treating children's scalps with radiation for ringworms and subsequent development of leukemia, thyroid malignancies, and brain tumors). Hence, these past failures led to more cautious and limited use of radiation. The public feared cancer development from RT for a benign condition (Morris, 2007).

c) Many years ago, the International Commission on Radiological Protection (1984) documented the progressive decline in the use of RT for benign conditions. This report commented on the tremendous variation of the use of RT for benign conditions worldwide. These trends still prevail today in the United States. However, the German Cooperative Group on Radiotherapy for Benign Diseases has documented a global rise in RT use for benign disease (Seegenschmiedt, Micke, & Willich, 2004).

d) Interest still exists for offering RT for a variety of benign conditions. The radiation oncologist together with the entire multidisciplinary medical team decides whether to offer treatment in this clinical setting. The patient requires an understanding of the risks, benefits, side effects, and alternative treatments to make an informed decision to agree—or not—to RT for a benign condition. Treatment of benign conditions is subject to the same scrutiny and stringent clinical standards as the treatment of malignancies (Morris, 2007).

e) Radiation professionals are both theoretically and clinically trained to manage the administration, assessment, and side effect potential of ionizing radiation. The team knows how to assess the patient and prescribe, plan, and administer RT. Radiation oncology nurses have a pivotal role in managing treatment-related side effects and toxicities and predicting long-term sequelae. The team is held to the same accountability and evidence-based practice standards when treating both benign diseases and malignant tumors. Patients require a thorough initial assessment and teaching plan; the course of treatment must be expertly prescribed, planned, and verified; the course must be monitored closely during treatment; and short- and long-term follow-up must be planned. If even the slightest doubt about the provision of RT to manage benign conditions exists for the patient, family, or clinicians, additional professional opinions must be sought to determine the appropriateness and still meet the needs of the patient.

References

Alpert, T.E., Alpert, S.G., Bersani, T.A., Hahn, S.S., Bogart, J.A., & Chung, C.T. (2003). Radiotherapy for moderate-to-severe Graves' ophthalmopathy: Improved outcomes with early treatment. *Cancer Journal, 9,* 472–475.

Alster, T.S., & Tanzi, E.L. (2003). Hypertrophic scars and keloids: Etiology and management. *American Journal of Clinical Dermatology, 4,* 235–243.

Altschul, D., Smith, M.L., & Sinson, G.P. (2009, March 26). Intracranial arteriovenous malformations. Retrieved from http://www.emedicine.com/med/topic3469.htm

Bahn, R.S. (2003). Clinical review 157: Pathophysiology of Graves' ophthalmopathy: The cycle of disease. *Journal of Clinical Endocrinology and Metabolism, 88,* 1939–1946. doi:10.1210/jc.2002-030010

Bartalena, L., Marcocci, C.L., Gorman, C.A., Wiersinga, W.M., & Pinchera, A. (2003). Orbital radiotherapy for Graves' ophthalmopathy: Useful or useless? Safe or dangerous? *Journal of Endocrinological Investigation, 26,* 5–16.

Bartalena, L., Marcocci, C., & Pinchera, A. (2002). Graves' ophthalmopathy: A preventable disease? *European Journal of Endocrinology, 146,* 457–461. doi:10.1530/eje.0.1460457

Bartalena, L., Tanda, M.L., Piantanida, E., Lai, A., & Pinchera, A. (2004). Relationship between management of hyperthyroidism and course of the ophthalmopathy. *Journal of Endocrinological Investigation, 27,* 288–294.

Bekibele, C.O., Baiyeroju, A.M., & Ajayi, B.G. (2004). 5-fluorouracil vs. beta-irradiation in the prevention of pterygium recurrence. *International Journal of Clinical Practice, 58,* 920–923. doi:10.1111/j.1742-1241.2004.00007.x

Brisman, R. (2007). Microvascular decompression vs. gamma knife radiosurgery for typical trigeminal neuralgia: Preliminary findings. *Stereotactic and Functional Neurosurgery, 85,* 94–98. doi:10.1159/000097925

Bradley, E.A., Gower, E.W., Bradley, D.J., Meyer, D.R., Cahill, K.V., Custer, P.L., ... Woog, J.J. (2008). Orbital radiation for Graves ophthalmopathy: A report by the American Academy of Ophthalmology. *Ophthalmology, 115,* 398–409. doi:10.1016/j.ophtha.2007.10.028

Chang, B., & Timmerman, R.D. (2009). Stereotactic radiosurgery/stereotactic body radiation therapy. In B.G. Haffty & L.D. Wilson (Eds.), *Handbook of radiation oncology: Basic principles and clinical protocols* (pp. 143–158). Sudbury, MA: Jones and Bartlett.

Chopra, R., Kondziolka, D., Niranjan, A., Lunsford, L.D., & Flickinger, J.C. (2007). Long-term follow-up of acoustic schwannoma radiosurgery with marginal tumor doses of 12 to 13 Gy. *International Journal of Radiation Oncology, Biology, Physics, 68,* 845–851. doi:10.1016/j.ijrobp.2007.01.001

Dicker, A.P. (2003). The safety and tolerability of low-dose irradiation for the management of gynaecomastia caused by antiandrogen monotherapy. *Lancet Oncology, 4,* 30–36. doi:10.1016/S1470-2045(03)00958-6

Eng, T.Y., Boersma, M.K., Fuller, C.D., Luh, J.Y., Siddiqi, A., Wang, S., & Thomas, C.R., Jr. (2006). The role of radiation therapy in benign diseases. *Hematology/Oncology Clinics of North America, 20,* 523–557. doi:10.1016/j.hoc.2006.01.023

Foote, R.L., Coffey, R.J., Swanson, J.W., Harner, S.G., Beatty, C.W., Kline, R.W., ... Hu, T.C. (1995). Stereotactic radiosurgery using the gamma knife for acoustic neuromas. *International Journal of Radiation Oncology, Biology, Physics, 32,* 1153–1160. doi:10.1016/0360-3016(94)00454-S

Garg, M.K., Weiss, P., Sharma, A.K., Gorla, G.R., Jaggernauth, W., Yaparpalvi, R., ... Beitler, J.J. (2004). Adjuvant high dose brachytherapy (Ir-192) in the management of keloids which have recurred after surgical excision and external radiation. *Radiotherapy and Oncology, 73,* 233–236. doi:10.1016/j.radonc.2004.04.010

Guix, B. (2004). Radiotherapy concepts for keloids: Current options and clinical results [Symposium/proffered papers abstract]. *Radiotherapy and Oncology, 71*(Suppl. 1), S15.

Hall, E.J., Miller, R.C., & Brenner, D.J. (1999). Radiobiological principles in intravascular irradiation. *Cardiovascular Radiation Medicine, 1,* 42–47. doi:10.1016/S1522-1865(98)00004-3

International Commission on Radiological Protection. (1984). *Protection of the patient in radiation therapy: A report of the International Commission on Radiation Protection* [ICRP Publication No. 44]. New York, NY: Pergamon Press.

International RadioSurgery Association. (2009). Stereotactic radiosurgery for patients with intracranial arteriovenous malformations (AVM) [Radiosurgery Practice Guideline Report #2-03]. Retrieved from http://www.irsa.org/AVM%20Guideline.pdf

Jacobs, D., & Galetta, S. (2002). Diagnosis and management of orbital pseudotumor. *Current Opinion in Ophthalmology, 13,* 347–351.

Jürgenliemk-Schulz, I.M., Hartman, L.J., Roesink, J.M., Tersteeg, R.J., van Der Tweel, I., Kal, H.B., … Wyrdeman, H.K. (2004). Prevention of pterygium recurrence by postoperative single-dose beta-irradiation: A prospective randomized clinical double-blind trial. *International Journal of Radiation Oncology, Biology, Physics, 59,* 1138–1147. doi:10.1016/j.ijrobp.2003.12.021

Kaprealian, T., Mishra, K.K., Wang-Chesebro, A., & Quivey, J.M. (2010). Malignant and benign diseases of the eye and orbit. In E.K. Hansen & M. Roach III (Eds.), *Handbook of evidence-based radiation oncology* (2nd ed., pp. 75–94). New York, NY: Springer.

Kienapfel, H., Koller, M., Wüst, A., Sprey, C., Merte, H., Engenhart-Cabillic, R., & Griss, P. (1999). Prevention of heterotopic bone formation after total hip arthroplasty: A prospective randomised study comparing postoperative radiation therapy with indomethacin medication. *Archives of Orthopaedic and Trauma Surgery, 119,* 296–302. doi:10.1007/s004020050414

Kogelnik, H.D. (1998). [100 years radiotherapy. On the birth of a new specialty]. *Wiener Klinische Wochenschrift, 110,* 313–320.

Koh, E.S., Millar, B.A., Ménard, C., Michaels, H., Heydarian, M., Ladak, S., … Laperriere, N.J. (2007). Fractionated stereotactic radiotherapy for acoustic neuroma: Single-institution experience at the Princess Margaret Hospital. *Cancer, 109,* 1203–1210. doi:10.1002/cncr.22499

Leon, M.B., Teirstein, P.S., Moses, J.W., Tripuraneni, P., Lansky, A.J., Jani, S., … Kuntz, R.E. (2001). Localized intracoronary gamma-radiation therapy to inhibit the recurrence of restenosis after stenting. *New England Journal of Medicine, 344,* 250–256. doi:10.1056/NEJM200101253440402

Luh, J.Y., Cavanaugh, S.X., Eng, T.Y., & Thomas, C.R. (2004). A graphic retrospective analysis of 32 studies investigating optimal dose and fractionation schedules in the prevention of heterotopic ossification after hip arthroplasty. *International Journal of Radiation Oncology, Biology, Physics, 60*(Suppl. 1), S547. doi:10.1016/j.ijrobp.2004.07.517

Luis, A.M., de Lucas, R.H., Morón, A.H., Lizarbe, E.F., García, S.S., Ocaña, C.V., … Aguerri, A.R. (2008). Radiation therapy for the treatment of benign vascular, skeletal and soft tissue diseases. *Clinical and Translational Oncology, 10,* 334–346.

Luthra, R., Nemesure, B.B., Wu, S.Y., Xie, S.H., & Leske, M.C. (2001). Frequency and risk factors for pterygium in the Barbados Eye Study. *Archives of Ophthalmology, 119,* 1827–1832.

Maruyama, K., Kawahara, N., Shin, M., Tago, M., Kishimoto, J., Kurita, H., … Kirino, T. (2005). The risk of hemorrhage after radiosurgery for cerebral arteriovenous malformations. *New England Journal of Medicine, 352,* 146–153. doi:10.1056/NEJMoa040907

Micke, O., & Seegenschmiedt, M.H. (2005). Radiation therapy for aggressive fibromatosis (desmoid tumors): Results of a national Patterns of Care Study. German Cooperative Group on Radiotherapy for Benign Diseases. *International Journal of Radiation Oncology, Biology, Physics, 61,* 882–891. doi:10.1016/j.ijrobp.2004.07.705

Morris, B.J. (2007). Stereotactic radiosurgery for benign conditions. *eRADIMAGING.* Retrieved from http://www.eradimaging.com/site/article.cfm?ID=190

Neal, B., Gray, H., MacMahon, S., & Dunn, L. (2002). Incidence of heterotopic bone formation after major hip surgery. *ANZ Journal of Surgery, 72,* 808–821.

Nuyttens, J.J., Rust, P.F., Thomas, C.R., Jr., & Turrisi, A.T., III. (2000). Surgery versus radiation therapy for patients with aggressive fibromatosis or desmoid tumors: A comparative review of 22 articles. *Cancer, 88,* 1517–1523.

Pajic, B., & Greiner, R.H. (2005). Long term results of non-surgical, exclusive strontium-/yttrium-90 beta-irradiation of pterygia. *Radiotherapy and Oncology, 74,* 25–29. doi:10.1016/j.radonc.2004.08.022

Pokrajac, B., Pötter, R., Wolfram, R.M., Budinsky, A.C., Kirisits, C., Lileg, B., … Minar, E. (2005). Endovascular brachytherapy prevents restenosis after femoropopliteal angioplasty: Results of the Vienna-3 randomised multicenter study. *Radiotherapy and Oncology, 74,* 3–9. doi:10.1016/j.radonc.2004.08.015

Seegenschmiedt, M.H. (2007). Radiotherapy of non-malignant diseases. In E.C. Halperin, C.A. Perez, & L.W. Brady (Eds.), *Perez and Brady's principles and practice of radiation oncology* (5th ed., pp. 1933–1958). Philadelphia, PA: Lippincott Williams & Wilkins.

Seegenschmiedt, M.H., Makoski, H.B., & Micke, O. (2001). Radiation prophylaxis for heterotopic ossification about the hip joint—A multicenter study. German Cooperative Group on Radiotherapy for Benign Diseases. *International Journal of Radiation Oncology, Biology, Physics, 51,* 756–765. doi:10.1016/S0360-3016(01)01640-6

Seegenschmiedt, M.H., Micke, O., & Willich, N. (2004). Radiation therapy for nonmalignant diseases in Germany. Current concepts and future perspectives. *Strahlentherapie und Onkologie, 180,* 718–730. doi:10.1007/s00066-004-9197-9

Tripuraneni, P. (2009). Benign diseases. In B.G. Haffty & L.D. Wilson (Eds.), *Handbook of radiation oncology: Basic principles and clinical protocols* (pp. 755–761). Sudbury, MA: Jones and Bartlett.

Tyrrell, C.J., Payne, H., Tammela, T.L., Bakke, A., Lodding, P., Goedhals, L., … Carroll, K. (2004). Prophylactic breast irradiation with a single dose of electron beam radiotherapy (10 Gy) significantly reduces the incidence of bicalutamide-induced gynecomastia. *International Journal of Radiation Oncology, Biology, Physics, 60,* 476–483. doi:10.1016/j.ijrobp.2004.03.022

Urgosik, D., Liscak, R., Novotny, J., Jr., Vymazal, J., & Vladyka, V. (2005). Treatment of essential trigeminal neuralgia with gamma knife surgery. *Journal of Neurosurgery, 102*(Suppl.), 29–33.

Wakelkamp, I.M., Baldeschi, L., Saeed, P., Mourits, M.P., Prummel, M.F., & Wiersinga, W.M. (2005). Surgical or medical decompression as a first-line treatment of optic neuropathy in Graves' ophthalmopathy? A randomized controlled trial. *Clinical Endocrinology, 63,* 323–328. doi:10.1111/j.1365-2265.2005.02345.x

Waksman, R.L, Ajani, A.E., White, R.L., Chan, R., Bass, B., Pichard, A.D., … Lindsay, J. (2004). Five-year follow-up after intracoronary gamma radiation therapy for in-stent restenosis. *Circulation, 109,* 340–344. doi:10.1161/01.CIR.0000109488.62415.01

Yuen, S.J., & Rubin, P.A. (2003). Idiopathic orbital inflammation: Distribution, clinical features, and treatment outcome. *Archives of Ophthalmology, 121,* 491–499. doi:10.1001/archopht.121.4.491

VII. Oncologic emergencies

A. Oncologic emergencies such as SCC and superior vena cava syndrome (SVCS) are complications in patients with cancer that require expedited intervention to maintain quality of life and prevent long-term consequences (Brumbaugh, 2009). EBRT plays a critical role in palliation of these potentially life-threatening complications.
  1. SCC
    a) Definition: *Metastatic SCC* is the compression or displacement of the spinal cord's thecal sac or cauda equina by metastatic or locally advanced cancer (Prasad & Schiff, 2005).
    b) *Epidural spinal cord compression* (ESCC) refers to compression of the thecal sac by a tumor mass in the epidural space. Tumor invades the epidural space by the hematogenous spread of cancer cells into the bone marrow of the spine (Prasad & Schiff, 2005). It develops in one of three ways.
      (1) Continued growth and expansion of vertebral metastasis into the epidural space causing compression of the cord (Prasad & Schiff, 2005); treated with steroids and RT.
      (2) Extension of a paraspinal lymph node into the neural foramina (Prasad & Schiff, 2005); treated with steroids and RT.
      (3) Mechanical destruction of vertebral cortical bone causing vertebral body collapse and displacement of bony fragments into the epidural space (Kwok, DeYoung, Garofalo, Dhople, & Regine, 2006); requires surgical intervention to maintain neurologic function. This type of compression causes back pain that worsens with movement (Cole & Patchell, 2008).
    c) SCC is one of the most devastating complications of metastatic cancer. Evidence suggests that 5%–10% of all patients with cancer develop SCC during the course of their disease (Penas-Prado & Loghin, 2008).
    d) In the United States, an estimated 20,000 SCC cases develop each year (Nelson et al., 2000; Quinn & DeAngelis, 2000).
    e) Most frequently, metastatic seeding appears in the thoracic spine (70%), with the lumbar spine being the next common site (20%). The cervical spine is affected in approximately 10% of cases (Kaplan, 2006). Thirty percent of patients with spinal metastases have numerous sites of involvement (Huff, 2010).
    f) Cancers that commonly metastasize to the spine include breast, lung, and prostate cancers and multiple myeloma (Kaplan, 2006). Others include renal tumors, lymphoma, sarcoma, and unknown primary. GI and pelvic malignancies usually affect the lumbar spine, whereas breast and lung cancers are likely to affect the thoracic spine (Huff, 2010).
    g) In the pediatric population, neuroblastoma, sarcomas, germ cell tumors, and Hodgkin lymphoma can lead to SCC (Penas-Prado & Loghin, 2008).
    h) Risk factors for the development of metastatic SCC in patients with cancer (Lu, Gonzalez, Jolesz, Wen, & Talcott, 2005)
      (1) Abnormal neurologic examination
      (2) Pain in the middle or upper back
      (3) Definitive vertebral metastases
      (4) Metastatic disease at initial presentation
    i) Presentation and symptoms
      (1) Pain
        (a) A constant back pain is the most common presenting symptom of SCC, occurring in 83%–95% of patients (Cole & Patchell, 2008). This usually is localized at or near the site of spinal metastases (Cole & Patchell, 2008). It may be worse when lying down because of distension of the epidural venous plexus (Prasad & Schiff, 2005).
        (b) May be localized, radicular (where a dermatome is involved), referred, or a combination (Brumbaugh, 2009).
        (c) Localized: Near the site of ESCC (Brumbaugh, 2009; Kaplan, 2006)
          i. Usually the initial symptom
          ii. Constant, dull, progressive ache
          iii. Worsens in supine position; improves with sitting or standing

      iv. Greatest intensity upon awakening

      v. Worsens with increased intra-abdominal or intrathoracic pressure, such as with sneezing, coughing, or the Valsalva maneuver

  (d) Radicular pain: Occurs when spinal nerve roots or cauda equina is compressed (Brumbaugh, 2009; Kaplan, 2006)

      i. Less common than localized back pain

      ii. Variable presentation

         • Constant, dull ache difficult to pinpoint

         • Intermittent burning, shooting sensation; location easily identified; triggered by spinal movement

      iii. Location of the lesion influences presentation.

         • Cervical or lumbar lesion: Pain radiates down one (commonly) or both (over time) extremities

         • Thoracic spine lesion: Tight, bilateral, band-like pain that extends from back to front across the abdomen or chest

      iv. Worsens with increased intra-abdominal or intrathoracic pressure, such as with sneezing, coughing, or the Valsalva maneuver

  (e) Referred pain: Site of ESCC does not match location of pain (Kaplan, 2006)

      i. Involves multiple dermatomes

      ii. Nonradicular

      iii. Example: Lumbosacral pain from a thoracic cord compression

      iv. May be mistaken for a lesion at the site of pain perception

(2) Motor weakness

  (a) The second most common symptom of ESCC is motor weakness, which is present in 85% of cases (Kaplan, 2006).

  (b) Presentation (Brumbaugh, 2009; Kaplan, 2006)

      i. Feelings of heaviness or stiffness

      ii. Typically begins in the legs, despite the level of the ESCC

      iii. More proximal than distal

      iv. Difficulty with walking can progress to irreversible paralysis if not treated promptly.

(3) Sensory loss

  (a) Changes in sensory perception are detectable in approximately 50% of patients with ESCC (Bach et al., 1990).

  (b) Presentation (Brumbaugh, 2009; Kaplan, 2006)

      i. Paresthesias

      ii. Numbness

      iii. Loss of temperature sensation

      iv. Loss of proprioception

      v. Loss of vibratory sense

  (c) Most often bilateral, beginning in the toes and ascending in a stocking fashion, eventually reaching the level of the metastatic lesion (Brumbaugh, 2009; Kaplan, 2006)

  (d) May present at the same time as motor weakness or shortly thereafter (Brumbaugh, 2009; Kaplan, 2006)

(4) Autonomic dysfunction (Brumbaugh, 2009; Kaplan, 2006)

  (a) Indicative of bilateral cord damage

  (b) Common late finding with ESCC; associated with a poor prognosis

  (c) Presentation

      i. Bladder dysfunction (most common)

      ii. Bowel dysfunction

      iii. Impotence

  (d) In older adults with ESCC, urinary retention is a sign of autonomic sphincter dysfunction. This is a poor prognostic indicator for preservation of or improvement in ambulatory status (Cole & Patchell, 2008).

  (e) Horner syndrome

      i. Involvement of cervical and thoracic spines with cancer

      ii. Drooping eyelid, constricted pupil, and decreased sweating on the affected side of the face

  (f) Autonomic hyperreflexia (Brumbaugh, 2009; Kaplan, 2006)

      i. Tumor involvement at or above the sixth or seventh thoracic vertebra

      ii. Symptoms present above the level of ESCC

- Pounding headache
- Nasal congestion
- Bradycardia
- Hypertension
- Perfuse sweating
- Pilomotor erection (goose bumps)

j) Prognostic factors for functional recovery and survival following metastatic SCC (Kaplan, 2006)

(1) Favorable prognostic factors

(a) Early recognition and diagnosis of metastatic SCC

(b) Prompt initiation of therapy

(c) Able to ambulate at presentation

(d) Slow onset of motor weakness

(e) Radiosensitive tumors: Myeloma, lymphoma, breast, prostate

(f) Good performance status

(g) Responsive to steroid treatment

(h) Female sex

(i) Long interval between diagnosis of primary tumor and appearance of metastatic SCC

(2) Poor prognostic factors

(a) Paraplegia prior to treatment

(b) Urinary retention

(c) Sphincter incontinence

(d) Rapidly deteriorating neurologic function (in less than 72 hours)

(e) Radioresistant tumors: Lung, renal, GI, sarcoma, bladder

(f) Extensive disease

(g) Poor performance status

k) Diagnosis of ESCC (Brumbaugh, 2009; Kaplan, 2006)

(1) Medical history with thorough exploration of complaints of pain, specifically back pain

(2) Physical examination including a thorough CNS and detailed pain evaluation

(3) MRI is the gold standard for detecting ESCC with 93% sensitivity and 97% specificity ratio (Prasad & Schiff, 2005). Often, multiple levels of spinal vertebrae are involved; thus, imaging of the entire spine is recommended. For patients who are unable to have an MRI (e.g., those with metallic implants), conventional CT scans are acceptable substitutes, although soft tissue structures are not as visible as on MRI (Prasad & Schiff, 2005).

(4) Plain films have a low sensitivity and specificity and thus do not warrant routine use if ESCC is suspected, as they could delay diagnosis.

l) Management of ESCC

(1) The goal is to optimize the patient's quality of life (Kaplan, 2006).

(a) Provide relief from pain.

(b) Palliate symptoms.

(c) Prevent permanent disability.

(d) Preserve or recover motor and sphincter function.

(e) Extend the active portion of the patient's remaining life.

(f) Treatment is palliative, as life expectancy with ESCC is usually less than six months (Helweg-Larsen & Sørensen, 1994).

(2) Treatment approaches are divided into temporizing (corticosteroids) and definitive (RT, surgery, or combination) therapies (Kaplan, 2006).

(3) Corticosteroids (Brumbaugh, 2009; Kaplan, 2006)

(a) Initially given to all patients with ESCC

(b) Improve neurologic symptoms and provide pain relief by reducing spinal cord vasogenic edema and downregulating vascular endothelial growth factor expression.

(c) Dexamethasone is the most common steroid administered to patients with ESCC.

i. Optimal dose has not been determined.

ii. Currently, two perspectives exist (Vaillant & Loghin, 2009).
- High dose (100 mg loading, 96 mg/day maintenance)
- Moderate dose (10 mg loading, 16 mg/day maintenance)

iii. Some providers advocate titrating the dose of steroids to the severity of motor symptoms, with a high dose for patients with rapidly deteriorating motor function and a moderate dose for those with minimal or nonprogressive motor function loss (Vaillant & Loghin, 2009).

iv. For patients with more chronic and less severe neurologic symptoms, 8 mg orally twice daily may be a reasonable starting point (Vaillant & Loghin, 2009).

(d) Tumor swelling and inflammation can be decreased rapidly with the use of these agents. No optimal loading dose of dexamethasone has been determined to be superior (Vecht et al., 1989).

(4) RT is the standard treatment for patients with SCC.

(a) The goal of RT is to cause cancer cell death within the tumor. This reduces its size, decreases compression on the cord, and reduces the tumor growth rate (Vaillant & Loghin, 2009).

(b) Indications for RT as primary treatment: Radiosensitive tumors in a patient without surgical indications (lymphoma, SCLC, breast, prostate, multiple myeloma, seminoma, neuroblastoma, Ewing sarcoma); short life expectancy; high surgical risk; multilevel or diffuse spinal involvement; total neurologic deficit below the level of compression for greater than 24–48 hours; and subclinical SCC (imaging finding) (Penas-Prado & Loghin, 2008). RT is appropriate for patients without evidence of structural instability or epidural cord compression (Swift, 2009).

(c) Radiosensitive tumors have a better response to RT than do radioresistant tumors such as melanoma and renal cell carcinoma (Huff, 2010).

(d) RT usually is initiated within 24 hours of establishing an ESCC diagnosis and after corticosteroid therapy has begun (Kaplan, 2006).

(e) Dose and fractionation

  i. Optimum dosing and fractionation regimen is controversial (Brumbaugh, 2009; Kaplan, 2006). Comparison studies are needed (Kaplan, 2006).

  ii. Most common is a total dose of 30 Gy in 3 Gy fractions one to two spinal vertebrae above and below the affected region (Vaillant & Loghin, 2009).

  iii. Shorter courses of 4 Gy for seven days and very short courses of 8 Gy for two days one week apart have been effective in certain circumstances (Rades et al., 2009).

  iv. Prolonged courses of 25–40 Gy delivered over 10–20 fractions over a four-week period have also proved to be effective (Rades, Karstens, & Alberti, 2002).

  v. For debilitated patients with a short life expectancy and few therapeutic options, a single large fraction of 800 cGy may be best in order to reduce the number of hospital visits (Swift, 2009). Patients given single fractions, however, need retreatment more often than those receiving fractionated treatment.

(f) IMRT uses a specialized form of highly conformal three-dimensional RT that is planned with the use of sophisticated computer-based methods. This technique leads to a high degree of control by delivering radiation to different anatomic regions (Prasad & Schiff, 2005).

  i. IMRT minimizes dose delivered to the spinal cord while delivering therapeutic doses to the disease (Bartels, van der Linden, & van der Graaf, 2008).

  ii. Patients needing retreatment to a spinal lesion most often will receive treatment using an IMRT technique (Bartels et al., 2008).

  iii. Spinal cord irradiation tolerance appears to be in the range of 45–50 Gy, although in patients receiving radiosensitizing chemotherapy, spinal cord tolerance may be lower (Swift, 2009).

(g) Emerging RT treatment options

   i. SRS is the use of a single high dose of radiation delivered with stereotactic guidance to a well-defined target volume. It introduces a steep gradient of radiation into the surrounding tissue with a high level of biologic effectiveness (Prasad & Schiff, 2005).

     • SRS can be delivered in one or two sessions with a total dose of 8–18 Gy (Sun & Nemecek, 2009).

     • It has limited use because of the poor tolerance of the spinal cord to radiation.

     • Spinal cord irradiation tolerance appears to be in the range of 45–50 Gy, although in patients receiving radiosensitizing chemotherapy, spinal cord tolerance may be lower (Swift, 2009).

   ii. Brachytherapy is the implantation of radioactive seeds near the region of compression and is limited to a very small group of patients who have good performance status and expected long-term survival (Prasad & Schiff, 2005).

(5) Surgery is the preferred treatment for bony invasion, which will not respond to RT.

  (a) General indications for surgery (Penas-Prado & Loghin, 2008)

   i. Spinal instability

   ii. Spinal compression secondary to retropulsed bones (when a fractured fragment is pushed backward onto the spinal cord) or spinal deformity

   iii. Radiation-resistant tumors

   iv. Failure of radiation (progression during treatment or recurrence)

   v. Intractable pain unresponsive to medical treatment

   vi. Unknown primary tumor (histologic diagnosis)

   vii. Presence of paravertebral mass

   viii. Rapid progression of neurologic deficits

(b) Surgery is the only treatment method that leads to immediate cord decompression and stabilization of disease that has caused a weakened vertebral column (Prasad & Schiff, 2005).

(c) Historically, posterior decompression with a laminectomy for patients with ESCC was the initial approach in patients with neurologic compromise. Retrospective comparisons of patients treated with posterior laminectomy with or without RT versus RT alone revealed no advantage to a surgical approach (Findlay, 1984).

(d) Newer surgical techniques using an anterior approach (transthoracic or retroperitoneal) or lateral approach (transpedicular, costotransverse, or lateral extracavitary) have been developed (Penas-Prado & Loghin, 2008).

   i. Anterior approach: Provides direct access to the vertebral body (Vaillant & Loghin, 2009) for resection of tumor and installation of polymethyl methacrylate (bone cement) (Patchell et al., 2005)

   ii. Lateral approach: Used for diffuse bony involvement or multilevel disease (Vaillant & Loghin, 2009)

(e) In some cases, surgical intervention plus irradiation is required. A combination of techniques may be used for circumferential cord decompression (Bartels et al., 2008).

(6) Chemotherapy (Brumbaugh, 2009; Kaplan, 2006)

  (a) Indicated for chemosensitive tumors

   i. Breast

   ii. Lymphoma: HL, NHL

   iii. Multiple myeloma

   iv. Small cell carcinoma

   v. Germ-cell tumors

  (b) Other indications

   i. Previously irradiated patients who cannot tolerate additional RT

   ii. Nonsurgical candidates who have failed RT

  (c) Usually given with another therapy

       i. As combination therapy with RT

      ii. As adjunctive therapy with surgery

m) Side effects of RT: The side effects of RT delivered to the spine are generally mild.

(1) Esophagitis: Treatment to the cervical and/or upper thoracic spine can induce esophagitis typically occurring two to three weeks after initiation of RT and remitting two to three weeks after completion of treatment. Characteristic clinical features of acute radiation esophagitis include dysphagia, odynophagia, and substernal pain (Rose, Rodrigues, Yaremko, Lock, & D'Souza, 2009). (See also sections IV.G—Nutritional issues and V.B—Head and neck.)

    (a) Esophagitis is caused by irritation of the membranes lining the esophagus and throat.

    (b) A short course of analgesic medication may be necessary.

    (c) A temporary diet consisting of soft, bland foods and thick liquids can help support a patient through this short-term side effect.

    (d) Patient education should include known anecdotal therapies such as avoidance of extremely hot or cold food or drink and known irritants such as spicy foods, citrus foods, and alcohol.

    (e) Use of "magic" mouth rinse, a combination of lidocaine, diphenhydramine, and aluminum hydroxide, has proven to reduce symptoms of mucositis caused by RT (Harris, Eilers, Harriman, Cashavelly, & Maxwell, 2008; Rosenthal & Trotti, 2009).

(2) Nausea and vomiting: Treatment to the lower thoracic and upper lumbar spine can cause nausea and vomiting.

    (a) Occur as a result of the radiation beam exiting through the epigastrium

    (b) Antiemetics can aid in the reduction of these symptoms.

(3) Fatigue is a common treatment-related side effect of RT. (See section IV.B—Fatigue.)

    (a) Encourage short rest periods throughout the day.

    (b) Encourage modest exercise as tolerated (Segal et al., 2009).

(4) Radiodermatitis: Erythema and dry desquamation (see section IV.C—Skin reactions)

    (a) Caused by a decrease in stem cells of the basal layer of the epidermis as a result of ionizing radiation (Baney, 2011)

    (b) Personal hygiene habits and recommendations based on expert opinion (Baney et al., 2011)

      i. Gentle skin washing with water or mild soap and water

      ii. Encouragement of personal hygiene habits according to the patient's usual routine

      iii. Individualized management according to the severity of the skin toxicity in addition to generalized approaches noted previously

    (c) Application of emollients and moisturizers after RT is completed may aid in the healing of developed areas of desquamation (author's personal clinical experience).

2. SVCS

  a) Definition: SVCS results from any condition that leads to obstruction of blood flow through the superior vena cava (SVC). In the United States, SVCS occurs in approximately 15,000 people per year (Higdon & Higdon, 2006).

  b) Obstruction may be the result of invasion or external compression of the SVC by adjacent pathologic processes involving the right lung, lymph nodes, and other mediastinal structures.

(1) The thin walls of the SVC are easily compressed by tumors, which results in impaired venous drainage from the head, neck, and upper extremities (Halfdanarson, Hogan, & Moynihan, 2006).

(2) The obstruction of venous drainage in the upper thorax, along with increased venous pressure, may lead to

    (a) Dilation of collateral veins of the upper part of the chest and neck

    (b) Edema and plethora of the face, neck, and upper torso

    (c) Suffusion and edema of the conjunctiva.

(3) Transiently decreased cardiac output may be caused by acute SVC obstruction, but typically blood return is reestablished by increased venous pressure and collaterals. If hemodynam-

ic compromise is present, this more often results from mass effect on the heart rather than from SVC compression (Wilson, Detterbeck, & Yahalom, 2007).

 (4) SVCS may be caused by thrombosis within the SVC. Occasionally, thrombosis and external compression coexist (Mónaco et al., 2003).

c) More than 90% of all cases of SVCS are related to malignant disease (Beeson, 2010). Lung, breast, and mediastinal tumors are common causes (Rice, Rodriguez, & Light, 2006). The most common malignant causes of SVCS are NSCLC (approximately 50% of patients), SCLC (approximately 25% of patients), lymphoma, and metastatic lesions (each approximately 10% of patients) (Wilson et al., 2007).

d) Widespread use of permanent central venous access catheters and the increasing use of multilead implantable cardiac rhythm management devices have increased the incidence of SVCS not caused by direct tumor infiltration but by thrombosis (Schifferdecker, Shaw, Piemonte, & Eisenhauer, 2005).

e) Before the mid-20th century, SVCS was often the result of an infection such as tuberculosis, goiter, or a syphilitic aortic aneurysm (Nunnelee, 2007).

f) Risk factors (Brumbaugh, 2009; Kuzin, 2006)
 (1) Most common: Mediastinal cancer
 (2) Benign obstruction
 (3) Thrombosis from central line or pacemaker catheters
 (4) Mediastinal fibrosis
 (5) Histoplasmosis
 (6) Thoracic aortic aneurysm

g) Presentation of SVCS
 (1) Subtle but rapid onset, especially if the underlying cause is a rapidly growing tumor or thrombosis
 (2) Most common symptoms (Schifferdecker et al., 2005)
  (a) Dyspnea
  (b) Facial edema
  (c) Cough that may be exacerbated by bending forward or stooping
 (3) Most common signs (Kuzin, 2006; Schifferdecker et al., 2005)
  (a) Distended chest wall and neck veins
  (b) Facial swelling and plethora
  (c) Edema of the upper extremities

h) Diagnosis
 (1) Comprehensive history
 (2) Thorough physical examination
 (3) Histologic diagnosis to confirm cancer (Brumbaugh, 2009)
 (4) In patients who present without a known diagnosis of malignancy, biopsies should be performed before beginning therapy. Sputum cytology, thoracentesis, or mediastinoscopy may be helpful to definitively determine a cancer diagnosis (Kuzin, 2006).
 (5) The majority of patients with SVCS have an abnormal chest x-ray showing mediastinal widening and pleural effusion, as malignancy is the most common underlying disorder (Eren, Karaman, & Okur, 2006).
 (6) CT is often used for confirmation of SVCS (Higdon & Higdon, 2006).
 (7) Contrast venography is able to define the site and extent of SVC obstruction and visualize collateral pathways. Magnetic resonance venography may be used as an alternative for patients with a contrast allergy (Wilson et al., 2007).

i) Management
 (1) Acute SVCS is an emergency requiring immediate attention to alleviate obstructive symptoms (Brumbaugh, 2009). Treatment is determined by the underlying cause, the patient's prognosis and severity of symptoms, and the presence of a thrombosis (Brumbaugh, 2009; Kuzin, 2006). Patients have a very poor prognosis if SVCS is left untreated. Patients with SVCS typically have advanced disease, and less than 10% survive more than 30 months after treatment (Higdon & Higdon, 2006).
 (2) RT is the treatment of choice for SVCS caused by NSCLC and other malignancies (Brumbaugh, 2009; Kuzin, 2006).
  (a) Standard dose and schedule do not exist (Kuzin, 2006).

(b) Dose is determined by (Brumbaugh, 2009)
   i. Tumor type
   ii. Extent of disease
   iii. Previous radiation to the area
   iv. Patient's performance status.
(c) Options (Brumbaugh, 2009; Kuzin, 2006)
   i. High-dose fractions: 300–400 cGy for two to four treatments, then 180–200 cGy daily
   ii. Standard fractionation
   iii. Hypofractionated RT
(d) Most malignancies causing SVCS are radiosensitive, and improvement in symptoms may be apparent within 72 hours (Rowell & Gleeson, 2002).

(3) Chemotherapy: Chemotherapy has been an effective treatment for the management of SVCS when the underlying cause was small cell cancer or malignant lymphoma (Charokopos et al., 2007).

(4) Surgery: Because of the success of endovascular treatment, surgery is used less often in patients with malignant causes of SVCS. However, with malignant thymoma and thymic carcinoma, which are relatively resistant to chemotherapy and radiation, surgery could be considered (Charokopos et al., 2007).

(5) Stent placement: Placement of an endovascular stent restores venous return and sustains symptom control in patients with SVCS (Nagata et al., 2007).

(6) Pharmacologic therapy
(a) Diuretic therapy can provide symptomatic relief of edema (Wilson et al., 2007).
(b) Thrombolysis and anticoagulation may be indicated if thrombosis is the underlying cause of SVCS (Escribano et al., 2007).
(c) If lymphoma, which is responsive to steroids, is the cause of SVCS, steroids will be useful (Kuzin, 2006).

(7) Supportive therapy
(a) Oxygen can relieve dyspnea (Kuzin, 2006). Supportive therapy should include supplemental oxygen for hypoxia (Armstrong, Perez, Simpson, & Hederman, 1987).
(b) Elevation of the head of the bed reduces edema (Higdon & Higdon, 2006).

j) Side effects of SVCS treatment
   (1) Side effects of RT for SVCS vary depending on the areas included in the treatment field.
   (2) May include skin irritation, dyspnea, cough, pneumonitis, mucositis, appetite and taste changes, fatigue, and decrease in blood counts (Vachani, 2006).

B. SCC and SVCS are two common oncologic emergencies treated with RT. Rapid diagnosis can lead to early intervention resulting in symptom improvement and life extension.

References

Armstrong, B.A., Perez, C.A., Simpson, J.R., & Hederman, M.A. (1987). Role of irradiation in the management of superior vena cava syndrome. *International Journal of Radiation Oncology, Biology, Physics, 13*, 531–539. doi:10.1016/0360-3016(87)90068-X

Bach, F., Larsen, B.H., Rohde, K., Børgesen, S.E., Gjerris, F., Bøge-Rasmussen, T., … Sørensen, P.S. (1990). Metastatic spinal cord compression. Occurrence, symptoms, clinical presentations and prognosis in 398 patients with spinal cord compression. *Acta Neurochirurgica, 107*, 37–43.

Baney, T. (Ed.). (2011). Radiodermatitis. In L.H. Eaton, J.M. Tipton, & M. Irwin (Eds.), *Putting evidence into practice: Improving oncology patient outcomes, volume 2* (pp. 49–56). Pittsburgh, PA: Oncology Nursing Society.

Baney, T., McQuestion, M., Bell, K., Bruce, S., Feight, D., Weis-Smith, L., & Haas, M. (2011). ONS PEP resource: Radiodermatitis. In L.H. Eaton, J.M. Tipton, & M. Irwin (Eds.), *Putting evidence into practice: Improving oncology patient outcomes, volume 2* (pp. 57–75). Pittsburgh, PA: Oncology Nursing Society.

Bartels, R.H., van der Linden, Y.M., & van der Graaf, W.T. (2008). Spinal extradural metastasis: Review of current treatment options. *CA: A Cancer Journal for Clinicians, 58*, 245–259. doi:10.3322/CA.2007.0016

Beeson, M.S. (2010). Superior vena cava syndrome in emergency medicine. Retrieved from http://emedicine.medscape.com/article/760301-overview

Brumbaugh, H.L. (2009). Structural oncologic emergencies. In B.H. Gobel, S. Triest-Robertson, & W.H. Vogel (Eds.), *Advanced oncology nursing certification review and resource manual* (pp. 599–636). Pittsburgh, PA: Oncology Nursing Society.

Charokopos, N., Antonitsis, P., Klimatsidas, M., Giavroglou, C., Hatzibaloglou, A., & Papakonstantinou, C. (2007). Secondary endovascular repair of a reconstructed superior vena cava in a patient with a malignant thymic epithelial neoplasm. *Thoracic and Cardiovascular Surgeon, 55*, 267–270. doi:10.1055/s-2006-924701

Cole, J.S., & Patchell, R.A. (2008). Metastatic epidural spinal cord compression. *Lancet Neurology, 7*, 459–466. doi:10.1016/S1474-4422(08)70089-9

Eren, S., Karaman, A., & Okur, A. (2006). The superior vena cava syndrome caused by malignant disease. Imaging with multi-detector row CT. *European Journal of Radiology, 59*, 93–103. doi:10.1016/j.ejrad.2006.01.003

Escribano, J.F.G., Antón, R.F., Rubio, A.C., Cascos, L.S., González, F.S., & Rodríguez, R.A. (2007). Superior vena cava syndrome with central venous catheter for chemotherapy treated successfully with fibrinolysis. *Clinical and Translational Oncology, 9,* 198–200. doi:10.1007/s12094-007-0036-1

Findlay, G.F. (1984). Adverse effects of the management of malignant spinal cord compression. *Journal of Neurology, Neurosurgery, and Psychiatry, 47,* 761–768. doi:10.1136/jnnp.47.8.761

Halfdanarson, T.R., Hogan, W.J., & Moynihan, T.J. (2006). Oncologic emergencies: Diagnosis and treatment. *Mayo Clinic Proceedings, 81,* 835–848. doi:10.4065/81.6.835

Harris, D.J., Eilers, J., Harriman, A., Cashavelly, B.J., & Maxwell, C. (2008). Putting evidence into practice: Evidence-based intervention for the management of oral mucositis. *Clinical Journal of Oncology Nursing, 12,* 141–152. doi:10.1188/08.CJON.141-152

Helweg-Larsen, S., & Sørensen, P.S. (1994). Symptoms and signs in metastatic spinal cord compression: A study of progression from first symptom until diagnosis in 153 patients. *European Journal of Cancer, 30A,* 396–399.

Higdon, M.L., & Higdon, J.A. (2006). Treatment of oncologic emergencies. *American Family Physician, 74,* 1873–1880.

Huff, J.S. (2010). Spinal cord neoplasms. Retrieved from http://emedicine.medscape.com/article/779872-overview

Kaplan, M. (2006). Spinal cord compression. In M. Kaplan (Ed.), *Understanding and managing oncologic emergencies: A resource for nurses* (pp. 219–259). Pittsburgh, PA: Oncology Nursing Society.

Kuzin, E. (2006). Superior vena cava syndrome. In M. Kaplan (Ed.), *Understanding and managing oncologic emergencies* (pp. 261–284). Pittsburgh, PA: Oncology Nursing Society.

Kwok, Y., DeYoung, C., Garofalo, M., Dhople, A., & Regine, W. (2006). Radiation oncology emergencies. *Hematology/Oncology Clinics of North America, 20,* 505–522. doi:10.1016/j.hoc.2006.01.001

Lu, C., Gonzalez, R.G., Jolesz, F.A., Wen, P.Y., & Talcott, J. (2005). Suspected spinal cord compression in cancer patients: A multidisciplinary risk assessment. *Journal of Supportive Oncology, 3,* 305–312.

Mónaco, G.R., Bertoni, H., Pallota, G., Lastiri, R., Varela, M., Beveraggi, E.M., & Vassallo, B.C. (2003). Use of self-expanding vascular endoprostheses in superior vena cava syndrome. *European Journal of Cardio-Thoracic Surgery, 24,* 208–211. doi:10.1016/S1010-7940(03)00293-8

Nagata, T., Makutani, S., Uchida, H., Kichikawa, K, Maeda, M., Yoshioka, T., ... Yoshimura, H. (2007). Follow-up results of 71 patients undergoing metallic stent placement for the treatment of a malignant obstruction of the superior vena cava. *Cardiovascular and Interventional Radiology, 30,* 959–967. doi:10.1007/s00270-007-9088-4

Nelson, K.A., Walsh, D., Abdullah, O., McDonnell, F., Homsi, J., Komurcu, S., ... Zhukovsky, D.S. (2000). Common complications of advanced cancer. *Seminars in Oncology, 27,* 34–44.

Nunnelee, J.D. (2007). Superior vena cava syndrome. *Journal of Vascular Nursing, 25,* 2–5. doi:10.1016/j.jvn.2006.09.004

Patchell, R.A., Tibbs, P.A., Regine, W.F., Payne, R., Saris, S., Kryscio, R.J., ... Young, B. (2005). Direct decompressive surgical resection in the treatment of spinal cord compression caused by metastatic cancer: A randomised trial. *Lancet, 366,* 643–648. doi:10.1016/S0140-6736(05)66954-1

Penas-Prado, M., & Loghin, M.E. (2008). Spinal cord compression in cancer patients: Review of diagnosis and treatment. *Current Oncology Reports, 10,* 78–85.

Prasad, D., & Schiff, D. (2005). Malignant spinal-cord compression. *Lancet Oncology, 6,* 15–24. doi:10.1016/S1470-2045(04)01709-7

Quinn, J.A., & DeAngelis, L.M. (2000). Neurologic emergencies in the cancer patient. *Seminars in Oncology, 27,* 311–321.

Rades, D., Karstens, J.H., & Alberti, W. (2002). Role of radiotherapy in the treatment of motor dysfunction due to metastatic spinal cord compression: Comparison of three different fractionation schedules. *International Journal of Radiation Oncology, Biology, Physics, 54,* 1160–1164. doi:10.1016/S0360-3016(02)02979-6

Rades, D., Lange, M., Veninga, T., Rudat, V., Bajrovic, A., Stalpers, L.J., ... Schild, S.E. (2009). Preliminary results of spinal cord compression recurrence evaluation (score-1) study comparing short course versus long-course radiotherapy for local control of malignant epidural spinal cord compression. *International Journal of Radiation Oncology, Biology, Physics, 73,* 228–234. doi:10.1016/j.ijrobp.2008.04.044

Rice, T.W., Rodriguez, R.M., & Light, R.W. (2006). The superior vena cava syndrome: Clinical characteristics and evolving etiology. *Medicine, 85,* 37–42. doi:10.1097/01.md.0000198474.99876.f0

Rose, J., Rodrigues, G., Yaremko, B., Lock, M., & D'Souza, D. (2009). Systematic review of dose-volume parameters in the prediction of esophagitis in thoracic radiotherapy. *Radiotherapy and Oncology, 91,* 282–287. doi:10.1016/j.radonc.2008.09.010

Rosenthal, D.I., & Trotti, A. (2009). Strategies for managing radiation-induced mucositis in head and neck cancer. *Seminars in Radiation Oncology, 19,* 29–34. doi:10.1016/j.semradonc.2008.09.006

Rowell, N.P., & Gleeson, F.V. (2002). Steroids, radiotherapy, chemotherapy and stents for superior vena caval obstruction in carcinoma of the bronchus: A systematic review. *Clinical Oncology, 14,* 338–351.

Schifferdecker, B., Shaw, J.A., Piemonte, T.C., & Eisenhauer, A.C. (2005). Nonmalignant superior vena cava syndrome: Pathophysiology and management. *Catheterization and Cardiovascular Interventions, 65,* 416–423. doi:10.1002/ccd.20381

Segal, R.J., Reid, R.D., Courneya, K.S., Sigal, R.J., Kenny, G.P., Prud'Homme, D.G., ... D'Angelo, M.E.S. (2009). Randomized controlled trial of resistance or aerobic exercise in men receiving radiation therapy for prostate cancer. *Journal of Clinical Oncology, 27,* 344–351. doi:10.1200/JCO.2007.15.4963

Sun, H., & Nemecek, A.N. (2009). Optimal management of malignant epidural spinal compression. *Emergency Medicine Clinics of North America, 27,* 195–208. doi:10.1016/j.emc.2009.02.001

Swift, P.S. (2009). Radiation for spinal metastatic tumors. *Orthopedic Clinics of North America, 40,* 133–144. doi:10.1016/j.ocl.2008.09.001

Vachani, C. (2006). Superior vena cava syndrome. Retrieved from http://69.63.133.6/resources/article.cfm?c=16&s=46&ss=205&id=893

Vaillant, B., & Loghin, M. (2009). Treatment of spinal cord tumors. *Current Treatment Options in Neurology, 11,* 315–324.

Vecht, C.J., Haaxma-Reiche, H., van Putten, W.L., de Visser, M., Vries, E.P., & Twijnstra, A. (1989). Initial bolus of conventional versus high dose dexamethasone in metastatic spinal cord compression. *Neurology, 39,* 1255–1257.

Wilson, L.D., Detterbeck, F.C., & Yahalom, J. (2007). Superior vena cava syndrome with malignant causes. *New England Journal of Medicine, 356,* 1862–1869. doi:10.1056/NEJMcp067190

VIII. Modality-specific management

A. External beam (teletherapy)
1. History of EBRT (Bentel, 1996)
   a) Wilhelm Conrad Roentgen discovered invisible rays, which he later named x-rays, on November 8, 1895.
   b) Wilhelm Roentgen took a dramatic radiologic picture of his wife's hand on December 22, 1895.
   c) The first therapeutic application of x-rays was delivered on January 29, 1896, to a patient with carcinoma of the breast.
   d) Marie Curie and her husband, Pierre Curie, discovered the effect of radioactivity on the skin in July 1898. Fellow physicians conducted further research on the use of x-rays on malignant tumors.
   e) Basal cell epitheliomas became the first cancer to be cured by radiation in 1899.
   f) Severe tissue damage occurred after single high-dose radiation treatments because radiation was focused on eradicating the tumor. Tumor recurrences and adverse effects following RT dimmed the excitement of its usefulness in curing cancers. However, in the 1930s, Claude Regaud and Henri Coutard found that administering fractionated doses of radiation could achieve the same tumor response with decreased tissue injury.
   g) Surgeons and dermatologists were the first physicians to administer RT in the early 1900s, and determined the proper length of treatment based on the amount of skin erythema present.
   h) The "penometer" was introduced in 1901, which allowed direct measurement of the quality and quantity of x ray beams. A "chromoradiometer" and "radiometer" also were used to measure the quantity of radiation doses in the early 1900s.
   i) H. Geiger and W. Mueller developed an improved radiation detector in 1928. The Geiger counter was used well into the 1960s to measure the dose given to the patient.
   j) The roentgen was recognized as a unit of measurement of x-rays and gamma rays in 1928. ICRU recommended the rad as the measurement for radiation absorbed dose in 1953, which was later replaced by the gray (Gy).
   k) The first use of a megavoltage RT machine that created greater than one million volts occurred in 1937 at St. Bartholomew's Hospital in London. The high-dose delivery improved the skin-sparing effect and allowed radiation to be delivered to deep-seated tumors without causing significant skin erythema.
2. Electromagnetic radiation: Does not produce chemical or biologic damage until it passes through an agent, which causes the radiation to give up energy and produce fast-moving electrons (Hall & Cox, 2010).
   a) X-rays (Moore-Higgs, 2007)
      (1) 40–150 peak kilovolts (kVp)
          (a) Superficial penetration
          (b) Limited range
          (c) Used with skin cancers or other superficial lesions
      (2) 150–1,000 kVp
          (a) Deep penetration
          (b) High skin dose
          (c) High bone absorption
          (d) Limited usage because of increased probability of bone necrosis from high bone absorption
   b) Photons: X-ray and gamma ray interactions (Moore-Higgs, 2007)
      (1) 4–20 MeV
          (a) Deep penetration
          (b) Skin sparing
          (c) Versatile and allow for precise dose distribution
          (d) Used with deep-seated tumors and/or large treatment fields
          (e) Photons are delivered by a complex electronic machine, which has the potential for frequent downtime, thus causing delays in patient treatments.
      (2) 18–40 MeV
          (a) High-energy photons
          (b) Infrequently used with tumors because of the bulky size of the equipment
   c) Gamma rays (Moore-Higgs, 2007)
      (1) Cesium (600 kVp)
          (a) Has a long radioactive half-life
          (b) Low energy
          (c) Used with head and neck cancers

    (2) Cobalt (1.25–2 MeV)
       (a) Deep penetration
       (b) Skin sparing
       (c) Used with deep-seated tumors
       (d) As the source decays, treatment times are longer because of a slower dose being delivered.

3. Particulate radiation
  a) Electrons: Light, negatively charged particles, which can be accelerated to the speed of light by a betatron or linear accelerator (Hall & Cox, 2010).
    (1) 6–30 MeV
       (a) Penetrates a few centimeters below the surface and thus delivers maximum dose to skin surfaces
       (b) Used with skin lesions, chest wall recurrences, and superficial lymph nodes
    (2) 10–30 MeV (Moore-Higgs, 2007): Deep penetration of skin structures
  b) Protons: Positively charged particles; mass is 2,000 times the mass of an electron; requires expensive and complicated equipment to accelerate particles (Hall & Cox, 2010). Radiation dose is 600 MeV (Moore-Higgs, 2007).
    (1) Precise dose-delivery system
    (2) Delivers high doses to tumor while limiting the dose to adjacent normal tissue, which is referred to as the Bragg peak
    (3) Used with pituitary tumors, chondrosarcoma, chordoma, abdominal and pelvic tumors, soft tissue sarcomas, and head and neck tumors
  c) Neutrons: Mass is similar to a proton but it has no electrical charge. No advantage has been found over other sources. Radiation dose is 16–50 MeV (Moore-Higgs, 2007)
    (1) Uses a fixed field size and beam position
    (2) Absorbed dose decreases greatly with increased depth penetration
    (3) Currently, used only in clinical trials

4. Radioactive sources used in EBRT (Washington & Leaver, 2004)
  a) Cobalt-60 (1.25 MeV) uses
    (1) Gamma Knife
       (a) Multiple radionuclides
       (b) Radiosurgery with well-defined fields using collimated beams (shaped beams)
       (c) Most commonly used for CNS tumors
    (2) TBI: Given during bone marrow transplantation

5. Types of beams (Washington & Leaver, 2004)
  a) Two-dimensional conformal
    (1) Two-dimensional images of the body
    (2) Computerized digital radiography also used
    (3) Unable to differentiate soft tissue densities
    (4) Can be used for emergency cases, bone metastasis, and whole brain RT (J. Lowden, personal communication, May 24, 2011)
  b) Three-dimensional conformal
    (1) Treatments based on three-dimensional anatomic information
    (2) Includes the physical as well as the biologic response of the tumor
    (3) Can be used for any case (J. Lowden, personal communication, May 24, 2011)
  c) Intensity modulated (Meyer, 2007)
    (1) Precise delivery of RT dose (Meyer, 2007)
       (a) Static: Also known as "step and shoot." The MLCs do not move while the beams are on. Because numerous beams are used, the process can take up to 30 minutes to treat a patient (L. Grove-Narayan, personal communication, April 30, 2010).
       (b) Dynamic: The MLCs do move when the beam is on (L. Grove-Narayan, personal communication, April 30, 2010). Process as described in *(a)* but is fluid and without stops to move the gantry or reset the MLC.
    (2) Both TomoTherapy® (TomoTherapy Inc.) equipment and linear accelerators can use this technique (L. Grove-Narayan, personal communication, April 30, 2010).
    (3) MLCs became popular after 1996 (Meyer, 2007).
    (4) Indicated with head and neck and prostate cancers and some breast cancers (Meyer, 2007)
  d) Image-guided (Meyer, 2007)
    (1) Based on the knowledge that tumor and normal tissues move over time
    (2) Movement
       (a) Predictable—Respiratory motion (also known as 4D)
       (b) Unpredictable—Bowel peristalsis, gas, bladder movement
       (c) Permanent—Tumor shrinkage

(3) Attempts are made to image, track, and manage motion during treatment for more precise RT treatments.

    e) Stereotactic body RT (used to treat tumors in the body) and SRS (used to treat tumors in the brain)

        (1) Based on the same principles as stereotactic brain RT

        (2) Allow precise delivery of RT dose

        (3) Can be used in solitary tumors of the spine, lung, liver, prostate, and pancreas

        (4) Use MLCs or TomoTherapy

        (5) Doses of 7.7–45 Gy in one to four fractions

6. Equipment

    a) Betatrons (Bentel, 1996)

        (1) Developed by Kerst in 1941 and first used in the 1950s

        (2) Changing magnetic fields accelerate electrons in a circular path. The electrons are removed from this path to produce an electron beam that is used in RT.

        (3) Have largely been replaced by linear accelerators because of the betatron's inability to deliver low dose rates, limited field sizes, and limited motions, which lead to difficult patient setup. The size of the betatron is also very large.

    b) Linear accelerators (Khan, 2010)

        (1) Developed in 1928 by Wideroe to accelerate heavy ions such as neutrons and protons

        (2) Electron linear accelerators were first developed during the 1940s.

        (3) The linear accelerator became the radiation device of choice by 1970 (Khan, 2007).

7. Indications

    a) RT treats almost all cancers—an estimated 60% of patients will receive some type of RT during the course of their cancer treatment (Haas, 2010).

    b) Curative intent (Haas, 2010).

        (1) Definitive: Primary RT with or without chemotherapy (e.g., head and neck, lung, prostate, or bladder cancer)

        (2) Neoadjuvant: Given before primary treatment (e.g., esophageal, colon, or breast cancer)

        (3) Adjuvant: Given after primary treatment in order to increase disease-free survival (e.g., breast, lung, and high-risk rectal cancer)

        (4) Prophylactic: Given for asymptomatic patients with a high risk for occurrence (e.g., SCLC)

    c) Palliative intent (Haas, 2010): Given to control symptoms such as bleeding, pain, airway obstruction, neurologic compromise, and other structural emergencies (e.g., bone metastasis, increased intracranial pressure, SVCS, dyspnea, or SCC)

    d) May be given as a single modality or may be combined in a variety of therapies (e.g., surgery, chemotherapy)

    e) Patient must be able to lie still on the radiation treatment table during the treatment in order to decrease or eliminate movement of the treatment target. Immobilization devices as well as medication can be ordered to enable patients to lie still and remain calm during the treatment (Kahn, 2007).

    f) Individuals with multiple sites of disease typically are not candidates for radiation because their disease cannot be encompassed in an RT field.

8. Treatment preparation

    a) Simulation (Washington & Leaver, 2004)

        (1) Accurate positioning is imperative to replicate daily treatment fields.

        (2) May involve a simple radiographic unit attached to a treatment machine, fluoroscopy, or CT. Also, PET or MRI images can be fused with the treatment planning films.

        (3) Radiopaque markers (lead, copper, or solder wire) may be used to mark specific points on the patient to assist in calculations or mark critical structures for the treatment planning phase.

        (4) Contrast media are used to enhance anatomic structures that would normally be difficult to visualize.

            (a) Barium sulfate is used in the GI tract and is administered orally or rectally to visualize the esophagus, stomach, small bowel, colon, or oral cavity.

            (b) Barium paste can be used to visualize a tonsillar lesion.

            (c) Iodinated contrast (aqueous ionic or nonionic contrast) helps identify vessels and organs (e.g., kidneys, bladder, GI tract, prostate) and is administered intravenously, orally, or through catheters to enhance bladder or urethra images.

        (5) Selection of immobilization devices are determined (Washington & Leaver, 2004).

            (a) Simple (e.g., tape, plastic or cloth straps, arm pulls, rubber bands,

bite block). Bite blocks hold the jaw in place.

(b) Complex (e.g., plaster of paris, foaming agents, Vac-Lok™ [CIV-CO Medical Solutions], Aquaplast RT™ [WFR-Aquaplast Corp.])

9. Treatment planning (Washington & Leaver, 2004)

a) Treatment plan includes the number of treatments, dose per fraction, energy, prescription point location, and total dose.

b) Patient positioning

(1) Immobilization devices reproduce treatment positions daily.

(2) A three-point positioning technique is common, which allows the radiation therapist to align the treatment plane with the axis of the gantry rotation.

(3) The position is refined more with lasers and treatment field lights (crosshairs).

c) Localization

(1) Landmarks are used and can either be placed or already exist anatomically.

(2) Internal localization includes the use of ultrasound or electronic portal imaging devices.

(3) Planning includes GTV, which includes macroscopic disease; CTV, which includes the GTV and any microscopic disease; and the PTV, which includes the CTV and plans for motion and treatment setup variations.

d) Beam shaping

(1) Blocks: Used to shape photon or electron fields. Standardized lead blocks may be used, but customized blocks generally consist of cerrobend, a compound of bismuth, lead, tin, and cadmium.

(2) Process

(a) Area to be blocked is drawn on plain film.

(b) Blocked area image is transferred to a Styrofoam square.

(c) Area to be blocked is cut out of Styrofoam to create a mold.

(d) Molten cerrobend is poured into the mold and cooled.

(e) The block is inserted into the gantry to "block" beams from reaching area within the treatment field that should not be treated.

e) MLCs: Customize the field shape and size using "jaws" that have opposing leaves to form leaf pairs. Each leaf is independent and can produce multiple shapes and sizes.

f) Verification imaging

(1) Also known as portal imaging or electron portal imaging devices

(2) Images are taken at the beginning of treatment and at regular intervals during the treatment to ensure appropriate placement of radiation beam.

(3) The portal and simulation images are compared by the radiation oncologist, who either accepts or changes the daily treatment.

g) Beam-modifying devices

(1) Bolus

(a) Material that mimics tissue and brings radiation dose for target areas that are closer to the surface of the skin. Common materials are paraffin wax, Vaseline® (Unilever) gauze, wet gauze, towels, and water bags. Several commercially available products also may be used.

(b) May be used over scars, superficial nodes, variations in surface contours, or where there is a gap in tissue on the patient's body.

(2) Compensators: Used in places of tissue deficits on a patient. Tissue deficits occur in areas where the body is not a perfect geometric shape and can create "hot spots" or "cold spots". Common materials include copper, brass, cerrobend, and lead.

(3) Wedges

(a) Designed to change the angle of the beam at a specified depth

(b) Standard wedges are externally mounted on the machine. However, some treatment units have internal wedges.

h) Electron beam shields

(1) Cutouts that are used to shape the beam

(2) Can be used to protect the patient's nasal membranes, skin behind the ears,

optic lens, and gingiva. Electron beam shields typically are made of aluminum, tin, or paraffin wax.

   i) Patient comorbid factors

      (1) Smoking, recent surgery, concurrent or recent chemotherapy

      (2) Pretreatment nutritional assessment in patients with evidence of anorexia, significant weight loss, or obvious cachexia

      (3) For patients who have cardiac pacemakers or implantable defibrillators, contact the manufacturer before initiating radiation. Cardiac monitoring before, during, and after may be required (Haas & Kuehn, 2001).

10. Delivery (Moore-Higgs, 2007)

   a) Length of treatment depends on the type and stage of cancer.

   b) Most treatments are daily (Monday through Friday) for 2–10 weeks; some treatments are twice daily with six hours between doses. Reduces the probability of tumor regeneration and repair.

   c) Before the first treatment, verification or portal film is taken to confirm that setup is accurate. Port films are repeated on a weekly basis. The physician may check the patient on the treatment table before the first treatment is given.

   d) The patient lies on the table for approximately 15 minutes or longer depending on the complexity of the setup, although the beam is only on for a few minutes.

11. Side effects (Haas, 2010)

   a) Tissue and organ response to radiation

      (1) Dependant on total dose, fractionation schedule, and volume treated

      (2) Cells and structures in the direct path of radiation beam are subject to damage.

      (3) Most damage occurs in the gap 2 (or G2) and mitosis stages of the cell cycle.

      (4) Tissue and organs have variable tolerances to radiation.

      (5) Concurrent chemotherapy and RT changes the tissue and organ tolerance, which generally results in acute and chronic reactions at much lower doses of radiation.

   b) Side effects and symptom management

      (1) Fatigue (see section IV.B—Fatigue and ONS PEP Resource in Eaton & Tipton, 2009)

      (2) Radiodermatitis (see section IV.C—Skin reactions and ONS PEP Resource in Eaton & Tipton, 2009)

      (3) Pain (see section IV.D—Pain and ONS PEP Resource in Eaton & Tipton, 2009)

      (4) Distress (see section IV.E—Distress/coping and ONS PEP Resources on anxiety, depression, and sleep-wake disturbances in Eaton & Tipton, 2009)

      (5) Nutritional issues (see section IV.G—Nutritional issues and ONS PEP Resources on anorexia, diarrhea, and mucositis in Eaton & Tipton, 2009)

12. Patient and caregiver education (Haas, 2010)

   a) Sensory information

      (1) The treatment does not hurt. The machine will not touch the patient. The machine will make noise as it works and the gantry moves.

      (2) The patient is not radioactive.

      (3) The radiation beam cannot be seen, felt, or smelled.

   b) Procedural information

      (1) Provide an overview of the treatment plan.

      (2) Discuss the simulation procedure.

      (3) Tattoos or small marks will be made on the skin. These marks are important to align the radiation beams the same way every day.

      (4) A body or mask mold may be needed to ensure proper dose delivery.

      (5) Inform patients that while they are alone in treatment room, the radiation therapists can see them via camera and can hear them and speak to them via a speaker and microphone.

      (6) Laser lights will not damage the eyes if looked at directly.

      (7) Instruct the patient to wear loose, comfortable clothes.

      (8) The patient should plan on staying longer than usual at least once a week for an on-treatment visit with the healthcare provider.

   c) Expected outcomes: Cure, control, prevention, or palliation of cancer

   d) Address caregiver strain and burden (see ONS PEP Resource in Eaton & Lipton, 2009).

   e) Address any myths and misconceptions associated with RT.

References

Bentel, G.C. (1996). *Radiation therapy planning* (2nd ed.). New York, NY: McGraw-Hill.

Eaton, L.H., & Tipton, J.M. (Eds.). (2009). *Putting evidence into practice: Improving oncology patient outcomes.* Pittsburgh, PA: Oncology Nursing Society.

Haas, M.L. (2010). *Radiation therapy: Toxicities and management.* In C.H. Yarbro, D. Wujcik, & B.H. Gobel (Eds.), *Cancer nursing: Principles and practice* (7th ed., pp. 312–351). Sudbury, MA: Jones and Bartlett.

Haas, M.L., & Kuehn, E.F. (2001). Teletherapy: External radiation therapy. In D. Watkins-Bruner, G. Moore-Higgs, & M. Haas (Eds.), *Outcomes in radiation therapy: Multidisciplinary management* (pp. 55–66). Sudbury, MA: Jones and Bartlett.

Hall, E.J., & Cox, J.D. (2010). Physical and biologic basis of radiation therapy. In J.D. Cox & K.K. Ang (Eds.), *Radiation oncology: Rationale, technique, results* (9th ed., pp. 3–49). Philadelphia, PA: Elsevier Mosby.

Khan, F.M. (Ed.). (2007). *Treatment planning in radiation oncology* (2nd ed.). Philadelphia, PA: Lippincott Williams & Wilkins.

Khan, F.M. (2010). *The physics of radiation therapy* (4th ed.). Philadelphia, PA: Lippincott Williams & Wilkins.

Meyer, J.L. (Ed.). (2007). *IMRT, IGRT, SBRT: Advances in the treatment planning and delivery of radiotherapy.* Basel, Switzerland: S. Karger.

Moore-Higgs, G.J. (2007). Basic principles of radiotherapy. In M.L. Haas, W.P. Hogle, G.J. Moore-Higgs, & T.K. Gosselin-Acomb (Eds.), *Radiation therapy: A guide to patient care* (pp. 8–24). St. Louis, MO: Elsevier Mosby.

Washington, C.M., & Leaver, D. (Eds.). (2004). *Principles and practice of radiation therapy* (2nd ed.). St. Louis, MO: Mosby.

B. LDR and HDR brachytherapy
  1. Procedure description: Brachytherapy is the temporary or permanent placement of a radioactive source into a body cavity (intracavitary), into tissue (interstitial), or on the surface of the body (e.g., plaque, custom bolus). It is also used by placing catheters into the airway, GI tract, or a blood vessel (intraluminal or intravascular). Brachytherapy may be used by itself or as an adjunctive treatment in combination with EBRT to increase the total dose to a specified target. Brachytherapy is the optimum way of delivering conformal RT tailored to the shape of the tumor while sparing surrounding normal tissues (Lawrence, Ten Haken, & Giaccia, 2008). With temporary sealed sources, the patient is not radioactive; only the source is. Upon removal of the implanted source, no special precautions need to be used with the patient (Haas & Kuehn, 2001).
    a) LDR brachytherapy enhances radiation effect by taking advantage of repair, redistribution, and repopulation principles even in poorly oxygenated tissue (Gosselin, 2011). With LDR brachytherapy treatments, approximately 0.4–2 Gy is given in an hour, requiring treatment times of 24–144 hours.
    b) The advantage with HDR brachytherapy is that the dose is delivered quickly, resulting in improved patient comfort, more reliable positioning of the source, less dose to ancillary personnel, and an ability to perform the procedure on an outpatient basis (Gosselin & Waring, 2001; Haas & Kuehn, 2001). With HDR brachytherapy treatments, approximately 0.2 Gy is delivered per minute with a treatment time of a few minutes.
  2. Indications
    a) Brachytherapy delivers the radiation dose to a specified tumor volume with a rapid falloff in radiation dose to adjacent normal tissue (Fieler, 1997; Gosselin & Waring, 2001; Williamson & Brenner, 2008; Zeroski, Abel, Butler, Wallner, & Merrick, 2005).
    b) Common diseases treated with LDR/HDR brachytherapy are gynecologic cancers, such as cancers of the cervix, vulva, vagina, and endometrium; breast cancer; bronchogenic cancers; esophageal cancer; head and neck cancers; brain cancers; prostate cancer; choroidal melanoma; retinoblastoma; and others (Fieler, 1997; Gosselin & Waring, 2001).
    c) LDR/HDR brachytherapy may be used as a "boost" in conjunction with EBRT (Waring & Gosselin, 2010).
  3. Potential risks
    a) Acute and late effects of brachytherapy are those caused by effects of ionizing radiation (Zeroski et al., 2005).
      (1) Invasive brachytherapy procedures to various body sites such as the pelvis or lung carry risks of complications such as perforation, infection, or bleeding (Shah, Strauss, Gielda, & Zusag, 2010).
      (2) Complications associated with bed rest and catheterization, especially for LDR brachytherapy, include thrombophlebitis, pulmonary embolus, and urinary sepsis.
    b) Incidence: The majority of patients undergoing brachytherapy experience site-specific side effects related to the implant. In addition, the patient may have unresolved acute side effects of EBRT at the time of the implant because brachytherapy often is administered during or soon after the course of EBRT (Velji & Fitch, 2001). Older adult or debilitated patients are more vulnerable to complications.
    c) Assessment and management: See site-specific assessment and management for each implant site.
  4. Brachytherapy history and indications

a) Used since early 1900s following discovery of radium by Marie Curie (Eifel, 1997; Hogle, Quinn, & Heron, 2003; Moore-Higgs, 2007a; Wright, Jones, Whelan, & Lukka, 1994)

b) Has been used clinically for more than 100 years (Behrend, 2011)

c) First use of afterloaders was in 1905 (Nag, n.d.).
  (1) Source holders (applicators) are placed in an outpatient clinic or while in surgery.
  (2) Removable source or sources are loaded when the patient is in radiation procedure room or radiation-safe inpatient room.
  (3) Afterloaders reduce exposure to healthcare provider.

d) Use declined in 1960s–1970s because of the development of linear accelerators.

e) In the 1980s, interest was renewed (Nag, n.d.).
  (1) Single modality
  (2) Combined with other modalities (EBRT, hyperthermia)

f) Currently widely used (Nag, n.d.)
  (1) Knowledge of long-term effects
  (2) Reduced radiation exposure hazards
  (3) Increased positional accuracy
  (4) Superior optimized dose distribution
  (5) Increased knowledge regarding care of patients with implants (Lawrence et al., 2008). Brachytherapy requires the expertise of a team of trained personnel (physician, physicist, dosimetrist, radiation therapist, radiation nurse, and RSO) to implement the individualized treatment plan designed by the radiation oncologist.
    (a) Brachytherapy has a variety of current uses alone or in combination with other therapies and in specific cancers.
    (b) Brachytherapy is used to improve local tumor control.
      i. Gynecologic cancers (Eifel, 1992, 1997; Erickson et al., 2005; Gosselin & Waring, 2001; Gupta et al., 1999; Holland, 2001; Mock, Kucera, Fellner, Knocke, & Pötter, 2003; Moore-Higgs, 2007b; Velji & Fitch, 2001; Wright et al., 1994)
        • Vaginal cylinder/stump
        • Tandem and ovoids

        • Interstitial needles and template (e.g., Syed)
      ii. Head and neck cancers (Devine & Doyle, 2001; Kremer, Klimek, Andreopoulos, & Mösges, 1999)
        • Intracavitary catheters
        • Interstitial catheters
      iii. Lung cancer (Fieler, 1997; Powell, 1999)
        • Endobronchial catheters
        • Interstitial catheters
      iv. Breast cancer (Behrend, 2011; Hogle et al., 2003; Nelson et al., 2009)
        • Interstitial catheters
        • Applicators
        • Multichannel applicators
        • Inflatable catheters
        • See section V.C—Breast cancer for more information.
      v. Prostate cancer
        • Permanent interstitial radioactive seed implant (LDR) (Abel, Dafoe-Lambie, Butler, & Merrick, 2003; Behrend, 2011)
        • Temporary interstitial radioactive seed implant (HDR) (Waring & Gosselin, 2010)
        • See section V.G—Male pelvis/prostate for more information.

g) Brachytherapy irradiates small volumes and can potentially minimize complications (Nag, Shasha, Janjan, Petersen, & Zaider, 2001). Brachytherapy is used to preserve vital organ function.
  (1) Soft tissue sarcoma
  (2) Oropharyngeal cancers
  (3) Intraocular melanoma and retinoblastoma (Finger, Chin, & Yu, 2010; Halperin & Kirkpatrick, 2005; Shields, Naseripour, Shields, Freire, & Cater, 2003)

(4) Meningiomas

(5) Malignant brain tumors

h) Brachytherapy is used to treat recurrent or inoperable cancers.

(1) Lung cancer (bronchogenic)

(2) Esophageal cancer

i) Brachytherapy is used to control disease in previously irradiated sites.

(1) Recurrent gynecologic cancers

(2) Head and neck cancers

(3) GI malignancies

j) Isotopes and techniques used: Currently, most brachytherapy is performed with reactor-produced radionuclides.

(1) Isotopes used

(a) Cesium-137

(b) Iridium-192

(c) Iodine-125

(d) Palladium-103

(e) Gold-198

(2) Radiobiology (Gosselin, 2011; Hogle, 2006; Moore-Higgs, 2007a)

(a) Alpha, beta, and gamma rays transfer energy to living matter.

(b) Cellular reproduction process is altered (DNA is damaged).

(c) Irradiated cells are affected both directly and indirectly.

(d) Irradiated cell dies instantly or is rendered unable to divide.

(e) The extent of cell injury is related to the capabilities of the isotope and the amount of time the isotope is in place.

(3) Disease sites treated with brachytherapy (see Table 15)

k) LDR and HDR brachytherapy

(1) Conventional LDR brachytherapy involves an operative procedure with anesthesia for placement of a hollow applicator device or catheter into body tissues or cavities. Radioactive sources are manually afterloaded into the applicators after the patient has returned to the designated hospital room (Behrend, 2011). With postoperative soft tissue sarcomas, no radiation is administered for at least five days to allow for wound healing (Carrubba, Jankowski, & Kunsman, 1999).

(a) Hospitalization and specialized nursing care are required while the implant remains in place, which may be from one to several days.

(b) Bed rest is required for gynecologic, rectal, and some prostate implants.

(c) LDR brachytherapy can be performed using remote afterloading techniques.

(d) Strict room confinement is required for all inpatient brachytherapy (see section III—Radiation protection and safety).

(e) Invasive brachytherapy procedures to specific body sites such as the pelvis or lung carry risks of complications such as perforation, infection, and bleeding.

(2) HDR brachytherapy involves the use of an automated remote afterloading device for the placement of the radioactive source (e.g., iridium-192) into the applicators, which have been placed in the tumor or cavity (see Figure 21). Sources are remotely loaded from a storage safe that is in the afterloader and delivered via source guide tubes that connect the afterloader to the applicator in the tumor or body cavity (Behrend, 2011).

Table 15. Disease Sites, Techniques, and Isotopes Used for Brachytherapy

Disease Site	Technique	Isotope
Breast	Interstitial	Iridium-192, iodine-125
Central nervous system	Interstitial or intracavitary	Iodine-125, iridium-192
Cervical	Intracavitary or interstitial	Iridium-192, cesium-137, radium-226
Endometrial	Intracavitary	Cesium-137, iridium-192
Esophageal	Intraluminal	Iridium-192, cesium-137
Eye (melanoma)	Plaque	Iodine-125
Eye (pterygium)	Plaque	Strontium-90
Head and neck	Interstitial or intracavitary	Iridium-192, cesium-137, radium-226
Lung	Endobronchial or interstitial	Iridium-192
Prostate	Interstitial	Iodine-125, palladium-103
Rectal	Interstitial	Iridium-192, cesium-137

Note. Based on information from Behrend, 2011; Gosselin, 2011; Moore-Higgs, 2007a.

Figure 21. High-Dose-Rate Treatment Unit and Control Console

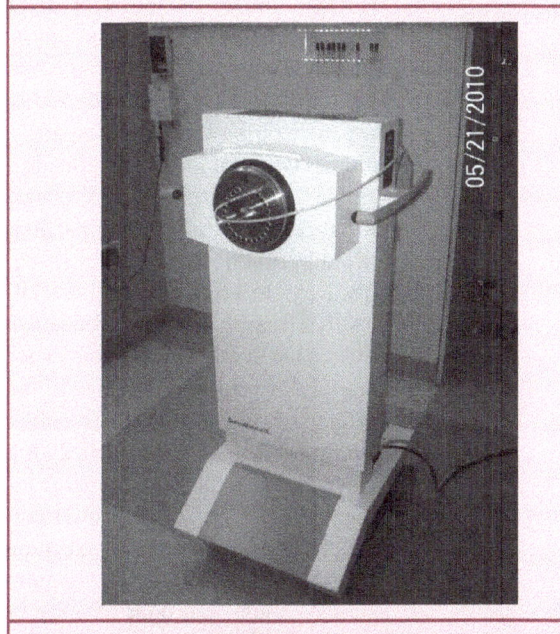

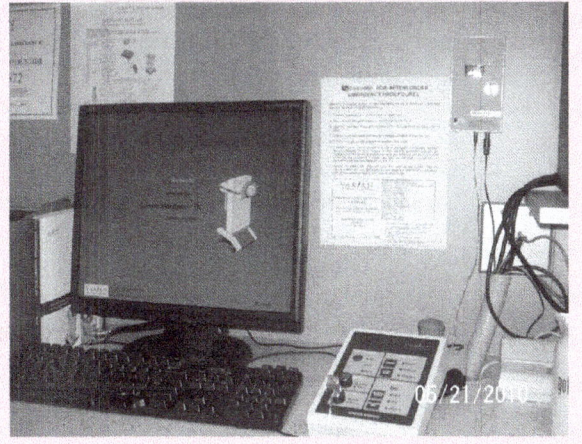

Note. Photos courtesy of Duke University Health System. Used with permission.

(3) HDR brachytherapy allows patients to be treated with a high dose of radiation in a short period of time on an outpatient basis, with minimal radiation exposure to healthcare providers (Gosselin & Waring, 2001; Waring & Gosselin, 2010). Generally, the HDR treatments are repeated until the desired dose has been delivered (Holland, 2001).

    (a) The use of HDR brachytherapy is possible in virtually all sites treated by conventional LDR brachytherapy and by intracavitary, interstitial, intravascular, mold, percutaneous, or intraoperative techniques

and has advantages for both pediatric and adult patients. In selected instances, HDR treatment appears to be well tolerated and as effective as LDR treatment (Mock et al., 2003). Patients state a variety of reasons (traveling distance is most often cited) for preferring LDR or HDR when given the option (Wright et al., 1994).

    (b) Anesthesia or sedation may be required depending on the site, applicator, and age or comprehension of the patient; however, these procedures generally are performed on an outpatient basis with or without sedation or anesthesia (Eifel, 1992; Waring & Gosselin, 2010).

    (c) Treatment times are shorter, but more treatments may be needed. Caregivers and visitors are not subject to radiation exposure after the patient is discharged (Brandt, 1991; Waring & Gosselin, 2010).

5. Collaborative management

    a) Gynecologic implants, LDR: Applicators include intracavitary tandem and ovoids, vaginal cylinders, and transperineal interstitial vaginal template and needles (for advanced gynecologic malignancies) (Gupta et al., 1999; Moore-Higgs, 2007b).

      (1) Follow pretreatment bowel preparation regimen per institution (i.e., enema on the morning of implantation).

      (2) Place a radiation precaution sign at the door to the patient's room according to institutional guidelines when the source is placed within the applicator. Refer to institutional radiation safety guidelines for exposure limits for staff, family, and other visitors (see section III—Radiation protection and safety). Use portable radiation shields at the patient's bedside according to institutional guidelines.

      (3) Strict bed rest with log roll for care is mandatory to prevent possible dislodgment of applicators. In addition, a Foley catheter is inserted prior to the procedure to allow the patient to remain on strict bed rest during the implant. Moistened vaginal packing is used to secure the position of the applicators and to pack the bladder and rectum away from the vaginal sources (Eifel, 1997). The applicator may be held in place with radiation briefs (see Figure 22) or by suturing. Bowel management with antidiar-

Figure 22. Radiation Implant Briefs™

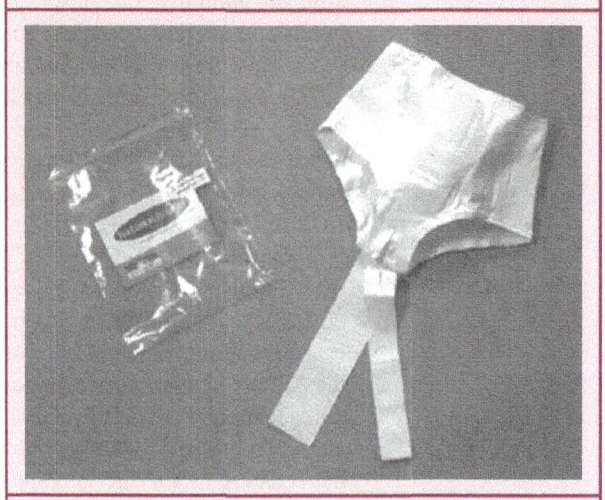

Note. From "Nursing Management of Patients Receiving Brachytherapy for Gynecologic Malignancies," by T.K. Gosselin and J.S. Waring, 2001, *Clinical Journal of Oncology Nursing, 5*, p. 60. Copyright 2001 by the Oncology Nursing Society. Reprinted with permission.

rheal medication is given; a low-residue diet (with finger foods) for nutrition is provided; and the head of the bed should be raised no higher than 30°. Check position of implant every shift and as necessary; modify bathing and linen change. Instruct the patient on care guidelines and rationale while on bed rest (Gosselin & Waring, 2001). The RSO or designee routinely inspects the patient's bed linens and surroundings for dislodged radioactive sources. Contact the RSO and the radiation oncologist if the applicator or radioactive source appears to be dislodged.

(4) Prevent complications of immobility by use of compression stockings, coughing and deep breathing postoperatively, isometric exercises, and anticoagulants, if ordered.

(5) Promote the patient's comfort and decrease procedure-related pain with use of analgesics (oral, IV, patient-controlled analgesia, transdermal, epidural). Evaluate pain control each shift and more frequently if needed. Analgesia is required a half hour to one hour prior to removal of applicators (especially with interstitial needles and templates, which could cause more pain during removal than other applicators). Apply pressure and ice to the perineum for five minutes or longer after removal of needles

to minimize bleeding and improve comfort (Gosselin & Waring, 2001).

(6) Decrease social isolation, keep items within reach (call bell, oral hydration, tissues), answer call light promptly and check on the patient often, and educate the patient on the rationale of isolation.

(7) Address issues of long-term effects of vaginal stenosis. Prescribe and educate the patient on the use of a vaginal dilator. Address concerns regarding sexuality. Refer to a therapist who specializes in sexual dysfunction if needed. Patients receiving brachytherapy have a variety of informational needs and prefer to be fully informed about their conditions (Brandt, 1991; Wolf, 2006).

(8) Provide the patient with discharge instructions and contact telephone numbers. Report any excessive bleeding from the bladder, vagina, or rectum; excessive pain; foul odor of urine or vaginal drainage; temperature above 101°F (38.3°C); increased urinary frequency or dysuria; inability to void after four hours; and diarrhea not controlled with diet or antidiarrheal medications (Gosselin & Waring, 2001).

(9) Educate staff caring for the patient about the applicator, source, and rationale. Lack of knowledge of staff members can contribute to fear on the caregiver's part (Gosselin & Waring, 2001; Stajduhar et al., 2000; Sticklin, 1994; Velji & Fitch, 2001).

b) Gynecologic implants, HDR: Applicators include tandem and ovoids and ring type or vaginal cylinders/stumps.

(1) Teach the patient and family what to expect during the treatment. Treatment context, symptomatology, and passage of time are important to address during and after brachytherapy (Velji & Fitch, 2001).

(2) Provide special instructions, if any, such as eat a light breakfast, take regular medications, and take antidiarrheal medication if necessary.

(3) Brachytherapy applicators need to be stabilized or anchored in place to ensure accuracy of source placement. There are several ways to accomplish this. With tandem and ovoid applicators, the applicators are stabilized after insertion with gauze packing to minimize movement while transporting the patient. After packing is com-

plete, the device should be further stabilized by suturing the labia or using a less invasive approach, such as Radiation Implant Briefs™ (DM Medical) (see Figure 22). With a vaginal cylinder applicator, a device that is secured to the treatment table can be attached to the applicator for stabilization of the applicator during treatment.

(4) Assess and prepare the patient upon arrival to the clinic. Have the patient put on a pair of Radiation Implant Briefs. A Foley catheter and rectal tube may be inserted prior to the applicator being placed. Premedicate with oral pain medication and antianxiety medication, if necessary.

(5) The patient's vital signs and pain level should be assessed throughout the preparation and procedure.

(6) Instruct the patient upon discharge about problems to report (e.g., increased urinary frequency or dysuria, foul odor of urine or vaginal discharge, fever, increased pain, heavy bleeding) (Gosselin & Waring, 2001) (see Table 16).

(7) Educate the patient on pelvic site-specific management, such as vaginal stenosis and sexuality issues (see Figure 23) (Bosserman, 2006; Wolf, 2006). Refer to a therapist who specializes in sexual dysfunction if needed.

c) Head and neck implants, LDR: Plastic catheters are afterloaded with iridium seeds.

(1) Prevent respiratory or cardiovascular complications by encouraging routine postoperative exercises (e.g., deep breathing, changing position in bed, ambulating inside room) if appropriate.

(2) Prior to implantation, the patient should follow an aggressive bowel regimen to decrease the chance of dislodging radioactive sources while straining during bowel movement (Devine & Doyle, 2001).

(3) Prior to implantation, assess the patient's ability to read and write. Provide tools for communication if needed (e.g., pen, paper, whiteboard with marker). If the patient is illiterate, provide alternative communication

Table 16. Acute Side Effects of Treatment

Side Effect	Symptoms	Nursing Interventions
Urinary tract infection or bladder/urethral inflammation	Dysuria, frequency, and foul odor	Obtain urine specimen for urinalysis and culture and sensitivity. Monitor and report results to physician or advanced practice nurse (APN). Consult with physician or APN regarding antibiotics or other medications.
Vaginal infection	Elevated temperature and pain, malodorous vaginal discharge	Patient should report to emergency department or clinic for evaluation.
Vaginal stenosis	Difficulty with sexual intercourse, difficulty with gynecologic examination	Review use of vaginal dilator and lubricant. Provide American Cancer Society booklet on sexuality.
Perineal discomfort	Pain, erythema, and moist desquamation	Consult with physician or APN regarding pain relief. Educate patient on pain medications and side effects. Review use of sitz baths. Review use of topical anesthetics in treatment field.
Constipation	Absence of bowel movement	Review laxative protocol. Provide and review dietary modifications.
Diarrhea	Increased frequency of liquid stool	Review dietary modifications. Provide and review with patient a low-residue diet sheet. Consult with physician or APN regarding use of antidiarrheal medications. Encourage oral fluids.
Fatigue	Decreased ability to perform activities of daily living	Monitor hematocrit and hemoglobin. Review energy-conservation techniques. Review dietary needs. Screen for depression, if chronic.

Note. From "Nursing Management of Patients Receiving Brachytherapy for Gynecologic Malignancies," by T.K. Gosselin and J.S. Waring, 2001, *Clinical Journal of Oncology Nursing, 5*, p. 63. Copyright 2001 by the Oncology Nursing Society. Reprinted with permission.

Figure 23. Vaginal Dilator and Patient Instruction Sheet

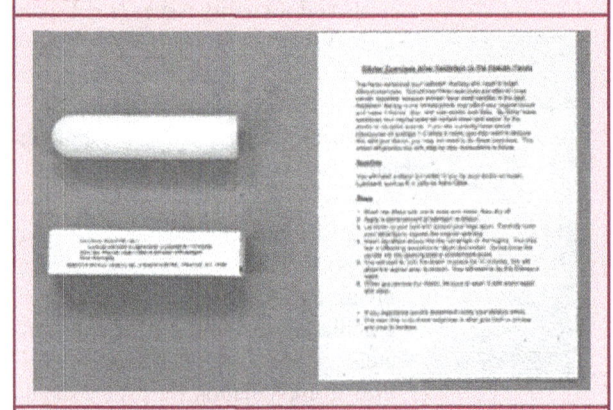

Note. From "Nursing Management of Patients Receiving Brachytherapy for Gynecologic Malignancies," by T.K. Gosselin and J.S. Waring, 2001, *Clinical Journal of Oncology Nursing, 5,* p. 63. Copyright 2001 by the Oncology Nursing Society. Reprinted with permission.

strategies (e.g., cards with commonly needed items or nursing care procedures pictured). Comprehensive patient and family education reduces stress about the procedure (Devine & Doyle, 2001).

(4) Have tracheostomy set in room; tracheostomy may be performed for airway obstruction resulting from edema. Have respiratory suctioning equipment and oxygen available.

(5) Prior to implantation, teach the patient techniques for self-suctioning, oral hygiene, and tracheostomy care if indicated (Devine & Doyle, 2001).

(6) Provide nutrition and fluids during the time period of the implant with a soft or liquid diet, nasogastric tube, or IV hydration. Although some patients with head and neck implants can be allowed to sip a liquid formula through a straw, most require feeding through a nasogastric tube (Montemaggi, Guerrieri, Federico, & Mortellaro, 2008).

(7) Promote comfort by medicating as needed with NSAIDs or narcotic analgesics. Avoid overmedication, which can result in suppression of cough reflex or respirations.

(8) Inspect the implant site at every shift for intactness. Discourage the patient from touching the site. Exact placement of the applicator is crucial for treatment efficacy.

(9) Instruct the patient that bleeding may occur during removal of catheters.

d) Lung implants, HDR or LDR: Endobronchial catheters are placed during fiber-optic bronchoscopy, and iridium-192 seed ribbons are temporarily applied (Behrend, 2011) (see Figure 24). Permanent brachytherapy is also utilized; a radioactive mesh with cesium-131 is placed intraoperatively in the tumor bed.

(1) HDR is an outpatient procedure.

   (a) The patient is NPO (nothing by mouth) for 8–12 hours before the procedure. Vital signs and oxygen saturation are monitored and an IV is started.

   (b) The nurse prepares the patient for bronchoscopy through which a catheter is guided to the tumor area.

   (c) IV sedation (e.g., diazepam, midazolam, fentanyl), a local anesthetic (e.g., topical lidocaine [aerosol or viscous]), and additional medications (atropine, epinephrine) may be administered to keep the patient comfortable and minimize gag reflex during procedure (Powell, 1999).

   (d) The patient may be discharged to a responsible party when vital signs are stable, gag reflex returns, and he or she is able to ambulate (Powell, 1999).

(2) LDR is an inpatient procedure.

   (a) The patient receiving LDR treatment requires hospitalization for two to seven days depending on the radioactive source strength (Behrend, 2011).

   (b) After bronchoscopy and placement of the catheter, the patient is placed in a radiation safety–approved room (see section III—Radiation protection and safety) where the radioactive source is loaded.

   (c) The nurse monitors for complications such as bleeding, infection, and respiratory compromise. Cough suppressant medication may be used to prevent coughing while the implant is in place.

   (d) The patient is discharged after the radioactive source and catheter are removed and the patient has recovered from the procedure. A follow-up appointment is scheduled with the radiation oncologist and pulmonologist the next day.

Figure 24. Localization Film of Endobronchial Iridium Seed Implant for Brachytherapy: Isodose Curves Superimposed

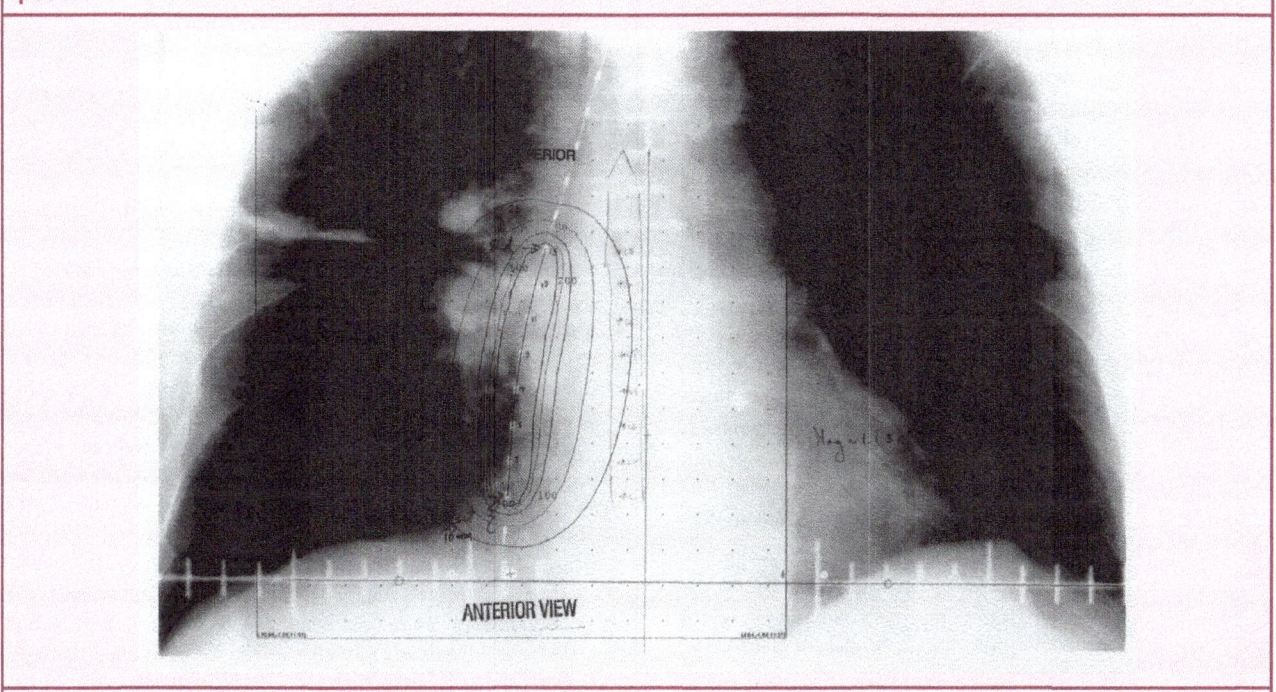

Note. Image courtesy of City of Hope Medical Center. Used with permission.

e) Eye plaques: Eye plaques are used to treat retinoblastoma, which is most common in pediatric patients and young adults; ocular/choroidal melanoma is most common in adults (Halperin & Kirkpatrick, 2005). Plaque RT is effective in the management of cases that otherwise would have been managed with enucleation (Finger et al., 2010; Shields et al., 2003).

   (1) Plaque RT is LDR and is performed in operating room by an ophthalmologic surgeon.

   (2) Radiation physicist is also present.

   (3) Equipment for iodine-125 ocular plaque construction and placement includes a dummy plaque to aid in the placement of the necessary retention sutures, a gold backing with lug holes for sutures, and a plastic insert to hold the radioactive iodine-125 seeds (Finger et al., 2010; Halperin & Kirkpatrick, 2005).

   (4) Other types of plaques using various isotopes are available.

   (5) Special care for both adult and pediatric patients: Protect the affected eye from trauma (e.g., creative, occlusive bandaging for pediatric patients).

   (6) Acute effects are pain and operative infection.

   (7) Long-term effects are cataracts.

6. Patient and family education

   a) Educate the patient and family on the type of implant, the rationale, the procedure, preparation, sensory information, availability of pain medication, and care during treatment specific to the implant used. Comprehensive patient and family education about the brachytherapy procedure, necessary visitation restrictions, and the anticipation of potential patient problems is instrumental in preventing complications. Patients receiving HDR brachytherapy experience side effects similar to those caused by external radiation treatments, with fatigue being the most often reported symptom (Fieler, 1997).

   b) Discuss the rationale and methods for radiation protection such as self-care while the implant is in place and limitations on staff and visitor time in room (see section III—Radiation protection and safety).

   c) Provide verbal and written discharge instructions with guidelines for activity, bathing, skin or wound care, diet, smoking restrictions (with bronchoscopy), alcohol restrictions, medication guidelines, and symptoms to report to the doctor or nurse. Patients and families need to be given telephone numbers to use for seeking help during after-hours.

   d) Instruct the patient on the early and late side effects, address specific questions and concerns, and provide follow-up appointment information.

7. Brachytherapy for benign disease
   a) Pterygium: A wedge-shaped membrane growing from the conjunctiva to the cornea, arising from the fissure between the eyelids (*Dorland's Illustrated Medical Dictionary,* 2007).
   b) Caused by repeated irritation to the eyes (e.g., welding, woodwork, sun, sand)
   c) Treatment
       (1) Beta-emitting applicator
       (2) Treatment dose is one single fraction of 20 Gy to multiple-fraction regimens of 8–10 Gy given immediately postoperatively followed by two more treatments at seven-day intervals (Pajic & Greiner, 2005).
       (3) Rationale (Luthra, Nemesure, Wu, Xie, & Leske, 2001)
           (a) Primary treatment is surgery.
           (b) Rate of regrowth with surgery is high (20%–30%) (Luthra et al., 2001).
           (c) Brachytherapy decreases recurrence rates to 20% or less (Tripuraneni, 2009).

8. Related Web sites
   a) American Brachytherapy Society: www.americanbrachytherapy.org
   b) ASTRO: www.astro.org
   c) ONS: www.ons.org

References

Abel, L., Dafoe-Lambie, J., Butler, W.M., & Merrick, G.S. (2003). Treatment outcomes and quality-of-life issues for patients treated with prostate brachytherapy. *Clinical Journal of Oncology Nursing, 7,* 48–54. doi:10.1188/03.CJON.48-54

Behrend, S.H. (2011). Radiation treatment planning. In C.H. Yarbro, D. Wujcik, & B.H. Gobel (Eds.), *Cancer nursing: Principles and practice* (7th ed., pp. 269–311). Sudbury, MA: Jones and Bartlett.

Bosserman, L.D. (2006). Strategies for helping patients manage the side effects of pelvic radiation therapy. *Community Oncology, 3,* 669–671.

Brandt, B. (1991). Informational needs and selected variables in patients receiving brachytherapy. *Oncology Nursing Forum, 18,* 1221–1227.

Carrubba, D.M., Jankowski, C.B., & Kunsman, J. (1999). Nursing management of soft tissue sarcomas of the extremities. *Clinical Journal of Oncology Nursing, 3,* 168–179.

Devine, P., & Doyle, T. (2001). Brachytherapy for head and neck cancer: A case study. *Clinical Journal of Oncology Nursing, 5,* 55–57.

Dorland's illustrated medical dictionary (31st ed.). (2007). Philadelphia, PA: Elsevier Saunders.

Eifel, P.J. (1992). High-dose-rate brachytherapy for carcinoma of the cervix: High tech or high risk? *International Journal of Radiation Oncology, Biology, Physics, 24,* 383–386.

Eifel, P.J. (1997). Intracavitary brachytherapy in the treatment of gynecologic neoplasms. *Journal of Surgical Oncology, 66,* 141–147.

Erickson, B., Eifel, P., Moughan, J., Rownd, J., Iarocci, T., & Owen, J. (2005). Patterns of brachytherapy practice for patients with carcinoma of the cervix (1996–1999): A patterns of care study. *International Journal of Radiation Oncology, Biology, Physics, 63,* 1083–1092. doi:10.1016/j.ijrobp.2005.04.035

Fieler, V.K. (1997). Side effects and quality of life in patients receiving high-dose rate brachytherapy. *Oncology Nursing Forum, 24,* 545–553.

Finger, P.T., Chin, K.J., & Yu, G.-P. (2010). Risk factors for radiation maculopathy after ophthalmic plaque radiation for choroidal melanoma. *American Journal of Ophthalmology, 149,* 608–615. doi:10.1016/j.ajo.2009.11.006

Gosselin, T.K. (2011). Principles of radiation therapy. In C.H. Yarbro, D. Wujcik, & B.H. Gobel (Eds.), *Cancer nursing: Principles and practice* (7th ed., pp. 249–268). Sudbury, MA: Jones and Bartlett.

Gosselin, T.K., & Waring, J.S. (2001). Nursing management of patients receiving brachytherapy for gynecologic malignancies. *Clinical Journal of Oncology Nursing, 5,* 59–63.

Gupta, A.K., Vicini, F.A., Frazier, A.J., Barth-Jones, D.C., Edmundson, G.K., Mele, E., … Martinez, A.A. (1999). Iridium-192 transperineal interstitial brachytherapy for locally advanced or recurrent gynecological malignancies. *International Journal of Radiation Oncology, Biology, Physics, 43,* 1055–1060. doi:10.1016/S0360-3016(98)00522-7

Haas, M.L., & Kuehn, E.F. (2001). Brachytherapy. In D. Watkins-Bruner, G. Moore-Higgs, & M. Haas (Eds.), *Outcomes in radiation therapy: Multidisciplinary management* (pp. 67–72). Sudbury, MA: Jones and Bartlett.

Halperin, E.C., & Kirkpatrick, J.P. (2005). Retinoblastoma. In E.C. Halperin, L.S. Constine, N.J. Tarbell, & L.E. Kun (Eds.), *Pediatric radiation oncology* (4th ed., pp. 135–177). Philadelphia, PA: Lippincott Williams & Wilkins.

Hogle, W.P. (2006). The state of the art in radiation therapy. *Seminars in Oncology Nursing, 22,* 212–220. doi:10.1016/j.soncn.2006.07.004

Hogle, W.P., Quinn, A.E., & Heron, D.E. (2003). Advances in brachytherapy: New approaches to target breast cancer. *Clinical Journal of Oncology Nursing, 7,* 324–328. doi:10.1188/03.CJON.324-328

Holland, J. (2001). New treatment modalities in radiation therapy. *Journal of Intravenous Nursing, 24,* 95–101.

Kremer, B., Klimek, L., Andreopoulos, D., & Mösges, R. (1999). A new method for the placement of brachytherapy probes in paranasal sinus and nasopharynx neoplasms. *International Journal of Radiation Oncology, Biology, Physics, 43,* 995–1000. doi:10.1016/S0360-3016(98)00521-5

Lawrence, T.S., Ten Haken, R.K., & Giaccia, A. (2008). Principles of radiation oncology. In V.T. DeVita Jr., T.S. Lawrence, & S.A. Rosenberg (Eds.), *Cancer: Principles and practice of oncology* (8th ed., pp. 307–336). Philadelphia, PA: Lippincott Williams & Wilkins.

Luthra, R., Nemesure, B.B., Wu, S.Y., Xie, S.H., & Leske, M.C. (2001). Frequency and risk factors for pterygium in the Barbados Eye Study. *Archives of Ophthalmology, 119,* 1827–1832.

Mock, U., Kucera, H., Fellner, C., Knocke, T.H., & Pötter, R. (2003). High-dose-rate (HDR) brachytherapy with or without external beam radiotherapy in the treatment of primary vaginal carcinoma: Long-term results and side effects. *International Journal of Radiation Oncology, Biology, Physics, 56,* 950–957. doi:10.1016/S0360-3016(03)00217-7

Montemaggi, P., Guerrieri, P., Federico, M., & Mortellaro, G. (2008). Clinical applications of brachytherapy: Low–dose-rate and pulse–dose-rate. In E.C. Halperin, C.A. Perez, & L.W. Brady (Eds.), *Perez and Brady's principles and practice of radiation oncology* (5th ed., pp. 476–539). Philadelphia, PA: Lippincott Williams & Wilkins.

Moore-Higgs, G.J. (2007a). Basic principles of radiation therapy. In M.L. Haas, W.P. Hogle, G.J. Moore-Higgs, & T.K. Gosselin-Acomb (Eds.), *Radiation therapy: A guide to patient care* (pp. 3–7). St. Louis, MO: Elsevier Mosby.

Moore-Higgs, G.J. (2007b). Gynecologic cancers. In M.L. Haas, W.P. Hogle, G.J. Moore-Higgs, & T.K. Gosselin-Acomb (Eds.), *Radiation therapy: A guide to patient care* (pp. 207–233). St. Louis, MO: Elsevier Mosby.

Nag, S. (n.d.). A brief history of brachytherapy. Retrieved from http://www.americanbrachytherapy.org/aboutbrachytherapy/history.cfm

Nag, S., Shasha, D., Janjan, N., Petersen, I., & Zaider, M. (2001). The American Brachytherapy Society recommendations for brachytherapy of soft tissue sarcomas. *International Journal of Radiation Oncology, Biology, Physics, 49,* 1033–1043. doi:10.1016/S0360-3016(00)01534-0

Nelson, J.C., Beitsch, P.D., Vicini, F.A., Quiet, C.A., Garcia, D., Snider, H.C., … Kuerer, H.M. (2009). Four-year clinical update from the American Society of Breast Surgeons MammoSite brachytherapy trial. *American Journal of Surgery, 198,* 83–91. doi:10.1016/j.amjsurg.2008.09.016

Pajic, B., & Greiner, R.H. (2005). Long term results of non-surgical, exclusive strontium-/yttrium-90 beta-irradiation of pterygia. *Radiotherapy and Oncology, 74,* 25–29. doi:10.1016/j.radonc.2004.08.022

Powell, G. (1999). High dose rate brachytherapy endobronchial treatments: Adjunctive medications and discharge instructions. *Canadian Oncology Nursing Journal, 9,* 143–144.

Shah, A.P., Strauss, J.B., Gielda, B.T., & Zusag, T.W. (2010). Toxicity associated with bowel or bladder puncture during gynecologic interstitial brachytherapy. *International Journal of Radiation Oncology, Biology, Physics, 77,* 171–179. doi:10.1016/j.ijrobp.2009.04.077

Shields, C.L., Naseripour, M., Shields, J.A., Freire, J., & Cater, J. (2003). Custom-designed plaque radiotherapy for nonresectable iris melanoma in 38 patients: Tumor control and ocular complications. *American Journal of Ophthalmology, 135,* 648–656. doi:10.1016/S0002-9394(02)02241-9

Stajduhar, K.I., Neithercut, J., Chu, E., Pham, P., Rohde, J., Sicotte, A., & Young, K. (2000). Thyroid cancer: Patients' experiences of receiving iodine-131 therapy. *Oncology Nursing Forum, 27,* 213–218.

Sticklin, L.A. (1994). Strategies for overcoming nurses' fear of radiation exposure. *Cancer Practice, 2,* 275–278.

Tripuraneni, P. (2009). Benign diseases. In B.G. Haffty & L.D. Wilson (Eds.), *Handbook of radiation oncology: Basic principles and clinical protocols* (pp. 755–761). Sudbury, MA: Jones and Bartlett.

Velji, K., & Fitch, M. (2001). The experience of women receiving brachytherapy for gynecologic cancer. *Oncology Nursing Forum, 28,* 743–751.

Waring, J., & Gosselin, T. (2010). Developing a high-dose-rate prostate brachytherapy program. *Clinical Journal of Oncology Nursing, 14,* 199–205. doi:10.1188/10.CJON.199-205

Williamson, J.F., & Brenner, D.J. (2008). Physics and biology of brachytherapy. In E.C. Halperin, C.A. Perez, & L.W. Brady (Eds.), *Perez and Brady's principles and practice of radiation oncology* (5th ed., pp. 423–475). Philadelphia, PA: Lippincott Williams & Wilkins.

Wolf, J.K. (2006). Prevention and treatment of vaginal stenosis resulting from pelvic radiation therapy. *Community Oncology, 3,* 665–671.

Wright, J., Jones, G., Whelan, T., & Lukka, H. (1994). Patient preference for high or low dose rate brachytherapy in carcinoma of the cervix. *Radiotherapy and Oncology, 33,* 187–194. doi:10.1016/0167-8140(94)90353-0

Zeroski, D., Abel, L., Butler, W.M., Wallner, K., & Merrick, G.S. (2005). Factors affecting patient selection for prostate brachytherapy: What nurses should know. *Clinical Journal of Oncology Nursing, 9,* 553–560. doi:10.1188/05.CJON.553-560

C. Intraoperative radiation therapy (IORT)
1. Procedure description: IORT is a single, large fraction of radiation that is given to an exposed solid tumor or resected tumor bed during a surgical procedure.
2. Indications
   a) IORT is most commonly used in the treatment of GI (anal, colorectal, pancreatic, stomach), gynecologic (cervical, ovarian, uterine), and genitourinary (bladder, kidney, prostate) cancers, as well as in the treatment of soft tissue sarcomas. Its use has been reported in the treatment of head and neck and brain tumors and, more recently, in women with breast cancer undergoing breast-conserving surgery (Vaidya et al., 2010).
   b) Patients who are candidates for IORT may receive it before or after EBRT and as part of a combined-modality treatment plan (Willett, Czito, & Tyler, 2007).
   c) It is used when vital structures are close by or are attached to the tumor and in the setting of certain locally advanced (e.g., rectal) or recurrent tumors (e.g., soft tissue sarcomas).
   d) In the pediatric setting, IORT represents an attractive method to increase the dose to the tumor bed while minimizing the long-term risks of radiation exposure to normal tissue, such as growth retardation and secondary malignancies (Hu, Enker, & Harrison, 2002).
3. Treatment
   a) The use of IORT was first reported in the 1900s and was further developed in clinical trials (Gosselin, 2011).
   b) Calvo, Meirino, and Orecchia (2006a) and Willett et al. (2007) identified the following with the use of IORT.
      (1) Radiobiologic advantage (increased dose to tumor bed)
      (2) Better dose distribution
      (3) Potential to limit tumor seeding
      (4) Avoidance of trauma to normal tissues associated with interstitial implantation
      (5) No dose to surrounding normal structures because of mobilization and direct shielding
   c) IORT can be delivered with high-energy electrons or an HDR gamma-emitting isotope.
   d) Each of these treatment units has specially designed applicators that come in different sizes that are attached to the unit. Cones that are used for other types of radiation treatment may be used on the linear accelerator or on the mobile electron linear accelerator. The Harrison-Anderson-

Mick applicator was developed at Memorial Sloan-Kettering Cancer Center and is a 1-cm-thick pad made of flexible material ("super flab") with source guide tubes running through the center and a cap at the end that secures the source guide tubes, which then attach to the remote afterloader (Harrison, Enker, & Anderson, 1995).

e) If IORT is going to be given in the operating room via a traditional linear accelerator or an HDR unit, then the operating room staff needs to be shielded and another set of monitoring equipment needs to be outside of the room to be used during IORT. Two challenges exist with a fixed linear accelerator–based program (Harrison et al., 1995).

(1) Transferring of the patient from the operating room to the radiation department and the various associated risks

(2) Often cost-prohibitive to have a dedicated accelerator in an operating room based on patient treatment volumes

f) Newer technology for IORT has been developed and used in practice.

(1) Mobetron (IntraOp Medical Corp.) is a mobile linear accelerator that uses electrons and therefore requires no additional operating room shielding. The unit is portable and thereby increases flexibility of use. With this being a newer technology, it is essential for centers to develop a quality assurance program (Beddar et al., 2006).

(2) Intrabeam is a mobile system that can be used in the treatment of breast cancer and delivers a spherical treatment dose with low-energy x-rays and, like the Mobetron, requires no additional operating room shielding.

g) Preoperative care

(1) In an effort to determine the tumor size, location, and extent of disease preoperatively, the patient may need to undergo numerous invasive and/or non-invasive procedures.

(2) The patients will undergo all routinely required preoperative studies, including chest x-ray, electrocardiogram, and other laboratory studies, as deemed necessary.

(3) The multidisciplinary team should obtain informed consent from the patient for the procedure prior to the day of surgery.

(4) The patient will have necessary catheters, tubes, and IV lines started prior to surgery.

h) Intraoperative care

(1) The surgical team (e.g., physician, nurse) provides status updates to the radiation oncologist about the patient and what time he or she will be ready for the radiation oncologist and medical dosimetrist in the operating room. It is important for all team members to understand the procedure, their specific role, and care needs of the patient (Gao, Delclos, Tomas, Crane, & Beddar, 2007).

(2) During the operation, the normal organs are physically moved out of the pathway of the radiation beam whenever possible (Skandarajah, Lynch, Mackay, Ngan, & Heriot, 2009; Willett et al., 2007).

(3) If the patient is to be transported to the radiation oncology department to receive radiation, the following need to occur (Willett et al., 2007).

   (a) Incisions are temporarily closed with a running continuous suture or clamps, and the wound is covered with a sterile adhesive dressing.

   (b) The patient is placed on a stretcher and transported to the department with portable anesthesia.

   (c) The patient then is transferred to the treatment couch and again is prepared and draped.

   (d) After involved personnel put on new gloves and new gowns, the surgeon reopens the incision, and the treatment applicator is placed.

(4) When the radiation oncologist and medical physicist arrive, they will examine the area that is to be treated. The resected specimen is reviewed with the pathologist, who analyzes the margins by frozen section. The team selects and secures in place the desired treatment applicator and

places appropriate shielding to protect the normal tissue.

(5) The radiation oncologist prescribes the treatment dosage, and the medical physicist performs the dose calculations. Depending on the type of treatment delivery system, appropriate treatment devices and applicators are selected and connected.

(6) The team leaves the room and monitors the patient on another set of equipment outside of the operating room when the treatment is delivered.

(7) Depending on the total dose to be delivered and the activity of the source, treatment time will vary. For HDR, it is approximately 10–20 minutes (Gao et al., 2007; Skandarajah et al., 2009).

(8) Although not done frequently, the patient may receive more than one fraction during the procedure because of the size of the area that needs to be treated (Domanovic, Ouzidane, Ellis, Kinsella, & Beddar, 2003; Willett et al., 2007).

(9) Surgical clips may be placed around the irradiated site so that it can be visualized in the future (Calvo et al., 2006a).

(10) Once treatment is completed, the surgeon removes the treatment applicator and lead shields (if HDR). The surgeon closes the incision, and the nurses complete the closing sharps, sponge, and instrument counts (Domanovic et al., 2003) while the physicist surveys the patient and room to ensure no radioactive materials remain in the patient or the room (Gao et al., 2007).

(11) Prior to transferring the patient, a report is called to the RN in the postanesthesia care unit.

i) Postoperative care

(1) Once the patient is in the postanesthesia care unit and has stabilized, he or she will be transferred to an intermediate or intensive care unit.

(2) The nurse caring for the patient who received IORT needs to be knowledgeable about the surgical procedure performed, the typical complications that arise, and issues related to the surgical resection and any anastomoses performed.

(3) A plan of care with nursing interventions should be developed that supports optimal patient outcomes.

4. Collaborative management

a) Acute effects

(1) Postoperative issues that could arise in any patient receiving a major surgical procedure include abscess formation, bleeding, fistula, infection, obstruction, seroma formation, and wound complications.

(2) Patients may experience pain, altered bowel patterns, and nutritional issues related to the surgical procedure.

b) Late effects

(1) Patients with pelvic/GI tumors may have sexuality issues related to the surgical intervention and IORT, the use of pre- or postoperative radiation, and/or chemotherapy (see section I V.F—Sexual dysfunction).

(2) Azinovic, Calvo, Puebla, Aristu, and Martínez-Monge (2001) found that the incidence of severe toxicity was lower in patients with gynecologic, head and neck, and genitourinary cancers, whereas toxicity was higher in patients with bone sarcomas and soft tissue sarcomas.

(3) Peripheral nerve injury was the dominant event in long-term survivors of extremity, thoracic, and pelvic malignancies who had a peripheral nerve in the surgical bed (Azinovic et al., 2001; Calvo, Meirino, & Orecchia, 2006b).

(4) Other side effects that may arise, depending on the treatment area, include ureteral and bile duct stenosis and fibrosis, hydronephrosis, pelvic fibrosis, limb edema, and cystitis (Azinovic et al., 2001; Calvo et al., 2006b).

5 Patient and family education (Domanovic et al., 2003; Gao et al., 2007)

a) Teach the patient and family about the required studies prior to surgery and the length of time required for the studies.

b) Teach the patient and family about the surgical procedure and the radiation treatment. Review with them NPO status, GI prep if ordered, and where and when to arrive for surgery if the patient is not to be admitted the evening before.

c) Teach the patient and family about discharge care, which may include wound care, dietary needs, and ostomy care, and whom to contact if issues arise. Surgical supplies may be purchased at a surgical supply store or local pharmacy.

d) Provide the patient and family, if applicable, with counseling on sexuality as well as reputable resources, such as ACS's Web site for information related to male and female sexual side effects, www.cancer.org/Treatment/TreatmentsandSideEffects/PhysicalSide Effects/index (see section IV.F—Sexual dysfunction).

e) Provide appropriate referrals to services that may include social work, vocational counseling, and pastoral support.

f) Teach the patient about treatment planning, EBRT, and acute and late side effects if he or she is to receive postoperative radiation.

g) Teach the patient and family the signs and symptoms of peripheral neuropathy and how to manage this side effect.

h) Teach the patient and family the importance of follow-up care to assess for acute and late effects.

6. Follow-up

a) Patients may be seen frequently during the first few months following treatment for assessments and to determine their response to treatment.

b) The surgical oncologist in conjunction with the radiation oncologist may follow patients.

7. Related Web sites

a) ACS: www.cancer.org

b) Intrabeam: www.zeiss.de/C125679E00 51C774/Contents-Frame/9A7F82907E13 38A28825724C007C73D0

c) Mobetron: www.intraopmedical.com/ ?q=node/2

References

Azinovic, I., Calvo, F.A., Puebla, F., Aristu, J., & Martínez-Monge, R. (2001). Long-term normal tissue effects of intraoperative electron radiation therapy (IOERT): Late sequelae, tumor recurrence, and second malignancies. *International Journal of Radiation Oncology, Biology, Physics, 49,* 597–604. doi:10.1016/S0360 -3016(00)01475-9

Beddar, A.S., Biggs, P.J., Chang, S., Ezzell, G.A., Faddegon, B.A., Hensley, F.W., & Mills, M.D. (2006). Intraoperative radiation therapy using mobile electron linear accelerators: Report of AAPM Radiation Therapy Committee Task Group No. 72. *Medical Physics, 33,* 1476–1489.

Calvo, F.A., Meirino, R.M., & Orecchia, R. (2006a). Intraoperative radiation therapy: First part: Rationale and techniques. *Critical Reviews in Oncology/Hematology, 59,* 106–115. doi:10.1016/j .critrevonc.2005.11.004

Calvo, F.A., Meirino, R.M., & Orecchia, R. (2006b). Intraoperative radiation therapy: Part 2. Clinical results. *Critical Reviews in Oncology/Hematology, 59,* 116–127. doi:10.1016/j.critrevonc .2006.04.004

Domanovic, M.A., Ouzidane, M., Ellis, R.J., Kinsella, T.J., & Beddar, A.S. (2003). Using intraoperative radiation therapy—A case study. *AORN Journal, 77,* 412, 414–417. doi:10.1016/S0001 -2092(06)61208-8

Gao, S., Delclos, M.E., Tomas, L.C., Crane, C.H., & Beddar, S. (2007). High-dose-rate remote afterloaders for intraoperative radiation therapy. *AORN Journal, 86,* 827–836. doi:10.1016/j. aorn.2007.07.002

Gosselin, T.K. (2011). Principles of radiation therapy. In C.H. Yarbro, D. Wujcik, & B.H. Gobel (Eds.), *Cancer nursing: Principles and practice* (7th ed., pp. 249–268). Sudbury, MA: Jones and Bartlett.

Harrison, L.B., Enker, W.W., & Anderson, L.L. (1995). High-dose-rate intraoperative radiation therapy for colorectal cancer, part 1. *Oncology, 9,* 679–683.

Hu, K.S., Enker, W.E., & Harrison, L.B. (2002). High-dose-rate intraoperative irradiation: Current status and future directions. *Seminars in Radiation Oncology, 12,* 62–80. doi:10.1053/srao.2002.28666

Skandarajah, A.R., Lynch, A.C., Mackay, J.R., Ngan, S., & Heriot, A.G. (2009). The role of intraoperative radiotherapy in solid tumors. *Annals of Surgical Oncology, 16,* 735–744. doi:10.1245/ s10434-008-0287-

Vaidya, J.S., Joseph, D.J., Tobias, J.S., Bulsara, M., Wenz, F., Saunders, C., … Baum, M. (2010). Targeted intraoperative radiotherapy versus whole breast radiotherapy for breast cancer (TARGIT-A trial): An international, prospective, randomized, non-inferiority phase 3 trial. *Lancet, 376,* 91–102. doi:10.1016/S0140-6736(10)60837-9

Willett, C.G., Czito, B.G., & Tyler, D.S. (2007). Intraoperative radiation therapy. *Journal of Clinical Oncology, 25,* 971–977. doi:10.1200/JCO.2006.10.0255

D. Stereotactic radiosurgery

1. Procedure description

a) SRS is a technique to deliver precisely directed, high-dose ionizing radiation to a target with the purpose of complete destruction while minimizing radiation dose to the surrounding normal tissue (Flickinger & Niranjan, 2008). Stereotactic describes using three-dimensional guidance to precisely perform a procedure. Radiosurgery describes delivery of the stereotactically guided radiation treatment to the defined target volume in a single session (Flickinger & Niranjan, 2008). The evolution of SRS has included delivery of this high-dose, precise radiation in more than one session. In 2006, members of the American Association of Neurological Surgeons/Congress of Neurological Surgeons Washington Committee Stereotactic Radiosurgery Task Force, in conjunction with ASTRO, approved a contemporary definition of SRS to include delivery of the intended dose in one to five sessions (Barnett et al., 2007).

b) Lars Leksell, MD, PhD, a Swedish neurosurgeon, was the first to describe the concept of using single-fraction irradiation of intracranial targets to replace surgery in selected patients in 1951 (Slotman, Solberg, Wurm, & Verellen, 2006).

c) Radiobiologic advantages (Kirkpatrick, Meyer, & Marks, 2008)

(1) SRS technique allows delivery of high-dose ionizing radiation to the intended target, while exposing surrounding normal tissues to a much lower dose.

(2) The biologically effective dose of single-fraction SRS appears to be more clinically efficacious than predicted using the linear-quadratic model. The linear-quadratic model is the most widely accepted mathematical model for describing the damaging effects of conventionally fractionated ionizing radiation on normal and neoplastic tissue.

(3) High-dose-per-fraction ionizing radiation causes direct cytotoxic damage related to DNA damage as is seen in conventional low-dose fractionation. Additionally, it also causes damage to supporting tissues of the neoplasm, such as microvasculature and stromal tissues, which is specific to high doses.

(4) SRS may be more effective against radioresistant tumor stem cells, which may enhance tumor eradication.

d) Optimal requirements for use of SRS (Flickinger & Niranjan, 2008)

(1) Small target/treatment volume—Improves the tolerance of surrounding normal tissues

(2) Sharply defined target—Allows irradiation with minimal margin of surrounding normal tissue without underdosing the target (marginal miss)

(3) Accurate radiation delivery—Minimal potential for setup error, which would require a margin of normal tissue to prevent underdosing of the target

(4) High conformity—The delivered treatment volume is able to be matched to the planned target volume.

(5) Sensitive structures are excluded from the target—Radiation dose-limiting structures (such as optic chiasm and spinal cord) are able to be excluded from the planned target volume to limit the risk of radiation injury.

2. Indications

a) Intracranial metastases

(1) SRS plus whole brain RT: RTOG 95-08 trial demonstrated significant survival advantage in patients with a solitary lesion treated with combination therapy; patients with two to three lesions had significantly improved local control without survival advantage (Andrews et al., 2004).

(2) SRS as monotherapy

(a) Appropriate treatment for patients with one to four lesions, with none larger than 4 cm in diameter. Advantages over surgical management include that SRS is able to treat lesions in deep or eloquent regions of the brain; it is a noninvasive, outpatient procedure without anesthesia risk; and it has a short recovery time and allows rapid initiation of systemic therapies (Suh, 2010).

(b) SRS as monotherapy is a reasonable treatment option but carries a higher risk of developing distant brain recurrence. Thus, it requires careful, active surveillance to ensure early identification of intracranial recurrence and initiation of salvage therapy (Linskey et al., 2010).

b) Primary malignant brain tumor

(1) SRS with a median dose of 14 Gy has been investigated as salvage therapy for locally recurrent GBM after standard fractionated RT and as consolidation therapy following conventional RT (Biswas et al., 2009).

(2) The efficacy of SRS as a boost in the initial treatment of malignant gliomas was not established in randomized trials (Souhami et al., 2004).

(3) Further studies are needed to determine the best use of SRS in patients with malignant gliomas (Biswas et al., 2009).

c) Benign tumors

(1) Acoustic neuroma (also known as vestibular schwannoma)

(a) Multiple studies have demonstrated comparable tumor control rates compared to surgical resection for small to medium lesions (Flickinger & Niranjan, 2008).

(b) Advantages of SRS over microsurgery include higher rate of hearing preservation, decreased incidence of facial and trigeminal neuropathy, and fewer postoperative complications (Karpinos et al., 2002).

(2) Meningioma

(a) Multiple studies have demonstrated a five-year local control rate of 86%–99%. SRS is appropriate for incompletely resected or inoperable meningiomas 3 cm or smaller (Elia, Shih, & Loeffler, 2007).

(b) Cavernous sinus and base-of-skull meningiomas have high surgical morbidity including vascular and cranial nerve morbidity. SRS is a much less morbid option for treatment for lesions smaller than 3 cm (Metellus et al., 2005).

(c) SRS is not indicated for tumors involving the optic apparatus, those substantially compressing the brain stem, or those that are large (Torres et al., 2003).

(3) Pituitary adenoma—SRS has an 85% overall response rate (volume reduction) for patients with nonsecretory adenomas, 54% hormonal normalization in acromegaly and Cushing disease, and 24% remission for prolactinomas (Jagannathan, Yen, Pouratian, Laws, & Sheehan, 2009).

(4) Glomus jugulare tumors

(a) Glomus jugulare tumors are a common site of paraganglioma involving the jugular bulb that cause lower cranial nerve symptoms including loss of hearing, tinnitus, hoarseness, vertigo, and facial weakness/numbness (Chino, Sampson, Tucci, Brizel, & Kirkpatrick, 2009).

(b) SRS achieved excellent tumor control with low risk of morbidity and 60% reported improvement in one or more of their presenting symptoms (Foote et al., 2002).

d) AVM

(1) SRS has been widely used to treat AVM over the past two decades. Angiographic evidence of cure (obliteration) occurs in 80%–95% of patients after a latency period of three to five years (Maruyama et al., 2005).

(2) The risk of hemorrhage from AVM decreases significantly during the latency period (after radiosurgery and before angiographic obliteration) and further decreases after obliteration (Maruyama et al., 2005). The risk reduction appears greatest in patients presenting with hemorrhage (Maruyama et al., 2005).

(3) The risks of developing permanent symptomatic sequelae (necrosis) from SRS treatment for AVM are significantly correlated with intracranial location and the volume of brain tissue receiving 12 Gy (Flickinger et al., 2000). Highest to lowest risk locations are

pons/midbrain, basal ganglia, thalamus, medulla, occipital lobe, corpus callosum, cerebellum, parietal lobe, and intraventricular, temporal, and frontal lobes (Flickinger et al., 2000).

(4) Management of large AVMs may include the addition of pre-SRS embolization and staged SRS where the lesion is treated in two to three sections separated by several months (Flickinger & Niranjan, 2008).

(5) One recent study concluded that SRS was effective in improving AVM headaches but not in improving the performance status of treated patients as measured by modified Rankin score (Sun et al., 2011). Modified Rankin score is a widely accepted six-point measure of functional outcome after stroke, which reflects limitations in activity and changes in lifestyle (Wilson et al., 2002).

e) Trigeminal neuralgia

(1) SRS is used for typical trigeminal neuralgia refractory to medical therapy. Maximum dose is 80 Gy to a 4 mm target area (Flickinger & Niranjan, 2008).

(2) Initial response rate is high (70%–85%) but deteriorates over years. (Dhople et al., 2009; Riesenburger et al., 2010). Re-treatment may need to be considered including repeat SRS, microvascular decompression, or rhizotomy (Dhople et al., 2009).

f) Spinal metastasis—A large, single-institution, prospective study using SRS (12.5–20 Gy) for spinal metastasis from multiple pathologic histologies reported that 86% of patients had improvement in pain (Gerszten, Burton, Ozhasoglu, & Welch, 2007). Of those with pretreatment neurologic deficits, 35% noted some improvement (Gerszten et al., 2007).

g) Extracranial sites: SBRT

(1) Lung

(a) Medically inoperable early-stage NSCLC—A recent large, multicenter, prospective trial (RTOG 02-36) demonstrated a survival rate of approximately 55% at three years with a 97% rate of tumor control (Timmerman et al., 2010). Dose delivered was 18 Gy for three fractions (54 Gy total) over 1.5–2 weeks (Timmerman et al., 2010).

(b) Lung metastasis—Safety and efficacy of SBRT for treatment of one

to three lesions has been shown with two-year local control of 96% and a low incidence of grade 3 toxicity (Rusthoven et al., 2009).

(2) Liver

   (a) Primary hepatocellular carcinoma—Early feasibility studies used doses of 14–45 Gy given in one to three fractions (Kavanagh, Bradley, & Timmerman, 2008). SBRT is effective treatment for small hepatocellular carcinoma (smaller than 5 cm) with up to 80% overall response rate (Choi et al., 2008). SBRT can be combined with transarterial chemoembolization for advanced hepatocellular carcinoma with portal vein tumor thrombosis with minimal side effects and a response rate comparable to invasive local therapies (Choi et al., 2008).

   (b) Liver metastasis—SBRT was given as a well-tolerated noninvasive therapy with 12-month tumor control of 71% in one prospective study using 27–60 Gy in six fractions (Lee et al., 2009). Long-term survivors of unresected liver metastasis treated with SBRT (25–45 Gy in two to five fractions) have been documented (Gunvén, Blomgren, Lax, & Levitt, 2009).

(3) Pancreatic cancer—SBRT has been used to treat locally advanced unresectable and recurrent pancreatic adenocarcinoma. Didolkar et al. (2010) demonstrated low morbidity and high local tumor control rate with significant pain relief that generally lasted 18–24 weeks. Most patients, however, died of distant disease progression.

(4) Prostate cancer—Typically is a slowly proliferating cancer, which radiobiologically is thought to be more sensitive to hypofractioned RT (Brenner, 2003). Katz, Santoro, Ashley, Diblasio, & Witten (2010) used SBRT, 35–36.25 Gy in five fractions, to treat 304 patients with clinically localized prostate cancer. No patients experienced RTOG grade III or IV acute toxicities. At a median follow-up of 30 months, long-term urinary and rectal toxicities were low at less than 5% RTOG grade II occurrences and only 0.5 % RTOG grade III urinary occurrence. At a 17-month median follow-up, only

four patients had biochemical failure (Katz et al., 2010).

(5) Renal cell carcinoma—Traditionally thought to be radioresistant to conventionally fractionated RT. SBRT is being investigated by multiple practitioners for both primary and metastatic renal cell carcinoma with early evidence of efficacy for pain relief and local control (Teh et al., 2010).

3. SRS delivery systems

  a) Gamma Knife

   (1) The first prototype developed by Leksell and Larson in 1967 used a hemispherical array of 201 fixed cobalt-60 beams to create spherical treatment volumes of varied diameter (Flickinger & Niranjan, 2008).

   (2) Multiple upgrades have produced the ability to treat a wider range of lesion sizes and reduced treatment time.

  b) Positively charged particles (protons)

   (1) Advantage is the beam's ability to stop at a depth related to the beam's energy; hence, it lacks an exit dose. Increased ionization at the distal aspect of the beam causes increased radiobiologic (cell kill) effect. This is termed Bragg peak (Flickinger & Niranjan, 2008).

   (2) Disadvantages include that it is currently available at few treatment centers and the high cost of equipment and maintenance.

  c) Linear accelerator–based system: Modification of a linear accelerator designed for conventional RT to be used for SRS includes hardware and software advances for improved beam shaping with circular secondary and micromultileaf collimators, stereotactic guidance systems, increased conformity dose planning, and improved immobilization/position verification. Commercially available systems include Novalis TX™ (BrainLAB AG and Varian Medical Systems, Inc.) and the XKnife™ (Radionics Inc.).

d) CyberKnife® (Accuray Inc.) combines a miniaturized linear accelerator mounted on a robotic arm with continual image guidance to track target motion throughout the multiple-beam treatment.

4. Immobilization

a) SRS delivery systems have specialized immobilization devices that coordinate with each system's treatment device and planning software to define the target and ensure precise patient positioning during treatment.

b) Cranial systems may have a head frame that attaches to the skull with screws (e.g., Gamma Knife, XKnife) or a frameless system using a custom-fitted thermoplastic face mask (e.g., Novalis TX, CyberKnife).

c) SBRT mobilization devices include custom-fitted, foam-based body molds (e.g., Alpha Cradle®, Smithers Medical Products, Inc.) and customized external vacuum-type body molds (e.g., Vac-Lok, Body-FIX® [Elekta, Inc.]). The CyberKnife system uses a custom-designed vest worn by the patient (Synchrony System).

5. Planning (Benedict et al., 2008; Potters et al., 2010)

a) SRS delivery systems have complex, integrated software planning systems that coordinate all SRS treatment steps: imaging for target definition, development of a treatment plan using many radiation beams, and successful delivery of the planned treatment with very precise accuracy.

b) SRS treatment planning systems integrate diagnostic imaging including CT, MRI, and angiogram to define target volumes.

c) SRS/SBRT requires intensive medical physics support and collaboration with multiple disciplines. Generally for cranial SRS, neurosurgery is involved to help define the target volume, assess the dose to critical structures, and approve the final treatment plan. For SBRT, a surgical procedure or endoscopy may be needed for placement of small metallic internal (fiducial) markers, which assist with defining and tracking the treatment target (e.g., in lung or liver tumors). Hence, the treatment planning period can take days or longer depending on individual institution policies and procedures (e.g., if fiducials are needed for CyberKnife treatment, at least a week is recommended before treatment to ensure stability of placement) (Accuray Inc., n.d.).

6. Localization—IGRT (Benedict et al., 2008; Potters et al., 2010)

a) A variety of technologies are used to localize and track the target as well as to ensure reproducibility of the treatment plan during delivery of the actual treatment. This includes use of real-time CT scan during therapy (cone beam CT), sophisticated kilovoltage imaging, fluoroscopy, and use of infrared camera with skin markers.

b) For SBRT, multiple methods are used to track target movement due to respiratory motion, including four-dimensional CT scan. The end result is the ability to match a particular respiratory phase (and target position) with treatment beam-on time (called respiratory gating). This can be done with controlled breathing or free breathing techniques.

7. Collaborative management

a) Acute effects

(1) Cranial SRS effects are generally minimal and include nausea, vomiting, and headache. Less frequent are vertigo and seizures (Hong et al., 2004). Lawrence et al. (2010) reported 34.1% acute sequelae (95% were mild to moderate in severity) in a large, single-institution series. Most frequently seen in descending frequency were headache, seizures, fluid retention and other steroid effects, and neurologic changes (Lawrence et al., 2010).

(2) For invasive frame-based SRS, effects include possible discomfort, bleeding, or infection at insertion site of fixation pins (Suh, 2010).

b) Late effects

(1) Cranial SRS: Principal concerns are radiation necrosis and cognitive deterioration. The risk of complications increase with the size of the target (expressed as volume cm^3). Toxicity rapidly increases once volume of brain exposed to more than 12 Gy is larger than $5–10\,cm^3$ (Lawrence et al., 2010).

(2) Brain stem: Maximum dose of 12.5 Gy is associated with less than 5% risk (Mayo, Yorke, & Merchant, 2010). Higher doses of 15–20 Gy have been used in patients with poor prognosis with low reported incidence of complications (Mayo, Yorke, et al., 2010).

(3) Optic nerves/chiasm: Radiation-induced optic neuropathy is a painless, rapid visual loss likely caused by vasculature injury. Incidence is unlikely in dose range of 8–12 Gy but becomes greater than 10% in doses of 12–15 Gy (Mayo, Martel, et al., 2010).

(4) Cochlea: Dose should be limited to 12–14 Gy to the cochlea, such as when treating an acoustic neuroma to minimize risk of SNHL (Bhandare et al., 2010).

(5) Spine: Radiation-induced myelopathy is rare (less than 1%) with doses of 13 Gy or less in one fraction or 20 Gy or less in three fractions to the full-thickness spinal cord (Kirkpatrick, van der Kogel, & Schultheiss, 2010). Long-term data are insufficient to calculate the risk of myelopathy for partial cord radiation exposure in a hypofractionated regimen (Kirkpatrick et al., 2010).

c) Lung: Toxicities include radiation pneumonitis, bronchial injury or stenosis, chest wall pain, and rib fracture.

(1) Radiation pneumonitis incidence is less than 10% in most series but has been reported as high as 25% in one study (Marks et al., 2010). Radiation pneumonitis symptoms include shortness of breath and decline in functional tests (pulmonary function test, six-minute walk, exercise capacity).

(2) Bronchial injury or stenosis has been associated with SBRT of perihilar and central tumors. Recommended SBRT dose limit to central airways is 80 Gy to minimize this risk (Marks et al., 2010).

(3) Chest wall toxicity causing severe pain or rib fracture is strongly correlated with the volume of chest wall receiving 30 Gy in three to five fractions (30% risk for chest wall volume of 35 cm³) (Dunlap et al., 2010). Recommended chest wall volume receiving 30 Gy should be limited to 30 cm³ (Dunlap et al., 2010).

d) Liver: Radiation-induced liver disease involves anicteric hepatomegaly, ascites, and elevated liver transaminases or alkaline phosphatase.

(1) Pathology involves occlusion and injury to central hepatocyte lobules, retrograde congestion, and secondary hepatocyte necrosis (Pan et al., 2010).

(2) Broad guidelines for less than 5% risk of radiation-induced liver disease include SBRT dose less than 13 Gy in three fractions and less than 18 Gy in six fractions for primary liver cancer, and less than 15 Gy in three fractions and less than 20 Gy in six fractions for liver metastases (Pan et al., 2010).

8. Patient and family education: Review multiple procedures required for treatment planning and delivery.

a) Type of diagnostic imaging needed for treatment planning, which may include CT, MRI, PET, angiography, or surgical or interventional radiologic placement of fiducial markers

b) Type of immobilization device required
   (1) Invasive, fixed head frame is placed on the same day of SRS treatment. Local anesthetic is used for pin placement.
   (2) Frameless devices such as foam or vacuum are fashioned days before SRS treatment.

c) Consider patient body position and the amount of time required for fashioning of the immobilization device. Pain or anti-anxiety medication may be required.

d) Assess for any barriers to completing treatment, including physical, cognitive, emotional, and psychological.

e) Treatment time itself is highly variable and depends on the number of targets to be treated (e.g., can be multiple for brain metastases), complexity of the tracking, and position verification techniques required, as well as which treatment delivery system is used. Overall, the complexity of SRS/SBRT generally results in a longer treatment time compared to standard RT.

9. Follow-up

a) Review potential acute and late effects with the patient and family. Possible symptoms will depend on the area (normal tissues) treated.

b) Ensure that the patient and family understand when and how to contact appropriate healthcare personnel for reporting of symptoms, questions, or concerns. Consider that much less time is required in the radiation department for delivery of SRS/SBRT compared to conventional RT.

c) The follow-up required for monitoring disease response to therapy and management of potential treatment sequelae is dependent on the disease and site treated.

References

Accuray Inc. (n.d.). CyberKnife®: How does the CyberKnife System treat lung cancer? Retrieved from http://www.cyberknife.com/cyberknife-treatments/lung/how-used-treat-cancer.aspx?terms=lung+cancer

Andrews, D.W., Scott, C.B., Sperduto, P.W., Flanders, A.E., Gaspar, L.E., Schell, M.C., ... Curran, W.J., Jr. (2004). Whole brain radiation therapy with or without stereotactic radiosurgery boost for patients with one to three brain metastases: Phase III results of the RTOG 9508 randomised trial. Lancet, 363, 1665–1672. doi:10.1016/s0140-6736(04)16250-8

Barnett, G.H., Linskey, M.E., Adler, J.R., Cozzens, J.W., Friedman, W.A., Heilbrun, M.P., ... Sloan, A.E. (2007). Stereotactic radiosurgery—An organized neurosurgery-sanctioned definition. *Journal of Neurosurgery, 106,* 1–5. doi:10.3171/jns.2007.106.1.1

Benedict, S.H., Bova, F.J., Clark, B., Goetsch, S.J., Hinson, W.H., Leavitt, D.D., ... Yenice, K.M. (2008). Anniversary paper: The role of medical physicists in developing stereotactic radiosurgery. *Medical Physics, 35,* 4262–4277.

Bhandare, N., Jackson, A., Eisbruch, A., Pan, C.C., Flickinger, J.C., Antonelli, P., & Mendenhall, W.M. (2010). Radiation therapy and hearing loss. *International Journal of Radiation Oncology, Biology, Physics, 76*(Suppl. 3), S50–S57. doi:10.1016/j.ijrobp.2009.04.096

Biswas, T., Okunieff, P., Schell, M.C., Smudzin, T., Pilcher, W.H., Bakos, R.S., ... Milano, M.T. (2009). Stereotactic radiosurgery for glioblastoma: Retrospective analysis. *Radiation Oncology, 4,* 11. doi:10.1186/1748-717x-4-11

Brenner, D.J. (2003). Hypofractionation for prostate cancer radiotherapy—What are the issues? *International Journal of Radiation Oncology, Biology, Physics, 57,* 912–914. doi:10.1016/S0360-3016(03)01456-1

Chino, J.P., Sampson, J.H., Tucci, D.L., Brizel, D.M., & Kirkpatrick, J.P. (2009). Paraganglioma of the head and neck: Long-term local control with radiotherapy. *American Journal of Clinical Oncology, 32,* 304–307. doi:10.1097/COC.0b013e318187dd94

Choi, B.O., Choi, I.B., Jang, H.S., Kang, Y.N., Jang, J.S., Bae, S.H., ... Kang, K.M. (2008). Stereotactic body radiation therapy with or without transarterial chemoembolization for patients with primary hepatocellular carcinoma: Preliminary analysis. *BMC Cancer, 8,* 351. doi:10.1186/1471-2407-8-351

Dhople, A.A., Adams, J.R., Maggio, W.W., Naqvi, S.A., Regine, W.F., & Kwok, Y. (2009). Long-term outcomes of Gamma Knife radiosurgery for classic trigeminal neuralgia: Implications of treatment and critical review of the literature. Clinical article. *Journal of Neurosurgery, 111,* 351–358. doi:10.3171/2009.2.jns08977

Didolkar, M.S., Coleman, C.W., Brenner, M.J., Chu, K.U., Olexa, N., Stanwyck, E., ... Rabinowitz, S. (2010). Image-guided stereotactic radiosurgery for locally advanced pancreatic adenocarcinoma results of first 85 patients. *Journal of Gastrointestinal Surgery, 14,* 1547–1559. doi:10.1007/s11605-010-1323-7

Dunlap, N.E., Cai, J., Biedermann, G.B., Yang, W., Benedict, S.H., Sheng, K., ... Larner, J.M. (2010). Chest wall volume receiving > 30 Gy predicts risk of severe pain and/or rib fracture after lung stereotactic body radiotherapy. *International Journal of Radiation Oncology, Biology, Physics, 76,* 796–801. doi:10.1016/j.ijrobp.2009.02.027

Elia, A.E., Shih, H.A., & Loeffler, J.S. (2007). Stereotactic radiation treatment for benign meningiomas. *Neurosurgical Focus, 23*(4), E5. doi:10.3171/foc-07/10/e5

Flickinger, J.C., Kondziolka, D., Lunsford, L.D., Kassam, A., Phuong, L.K., Liscak, R., & Pollock, B. (2000). Development of a model to predict permanent symptomatic postradiosurgery injury for arteriovenous malformation patients. Arteriovenous Malformation Radiosurgery Study Group. *International Journal of Radiation Oncology, Biology, Physics, 46,* 1143–1148.

Flickinger, J.C., & Niranjan, A. (2008). Stereotactic radiosurgery and radiotherapy. In E.C. Halperin, C.A. Perez, & L.W. Brady (Eds.), *Perez and Brady's principles and practice of radiation oncology* (5th ed., pp. 378–388). Philadelphia, PA: Lippincott Williams & Wilkins.

Foote, R.L., Pollock, B.E., Gorman, D.A., Schomberg, P.J., Stafford, S.L., Link, M.J., ... Olsen, K.D. (2002). Glomus jugulare tumor: Tumor control and complications after stereotactic radiosurgery. *Head and Neck, 24,* 332–338. doi:10.1002/hed.10005

Gerszten, P.C., Burton, S.A., Ozhasoglu, C., & Welch, W.C. (2007). Radiosurgery for spinal metastases: Clinical experience in 500 cases from a single institution. *Spine, 32,* 193–199. doi:10.1097/01.brs.0000251863.76595.a2

Gunvén, P., Blomgren, H., Lax, I., & Levitt, S.H. (2009). Curative stereotactic body radiotherapy for liver malignancy. *Medical Oncology, 26,* 327–334. doi:10.1007/s12032-008-9125-4

Hong, T.S., Tomé, W.A., Hayes, L., Yuan, Z., Badie, B., Rao, R., & Mehta, M.P. (2004). Acute sequelae of stereotactic radiosurgery. *Radiosurgery, 5,* 38–45. doi:10.1159/000078135

Jagannathan, J., Yen, C.P., Pouratian, N., Laws, E.R., & Sheehan, J.P. (2009). Stereotactic radiosurgery for pituitary adenomas: A comprehensive review of indications, techniques and long-term results using the Gamma Knife. *Journal of Neuro-Oncology, 92,* 345–356. doi:10.1007/s11060-009-9832-5

Karpinos, M., Teh, B.S., Zeck, O., Carpenter, L.S., Phan, C., Mai, W.Y., ... Woo, S.Y. (2002). Treatment of acoustic neuroma: Stereotactic radiosurgery vs. microsurgery. *International Journal of Radiation Oncology, Biology, Physics, 54,* 1410–1421. doi:10.1016/S0360-3016(02)03651-9

Katz, A.J., Santoro, M., Ashley, R., Diblasio, F., & Witten, M. (2010). Stereotactic body radiotherapy for organ-confined prostate cancer. *BMC Urology, 10,* 1. doi:10.1186/1471-2490-10-1

Kavanagh, B.D., Bradley, J.D., & Timmerman, R.D. (2008). Stereotactic irradiation of tumors outside the central nervous system. In E.C. Halperin, C.A. Perez, & L.W. Brady (Eds.), *Perez and Brady's principles and practice of radiation oncology* (5th ed., pp. 389–396). Philadelphia, PA: Lippincott Williams & Wilkins.

Kirkpatrick, J.P., Meyer, J.J., & Marks, L.B. (2008). The linear-quadratic model is inappropriate to model high dose per fraction effects in radiosurgery. *Seminars in Radiation Oncology, 18,* 240–243. doi:10.1016/j.semradonc.2008.04.005

Kirkpatrick, J.P., van der Kogel, A.J., & Schultheiss, T.E. (2010). Radiation dose-volume effects in the spinal cord. *International Journal of Radiation Oncology, Biology, Physics, 76*(Suppl. 3), S42–S49. doi:10.1016/j.ijrobp.2009.04.095

Lawrence, Y.R., Li, X.A., el Naqa, I., Hahn, C.A., Marks, L.B., Merchant, T.E., ... Dicker, A.P. (2010). Radiation dose-volume effects in the brain. *International Journal of Radiation Oncology, Biology, Physics, 76*(Suppl. 3), S20–S27. doi:10.1016/j.ijrobp.2009.02.091

Lee, M.T., Kim, J.J., Dinniwell, R., Brierley, J., Lockwood, G., Wong, R., ... Dawson, L.A. (2009). Phase I study of individualized stereotactic body radiotherapy of liver metastases. *Journal of Clinical Oncology, 27,* 1585–1591. doi:10.1200/jco.2008.20.0600

Linskey, M.E., Andrews, D.W., Asher, A.L., Burri, S.H., Kondziolka, D., Robinson, P.D., ... Kalkanis, S.N. (2010). The role of stereotactic radiosurgery in the management of patients with newly diagnosed brain metastases: A systematic review and evidence-based clinical practice guideline. *Journal of Neuro-Oncology, 96,* 45–68. doi:10.1007/s11060-009-0073-4

Marks, L.B., Bentzen, S.M., Deasy, J.O., Kong, F.M., Bradley, J.D., Vogelius, I.S., ... Jackson, A. (2010). Radiation dose-volume effects in the lung. *International Journal of Radiation Oncology, Biology, Physics, 76*(Suppl. 3), S70–S76. doi:10.1016/j.ijrobp.2009.06.091

Maruyama, K., Kawahara, N., Shin, M., Tago, M., Kishimoto, J., Kurita, H., ... Kirino, T. (2005). The risk of hemorrhage after radiosurgery for cerebral arteriovenous malformations. *New England Journal of Medicine, 352,* 146–153. doi:10.1056/NEJMoa040907

Mayo, C., Martel, M.K., Marks, L.B., Flickinger, J., Nam, J., & Kirkpatrick, J. (2010). Radiation dose-volume effects of optic nerves and chiasm. *International Journal of Radiation Oncology, Biology, Physics, 76*(Suppl. 3), S28–S35. doi:10.1016/j.ijrobp.2009.07.1753

Mayo, C., Yorke, E., & Merchant, T.E. (2010). Radiation associated brainstem injury. *International Journal of Radiation Oncol-*

ogy, Biology, Physics, 76(Suppl. 3), S36–S41. doi:10.1016/j.ijrobp.2009.08.078

Metellus, P., Regis, J., Muracciole, X., Fuentes, S., Dufour, H., Nanni, I., ... Grisolo, F. (2005). Evaluation of fractionated radiotherapy and gamma knife radiosurgery in cavernous sinus meningiomas: Treatment strategy. *Neurosurgery, 57,* 873–886. doi:10.1227/01.NEU.0000179924.76551.cd

Pan, C.C., Kavanagh, B.D., Dawson, L.A., Li, X.A., Das, S.K., Miften, M., & Ten Haken, R.K. (2010). Radiation-associated liver injury. *International Journal of Radiation Oncology, Biology, Physics, 76*(Suppl. 3), S94–S100. doi:10.1016/j.ijrobp.2009.06.092

Potters, L., Kavanagh, B., Galvin, J.M., Hevezi, J.M., Janjan, N.A., Larson, D.A., ... Rosenthal, S.A. (2010). American Society for Therapeutic Radiology and Oncology (ASTRO) and American College of Radiology (ACR) practice guideline for the performance of stereotactic body radiation therapy. *International Journal of Radiation Oncology, Biology, Physics, 76,* 326–332. doi:10.1016/j.ijrobp.2009.09.042

Riesenburger, R.I., Hwang, S.W., Schirmer, C.M., Zerris, V., Wu, J.K., Mahn, K., ... Yao, K.C. (2010). Outcomes following single-treatment Gamma Knife surgery for trigeminal neuralgia with a minimum 3-year follow-up. *Journal of Neurosurgery, 112,* 766–771. doi:10.3171/2009.8.jns081706

Rusthoven, K.E., Kavanagh, B.D., Burri, S.H., Chen, C., Cardenes, H., Chidel, M.A., ... Schefter, T.E. (2009). Multi-institutional phase I/II trial of stereotactic body radiation therapy for lung metastases. *Journal of Clinical Oncology, 27,* 1579–1584. doi:10.1200/jco.2008.19.6386

Slotman, B.J., Solberg, T., Wurm, R., & Verellen, D. (2006). Introduction. In B.J. Slotman, T. Solberg, & D. Verellen (Eds.), *Extracranial stereotactic radiotherapy and radiosurgery* (pp. 1–4). Boca Raton, FL: Taylor & Francis.

Souhami, L., Seiferheld, W., Brachman, D., Podgorsak, E.B., Werner-Wasik, M., Lustig, R., ... Curran, W.J., Jr. (2004). Randomized comparison of stereotactic radiosurgery followed by conventional radiotherapy with carmustine to conventional radiotherapy with carmustine for patients with glioblastoma multiforme: Report of Radiation Therapy Oncology Group 93-05 protocol. *International Journal of Radiation Oncology, Biology, Physics, 60,* 853–860. doi:10.1016/j.ijrobp.2004.04.011

Suh, J.H. (2010). Stereotactic radiosurgery for the management of brain metastases. *New England Journal of Medicine, 362,* 1119–1127. doi:10.1056/NEJMct0806951

Sun, D.Q., Carson, K.A., Raza, S.M., Batra, S., Kleinberg, L.R., Lim, M., ... Rigamonti, D. (2011). The radiosurgical treatment of arteriovenous malformations: Obliteration, morbidities, and performance status. *International Journal of Radiation Oncology, Biology, Physics, 80,* 354–361. doi:10.1016/j.ijrobp.2010.01.049

Teh, B.S., Ishiyama, H., Mathews, T., Xu, B., Butler, E.B., Mayr, N.A., ... Timmerman, R.D. (2010). Stereotactic body radiation therapy (SBRT) for genitourinary malignancies. *Discovery Medicine, 10,* 255–262.

Timmerman, R., Paulus, R., Galvin, J., Michalski, J., Straube, W., Bradley, J., ... Choy, H. (2010). Stereotactic body radiation therapy for inoperable early stage lung cancer. *JAMA, 303,* 1070–1076. doi:10.1001/jama.2010.261

Torres, R.C., Frighetto, L., De Salles, A.A., Goss, B., Medin, P., Solberg, T., ... Selch, M. (2003). Radiosurgery and stereotactic radiotherapy for intracranial meningiomas. *Neurosurgical Focus, 14*(5), e5. doi:10.3171/foc.2003.14.5.6

Wilson, J.T., Hareendran, A., Grant, M., Baird, T., Schulz, U.G., Muir, K.W., & Bone, I. (2002). Improving the assessment of outcomes in stroke: Use of a structured interview to assign grades on the modified Rankin scale. *Stroke, 33,* 2243–2246. doi:10.1161/01.STR.0000027437.22450.BD

E. Hyperthermia
   1. Procedure description: Hyperthermia generally is defined as a modest elevation of temperature to a range of 40°–43°C (approximately 106°F) (Gosselin-Acomb, 2007; Jones, Samulski, Vujaskovic, Prosnitz, & Dewhirst, 2008). When tumor cells are heated, a number of events occur that have significant biologic consequences for cancer therapy. Hyperthermia causes direct cytotoxicity and acts as a radiosensitizer, sensitizing tumor cells to other forms of therapy, including RT and chemotherapy.
   2. Indications
      a) The physiologic consequences of hyperthermia have implications for RT, such as thermally induced reoxygenation. Mechanisms of action appear to be complementary to radiation effects with regard to inhibition of potential lethal damage, sublethal damage repair, cell-cycle sensitivity, and effects of hypoxia and nutrient deprivation.
      b) Hyperthermia has effects on blood flow and tumor physiology, which may be of interest with regard to tumor oxygenation and combination therapy with liposomal agents.
      c) Thermotolerance is the adaptive response to hyperthermia and may augment host immune responses against tumor cells.
      d) Hyperthermia has been used to treat a variety of diseases including breast cancer, rectal cancer, cervical cancer, and superficial tumors. Clinical trials continue to explore new disease sites and combination therapies (Gosselin-Acomb, 2007).
   3. Implementation of hyperthermia (Jones et al., 2008)
      a) Hyperthermia techniques include superficial, regional, and interstitial heating.
      b) Hyperthermia is a treatment that generally uses microwave or radiofrequency energy and ultrasound applicators to heat the area of the tumor.
      c) Several approaches and applicator devices have been developed to deliver hyperthermia treatments. It remains a challenge to heat tumor tissue volumes uniformly and with precision.
   4. Treatment
      a) Microwaves and ultrasound pass through water before entering the body. Deionized water–filled pillows or other devices are placed around the tumor area being treated.
      b) Hyperthermia treatments generally take about 60–90 minutes and are given once or twice weekly. When hyperthermia is

combined with other treatments, such as chemotherapy or RT, additional time and scheduling are required.

   c) Prior to the treatments, a small, plastic catheter is inserted into the tumor while the patient is under local anesthesia. Instruments for determining the tumor temperature are placed inside the catheters to provide critical information during treatment. The proper amount of heat can then be applied to obtain the desired tumor temperature based on this information.

   d) Conscious sedation may be given for patient tolerance; however, patients usually are awake enough to provide critical feedback during the treatments.

  5. Contraindications

   a) Patients with widely metastatic cancer are not eligible for regional hyperthermia treatments.

   b) Because of the microwave and ultrasound equipment used, patients with cardiac pacemakers, orthopedic metal rods, plates, or prostheses are not eligible.

   c) Patients with unstable cardiac disease, severe neuropathy, skin grafts or flaps, surgical implants or implanted devices, or pregnancy are not eligible.

   d) Patients with inadequate blood counts are not eligible.

  6. Collaborative management

   a) Acute effects

    (1) Thermal burns—The most significant side effect is a thermal injury. These may be first-, second-, or third-degree burns. They typically involve a small area of redness, usually about an inch or less in diameter, and occur in approximately 5% of all hyperthermia treatment sessions (Jones et al., 2008).

    (2) Pain—Pain during treatments may occur from the amount of heat directed to the treatment area. Narcotics are given during treatments, and pain usually resolves after power is turned off (see section IV.D—Pain).

    (3) Bleeding and infection—May occur from the insertion of the sterile catheters into the tumor to monitor temperatures during treatment.

    (4) Dehydration—May occur from a combination of chemotherapy, RT, and hyperthermia or may be induced by the hyperthermia treatment alone. During the treatment, patients usually will become diaphoretic, flushed, and thirsty.

    (5) Nausea and vomiting—May occur from a combination of chemotherapy, RT, and hyperthermia or may be induced by the hyperthermia treatment alone. Nausea and vomiting associated with this large amount of heat given in a short period of time usually will be short term and resolves after the power is turned off and the treatment has stopped.

    (6) Fatigue—May occur from a combination of chemotherapy, RT, and hyperthermia or may be induced by the hyperthermia treatment alone. The patient usually will feel "wiped out" after the hyperthermia treatment and will require a short nap or rest period afterward. Usually within 24 hours the patient is back to his or her baseline activities (see section IV.B—Fatigue).

   b) Late effects

    (1) Fat necrosis—Area of subcutaneous tissue burned during treatment may become firm and sore. Because of firmness, patient may be mistakenly alarmed of tumor recurrence. It routinely feels like a bruise and takes weeks to months to resolve. No treatment is necessary to expedite the healing process.

    (2) Thermal injury—Skin surface burn; third-degree burn requires a skin graft.

  7. Patient and family education

   a) Educate the patient and family about treatments, including procedure and time required to receive treatments. Discuss treatment scheduling, including total time involved for hyperthermia, RT, and/or chemotherapy treatments.

   b) Teach the patient and family about side effects directly from the hyperthermia treatments and the increased sensitivity that heat adds to RT and chemotherapy.

   c) Teach the patient and family how to recognize the degree of skin burn.

d) Instruct the patient and family to assess skin area and to report any new skin breakdown or changes.

e) Inform the patient and family about the use of skin care products to minimize discomfort if burn arises.

f) Teach the patient and family to report fever, chills, redness, swelling, pain, bleeding, and drainage from skin breakdown.

g) Teach the patient and family to comply with monitoring blood counts frequently, as adding hyperthermia to existing treatment therapies may increase hematologic toxicities.

h) Teach the patient and family to take medications needed prior to hyperthermia treatments. These medications include those for pain, nausea, and anxiety.

i) Teach the patient and family relaxation and distraction techniques to help the patient tolerate anticipated treatment sessions.

j) Instruct the patient and family to eat small, bland meals prior to treatment and to drink plenty of liquids, including water, juices, decaffeinated beverages, and/or sports drinks with electrolytes.

k) Teach the patient and family to decrease fatigue by saving energy for more important activities, alternating activity with rest periods, using relaxation techniques, and exercising regularly.

l) Emphasize to the patient and family the importance of follow-up care for assessment and management of side effects of treatment.

8. Follow-up

a) Patients are to be seen frequently over the first year after treatment by surgical, medical, and radiation oncology specialists for assessment and evaluation to determine their response to treatment.

b) Patients who have skin grafts associated with a third-degree burn will be followed by radiation oncologists and plastic reconstructive surgery specialists.

References

Gosselin-Acomb, T.K. (2007). Hyperthermia. In M.L. Haas, W.P. Hogle, G.J. Moore-Higgs, & T.K. Gosselin-Acomb (Eds.), *Radiation therapy: A guide to patient care* (pp. 488–495). Philadelphia, PA: Saunders.

Jones, E.L., Samulski, T.V., Vujaskovic, Z., Prosnitz, L.R., & Dewhirst, M. (2008). Hyperthermia. In E. Halperin, C. Perez, & L. Brady (Eds.), *Perez and Brady's principles and practice of radiation oncology* (5th ed., pp. 637–668). Philadelphia, PA: Lippincott Williams & Wilkins.

F. TBI and hematopoietic stem cell transplantation (HSCT)

1. TBI is the delivery of a homogenous dose of radiation to the entire body. It is myeloablative and immunosuppressive and therefore is used in conditioning regimens for some HSCT recipients (Copelan, 2006).

a) TBI was originally delivered in one fraction, which increased toxicities, especially pulmonary toxicity. Fractionated doses have been found to be better tolerated with decreased toxicities (Copelan, 2006).

b) TBI can more easily treat areas where blood flow is impaired (Copelan, 2006).

c) At higher doses, TBI works in conjunction with chemotherapy to eradicate cancer cells (Copelan, 2006).

d) TBI is immunosuppressive, allowing infused bone marrow, stem cells, or umbilical cord blood to engraft in allogeneic transplant recipients (Copelan, 2006).

e) Certain organs, such as the lungs or kidneys, can be blocked to decrease the total dose to those organs and decrease toxicity (Copelan, 2006).

f) Areas such as the testes and the CNS can be boosted with additional radiation in conjunction with TBI.

g) A single dose of 2 Gy is used in nonmyeloablative HSCT.

h) Doses of 12–15 Gy, delivered in 1.5–2 Gy fractions, are used in myeloablative HSCT. Fractionated radiation delivered in two to three doses per day is better tolerated with decreased toxicity. Total doses and fractions vary with treating institutions and treatment protocols (Harden et al., 2001).

i) Dose rates of TBI may range from very low rates of 0.04 Gy/minute to more common rates of 0.2–0.3 Gy/minute (Firat & Lawton, 2010). Treatment times may take 20–30 minutes or longer.

j) Patients may be treated in a standing position on a specially designed stand (see Figure 25), in a side-lying position, or in a supported lying position with arms positioned to shield the lungs (Harden et al., 2001).

k) Infants and very young children require general anesthesia for treatment.

2. A team approach with coordination among the medical and radiation oncologists, physicists, dosimetrists, radiation therapists, and nurses is key to successful TBI treatment.

a) Full evaluation of the patient prior to transplant is necessary to determine if there is organ dysfunction that could affect the outcome of the proposed transplant. Any previous RT needs to be taken into consideration to determine safety, additional risks, or toxicities with TBI.

Figure 25. Total Body Irradiation Stand and Seat

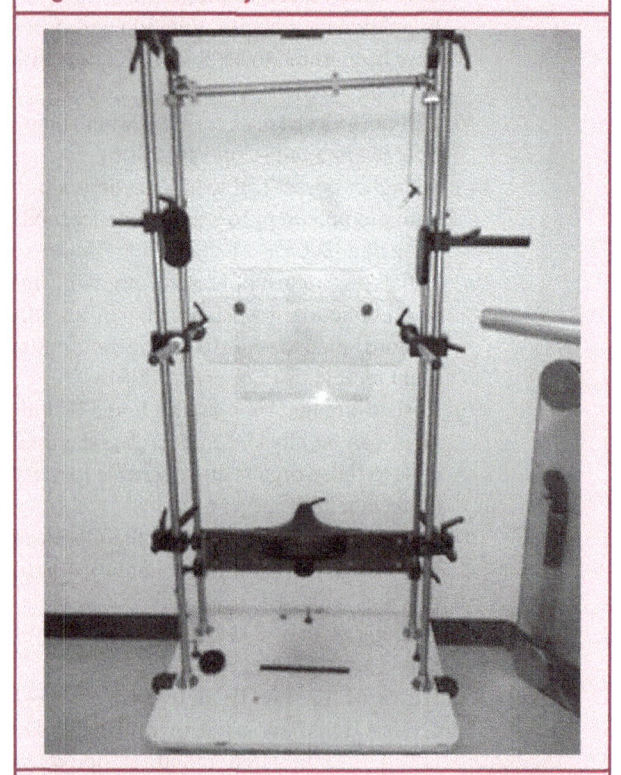

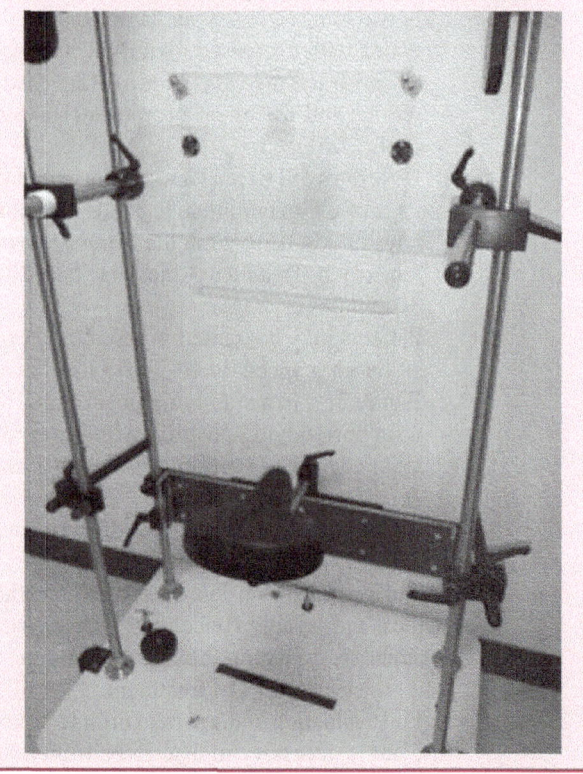

b) Dose calculations are performed by a medical physicist and confirmed by either another physicist or dosimetrist (ACR & ASTRO, 2006).

c) Radiation therapists execute TBI and are responsible for treating patients according to the treatment protocol and prescription. They are responsible for patient positioning and verifying any organ blocks, if applicable (ACR & ASTRO, 2006).

d) Nurses monitor patients during treatment, inform patients about what will be happening, provide supportive care, and communicate patient side effects with other team members.

e) Nurse practitioners and physician assistants may provide patient care along with oncologists during the HSCT process.

3. TBI side effects are evident in the short and long term. Mucositis/esophagitis and pancytopenia are discussed later in this section, although they may also manifest as short-term side effects. Other typical short-term side effects of TBI may include the following.

a) Nausea and vomiting may occur during or after treatment.

(1) Premedicate with 5-HT$_3$ receptor antagonists such as ondansetron, granisetron, or dolasetron. Additional antiemetics may be added as needed.

(2) Monitor fluids and electrolytes. Maintain adequate hydration by oral or IV route. Replace electrolytes as needed.

(3) Cold and bland foods may be better tolerated.

b) Diarrhea usually occurs three to seven days after treatment.

(1) Probiotic supplementation with VSL#3, *Lactobacillus acidophilus* NDCO 1748, and *Lactobacillus rhamnosus* may prevent diarrhea associated with RT to the pelvis (Muehlbauer et al., 2009); however, additional research is needed to specify strains, doses, and timing.

(2) Determine if there is an infectious cause of diarrhea such as *Clostridium difficile* (*C. difficile*).

(3) Oral opiates such as loperamide and diphenoxylate are effective in treating mild symptoms and recommended for clinical practice. Psyllium fiber supplementation and octreotide 100 mcg subcutaneously three times daily are both considered likely to be effective in treating radiation-induced diarrhea. The effectiveness of glutamine

and vitamins E and C for the prevention or treatment of radiation-induced diarrhea has not been established. The use of sucralfate to prevent diarrhea is not recommended (Muehlbauer et al., 2009).

(4) Monitor fluids and electrolytes and replace as needed.

(5) Maintain strict personal hygiene to prevent infection.

c) Fatigue is common after each fraction of TBI and is cumulative with three to four days of TBI.

(1) Allow for rest following TBI.

(2) Maintaining physical activity and engaging in exercise as able is recommended (Mitchell, Beck, Hood, Moore, & Tanner, 2009).

(3) Maintaining a balanced diet with an adequate intake of fluid, calories, protein, electrolytes, vitamins, minerals, and fats is supported by expert opinion (Mitchell et al., 2009).

d) Radiodermatitis or radiation skin reaction with generalized erythema or hyperpigmentation can occur early, whereas fibrosis and delayed wound healing may occur months to years after treatment (Baney, 2011). Ionizing radiation decreases stem cells to the basal layer of the epidermis and disrupts regeneration of skin cells (Baney, 2011).

(1) Gently cleanse the skin and hair with a mild pH-neutral soap (Baney et al., 2011).

(2) Avoid lotions, creams, powders, and deodorant prior to and during treatment. The effectiveness of a variety of topical agents, dressings, and oral agents has not been established (Baney et al., 2011). The use of gentian violet is not recommended. Lotions or gels may be used after treatments according to radiation oncology treatment center guidelines.

(3) Avoid using tape or adhesive in the treatment field (Baney et al., 2011).

(4) Advise the patient to wear loose-fitting clothing for comfort (Baney et al., 2011).

(5) Do not use ice packs or heating pads on the skin in the treatment field (Baney et al., 2011).

(6) Instruct the patient to not use cosmetics such as aftershave, makeup, and perfume on the skin in the treatment field (Baney et al., 2011).

(7) Instruct the patient to avoid submerging in lakes, chlorinated pools, and hot tubs if skin had dry desquamation (Baney et al., 2011).

e) Parotitis, painful swelling of the parotid glands, may occur 12–48 hours after the initial dose of TBI. It is self-limiting with resolution within 48 hours (Rimkus, 2009). Analgesics, including narcotic analgesics, may be necessary.

f) Alopecia will occur with doses of 12–15 Gy.

(1) Inform the patient that hair loss can occur.

(2) Wigs, scarves, or hats can be used.

4. HSCT is used in the treatment of malignant and nonmalignant diseases including, but not limited to, those listed here (Copelan, 2006). TBI is often included in the conditioning regimen for lymphoid cancers (Harris, 2010).

a) Select leukemias

b) Breast cancer

c) Ovarian cancer

d) Myelodysplastic syndrome

e) Multiple myeloma

f) HL and NHL

g) Germ-cell tumors

h) Aplastic anemia

i) Fanconi anemia

j) Thalassemia major

k) Sickle-cell anemia

l) Severe combined immunodeficiency

m) Neuroblastoma

n) Amyloidosis

o) Multiple sclerosis

p) Rheumatoid arthritis

5. Hematopoietic stem cells are undifferentiated cells that have the ability to reproduce themselves (self-renewal) and produce multipotent progenitor cells that are capable of differentiating into the full range of blood cells (Copelan, 2006). Progenitor cells differentiate into lymphoid or myeloid precursors.

a) Lymphoid precursors become T cells, B cells, and natural killer cells.

b) Myeloid progenitors differentiate into granulocyte and monocyte progenitors that mature into granulocytes, monocytes, and dendritic cells.

c) Myeloid progenitors also differentiate into megakaryocytic and erythrocyte progenitors that become platelets and erythrocytes.

6. Sources of stem cells

a) Bone marrow: Multiple aspirations of small amounts of bone marrow are taken from the donor's posterior iliac crests under general or regional anesthesia.

b) Peripheral blood by apheresis
  (1) Stem cells reside in the bone marrow and can be induced to replicate and release into the peripheral blood stream. Chemotherapy and granulocyte–colony-stimulating factor or granulocyte macrophage–colony-stimulating factor injections increase circulating hematopoietic stem cells. This method is used in autologous HSCT (Copelan, 2006).
  (2) Plerixafor is used in combination with granulocyte–colony-stimulating factor to mobilize stem cells in autologous HSCT (Kessans, Gatesman, & Kockler, 2010).
  (3) Granulocyte–colony-stimulating factor alone is used to stimulate stem cell production in bone marrow and peripheral blood stem cell donors (Copelan, 2006).
  (4) Cluster of designation 34+ cells are markers for stem cells.
c) Umbilical cord blood is used when there is no suitable unrelated human leukocyte antigen–matched donor. Umbilical cord blood units yield fewer stem cells; the number is usually sufficient for children. Adults typically require two umbilical cord blood units (Brunstein & Weisdorf, 2009).

7. Types of HSCT
  a) Autologous—Use of the patient's own bone marrow or stem cells
  b) Syngeneic—Bone marrow or stem cells from an identical twin who is human leukocyte antigen identical
  c) Allogeneic—Use of a related or unrelated donor bone marrow, stem cells, or umbilical cord blood
    (1) Transplant may be human leukocyte antigen–matched or have minor histocompatibility antigen mismatch.
    (2) Haploidentical transplants may come from siblings, parents, or children (Copelan, 2006).

8. Informed consent for HSCT is mandatory for patients to understand the risks and benefits of each aspect of the proposed treatment, including TBI, expected side effects and toxicities of treatment, management of side effects and toxicities, and treatment options other than HSCT.

9. Short- and long-term toxicities and side effects of TBI often are difficult to distinguish among TBI, conditioning chemotherapy, and previous treatment regimens.

a) Mucositis is the most common complication of preparative regimens for HSCT (Copelan, 2006), occurs 4–10 days after TBI, and resolves with engraftment of stem cells.
  (1) Pretransplant oral evaluation, cleaning, and treatments are performed to avoid dental problems likely to lead to oral infection (Epstein & Schubert, 2004).
  (2) Palifermin is a recombinant human keratinocyte growth factor that stimulates growth of epithelial cells and reduces the severity and duration of mucositis in patients with hematologic malignancies receiving chemotherapy and TBI or HSCT (Harris, Eilers, Cashavelly, Maxwell, & Harriman, 2009). Its use is likely to be effective; effectiveness has been demonstrated by supportive evidence from a single rigorously conducted controlled trial, consistent supportive evidence from well-designed controlled trials using small samples, or guidelines developed from evidence and supported by expert opinion (Harris et al., 2009).
    (a) Palifermin is given at a dose of 60 mcg/kg IV daily for three days prior to the start of the conditioning regimen and 60 mcg/kg IV daily for three days after stem cell infusion (Harris et al., 2009; Hensley et al., 2009).
    (b) A multicenter study of 30 patients with acute or chronic leukemia undergoing a matched related or unrelated allogeneic transplant showed a significant reduction in the incidence, severity, and duration of grade 2–4 oral mucositis with palifermin. The patients who received palifermin spent 15 days on TPN, whereas those in the control group were on TPN for 26 days. The total dose of morphine-equivalent narcotic pain medication was 150 mg in the palifermin group and 375 mg in the control group (Langner et al., 2008).
  (3) The effectiveness of low-level laser therapy has not been established (Harris et al., 2009).
  (4) Meticulous oral care is important to decrease the risk of infection. Mouth rinses with normal saline, sodium bi-

carbonate, and water or a combination of saline and sodium bicarbonate help to soothe and keep oral mucosa moist, while decreasing oral fluid acidity, diluting mucus, and dissuading yeast colonization (Harris et al., 2009). The use of chlorhexidine, granulocyte macrophage–colony-stimulating factor mouthwash, and sucralfate are not recommended.

b) Pancytopenia develops 7–10 days after TBI and high-dose chemotherapy. Patients are at risk for infection and bleeding until engraftment and recovery of blood counts.

(1) Patients are red blood cell and platelet transfusion dependent.

(2) Blood products must be leukoreduced and irradiated to prevent graft-versus-host disease (GVHD) from a small number of transfused lymphocytes in the blood product.

(3) The threshold for red blood cell transfusions vary by institution. A general threshold is hemoglobin less than 8 g/dl. A higher threshold may be necessary for a specific patient situation.

(4) Maintaining a platelet threshold at $10,000$ (10×10^3/mcl) for patients undergoing stem cell transplantation is recommended (Damron et al., 2009). Platelet transfusions are recommended for a platelet count less than 10,000 (Hensley et al., 2009). A higher threshold is necessary for patients who experience bleeding with a platelet count of 10,000. A platelet count of 20,000 is recommended before minor surgical procedures, and 40,000–50,000 is needed for major surgical procedures (Hensley et al., 2009). Platelet transfusion is recommended for patients with thrombocytopenia who are experiencing active bleeding (Damron et al., 2009).

(5) Epistaxis, gingival bleeding, or blood blisters indicate a low platelet count. Findings of petechiae on examination of the skin are another indication of low platelets.

(6) Follow institutional guidelines to prevent transfusion errors.

c) Patients are vulnerable to developing bacterial, viral, and fungal infections.

(1) Hand hygiene with soap and water or an antiseptic hand rub is recommended for all patients with cancer and their caregivers (Zitella et al., 2009).

(2) Supportive care is provided with prophylactic antibacterial, antiviral, and antifungal medications.

(a) Fluoroquinolones (NCCN, 2011) or quinolones such as ciprofloxacin or levofloxacin are recommended for antibacterial prophylaxis in patients at high risk for infection, such as HSCT recipients (Zitella et al., 2009).

(b) Trimethoprim-sulfamethoxazole is recommended to prevent *Pneumocystis jiroveci* pneumonia in HSCT recipients (Zitella et al., 2009).

(c) Antifungal prophylaxis with fluconazole (NCCN, 2011), posaconazole, voriconazole, echinocandins, oral itraconazole suspension, IV itraconazole, or IV amphotericin B is recommended for high-risk patients such as those undergoing HSCT (Zitella et al., 2009).

(d) Herpes virus prophylaxis with acyclovir and valacyclovir (NCCN, 2011) is recommended for selected seropositive patients with cancer during HSCT and until post-transplant day 30 (NCCN, 2011; Zitella et al., 2009).

(3) Risks may be prolonged because of immunosuppression for GVHD.

(4) Types of infections vary with time over the transplant period.

(a) Early bacterial infections occur in the first two to four weeks after transplant.

i. Gram-negative bacteria because of neutropenia and injury to mucosa

ii. Gram-positive bacteria related to central venous catheters

iii. *C. difficile* because of neutropenia, antibiotic therapy, and antacid medications *(b)* Early fungal infections are typically *Candida* infections resulting from neutropenia and mucosal injury.

(c) Early viral infection is typically herpes simplex reactivation.

(d) Bacterial infections can occur two to three months after transplant and after engraftment.

    i. Gram-positive bacteria related to central venous catheters

    ii. Gram-negative bacteria from gut-related GVHD and central venous catheters

(e) Fungal infections after engraftment often are related to GVHD.

    i. *Aspergillus* and other molds

    ii. *Pneumocystis jiroveci* (previously *Pneumocystis carinii*)

(f) Herpes viruses in the postengraftment period

    i. Cytomegalovirus (CMV) related to GVHD and impaired cellular immunity

    ii. Epstein-Barr virus (EBV)

(g) Other viruses in the early postengraftment stage include the BK virus (type of polyomavirus) related to GVHD and conditioning with cyclophosphamide, community-related respiratory viruses, and adenoviruses.

(h) Late postengraftment bacterial infections, more than two to three months after transplant, often are associated with GVHD, such as encapsulated bacteria and nocardia.

(i) Late fungal infections include *Aspergillus,* other molds, and *P. jiroveci* associated with GVHD.

(j) Late herpes viruses include CMV and varicella zoster virus related to GVHD and impaired cellular immunity. Patients who have T-cell depleted stem cells or have received antithymocyte globulin are at risk for EBV (Wingard, Hsu, & Hiemenz, 2010).

(k) Sites of infection

    i. Oral cavity

    ii. Skin

    iii. Central venous catheters

    iv. Lungs

    v. GI tract

    vi. Genitourinary tract

(l) Monitoring of the potential sites of infection and knowledge of the types of infections that can occur over the post-transplant period can lead to early detection and treatment.

d) GVHD is a major complication of allogeneic HSCT. Current thought is that donor T cells are activated in response to recognition of the recipient's major or minor histocompatibility antigens and attack target organs (Antin, 2002; Wolff, Steiner, Hildebrandt, Edinger, & Holler, 2009).

(1) Acute GVHD occurs within the first few weeks of transplant, whereas GVHD occurring 3–24 months after 100 days is considered chronic GVHD (Harris, 2010).

(2) Symptoms of acute GVHD include diffuse maculopapular rash, nausea, vomiting, anorexia, and diarrhea. Similar symptoms that occur after 100 days are considered persistent or late-onset acute GVHD (Lee & Flowers, 2008).

(3) Standard treatment of acute GVHD consists of short-term methotrexate or mycophenolate mofetil with longer-term treatment with a calcineurin inhibitor such as cyclosporine (Copelan, 2006; Wolff et al., 2009).

(4) Risk factors associated with chronic GVHD include previous acute GVHD, an unrelated or mismatched donor, peripheral blood stem cells as donor source, female donor for a male recipient, older age at transplant, a CMV-positive donor, and TBI used in the HSCT conditioning regimen (Antin, 2002; Baird, Cooke, & Schultz, 2010; Copelan, 2006).

(5) The most common sites of chronic GVHD are the skin, eyes, and oral cavity. Other organs affected include the GI tract, liver, lungs, esophagus, female genital tract, and joints. Less frequently, the heart and kidneys are affected (Lee & Flowers, 2008).

(6) Clinical findings of chronic GVHD are lichenoid changes of the skin and mucous membranes, scleroderma, alopecia, keratoconjunctivitis sicca, xerostomia, odynophagia, nail dysplasia, and increased risk of infection. Women can develop vaginal strictures and dyspareunia. Weight loss and joint contractures decrease mobility (Antin, 2002).

(7) Some degree of GVHD provides a graft-versus-tumor effect that reduces the risk of relapse of disease (Copelan, 2006; Miller et al., 2010).

(8) Standard initial treatment of GVHD consists of prednisone or prednisolone at a dose of 1 mg/kg/day. This often is combined with a calcineurin inhibitor (Wolff et al., 2009).

e) Liver dysfunction

(1) Sinusoidal obstruction syndrome, previously called veno-occlusive disease, is an early complication of allogeneic transplant and may occur within three weeks of transplant (Tabbara, Zimmerman, Morgan, & Nahleh, 2002).

(a) Sinusoidal obstruction syndrome is thought to be due to endothelial damage causing deposits of fibrinogen and collagen in blood vessel walls leading to obstruction (Childs, 2001; Tabbara et al., 2002).

(b) Sinusoidal obstruction syndrome is thought to be related to HSCT conditioning regimens, including TBI, cyclophosphamide, and other preparative agents (Copelan, 2006; Harris, 2010).

(c) Signs and symptoms include right upper quadrant pain, abnormal liver function tests, hepatomegaly, jaundice, fluid retention and weight gain, and ascites (Childs, 2001; Copelan, 2006).

(d) Sinusoidal obstruction syndrome may be self-limiting, but severe disease with hepatocyte necrosis can be fatal (Harris, 2010).

(e) Treatment of sinusoidal obstruction syndrome is supportive care in mild cases, and defibrotide, an antithrombotic and thrombolytic agent, is used (Harris, 2010).

(2) Hepatitis B and C may develop from blood transfusions.

(3) Iron overload causing liver damage can occur from multiple blood transfusions (Baker, Bresters, & Sande, 2010).

f) Pulmonary complications of TBI and HSCT

(1) Pulmonary function testing is routine prior to HSCT to determine adequate respiratory function to undergo transplantation.

(2) Infectious complications are common in the early post-transplant period because of neutropenia and immunosuppression.

(a) Fungal infections may occur with prolonged neutropenia, steroid therapy, and prior fungal infec-

tion. *Aspergillus* is the most common fungus, but molds and other fungal species may cause infection (Wingard et al., 2010).

(b) *P. jiroveci* incidence has been reduced with the use of trimethoprim-sulfamethoxazole, dapsone, and aerosolized pentamidine (Wingard et al., 2010).

(c) CMV symptoms include low-grade fever, nonproductive cough, and dyspnea. Bronchoalveolar lavage may be necessary to establish a diagnosis by viral culture or polymerase chain reaction of fluid obtained (Wingard et al., 2010).

i. Testing with anti-CMV immunologlobulin G antibodies is done prior to treatment to determine risk for reactivation.

ii. CMV is treated with IV ganciclovir or foscarnet and IV immunoglobulin (Childs, 2001).

(d) Respiratory syncytial virus has a high mortality rate in both children and adults after HSCT. The peak incidence is between January and March (Kaner, 2010).

(3) Bronchiolitis obliterans is a pulmonary complication that causes nonspecific inflammatory injury mainly affecting small airways. In early stages, bronchiolitis obliterans has pulmonary obstructive features, but late stages can cause both obstructive and restrictive changes (Tichelli, Rovó, & Gratwohl, 2008).

(a) Bronchiolitis obliterans is associated with chronic GVHD, older age of the stem cell donor or recipient, use of methotrexate for GVHD prophylaxis, use of peripheral blood stem cells for the transplant, use of busulfan in the conditioning regimen, decreased lung function prior to transplant, and respiratory infection within the first 100 days of transplant (Chien, Duncan, Williams, & Pavletic, 2010; Tichelli et al., 2008).

(b) Symptoms of dry cough, dyspnea, and wheezing are nonspecific but may indicate bronchiolitis obliterans.

(4) Bronchiolitis obliterans organizing pneumonia can occur from 1–12

months after transplant, although it can occur years after transplant (Tichelli et al., 2008).

- (a) Bronchiolitis obliterans organizing pneumonia generally occurs acutely with a fever, nonproductive cough, and dyspnea.
- (b) Bronchoscopy with bronchoalveolar lavage may be necessary for diagnosis.
- (c) It is associated with acute and chronic GVHD.
- (d) It usually is treated with steroid therapy (Tichelli et al., 2008). Azithromycin also may be used (Kaner, 2010).

(5) Idiopathic pneumonia syndrome generally occurs within the first four months of transplant (Tichelli et al., 2008). Contributing factors are thought to be pretransplant chemotherapy, TBI, GVHD, and older age at transplant (Tichelli et al., 2008).

(6) In children, pulmonary function abnormalities may persist for years, although mild to moderate impairments often are asymptomatic (Baker et al., 2010).

(7) Screening for pulmonary complications should be done routinely following allogeneic HSCT with pulmonary function testing. Complete additional testing with CT scan, bronchoscopy, bronchoalveolar lavage, and biopsy as clinically indicated (Tichelli et al., 2008).

(8) Patients should be counseled to quit smoking tobacco and marijuana if HSCT is planned because of the increased risk of pulmonary complications.

g) Cataracts are commonly attributed to TBI and can occur about 12 months after TBI treatment (Harris, 2010). Corticosteroids were found to increase the incidence of cataracts.

(1) Patients who have TBI should have regular eye examinations.

(2) Promote the use of sunglasses to protect against UV damage to the eyes.

(3) Artificial lens implantation after lens extraction is the recommended treatment for cataracts secondary to transplantation (Harris, 2010).

h) Endocrine dysfunction

(1) Thyroid disorders have been associated with TBI but also occur in patients who have had non-TBI conditioning regimens.

- (a) GVHD and prolonged immunosuppressive therapy may increase the risk of thyroid dysfunction (Savani et al., 2009).
- (b) Estimates of the incidence of hypothyroidism following allogeneic HSCT vary. Al-Hazzouri, Cao, Burns, Weisdorf, and Majhail (2009) found a 9%–15% incidence in adults, whereas Savani et al. (2009) found a 40% incidence.
  - i. Thyroid dysfunction in children following HSCT may reach 50% (Baker et al., 2010).
  - ii. Risk factors for hypothyroidism include TBI, older age at transplant, and GVHD (Al-Hazzouri et al., 2009; Savani et al., 2009).
  - iii. Patients undergoing nonmyeloablative conditioning regimens have similar rates of hypothyroidism (Al-Hazzouri et al., 2009). This is more likely to be an older group of patients.
- (c) In children, late effects of HSCT on thyroid function can include sick euthyroid syndrome, hypothyroidism, compensated hypothyroidism, rare thyrotoxicosis, and secondary thyroid cancer (Baker et al., 2010).

(2) Infertility and sexuality

- (a) Changes in sexual function, menopausal symptoms, and possible post-HSCT hormone therapy should be discussed prior to transplant.
- (b) TBI doses of 12 Gy cause permanent infertility in most men. Testosterone is unlikely to be affected. Sperm production may return

over time in 10%–17% of men (Simon, Lee, Partridge, & Runowicz, 2005).

(c) Azoospermia may occur with a dose of 1.5 Gy, and low sperm counts may last for four to six months after treatment (Simon et al., 2005).

(d) TBI or chronic GVHD can lead to decreased blood flow to the penis resulting in decreased libido and erectile dysfunction (Yi & Syrjala, 2009). Erectile dysfunction medications such as sildenafil may be used to improve sexual functioning.

(e) In women older than 40 years of age, radiation doses of 5–6 Gy will cause permanent ovarian failure (Simon et al., 2005). In women younger than 40, regular menses may return, but the risk of infertility remains. TBI for HSCT results in greater than 90% permanent ovarian failure (Simon et al., 2005).

(f) Patients undergoing HSCT need pretransplant referral to clinics that specialize in fertility for information about measures to preserve fertility, such as sperm banking and egg retrieval. In vitro fertilization with frozen embryos has an approximately 20% success rate (Simon et al., 2005). Preserving oocytes may result in pregnancy in a small number of women (Simon et al., 2005).

(g) Vaginal atrophy, dryness, and irritation can lead to dyspareunia. Chronic GVHD can affect vaginal and vulvar tissue, causing vaginal strictures and stenosis with resulting sexual dysfunction (Yi & Syrjala, 2009).

   i. Topical estrogen may improve vaginal dryness.

   ii. Vaginal dilators may be helpful for vaginal stenosis (Yi & Syrjala, 2009).

(h) Younger women may be more affected by ovarian failure and changes in sexual function (Yi & Syrjala, 2009).

(i) Girls who are treated with high-dose chemotherapy and fractionated radiation before puberty may have a normal progression through puberty. Boys who receive the same treatment before puberty may have delayed puberty. Girls who have gone through puberty often develop amenorrhea, although some may recover ovarian function (Baker et al., 2010).

(3) TBI for HSCT and cranial irradiation can result in growth retardation in children. The hypothalamic-pituitary axis can be affected, causing decreased growth hormone production. In addition, radiation damage to epiphyseal growth plates in bone can lead to premature fusion and stunted growth (Baker et al., 2010). Growth hormone replacement may improve growth in children with documented growth hormone deficiency (Baker et al., 2010).

(4) Bone mineral density loss

   (a) This is a risk following HSCT and is likely due to several factors, such as

      i. Pretransplant treatment with TBI and chemotherapy

      ii. Steroid treatment

      iii. Inactivity due to transplant

      iv. Use of TPN.

   (b) Treatment with bisphosphonates, calcium, and vitamin D may improve bone mineral density (Baker et al., 2010).

   (c) Bone health in adults and children needs to be evaluated routinely following HSCT and treated when indicated.

i) Cardiovascular complications are typically late complications of HSCT and include cardiomyopathy, congestive heart failure, valvular damage, and arrhythmias (Tichelli et al., 2008).

(1) Patients should be evaluated for cardiovascular risk factors that include family history, hyperlipidemia, hypertension, type 2 diabetes mellitus, smoking, and obesity.

(2) Anthracycline doses of 550 mg/m^2 or higher in patients older than 18 years of age, and 300 mg/m^2 in those younger, and mediastinal irradiation are risk factors (Tichelli et al., 2008).

(3) High-dose cyclophosphamide is reported as cardiotoxic (Baker et al., 2010).

(4) Because of GVHD, patients who have undergone an allogeneic HSCT may have a higher incidence of cardiovascular events compared to those who undergo an autologous HSCT (Tichelli et al., 2008).

(5) Childhood HSCT survivors may be at increased risk for development of metabolic syndrome, which consists of central obesity, insulin resistance, glucose intolerance, hypertension, and dyslipidemia. Metabolic syndrome increases the risks of type 2 diabetes mellitus and cardiovascular disease (Baker et al., 2010). TBI has been reported in the development of insulin resistance (Baker et al., 2010).

(6) Long-term follow-up should include an electrocardiogram and echocardiogram to screen for cardiac dysfunction. Additional testing can be done for symptomatic or high-risk patients (Tichelli et al., 2008).

j) Kidney dysfunction

(1) Chronic kidney disease may affect 15%–40% of patients who have had an allogeneic transplant. The incidence may be the same for myeloablative and nonmyeloablative regimens (Abboud et al., 2009; Al-Hazzouri, Cao, Burns, Weisdorf, & Majhail, 2008). Chronic kidney disease is defined as a glomerular filtration rate of less than 60 ml/min/1.73 m^2 (Abboud et al., 2009).

(2) Risk factors include older age at transplantation, female sex, acute and chronic GVHD, TBI, and use of cyclosporine for immunosuppression (Al-Hazzouri et al., 2008; Tichelli et al., 2008).

(3) Ongoing monitoring of kidney function is necessary for patients who have had either a myeloablative or nonmyeloablative HSCT with annual creatinine, glomerular filtration rate, and urine protein analysis. Additional testing with abdominal ultrasound to evaluate the kidneys or a kidney biopsy may be indicated for diagnosis of chronic kidney disease (Tichelli et al., 2008).

k) Patients undergoing HSCT with or without TBI are at an increased risk for secondary malignancies.

(1) Chronic GVHD and male sex increases the risk for squamous cell cancer of the skin and oral cavity (Ghelani, Saliba, & Lima, 2005; Leisenring, Friedman, Flowers, Schwartz, & Deeg, 2006).

(2) TBI increases the risk for basal cell carcinoma of the skin but not squamous cell carcinoma (Leisenring et al., 2006).

(3) TBI increases the risks for melanoma, thyroid cancer, and salivary gland cancer (Ghelani et al., 2005).

(4) Cranial irradiation increases the risks for thyroid and brain tumors (Ghelani et al., 2005).

(5) Post-transplant lymphoproliferative disease is caused by infection with EBV. If the stem cell donor has been infected with EBV, a small number of B cells carrying the virus can be infused during the transplant process. The recipient lacks cellular immunity to fight the infection. If the recipient has had a previous EBV infection, it can be reactivated because of immunosuppression and lack of T-cell immunity (Childs, 2001).

(6) Autologous HSCT recipients have a 5%–15% risk of secondary myelodysplastic syndrome and acute myeloid leukemia two to five years after transplant. Risk factors include older age at transplant, use of TBI, and use of alkylating agents in pretransplant treatment (Majhail, 2008).

(7) A study of more than 3,300 children and adults who had undergone bone marrow or peripheral blood stem cell transplantations at one transplant center found an eightfold increased risk over the general population of developing a secondary cancer. Treatment-related cancers included solid tumors of the brain, breast, thyroid, lung, oral cavity, and soft tissue sarcomas, as well as myelodysplastic syndrome and acute myeloid leukemia. Some of the secondary malignancies occurred 20 years after transplant (Baker et al., 2003).

(8) In children, the most common secondary cancers are brain tumors and thyroid cancer associated with craniospinal irradiation (Baker et al., 2010).

(9) HSCT in patients younger than 10 years old increased the risk of both

basal cell and squamous cell carcinoma of the skin (Leisenring et al., 2006).

(10) Long-term screening for secondary malignancies is necessary in the post-transplant population. Early diagnosis of some secondary malignancies can lead to cure. Screening includes

    (a) Patient education regarding the signs and symptoms to be aware of and to report

    (b) Regular oral and skin examination for squamous cell, basal cell carcinomas, and melanoma

    (c) Patient education regarding avoiding sun exposure and using sunscreen with an SPF of 30 or higher

    (d) Regular monitoring of the complete blood count.

l) Treatment options for disease relapse after HSCT to promote graft-versus-tumor effect

(1) Decrease of immunosuppression

(2) Additional treatment with chemotherapy or RT

(3) Donor lymphocyte infusion

(4) Second HSCT with nonmyeloablative protocol

(5) Palliative care or hospice care

10. Post-transplant care

a) Following myeloablative HSCT, patients are hospitalized until engraftment occurs and require monitoring for infectious complications, bleeding, sinusoidal obstruction syndrome, acute GVHD, pain, and nutritional complications.

(1) Patients require antibiotic, antifungal, and antiviral treatment.

(2) Patients are red blood cell and platelet transfusion dependent.

(3) TPN and narcotic pain medication are usually needed.

b) After hospital discharge, patients are immunosuppressed and remain on multiple medications for prophylaxis of GVHD and bacterial, viral, and fungal infections. Family or other caregivers have responsibility for providing care of the central venous catheter, administering medications, IV fluids, or TPN, and monitoring for signs and symptoms of infections or other complications of the transplant.

(1) Patients are followed as outpatients three or more times a week.

(2) Patients need to avoid crowds and contact with small children and pets to decrease the risk of infection.

(3) Over time, clinic visits can be decreased as patients recover.

c) Patients may require physical therapy for strengthening and to increase physical activity to help maintain bone, cardiovascular, and respiratory health.

d) Patients and family members/caregivers may need support and counseling to deal with the stress of a life-threatening disease, the HSCT process, and coping with short- and long-term side effects and uncertainty of the future.

e) Reimmunization to reconstitute immunity begins 12–24 months after transplantation.

f) Ongoing monitoring for late effects of treatment

(1) Pulmonary function tests for pulmonary complications

(2) Cardiovascular risk assessment

    (a) Dietary counseling to decrease the risks of type 2 diabetes mellitus and obesity

    (b) Blood pressure screening and treatment for hypertension

    (c) Screening for hyperlipidemia and treatment as indicated

(3) Thyroid testing

(4) Bone mineral density testing

    (a) Calcium and vitamin D

    (b) Possible treatment with bisphosphonates

(5) Assessment of kidney function with blood urea nitrogen, creatinine, and urine protein testing

(6) Evaluation of liver function and serum ferritin for iron overload

(7) Sexual function and hormonal deficiencies

(8) Psychosocial functioning

(9) Evaluation of growth and cognitive function in children

(10) Screening for secondary malignancies

11. Patient and family education, and evaluation of their understanding, is a continuous process.

a) Patients and families need to understand the disease process.

b) Patients need to understand the indications for the proposed transplant as well as specifics, including

(1) Transplant team members and their roles

(2) Chemotherapy treatments, number of treatments, and potential short- and long-term side effects

(3) The role of TBI, if planned, along with how it will be delivered, the potential short- and long-term side effects, and when they are likely to occur

(4) Management of side effects of treatment.

c) Family members or caregivers require extensive education about medications, the signs and symptoms they should report, and management of central venous catheters and IV pumps.

d) Resources for patients and families
   (1) Financial
   (2) Psychosocial
   (3) Spiritual

e) Web site resources for patients and families
   (1) ACS: www.cancer.org
   (2) Association of Cancer Resources: www.acor.org
   (3) International Myeloma Foundation: www.myeloma.org
   (4) Leukemia and Lymphoma Society: www.lls.org
   (5) National Marrow Donor Program: www.marrowdonor.org
   (6) NCI: www.cancer.gov
   (7) OncoLink: www.oncolink.org

References

Abboud, I., Porcher, R., Robin, M., de Latour, R.P., Glotz, D., Socié, G., & Peraldi, M.N. (2009). Chronic kidney dysfunction in patients alive without relapse 2 years after allogeneic hematopoietic stem cell transplantation. *Biology of Blood and Marrow Transplantation, 15,* 1251–1257. doi:10.1016/j.bbmt.2009.05.016

Al-Hazzouri, A., Cao, Q., Burns, L.J., Weisdorf, D.J., & Majhail, N.S. (2008). Similar risks for chronic kidney disease in long-term survivors of myeloablative and reduced-intensity allogeneic hematopoietic cell transplantation. *Biology of Blood and Marrow Transplantation, 14,* 658–663. doi:10.1016/j.bbmt.2008.03.008

Al-Hazzouri, A., Cao, Q., Burns, L.J., Weisdorf, D.J., & Majhail, N.S. (2009). Similar risks for hypothyroidism after allogeneic hematopoietic cell transplantation using TBI-based myeloablative and reduced-intensity conditioning regimens. *Bone Marrow Transplantation, 43,* 949–951. doi:10.1038/bmt.2008.413

American College of Radiology & American Society for Radiation Oncology. (2006). *ACR–ASTRO practice guideline for the performance of total body irradiation.* Retrieved from http://www.acr.org/SecondaryMainMenuCategories/quality_safety/guidelines/ro/total_body_irradiation.aspx

Antin, J.H. (2002). Clinical practice. Long-term care after hematopoietic cell transplantation in adults. *New England Journal of Medicine, 347,* 36–42. doi:10.1056/NEJMcp010518

Baird, K., Cooke, K., & Schultz, K.R. (2010). Chronic graft-versus-host disease (GVHD) in children. *Pediatric Clinics of North America, 57,* 297–322. doi:10.1016/j.pcl.2009.11.003

Baker, K.S., Bresters, D., & Sande, J.E. (2010). The burden of cure: Long-term effects following hematopoietic stem cell transplantation (HSCT) in children. *Pediatric Clinics of North America, 57,* 323–342. doi:10.1016/j.pcl.2009.11.008

Baker, K.S., DeFor, T.E., Burns, L.J., Ramsay, K.C., Neglia, J.P., & Robison, L.L. (2003). New malignancies after blood or marrow stem-cell transplantation in children and adults: Incidence and risk factors. *Journal of Clinical Oncology, 21,* 1352–1358. doi:10.1200/JCO.2003.05.108

Baney, T. (Ed.) (2011). Radiodermatitis. In L.H. Eaton, J.M. Tipton, & M. Irwin (Eds.), *Putting evidence into practice: Improving oncology patient outcomes, volume 2* (pp. 49–54). Pittsburgh, PA: Oncology Nursing Society.

Baney, T., McQuestion, M., Bell, K., Bruce, S., Feight, D., Weis-Smith, L., & Haas, M. (2011). ONS PEP resource: Radiodermatitis. In L.H. Eaton, J.M. Tipton, & M. Irwin (Eds.), *Putting evidence into practice: Improving oncology patient outcomes, volume 2* (pp. 57–75). Pittsburgh, PA: Oncology Nursing Society.

Brunstein, C.G., & Weisdorf, D.J. (2009). Future of cord blood for oncology uses. *Bone Marrow Transplantation, 44,* 699–707. doi:10.1038/bmt.2009.286

Chien, J.W., Duncan, S., Williams, K.M., & Pavletic, S.Z. (2010). Bronchiolitis obliterans syndrome after allogeneic hematopoietic stem cell transplantation—An increasingly recognized manifestation of chronic graft-versus-host disease. *Biology of Blood and Marrow Transplantation, 16*(Suppl. 1), S106–S114. doi:10.1016/j.bbmt.2009.11.002

Childs, R.W. (2001). Allogeneic stem cell transplantation. In V.T. DeVita Jr., S. Hellman, & S.A. Rosenberg (Eds.), *Cancer: Principles and practice of oncology* (pp. 2779–2798). Philadelphia, PA: Lippincott Williams & Wilkins.

Copelan, E.A. (2006). Hematopoietic stem-cell transplantation. *New England Journal of Medicine, 354,* 1813–1826. doi:10.1056/NEJMra052638

Damron, B.I., Samsonow, S.M., Brant, J.M., Friend, P.J., Lacher, M., & Schaal, A.D. (2009). ONS PEP resource: Prevention of bleeding. In L.H. Eaton & J.M. Tipton (Eds.), *Putting evidence into practice: Improving oncology patient outcomes* (pp. 257–265). Pittsburgh, PA: Oncology Nursing Society.

Epstein, J.B., & Schubert, M.M. (2004). Managing pain in mucositis. *Seminars in Oncology Nursing, 20,* 30–37.

Firat, S.Y., & Lawton, C. (2010). Radiation technique results. In J.D. Cox & K.K. Ang (Eds.), *Radiation oncology* (9th ed.). New York, NY: Elsevier.

Ghelani, D., Saliba, R., & Lima, M. (2005). Secondary malignancies after hematopoietic stem cell transplantation. *Critical Reviews in Oncology/Hematology, 56,* 115–126. doi:10.1016/j.critrevonc.2005.03.014

Harden, S.V., Routsis, D.S., Geater, A.R., Thomas, S.J., Coles, C., Taylor, P.J., … Williams, M.V. (2001). Total body irradiation using a modified standing technique: A single institution 7 year experience. *British Journal of Radiology, 74,* 1041–1047.

Harris, D.J. (2010). Transplantation. In J. Eggert (Ed.), *Cancer basics* (pp. 317–342). Pittsburgh, PA: Oncology Nursing Society.

Harris, D.J., Eilers, J.G., Cashavelly, B.J., Maxwell, C.L., & Harriman, A. (2009). ONS PEP resource: Mucositis. In L.H. Eaton & J.M. Tipton (Eds.), *Putting evidence into practice: Improving oncology patient outcomes* (pp. 201–213). Pittsburgh, PA: Oncology Nursing Society.

Hensley, M.L., Hagerty, K.L., Kewalramani, T., Green, D.M., Meropol, N.J., Wasserman, T.H., ... Schuchter, L.M. (2009). American Society of Clinical Oncology 2008 clinical practice guideline update: Use of chemotherapy and radiation therapy protectants. *Journal of Clinical Oncology, 27,* 127–145. doi:10.1200/JCO.2008.17.2627

Kaner, R.J. (2010). Pulmonary complications after allogeneic hematopoietic cell transplantation. Retrieved from http://www.uptodate.com

Kessans, M.R., Gatesman, M.L., & Kockler, D.R. (2010). Plerixafor: A peripheral blood stem cell mobilizer. *Pharmacotherapy, 30,* 485–492. doi:10.1592/phco.30.5.485

Langner, S., Staber, P., Schub, N., Gramatzki, M., Grothe, W., Behre, G., ... Neumeister, P. (2008). Palifermin reduces incidence and severity of oral mucositis in allogeneic stem-cell transplant recipients. *Bone Marrow Transplantation, 42,* 275–279. doi:10.1038/bmt.2008.157

Lee, S.J., & Flowers, M.E.D. (2008). Recognizing and managing chronic graft-versus-host disease. *Hematology: American Society of Hematology Education Program Book, 2008,* 134–141. doi:10.1182/asheducation-2008.1.134

Leisenring, W., Friedman, D.L., Flowers, M.E.D., Schwartz, J.L., & Deeg, H.J. (2006). Nonmelanoma skin and mucosal cancers after hematopoietic cell transplantation. *Journal of Clinical Oncology, 24,* 1119–1126. doi:10.1200/JCO.2005.02.7052

Majhail, N.S. (2008). Old and new cancers after hematopoietic-cell transplantation. *Hematology: American Society of Hematology Education Program Book, 2008,* 142–149. doi:10.1182/asheducation-2008.1.142

Miller, J.S., Warren, E.H., van den Brink, M.R., Ritz, J., Shlomchik, W.D, Murphy, W.J., ... Falkenburg, J.H. (2010). NCI first international workshop on the biology, prevention, and treatment of relapse after allogeneic hematopoietic stem cell transplantation: Report from the committee on the biology underlying recurrence of malignant disease following allogeneic HSCT: Graft-versus-tumor/leukemia reaction. *Biology of Blood and Marrow Transplantation, 16,* 565–596. doi:10.1016/j.bbmt.2010.02.005

Mitchell, S.A., Beck, S.L., Hood, L.E., Moore, K., & Tanner, E.R. (2009). ONS PEP resource: Fatigue. In L.H. Eaton & J.M. Tipton (Eds.), *Putting evidence into practice: Improving oncology patient outcomes* (pp. 155–174). Pittsburgh, PA: Oncology Nursing Society.

Muehlbauer, P., Thorpe, D., Davis, A.B., Drabot, R.C., Kiker, E.S., & Rawlings, B.L. (2009). ONS PEP resource: Diarrhea. In L.H. Eaton & J.M. Tipton (Eds.), *Putting evidence into practice: Improving oncology patient outcomes* (pp. 125–134). Pittsburgh, PA: Oncology Nursing Society.

National Comprehensive Cancer Network. (2011). *NCCN Clinical Practice Guidelines in Oncology: Prevention and treatment of cancer-related infections* [v.1.2011]. Retrieved from http://www.nccn.org/professionals/physician_gls/pdf/infections.pdf

Rimkus, C. (2009). Acute complications of stem cell transplant. *Seminars in Oncology Nursing, 25,* 129–138. doi:10.1016/j.soncn.2009.03.007

Savani, B.N., Koklanaris, E.K., Le, Q., Shenoy, A., Goodman, S., & Barrett, A.J. (2009). Prolonged chronic graft-versus-host disease is a risk factor for thyroid failure in long-term survivors after matched sibling donor stem cell transplantation for hematologic malignancies. *Biology of Blood and Bone Marrow Transplantation, 15,* 377–381. doi:10.1016/j.bbmt.2008.11.032

Simon, B., Lee, S.J., Partridge, A.H., & Runowicz, C. (2005). Preserving fertility after cancer. *CA: A Cancer Journal for Clinicians, 55,* 211–228. doi:10.3322/canjclin.55.4.211

Tabbara, I.A., Zimmerman, K., Morgan, C., & Nahleh, Z. (2002). Allogeneic hematopoietic stem cell transplantation: Complications and results. *Archives of Internal Medicine, 162,* 1558–1566.

Tichelli, A., Rovó, A., & Gratwohl, A. (2008). Late pulmonary, cardiovascular, and renal complications after hematopoietic stem cell transplantation and recommended screening practices. *Hematology: American Society of Hematology Education Program Book, 2008,* 125–133. doi:10.1182/asheducation-2008.1.125

Wingard, J.R., Hsu, J., & Hiemenz, J.W. (2010). Hematopoietic stem cell transplantation: An overview of infection risks and epidemiology. *Infectious Disease Clinics of North America, 24,* 257–272. doi:10.1016/j.idc.2010.01.010

Wolff, D., Steiner, B., Hildebrandt, G., Edinger, M., & Holler, E. (2009). Pharmaceutical and cellular strategies in prophylaxis and treatment of graft-versus-host disease. *Current Pharmaceutical Design, 15,* 1974–1997.

Yi, J.C., & Syrjala, K.L. (2009). Sexuality after hematopoietic stem cell transplantation. *Cancer Journal, 15,* 57–64. doi:10.1097/PPO.0b013e318198c758

Zitella, L., Gobel, B.H., O'Leary, C., Friese, C.R., Woolery, M., Hauser, J., & Andrews, F. (2009). ONS PEP resource: Prevention of infection. In L.H. Eaton & J.M. Tipton (Eds.), *Putting evidence into practice: Improving oncology patient outcomes* (pp. 273–283). Pittsburgh, PA: Oncology Nursing Society.

G. Total lymphoid irradiation
1. Total lymphoid irradiation (TLI) or total nodal irradiation involves treatment to all lymph node regions above and below the diaphragm including the thymus and spleen. TLI combines mantle fields and inverted Y fields (Lowsky et al., 2005).
   a) Extended field or mantle irradiation includes the submandibular, cervical, supraclavicular, infraclavicular, axillary, mediastinal, subcarinal, and hilar lymph nodes (Diehl, Mauch, & Harris, 2001).
   b) The inverted Y field includes the para-aortic lymph nodes, spleen, inguinal, and femoral nodes (Diehl et al., 2001).
2. TLI was originally used for curative intent in HL (Kohrt & Lowsky, 2009).
3. TLI has been used in the treatment of early-stage follicular NHL, as have other types of radiation treatment such as involved-field irradiation, extended-field irradiation, and total nodal irradiation, with good response with each treatment. Relapse of disease tends to occur in areas outside the RT fields (Heinzelmann, Engelhard, Ottinger, Bamberg, & Weinmann, 2010).
   a) Previous treatment for stages III and IV follicular NHL included TLI and chemotherapy, although no survival advantage exist-

ed compared with chemotherapy and involved-field irradiation (Hoppe, 2007).

b) Both follicular NHL and HL are commonly treated with chemotherapy for systemic disease and involved-field radiation to all areas of clinically identified disease (Heinzelmann et al., 2010; Hoppe, 2007). Some patients who had relapse of disease or disease refractory to conventional treatment underwent autologous or allogeneic HSCT.

c) Standard doses of extended-field or involved-field radiation are 20–30 Gy in low-risk, early-stage patients without bulky disease and 30–40 Gy in those at high risk and/or with bulky disease (Diehl et al., 2001).

4. Side effects of TLI may include pancytopenia with increased risk of infection, odynophagia, esophagitis, and fatigue. Teach the patient and family about the purpose and duration of treatment, lung shielding, potential side effects, potential long-term toxicities of treatment, and management of side effects.

a) Decreased blood counts will be present in 7–10 days. The patient and family need to report temperatures of 100.5°F or higher or signs of infection.

b) Maintain hydration and nutrition with soft foods and liquid supplements.

c) Pain medication and IV hydration may be necessary for pain with swallowing and eating.

5. Evens et al. (2007) reported on a clinical trial of 48 patients with relapsed or refractory HL. Thirty-two patients received TLI and high-dose chemotherapy conditioning for autologous HSCT. Doses of TLI were 15 Gy to previously uninvolved nodal areas and 30 Gy to areas of current or previous disease. Median follow-up at 27 months found an event-free survival of 4% and overall survival of 48%, which compared favorably with patients treated with chemotherapy conditioning alone (Evens et al., 2007).

6. GVHD is a major cause of morbidity and mortality in allogeneic HSCT.

a) The skin, mouth, liver, and eyes are the most commonly involved areas at initial diagnosis of chronic GVHD. Other sites less commonly involved are the GI tract, lung, esophagus, female genital tract, and joints (Lee & Flowers, 2008).

b) GVHD increases the risks for infection and pulmonary complications of HSCT (Tichelli, Rovó, & Gratwohl, 2008).

c) GVHD negatively affects quality of life following HSCT.

7. Attempts to improve the results in HSCT led to studies to prevent or alleviate the occurrence of GVHD. GVHD is thought to be due to activation of donor T cells when they interact with recipient major or minor histocompatibility antigens and attack target organs (Antin, 2002; Wolff, Steiner, Hildebrandt, Edinger, & Holler, 2009).

a) T-cell depletion of donor stem cells prior to HSCT has been found to reduce GVHD but also has led to relapse of disease and graft rejection (Fowler & Griess, 2000; Miller et al., 2010).

b) Kohrt et al. (2009) reported on a clinical trial of 111 patients enrolled between 2001 and 2007 with a variety of malignancies (HL and NHL, pre-B-cell acute lymphoblastic leukemia, small lymphocytic leukemia/chronic lymphocytic leukemia, acute myeloid leukemia, chronic myeloid leukemia, and myelodysplastic syndrome) who underwent reduced-intensity allogeneic HSCT from matched related and unrelated donors with TLI and antithymocyte globulin conditioning.

(1) The dose of TLI was 80 cGy daily for 10 days for a total dose of 800 cGy.

(2) The blood of HSCT recipients was checked after TLI with findings of substantial decreases in CD3+, CD4+, and CD8+ T cells that mediate GVHD and an increased percentage of natural killer cells that are protective against GVHD.

(3) The rate of acute GVHD by post-transplant day 100 was 2% in related donor transplants and 10% in unrelated donor transplants, which were lower than rates reported in reduced-intensity HSCT that included chemotherapy and low-dose TBI.

(4) Overall survival after transplant was higher in younger patients (younger than 60 years old) and in those who were in first or second complete remission prior to transplant (Kohrt et al., 2009).

8. Organ rejection is a serious complication after transplantation of kidneys, lungs, heart, or any organ. Transplant recipients require long-term immunosuppressive therapy to prevent rejection. A small number of reports exist on the use of TLI to treat rejection.

a) Kawai and Cosimi (2010) reported on five patients at Massachusetts General Hospital who underwent combined kidney and bone marrow transplantation from a sibling or parent. A dose of 800 cGy TLI was used to induce tolerance for the transplant.

b) Ghadjar et al. (2010) used TLI in seven patients who had recurrent episodes of rejection of heart transplants over a 10-year period. The dose of TLI was 1.6–8.8 Gy. The rate of rejection episodes was significantly reduced with TLI. At a follow-up of seven years, one patient had died from coronary artery disease. TLI was considered to be well tolerated.

c) TLI has also been used in pediatric heart transplant patients who had multiple episodes of rejection (Asano et al., 2002).

d) Bronchiolitis obliterans is thought to be due to organ rejection and is a leading cause of morbidity and late mortality in lung and heart-lung transplant recipients. TLI has been used in a small number of patients to improve pulmonary function in patients with difficult-to-treat bronchiolitis obliterans (Verleden et al., 2009).

e) These reports of TLI use in heart and lung rejection included only a small number of patients, with TLI used only in severe cases of organ rejection after standard methods had failed.

9. Most studies of TLI in modifying recipient T-cell response to GVHD have been performed in mice or rats. Clinical trials of human subjects seem promising, but only a small number of patients have been treated. Use of TLI and antithymocyte globulin in nonmyeloablative HSCT may be a feasible alternative to chemotherapy and low-dose TBI, but more studies are necessary to determine whether one conditioning regimen is better than another.

10. Further studies are necessary to determine the best methods to reduce GVHD while preserving graft-versus-tumor/graft-versus-leukemia effect.

References

Antin, J.H. (2002). Clinical practice. Long-term care after hematopoietic cell transplantation in adults. *New England Journal of Medicine, 347,* 36–42. doi:10.1056/NEJMcp010518

Asano, M., Gundry, S.R., Razzouk, A.J., del Rio, M.J., Thomas, M., Chinnock, R.E., & Bailey, L.L. (2002). Total lymphoid irradiation for refractory rejection in pediatric heart transplantation. *Annals of Thoracic Surgery, 74,* 1979–1985.

Diehl, V., Mauch, P.M., & Harris, N.L. (2001). Hodgkin's disease. In V.T. DeVita Jr., S. Hellman, & S.A. Rosenberg (Eds.), *Cancer: Principles and practice of oncology* (6th ed., pp. 2339–2387). Philadelphia, PA: Lippincott Williams & Wilkins.

Evens, A.M., Altman, J.K., Mittal, B.B., Hou, N., Rademaker, A., Patton, D., ... Gordon, L.I. (2007). Phase I/II trial of total lymphoid irradiation and high-dose chemotherapy with autologous stem-cell transplantation for relapsed and refractory Hodgkin's lymphoma. *Annals of Oncology, 18,* 679–688. doi:10.1093/annonc/mdl496

Fowler, D.H., & Gress, R.E. (2000). Th2 and Tc2 cells in the regulation of GVHD, GVL, and graft rejection: Considerations for the allogeneic transplantation therapy of leukemia and lymphoma. *Leukemia and Lymphoma, 38,* 221–234. doi:10.3109/10428190009087014

Ghadjar, P., Joos, D., Martinelli, M., Hullin, R., Zwahlen, M., Lössl, K., ... Mohacsi, P. (2010). Tailored total lymphoid irradiation in heart transplant patients: 10-years experience of one center. *Radiation Oncology, 5,* 1–6. doi:10.1186/1748-717X-5-3

Heinzelmann, F., Engelhard, M., Ottinger, H., Bamberg, M., & Weinmann, M. (2010). Nodal follicular lymphoma: The role of radiotherapy for stages I and II. *Strahlentherapie und Onkologie, 186,* 191–196. doi:10.1007/s00066-010-2090-9

Hoppe, R.T. (2007). Hodgkin's lymphoma: The role of radiation in the modern combined strategies of treatment. *Hematology/Oncology Clinics of North America, 21,* 915–927. doi:10.1016/j.hoc.2007.06.013

Kawai, T., & Cosimi, A.B. (2010). Induction of tolerance in clinical kidney transplantation. *Clinical Transplantation, 24*(Suppl.), 2–5. doi:10.1111/j.1399-0012.2010.01268.x

Kohrt, H., & Lowsky, R. (2009). Total lymphoid irradiation for graft-versus-host disease protection. *Current Opinion in Oncology, 21*(Suppl. 1), S23–S26. doi:10.1097/01.cco.0000357471.68713.35

Kohrt, H.E., Turnbull, B.B., Heydari, K., Shizuru, J.A., Laport, G.G., Miklos, D.B., ... Lowsky, R. (2009). TLI and ATG conditioning with low risk of graft-versus-host disease retains antitumor reactions after allogeneic hematopoietic cell transplantation from related and unrelated donors. *Blood, 114,* 1099–1109. doi:10.1182/blood-2009-03-211441

Lee, S.J., & Flowers, M.E.D. (2008). Recognizing and managing chronic graft-versus-host disease. *Hematology: American Society of Hematology Education Program Book, 2008,* 134–141. doi:10.1182/asheducation-2008.1.134

Lowsky, R., Takahasi, T., Liu, Y.P., Dejbakhsh-Jones, S., Grumet, F.C., Shizuru, J.A., ... Strober, S. (2005). Protective conditioning for acute graft-versus-host disease. *New England Journal of Medicine, 353,* 1321–1331. doi:10.1056/NEJMoa050642

Miller, J.S., Warren, F.H., van den Brink, M.R., Ritz, J., Shlomchik, W.D, Murphy, W.J., ... Falkenburg, J.H. (2010). NCI first international workshop on the biology, prevention, and treatment of relapse after allogeneic hematopoietic stem cell transplantation: Report from the committee on the biology underlying recurrence of malignant disease following allogeneic HSCT: Graft-versus-tumor/leukemia reaction. *Biology of Blood and Marrow Transplantation, 16,* 565–596. doi:10.1016/j.bbmt.2010.02.005

Tichelli, A., Rovó, A., & Gratwohl, A. (2008). Late pulmonary, cardiovascular, and renal complications after hematopoietic stem cell transplantation and recommended screening practices. *Hematology: American Society of Hematology Education Program Book, 2008,* 125–133. doi:10.1182/asheducation-2008.1.125

Verleden, G.M., Lievens, Y., Dupont, L.J., Van Raemdonck, D.E., De Vleeschauwer, S.I., Vos, R., & Vanaudenaerde, B.M. (2009). Efficacy of total lymphoid irradiation in azithromycin nonresponsive chronic allograft rejection after lung transplantation. *Transplantation Proceedings, 41,* 1816–1820. doi:10.1016/j.transproceed.2009.03.070

Wolff, D., Steiner, B., Hildebrandt, G., Edinger, M., & Holler, E. (2009). Pharmaceutical and cellular strategies in prophylaxis and treatment of graft-versus-host disease. *Current Pharmaceutical Design, 15,* 1974–1997.

H. Total skin irradiation
1. Procedure description: Total skin irradiation is a type of RT that is delivered to the entire skin surface with electrons and is referred to as total skin electron beam therapy.
2. Indications (Diamantopoulos et al., 2011; Heese, Beriwal, Brady, & Vonderheid, 2008)
   a) Total skin irradiation is most commonly used in the treatment of cutaneous T-cell lymphoma, which incorporates two major subgroups.
      (1) Mycosis fungoides
      (2) Sézary syndrome
   b) Total skin irradiation may be a localized treatment in patients with unilateral or localized mycosis fungoides, lymphoma cutis, and Kaposi sarcoma.
   c) Total skin irradiation may be part of a non-myeloablative allogeneic HSCT (Duvic et al., 2010).
3. Treatment
   a) Treatment is often complex; positioning and dosing vary based on institutional guidelines and protocols.
   b) A variety of treatments for mycosis fungoides exist that can be used alone or in combination with chemotherapy, biotherapy, RT, or photochemotherapy.
   c) The role of total skin irradiation was first described in 1953 and historically is considered the single most effective method in treating cutaneous T-cell lymphoma (Becker, Hoppe, & Knox, 1995).
   d) Procedure
      (1) Boost treatment may be given to areas of ulceration prior to total skin irradiation (Gosselin-Acomb, 2007).
      (2) Treatment typically is delivered via a 6 MeV electron beam, and the patient is placed in a standing position in front of the beam.
      (3) A two-day, six-field treatment approach is used that encompasses the following fields on day 1: straight anterior, right posterior oblique, and the left posterior oblique. On the following day, the patient receives treatment to the straight posterior, right anterior oblique, and left anterior oblique.
         (a) Patient positioning is important so that skin folds are minimized. Typically this includes special care for the breasts, perineum, and the panniculi of obese patients.
         (b) Patients may have their hands and feet shielded during the six-field approach and then receive supple-mental therapy to these sites and the scalp, if warranted.
      (4) External or internal eye shields may be used to protect the cornea and lens.
      (5) Treatment typically is delivered four days a week for 30–45 minutes over the course of six to eight weeks for a total dose of 36–40 Gy to the skin and 18–20 Gy to the hands and feet.
4. Collaborative management
   a) Acute effects
      (1) Patients will experience epithelial reactions, including pruritus, erythema, dry desquamation, and moist desquamation (see section IV.C—Skin reactions).
      (2) Superficial atrophy with wrinkling, telangiectasia, xerosis, and uneven pigmentation are the most common changes (Chao, Perez, & Brady, 2002).
      (3) Patients may experience pain related to skin changes.
      (4) Patients will experience alopecia, which is reversible in four to six months (Reavely & Wilson, 2004).
      (5) Patients will experience nail loss.
      (6) At higher doses (greater than 25 Gy), some patients may develop transient swelling of the hands, edema of the ankles, and occasionally large blisters, necessitating local shielding or temporary discontinuation of therapy (Chao et al., 2002) (see section IV.C—Skin reactions).
      (7) Patients may report an inability to sweat properly for the first 6–12 months following therapy (Reavely & Wilson, 2004).
      (8) Gynecomastia may develop; the mechanism for this is unknown (Heese et al., 2008).
   b) Late effects ("Total-Skin Electron-Beam Irradiation," n.d.)
      (1) Superficial atrophy with wrinkling, telangiectasia, xerosis, and uneven pigmentation are the most common changes.
      (2) Although rare, higher doses may cause permanent alopecia, frank poikiloderma (mottled skin appearance), skin fragility, and subcutaneous fibrosis.
5. Patient and family education
   a) Teach the patient and family about the treatment procedure and the time required for the treatment each day, as well as positioning used for the treatment (Reavely & Wilson, 2004).

b) Inform the patient and family that the majority of the treatment area will be exposed during the treatment, and measures will be implemented to protect the patient's privacy.

c) Teach male patients about the potential risk of infertility caused by the dose received to the testes and options such as sperm banking (Jones et al., 2002; Reavely & Wilson, 2004).

d) Teach the patient about eye rinses to minimize irritation from eye shields.

e) Teach the patient and family about the use of skin products to minimize dry pruritus and dry desquamation (see section IV.C—Skin reactions).

f) Teach the patient and family about skin care if blisters or moist desquamation arises (see section IV.C—Skin reactions).

g) Teach the patient and family to elevate the extremity if swelling or edema arises.

h) Teach the patient and family about performing skin checks and to report any new lesions or changes in lesions.

i) Emphasize to the patient and family the importance of follow-up care to assess for late effects.

6. Follow-up

a) Patients may be seen frequently over the first few months after treatment for skin assessments and to determine their response to treatment.

b) Patients may be followed by a dermatologist in conjunction with the radiation oncologist.

References

Becker, M., Hoppe, R.T., & Knox, S.J. (1995). Multiple courses of high-dose total skin electron beam therapy in the management of mycosis fungoides. *International Journal of Radiation Oncology, Biology, Physics, 32,* 1445–1449. doi:10.1016/0360-3016(94)00590-H

Chao, K.S.C., Perez, C.A., & Brady, L.W. (Eds.). (2002). *Radiation oncology: Management decisions* (2nd ed.). Philadelphia, PA: Lippincott Williams & Wilkins.

Diamantopoulos, S., Platoni, K., Dilvoi, M., Nazos, I., Geropantas, K., Maravelis, G., ... Kouloulias, V. (2001). Clinical implementation of total skin electron beam (TSEB) therapy: A review of the relevant literature. *Physica Medica, 27,* 62–68. doi:10.1016/j.ejmp.2010.09.001

Duvic, M., Donato, M., Dabaja, B., Richmond, H., Singh, L., Wei, W., ... Hosing, C. (2010). Total skin electron beam and non-myeloablative allogeneic hematopoietic stem-cell transplantation in advanced mycosis fungoides and Sézary syndrome. *Journal of Clinical Oncology, 28,* 2365–2372. doi:10.1200/JCO.2009.25.8301

Gosselin-Acomb, T.K. (2007). Total skin electron beam therapy. In M.L. Haas, W.P. Hogle, G.J. Moore-Higgs, & T.K. Gosselin-Acomb (Eds.), *Radiation therapy: A guide to patient care* (pp. 503–507). St. Louis, MO: Elsevier Mosby.

Heese, C., Beriwal, S., Brady, L.W., & Vonderheid, E. (2008). Cutaneous T-cell lymphoma. In E.C. Halperin, C.A. Perez, & L.W.

Brady (Eds.), *Perez and Brady's principles and practice of radiation oncology* (5th ed., pp. 1766–1776). Philadelphia, PA: Lippincott Williams & Wilkins.

Jones, G.W., Kacinski, B.M., Wilson, L.D., Willemze, R., Spittle, M., Hohenberg, G., ... Knobler, R. (2002). Total skin electron radiation in the management of mycosis fungoides: Consensus of the European Organization for Research and Treatment of Cancer (EORTC) Cutaneous Lymphoma Project Group. *Journal of the American Academy of Dermatology, 47,* 364–370. doi:10.1067/mjd.2002.123482

Reavely, M.M., & Wilson, L.D. (2004). Total skin electron beam therapy and cutaneous T-cell lymphoma: A clinical guide for patients and staff. *Dermatology Nursing, 16,* 36, 39, 57.

Total-skin electron-beam irradiation. (n.d.). Retrieved from http://www.aboutcancer.com/tseb_0510.htm

I. Photodynamic therapy (PDT)

1. Definition: PDT is a treatment modality using a photosensitizing agent and light to kill cells in the presence of oxygen (Hahn et al., 2006). Individually, the photosensitizer and light have no effect, but together they induce a local cytotoxic reaction (Pinthus, Bogaards, Weersink, Wilson, & Trachtenberg, 2006). PDT has emerged as an important treatment modality in the management of cancer and noncancerous conditions.

a) The appeal of PDT in oncology is that the photosensitizer is retained in tumor tissues for a longer period of time than in normal tissues, resulting in a large therapeutic index (Chatterjee, Fong, & Zhang, 2008; Triesscheijn, Baas, Schellens, & Stewart, 2006).

b) The therapeutic response of PDT depends on a complex combination of parameters that include drug dose, drug-light interval, tissue oxygenation, light dose, and light intensity (Wildeman, Nyst, Karakullukcu, & Tan, 2009).

2. Procedure description: The patient is given the photosensitizer or it is applied topically. The tumor is illuminated through a fiber-optic scope with a visible light in a wavelength that matches the absorption characteristics of the photosensitizer. Light interacting with the photosensitizer triggers the release of free radicals that attack and destroy tumor cells. This chemical reaction causes a decrease in the size of the tumor and cuts off the blood supply. The dead cells begin sloughing and aid in debulking the tumor. PDT has several potential advantages over surgery and RT: It is comparatively noninvasive, it can be targeted accurately, repeated doses can be given without the total dose limitations associated with RT, and the healing process results in little or no scarring (Brown, Brown, & Walker, 2004).

3. Stages of PDT (Chatterjee et al., 2008)
    a) Stage I: Application of the photosensitizer, either locally or systemically
    b) Stage II: Accumulation of the photosensitizing agent in the tumor
    c) Stage III: Activation of the external illumination
    d) Stage IV: Induction of cell damage and apoptosis
4. Photosensitizers
    a) Photosensitizing agents have been used in medicine for several thousand years. The first clinical application was described by von Tappeiner and Jesionek in 1903 for basal cell carcinomas (Triesscheijn et al., 2006). It has just been in the past three decades or so that PDT has been used in the oncology setting with any success. In 1993, porfimer sodium (Photofrin®, Axcan Pharma US, Inc.) was approved for clinical use in Canada (see Table 17).
    b) First-generation photosensitizers are hematoporphyrin; its derivate, hematoporphyrin derivate; and the purified, commercially available Photofrin® (Nyst, Tan, Stewart, & Balm, 2009). The disadvantages associated with first-generation photosensitizers include prolonged skin photosensitivity and long illumination time. The skin photosensitivity lasts 4–12 weeks. Thirty minutes is required for illumination time to achieve curative PDT, which is a drawback in the clinical setting.

c) The primary second-generation photosensitizers include 5-aminolevulinic acid (Levulan®, DUSA Pharmaceuticals, Inc.), meta-tetra(hydroxyphenyl)chlorin (Foscan®, Biolitec Pharma), and Pd-bacteriopheophorbide (Tookad®, Steba Biotech). One of the advantages of these second-generation drugs is that a stronger absorption peak and longer light penetration enable deeper penetration into the tissues, leading to more effective tumor control. With Foscan, photosensitivity of the skin is much less prolonged than with Photofrin, 3 weeks compared to 6–12 weeks, respectively (Nyst et al., 2009). Tookad allows deep tissue penetration and is used mostly in prostate cancer.

d) Third-generation photosensitizers represent an emerging class of drugs. This group has delivery biomolecules, such as monoclonal antibodies, that specifically deliver photosensitizers to tumor tissue (O'Connor, Gallagher, & Byrne, 2009). The monoclonal antibody photosensitizer binds to tumor cells, facilitating photosensitization of tumor tissue and sparing normal tissue from damage. Nonporphyrin photosensitizers are being developed. Cationic photosensitizers have been one of the main areas of focus. Many cationic dyes accumulate selectively in transformed cells within the mitochondria as

Table 17. Photosensitizers Clinically Approved for Use in Oncology

Type of Cancer	Photosensitizer	Country
Actinic keratosis	ALA (Levulan®, Metvix®)	U.S., EU
Basal cell carcinoma	ALA (Metvix)	EU
Barrett's HGD	Porfimer sodium	U.S., Canada, EU, UK
Cervical cancer	Porfimer sodium	Japan
Endobronchial cancer	Porfimer sodium	Canada, Denmark, Finland, France, Germany, Ireland, Japan, The Netherlands, UK, U.S.
Esophageal cancer	Porfimer sodium	Canada, Denmark, Finland, France, Ireland, Japan, The Netherlands, UK, U.S.
Gastric cancer	Porfimer sodium	Japan
Head and neck cancer	Foscan®	EU, Norway, Iceland
Papillary bladder cancer	Porfimer sodium	Canada

ALA—5-aminolevulinic acid; EU—European Union; HGD—high-grade dysplasia; UK—United Kingdom

Note. From "Photodynamic Therapy in Oncology," by M. Triesscheijn, P. Baas, J.H. Schellens, and F.A. Stewart, 2006, Oncologist, 11, p. 1036. Copyright 2006 by AlphaMed Press. Reprinted with permission.

their main cellular target (O'Connor et al., 2009). This novel group of photosensitizers is now being developed and will be a new approach to the field of photodynamic therapy.

5. Light sources
   a) Diode lasers are ideal for routine use as clinical tools and need little technical expertise for use. They are small, portable, very reliable, and inexpensive (Brown et al., 2004).
   b) The BLU-U® Blue Light Photodynamic Therapy Illuminator (DUSA Pharmaceuticals, Inc.) is designed to be used with the photosensitizer Levulan Kerastick®. For more information, see www.dusapharma.com/blu-u1.html.
6. Clinical indications
   a) PDT with Photofrin (Axcan Pharma US, Inc., 2010b)
      (1) Esophageal cancer: Palliation of patients with complete or partially obstructing esophageal cancer who cannot be treated with Nd:YAG (neodymium-doped yttrium aluminum garnet) laser therapy
      (2) Endobronchial NSCLC
         (a) Treatment of patients with microinvasive endobronchial NSCLC who are not eligible for surgery or RT
         (b) Reduction of a complete or partial obstruction and palliation of symptoms in patients with obstructing NSCLC
      (3) Barrett esophagus: Ablation of high-grade dysplasia in patients with Barrett esophagus who are not treated with esophagectomy.
   b) PDT with Levulan Kerastick (DUSA Pharmaceuticals, Inc., 2011): Actinic keratosis of the face or scalp
      (1) Patients with a few to multiple minimally to moderately thick actinic keratoses of the face or scalp
      (2) Patients with actinic keratosis who are considered at risk for noncompliance with other therapies
   c) Investigational uses
      (1) PDT is currently being used in the treatment of liver metastases, cholangiocarcinoma, and prostate cancer (Harrod-Kim, 2006). Preliminary clinical data show the potential for benefit with the use of PDT in a neoadjuvant and adjuvant fashion to the minority of patients with cholangiocarcinoma currently considered resectable or of borderline resectability (Allison, Zervos, & Sibata, 2009). PDT affects interleukin-6 levels and may form the basis for a targeted therapy approach to cholangiocarcinoma.
      (2) Intraperitoneal PDT is a potential treatment for peritoneal carcinomatosis because of its relatively superficial treatment effect. This treatment approach is clinically well tolerated but is associated with substantial toxicity, indicating a narrow therapeutic index (Cengel, Glatstein, & Hahn, 2007). Responses were seen in heavily pretreated patients, suggesting clinical activity.
      (3) PDT has the potential to be a very effective local treatment modality for recurrent or persistent nasopharyngeal cancer and without the severe side effects seen with reirradiation (Wildeman et al., 2009).
      (4) The emergence of more potent and safer photosensitizers, portable light sources, dependable light delivery devices, and more accurate dosimetry and treatment planning renewed interest in PDT as a treatment for solid genitourinary tumors, such as prostate and renal cancers (Pinthus et al., 2006).
      (5) PDT is a minimally invasive treatment for cervical intraepithelial neoplasia. This can serve as a cervix-sparing treatment, which is particularly attractive to women desiring to preserve fertility (Yamaguchi et al., 2005). PDT is effective for treating cervical dysplasia and for the eradication of cervical human papillomavirus (Ichimura et al., 2003).
      (6) AIDS-related Kaposi sarcoma is the most common malignancy in patients with AIDS and presents as painful cutaneous lesions that are difficult to treat (Tardivo, Del Giglio, Paschoal, & Baptista, 2006). Bernstein et al. (1999) published a comprehensive study with 25 patients and concluded that Photofrin and laser illumination was effective as palliative treatment for AIDS-related Kaposi sarcoma.
7. Advantages of PDT (Chatterjee et al., 2008)
   a) Local treatment modality that uses a systemic photosensitizer
   b) Cost-effective when compared with other treatment options

c) Lengthened survival and improved quality of life (Brown et al., 2004)

d) Produces complete response in a very high percentage of patients (Detty, Gibson, & Wagner, 2004)

e) Spares extracellular tissue

f) Repetitive therapy without cumulative toxicity

g) Can be given in combination with debulking surgery for palliative treatment of larger tumors (Triesscheijn et al., 2006)

h) Can be repeated in case of recurrence or a new primary tumor in a previously treated area

8. Patient selection (Nyst et al., 2009)

a) Good nutritional status

b) Karnofsky performance score greater than 70%

c) Tumors must be easily accessible to laser light

9. Treatment: The sequence for a single PDT treatment covers a minimum of five days and is conducted in several stages (Axcan Pharma US, Inc., 2010a).

a) Day 1 involves the IV administration of Photofrin, a photosensitizing agent. PDT with Photofrin induces a photochemical effect, not a thermal effect (Axcan Pharma US, Inc., 2010a). The drug can be given in the outpatient setting or administered while the patient is in the hospital. The patient can eat and drink normally on the day of injection. Photosensitivity to the skin and eyes can begin within five minutes of the injection. The patient is instructed to wear protective clothing, dark sunglasses, and take special precautions (see later discussion of Patient and Family Education) that must be taken during the period of photosensitivity that lasts for one to three months (Axcan Pharma US, Inc., 2010a).

(1) The standard dose of Photofrin is 2 mg/kg. Photofrin is given via slow IV push over three to five minutes (Axcan Pharma US, Inc., 2010b). When the Photofrin freeze-dried cake or powder is reconstituted, it must be protected from bright light and used immediately (Axcan Pharma US, Inc., 2010b).

(2) Photofrin is classified as a miscellaneous antineoplastic agent. Although it is not a primary dermal irritant or vesicant, caution should be used to prevent extravasation of the drug. If extravasation occurs, protect the area from light and do not inject any additional substance into the area. The person preparing the Photofrin should wear gloves and protective eyewear to avoid contact with skin and eyes (Axcan Pharma US, Inc., 2010b).

b) On day 3, the patient is ready for the light activation step of the PDT process. The patient is NPO for eight hours before the laser light treatment. The application of the light is performed in the operating room, and the patient may receive a sedative, local anesthetic, or conscious sedation to provide comfort during the procedure. Some institutions may use general anesthesia and intubate the patient. The patient and staff are given protective eye goggles to wear during the procedure. The laser light is directed to the cancer cells through a fiber-optic guide that is passed through a scope (endoscope or bronchoscope). The instrument is positioned close to or into the tumor, and the precise amount of light is delivered. The light application takes 12½ minutes (Axcan Pharma US, Inc., 2010a), and the entire procedure takes approximately 30 minutes to complete. Recovery is brief unless the patient had general anesthesia and intubation, in which case the patient will go to the surgical intensive care unit or a step-down unit for close observation of the airway.

c) On day 5, another endoscopy or bronchoscopy is performed to remove necrotic tissue and exudates that could cause obstruction of the airway or esophagus (Axcan Pharma US, Inc., 2010a). This is an opportunity to evaluate the response to the PDT. The second-look procedure does not require another injection of Photofrin.

10. Collaborative management

a) Acute effects vary depending on tumor type and location.

(1) Photosensitivity is the main side effect that occurs immediately after administration of Photofrin and lasts for a minimum of 30 days. Side effects range from mild to moderate skin erythema to edema or blistering (Axcan Pharma US, Inc., 2010a). Other side effects directly related to the administration of Photofrin include nausea, mild constipation, and fever (Axcan Pharma US, Inc., 2010a).

(2) Ocular discomfort has been reported by patients as sensitivity to sunlight, car lights, and any bright light (Axcan Pharma US, Inc., 2010a).

(3) Respiratory distress as a result of tumor treatment–induced inflammation can block the airway or lead to coughing up large amounts of blood that can be life threatening.

(4) Bleeding can occur if enlarged veins are present in the esophagus or in patients with esophageal varices. Fatal hemoptysis can result with endobronchial tumors that are large, centrally located, cavitating, extensive, or extrinsic to the bronchus (Axcan Pharma US, Inc., 2010b).

(5) Post-PDT symptoms experienced include localized swelling and inflammation to the treated area, which may cause local discomfort (Axcan Pharma US, Inc., 2010b).

(6) Other common symptoms include mucositis, pharyngitis, nausea and vomiting, mild constipation, bleeding at the site, fever, infection (pneumonia or bronchitis), dyspnea, substernal chest pain caused by inflammation, and dysphagia.

b) Late effects: Essentially no chronic side effects occur with administration of Photofrin or the PDT process (Axcan Pharma US, Inc., 2010a).

11. Patient and family education (Axcan Pharma US, Inc., 2010a)

a) Teach the patient and family about Photofrin injection, side effects, photosensitivity, use of protective clothing and dark sunglasses, and strategies to protect against photosensitivity.

b) Photosensitivity begins immediately after injection of Photofrin and lasts for approximately one to three months.

c) Photofrin-induced photosensitivity reaction is characterized by mild to moderate erythema, swelling, pruritus, burning sensation, feeling hot, or blistering.

d) Protective clothing includes a tightly woven, light-colored, long-sleeve shirt and long pants, wide-brimmed hat, scarf, gloves, and dark sunglasses.

e) Sunscreen of any SPF offers no protective value against the photosensitivity because sunscreens protect against ultraviolet light. Photoactivation is caused by visible light, not UV light, which is invisible.

f) Teach the patient to avoid direct sunlight from skylights or undraped windows; the patient should remain at least six feet from windows.

g) Limit outdoor activities to after the sun has gone down.

h) Avoid helmet-type hair dryers to prevent burns on the scalp.

i) Teach the patient to not stay in a totally darkened room, as low levels of indoor light (ambient light) are necessary to help break down and inactivate (photo bleaching reaction) the Photofrin retained in the skin.

j) Patients requiring emergency or elective abdominal surgery need to tell their surgeon that they have had PDT so that special draping and operating room light filters can be used (Bruce, 2001).

k) Women of childbearing age should practice effective methods of birth control during use of Photofrin and PDT.

l) Fever, nausea, and constipation related to the Photofrin respond to conventional use of antipyretics, antiemetics, and a bowel regimen.

m) Teach the patient and family about the PDT procedure and recovery phase.

(1) Close monitoring during the procedure and immediately afterward on day 1 includes electrocardiogram, pulse oximetry, suction, oxygen, and IV access.

(2) Warn patients that substernal chest pain may occur (because of the inflammatory responses within the treatment area) during and after the procedure and that analgesics will be administered to reduce the discomfort.

n) Teach the patient and family how to test for photosensitivity on day 31 (Axcan Pharma US, Inc., 2010a).

(1) Have the patient place his or her hand in a paper bag with a two-inch hole in it.

    (2) Expose it to direct sunlight for 10 minutes.

    (3) If a reaction (erythema, edema, or blistering) occurs within 24 hours, continue with photosensitivity precautions for an additional two weeks, and then repeat the test.

    (4) If no reaction occurs within 24 hours, the patient may gradually increase exposure to sunlight while continuing to watch for skin reactions.

o) Signs and symptoms to report to the healthcare team

    (1) Red or blistered skin at any point following treatment

    (2) Bleeding

    (3) Respiratory distress

    (4) Chest pain

    (5) Infection

    (6) Mucositis, pharyngitis, and dysphagia

    (7) Unrelieved nausea, fever, or constipation

p) Follow-up

    (1) After discharge from the hospital, the patient will return initially for follow-up endoscopy or bronchoscopy one week after treatment, and then monthly for three months.

    (2) After treatment of high-grade dysplasia in Barrett esophagus, endoscopic biopsies are performed every three months until four consecutive negative evaluations have been recorded (Axcan Pharma US, Inc., 2010a).

12. Areas for research

a) This a field ripe for continued research in improved photosensitizers, light sources, and disease-specific indications.

b) More research is needed in the improvement of quality of life with PDT.

c) To date, no randomized phase III clinical trials have compared PDT with other treatment modalities (Nyst et al., 2009).

d) Researchers are exploring nanoparticles in PDT to develop a more optimal drug delivery system in which there is little or no uptake by nontarget cells (Chatterjee et al., 2008).

e) Self-lighting PDT is a combination of RT and PDT. Nanoparticles with attached photosensitizers are used. Upon exposure to ionizing radiation and activation of the photosensitizers, singlet oxygen (the most damaging reactive oxygen species generated during PDT, which can directly kill tumor cells by the induction of apoptosis and necrosis [Triesscheijn et al., 2006]) is produced to enhance the killing of cancer cells by ionizing radiation (Chatterjee et al., 2008). Supplementation of conventional RT with PDT would potentially allow the use of lower doses of radiation.

f) Combined therapy using PDT and antiangiogenic drugs such as bevacizumab or appropriately targeted research inhibitors of angiogenesis such as vascular endothelial growth factor and matrix metalloproteinases is also emerging as a focus of PDT (O'Connor et al., 2009).

g) The concept of photodynamic molecular beacons (PMBs) is recent in PDT. The aim of PMBs is to activate the photosensitizer only in the presence of a cancer cell–specific biomarker that is recognized by a disease-associated linker (O'Connor et al., 2009). The linker holds the photosensitizer in close proximity so that the phototoxicity of the photosensitizer is silenced in normal cells and activated only in diseased cells or tissue where the biomarker is expressed. These PMBs allow for an extra level of control within PDT, in addition to the preferential accumulation of a photosensitizer in tumor tissue. The fact that only diseased tissues are irradiated makes this a highly selective treatment modality for cancer. Work with these PMBs is ongoing.

References

Allison, R.R., Zervos, E., & Sibata, C.H. (2009). Cholangiocarcinoma: An emerging indication for photodynamic therapy. *Photodiagnosis and Photodynamic Therapy, 6,* 84–92. doi:10.1016/j.pdpdt.2009.05.001

Axcan Pharma US, Inc. (2010a). Patient guide to photodynamic therapy. Retrieved from http://www.photofrin.com

Axcan Pharma US, Inc. (2010b). *Photofrin®* [Package insert]. Retrieved from http://www.photofrin.com/pdf/prescribing-info.pdf

Bernstein, Z.P., Wilson, B.D., Oseroff, A.R., Jones, C.M., Dozier, S.E., Brooks, J.S., ... Dougherty, T.J. (1999). New photodynamic therapy protocol to treat AIDS-related Kaposi's sarcoma. *AIDS, 13,* 1697–1704.

Brown, S.B., Brown, E.A., & Walker, I. (2004). The present and future role of photodynamic therapy in cancer treatment. *Lancet Oncology, 5,* 497–508. doi:10.1016/S1470-2045(04)01529-3

Bruce, S. (2001). Photodynamic therapy: Another option in cancer treatment. *Clinical Journal of Oncology Nursing, 5,* 95–99.

Cengel, K.A., Glatstein, E., & Hahn, S.M. (2007). Intraperitoneal photodynamic therapy. *Cancer Treatment and Research, 134,* 493–514. doi:10.1007/978-0-387-48993-3_34

Chatterjee, D.K., Fong, L.S., & Zhang, Y. (2008). Nanoparticles in photodynamic therapy: An emerging paradigm. *Advanced Drug Delivery Reviews, 60,* 1627–1637. doi:10.1016/j.addr.2008.08.003

Detty, M.R., Gibson, S.L., & Wagner, S.J. (2004). Current clinical and preclinical photosensitizers for use in photodynamic therapy. *Journal of Medicinal Chemistry, 47,* 3897–3915. doi:10.1021/jm040074b

DUSA Pharmaceuticals, Inc. (2011). Levulan® Kerastick®. Retrieved from http://www.dusapharma.com/levulan-photodynamic-therapy.html

Hahn, S.M., Fraker, D.L., Mick, R., Metz, J., Busch, T.M., Smith, D., ... Glatstein, E. (2006). A phase II trial of intraperitoneal photodynamic therapy for patients with peritoneal carcinomatosis and sarcomatosis. *Clinical Cancer Research, 12,* 2517–2525. doi:10.1158/1078-0432.CCR-05-1625

Harrod-Kim, P. (2006). Tumor ablation with photodynamic therapy: Introduction to mechanism and clinical applications. *Journal of Vascular and Interventional Radiology, 17,* 1441–1448. doi:10.1097/01.RVI.0000231977.49263.DE

Ichimura, H., Yamaguchi, S., Kojima, A., Tanaka, T., Niiya, K., Takemori, M., ... Nishimura, R. (2003). Eradication and reinfection of human papillomavirus after photodynamic therapy for cervical intraepithelial neoplasia. *International Journal of Clinical Oncology, 8,* 322–325. doi:10.1007/s10147-003-0354-4

Nyst, H.J., Tan, I.B., Stewart, F.A., & Balm, A.J.M. (2009). Is photodynamic therapy a good alternative to surgery and radiotherapy in the treatment of head and neck cancer? *Photodiagnosis and Photodynamic Therapy, 6,* 3–11. doi:10.1016/j.pdpdt.2009.03.002

O'Connor, A.E., Gallagher, W.M., & Byrne, A.T. (2009). Porphyrin and nonporphyrin photosensitizers in oncology: Preclinical and clinical advances in photodynamic therapy. *Photochemistry and Photobiology, 85,* 1053–1074. doi:10.1111/j.1751-1097.2009.00585.x

Pinthus, J.H., Bogaards, A., Weersink, R., Wilson, B.C., & Trachtenberg, J. (2006). Photodynamic therapy for urological malignancies: Past to current approaches. *Journal of Urology, 175,* 1201–1207. doi:10.1016/S0022-5347(05)00701-9

Tardivo, J.P., Del Giglio, A., Paschoal, L.H., & Baptista, M.S. (2006). New photodynamic therapy protocol to treat AIDS-related Kaposi's sarcoma. *Photomedicine and Laser Surgery, 24,* 528–531. doi:10.1089/pho.2006.24.528

Triesscheijn, M., Baas, P., Schellens, J.H., & Stewart, F.A. (2006). Photodynamic therapy in oncology. *Oncologist, 11,* 1034–1044. doi:10.1634/theoncologist.11-9-1034

Wildeman, M.A., Nyst, H.J., Karakullukcu, B., & Tan, B.I. (2009). Photodynamic therapy in the therapy for recurrent/persistent nasopharyngeal cancer. *Head and Neck Oncology, 1,* 40. doi:10.1186/1758-3284-1-40

Yamaguchi, S., Tsuda, H., Takemori, M., Nakata, S., Nishimura, S., Kawamura, N., ... Nishimura, R. (2005). Photodynamic therapy for cervical intraepithelial neoplasia. *Oncology, 69,* 110–116. doi:10.1159/000087812

J. Proton beam RT
1. Procedure description: Protons, positively charged particles produced by cyclotrons or synchrocyclotrons (types of particle accelerators) deposit the majority of their energy at a designated depth, the Bragg peak. The Bragg peak is too narrow to treat most tumors. Therefore, several proton beams of various energies are superimposed to create a uniform dose that covers the depth of the tumor and produces a spread-out Bragg peak. Little energy is at the surface, less scattering occurs because of the sharp beam edges, and the dose falls off sharply beyond the peak (Durante & Loeffler, 2010; Schulz-Ertner, Jäkel, & Schlegel, 2006).
   a) Relative biologic effectiveness (RBE) is the ratio of x-ray and particle dose producing a similar biologic effect. It is influenced by LET and the rate of energy loss in tissue. RBE increases with increased LET. High LET radiation is less affected by tissue oxygenation, variations in cell cycle, and DNA repair (Durante & Loeffler, 2010).
      (1) Protons, with a low LET at entrance, lose a small amount of energy until reaching maximum penetration depth where the residual energy is deposited, thus delivering a high LET at the Bragg peak region where the tumor is located (Schulz-Ertner et al., 2006).
      (2) Biologic effects of protons and x-ray radiation in normal tissue are comparable, resulting in complications similar to conventional treatment (Durante & Loeffler, 2010; Halperin, 2006). However, the RBE of protons is 10% greater than for x-rays (Yock & Tarbell, 2004).
   b) Proton beam therapy has the potential to improve local control and decrease acute and long-term toxicity (DeLaney, 2008; Durante & Loeffler, 2010).
   c) Proton dose is reported as cobalt gray equivalent, which equals the photon dose measured in gray.
   d) Robert Wilson first proposed using protons for the treatment of cancer in 1946. A small number of patients were the first treated with protons in 1954 at Lawrence Berkeley National Laboratory in California. Fractionated proton treatment for patients began at the Harvard Cyclotron Laboratory in 1970 in collaboration with physicians at Massachusetts General Hospital (Hall, 2009). Hospital-based proton treatment facilities became available in 1990 (Smith, 2009).

e) In contrast to conventional x-ray radiation or photons, which deposit energy along their path from the point of entrance to exit beyond the tumor, proton beam RT reduces the entrance dose and eliminates an exit dose, sparing normal tissue (see Figure 26). Thus, improved dose distribution properties allow a higher dose to the tumor and a low dose to adjacent or surrounding tissues or critical structures.

2. Indications

a) Ocular tumors (uveal melanomas) (Levin, Kooy, Loeffler, & DeLaney, 2005)

b) Skull base and spinal sarcomas (Patel & DeLaney, 2008)

c) Head and neck tumors (paranasal sinus, nasal, and nasopharynx) because of their irregular configuration and proximity to critical and dose-limiting structures (i.e., optic nerves and chiasm, brain, and ocular globes) (Chan & Liebsch, 2008; Chera et al., 2009; Feng & Eisbruch, 2007)

d) For early-stage prostate cancer, protons may offer dose-sparing advantages to the rectum and bladder and reduce treatment-related morbidities. However, additional studies comparing protons to IMRT are needed (Nguyen, Trofimov, & Zietman, 2008; Trofimov et al., 2007; Vargas et al., 2008).

e) CNS benign lesions

(1) Unresectable acoustic neuromas and unresectable or irregularly shaped meningiomas

(2) Pituitary adenomas with treatment volumes greater than 2–3 cm or hormonally active tumors more than 5 mm from the optic chiasm (Shih, Chapman, Bussière, Chen, & Loeffler, 2008)

(3) AVMs when surgical resection is not possible (Shih et al., 2008)

f) Bone and soft tissue sarcomas (Ewing sarcoma, retroperitoneal, pelvic, and extremity sarcomas) (DeLaney & Kirsch, 2008)

g) Lung: Clinical trials with dose escalation using protons for localized NSCLC are ongoing (Georg, Hillbrand, Stock, Dieckmann, & Pötter, 2008).

h) In the pediatric setting, protons offer a method to deliver a highly conformal radiation dose to tumor while sparing dose to sensitive, growing normal tissue. This may significantly reduce treatment-related acute side effects related to tumor location and volume of normal tissue in treatment field and long-term morbidities (i.e., growth disturbance, neurocognitive and neuroendocrine dysfunction, hearing loss, and secondary treatment-related malignancies) (Halperin, 2006; Yock, DeLaney, Esty, & Tarbell, 2008; Yock et al., 2005) (see Figure 27).

i) Brain tumors (medulloblastoma, optic gliomas, craniopharyngiomas, ependymomas, meningiomas, chordomas, germinomas) (MacDonald et al., 2008; Merchant et al., 2004; Yock & Tarbell, 2004)

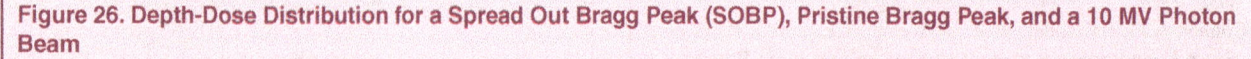

Figure 26. Depth-Dose Distribution for a Spread Out Bragg Peak (SOBP), Pristine Bragg Peak, and a 10 MV Photon Beam

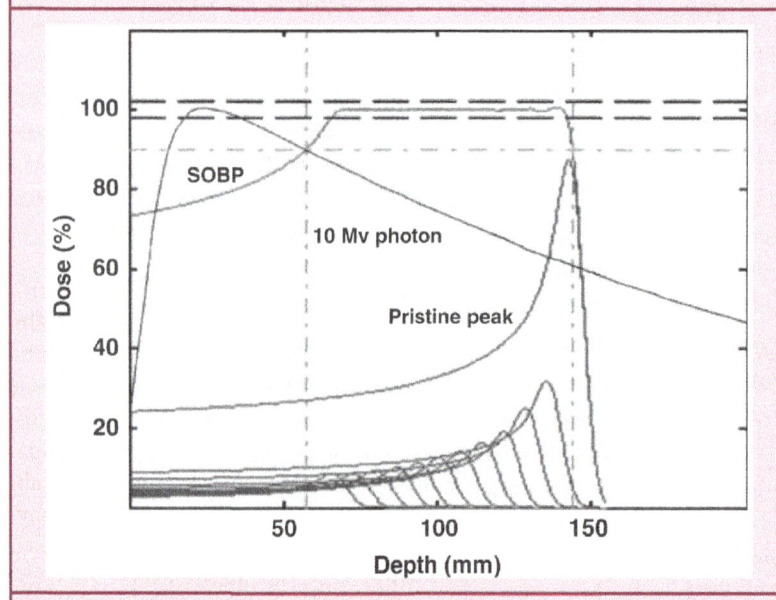

The SOBP dose distribution is created by adding the contributions of individually modulated pristine Bragg peaks. The penetration depth, or range, measured as the depth of the distal 90% of plateau dose, of the SOBP dose distribution is determined by the range of the most distal pristine peak (labeled "Pristine peak"). The modulation width, measured as the distance between the proximal and distal 90% of plateau dose values, of the SOBP dose distribution is controlled by varying the number and intensity of pristine Bragg peaks that are added, relative to the most distal pristine peak, to form the SOBP. The dashed lines indicate the clinical acceptable variation in the plateau dose of 72%. The dot–dashed lines indicate the 90% dose and spatial, range and modulation width, intervals. The SOBP dose distribution of even a single field can provide complete target volume coverage in depth and lateral dimensions, in sharp contrast to a single photon dose distribution; only a composite set of photon fields can deliver a clinical target dose distribution. Note the absence of dose beyond the distal falloff edge of the SOBP.

Note. From "Proton Beam Therapy," by W.P. Levin, H. Kooy, J.S. Loeffler, and T.F. DeLaney, 2005, *British Journal of Cancer, 93,* p. 850. Copyright 2005 by Macmillan Publishers Ltd. Reprinted with permission.

Figure 27. Coronal and Axial Photon Plan (left). Coronal and Axial Proton Plan (right).

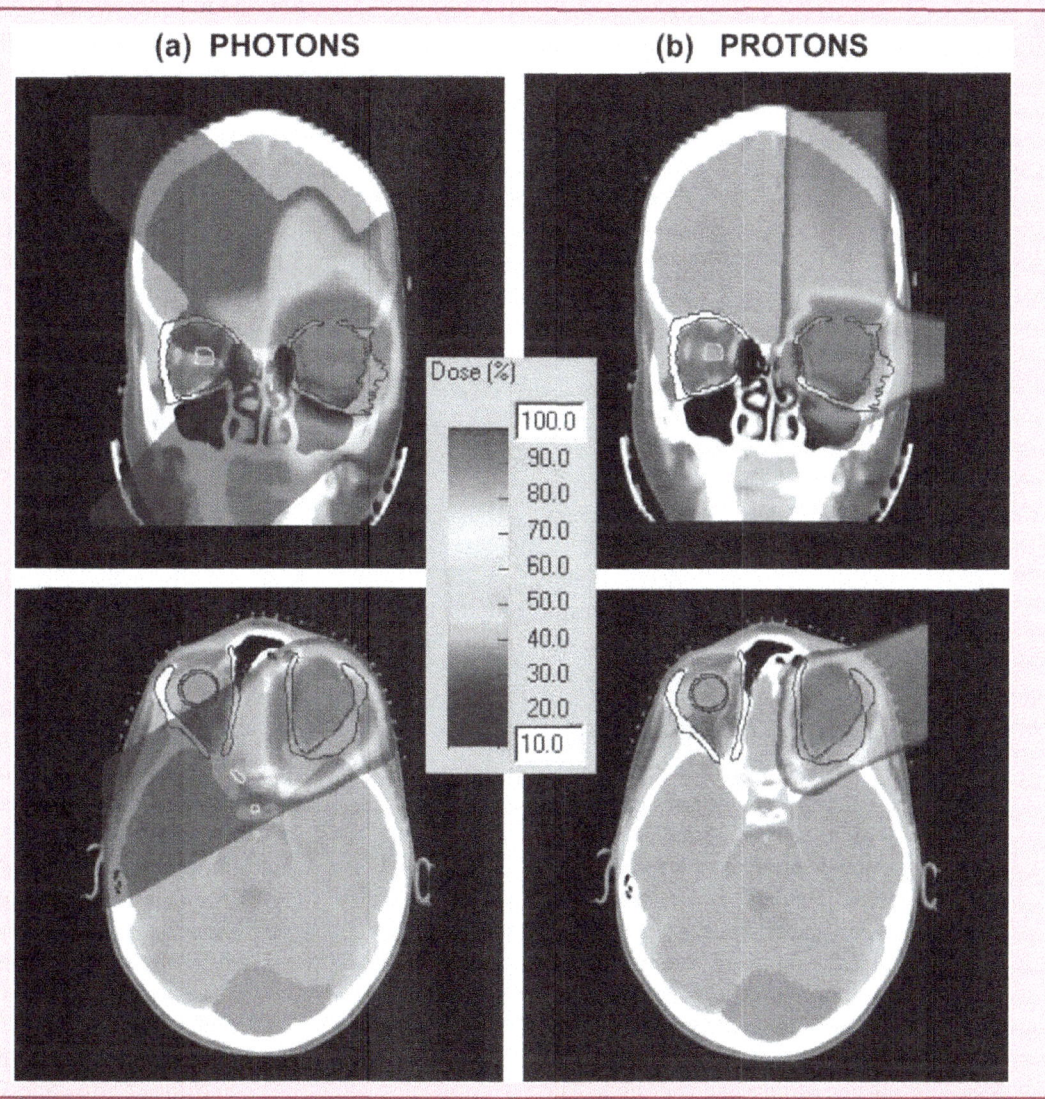

Note the absence of exit dose to the nontarget orbit, brain, and pituitary gland with protons.

Note. From "Proton Radiotherapy for Orbital Rhabdomyosarcoma: Clinical Outcome and a Dosimetric Comparison With Photons," by T. Yock, R. Schneider, A. Friedmann, J. Adams, B. Fullerton, and N. Tarbell, 2005, *International Journal of Radiation Oncology, Biology, Physics, 63,* p. 1163. Copyright 2005 by Elsevier. Reprinted with permission.

j) Retinoblastoma (Krengli et al., 2005; Lee et al., 2005)

k) Abdominal cancers (neuroblastoma and Wilms tumor) (Hillbrand, Georg, Gadner, Pötter, & Dieckmann, 2008)

l) Rhabdomyosarcoma (Yock et al., 2008)

3. Treatment setup and planning

a) Simulation is performed in the treatment position (i.e., prone, supine, or seated).

(1) An immobilization device is made to minimize patient motion during treatment, ensure accurate and precise daily treatment setup, and assist the patient in maintaining position. Because protons deposit dose at the distal edge of the spread-out Bragg peak, the thickness of the device must be kept to a minimum. Examples include thermoplastic face masks, bite blocks, head holders, vacuum bags, and body molds.

(2) A treatment planning CT scan is performed. Contrast may be used to help delineate normal structures or tumor volume.

(3) CT scan data are transferred to a treatment planning system. Tumor and normal tissue volumes are drawn on serial CT sections throughout the treatment volume using information from clinical reports and imaging studies (CT

and MRI) to accurately define the target and critical dose-limiting structures.

b) Beam application systems are used to shape and customize the beam to the target volume and minimize dose to defined normal tissues.

   (1) Passive beam shaping, most commonly used in proton treatment, uses a beam modulator to produce a depth-dose profile. The modulated Bragg peak, or spread-out Bragg peak, must cover the whole target homogeneously and match the distal end of the target volume. Patient-specific hardware is necessary (Gottschalk, 2008).

      (a) An aperture device customized for each treatment portal shapes the beam and eliminates protons outside the designed volume area.

      (b) A compensator accounts for differences in tissue depths within the field and the curvature of the patient's surface and is designed so that the distal end of the spread-out Bragg peak matches the end of the target volume.

   (2) Active beam shaping produces focused pencil beams, which allows three-dimensional scanning over the treatment/target field. The dose depth for the spread-out Bragg peak is set along each pencil beam to achieve 100% dose confined to the target (Gottschalk, 2008). Dose distributions can be conformed to irregular shapes without the use of patient-specific hardware, and treatment delivery is automatic via computer control systems (Gottschalk, 2008; Schulz-Ertner et al., 2006).

4. Treatment

   a) The patient is positioned using the same immobilization device used for the treatment planning CT.

   b) Radiographic verification of patient position and treatment fields is obtained.

   c) Treatment time varies according to the number of treatment fields and complexity of the setup.

   d) Treatments are given daily (fractionated) Monday through Friday; however, single high-dose treatment is used for benign lesions (AVMs and pituitary adenomas 5 mm or more from optic nerves and chiasm) (Shih et al., 2008).

5. Collaborative management

   a) Side effects: Site-specific side effects (acute and late) are determined by the area treated and may be reduced as a result of highly conformal dose distributions and lack of exit dose, thus minimizing the dose to normal tissues (see the specific treatment sites). For example, in craniospinal irradiation for medulloblastoma with protons, no exit dose reaches the heart, mediastinum, bowel, and bladder (Yock et al., 2008).

   b) Secondary malignancies: Protons may reduce the risk of secondary malignancies compared to photon treatment. This is especially important in pediatric patients (Durante & Loeffler, 2010; Yock et al., 2008).

   c) Multidisciplinary collaboration

      (1) Other treatment modalities (photon radiation, chemotherapy, and surgery) may be indicated depending on the disease, stage of the disease, treatment regimen, or clinical trial. Coordination of care, patient assessment, and symptom management are essential.

      (2) Anesthesia is necessary for daily treatment of young children to ensure precise treatment setup and maintenance of position. Coordination and timing of these treatments are essential.

      (3) Refer to support services (i.e., nutrition services, social services, patient navigator, and chaplain) as needed.

6. Patient and family education: Teach the patient and family about all aspects of proton treatment.

   a) Explain the difference between proton and photon radiation and how proton beam RT works.

   b) Provide information on the immobilization device and the importance of patient positioning and compliance.

   c) Describe simulation and daily treatment. Include the treatment schedule and any special instructions necessary for daily treatment (e.g., full bladder, NPO).

d) List possible side effects and symptom management strategies.

e) Provide information on communication with the treatment team (e.g., weekly status checks, telephone or contact numbers).

f) Provide information in various formats depending on patient preference and availability (written, audiovisual, verbal).

g) Confirm understanding by the patient and family and document.

7. Research

a) Particle Therapy Co-Operative Group (http://ptcog.web.psi.ch)

b) Proton Radiation Oncology Group (www.rtog.org): PROG's goal is to provide a centralized research base, not available elsewhere, for clinical trials employing proton therapy. PROG has been funded by NCI.

References

Chan, A.W., & Liebsch, N.J. (2008). Proton radiation therapy for head and neck cancer. *Journal of Surgical Oncology, 97,* 697–700. doi:10.1002/jso.21013

Chera, B.S., Malyapa, R., Louis, D., Mendenhall, W.M., Li, Z., Lanza, D.C., ... Mendenhall, N.P. (2009). Proton therapy for maxillary sinus carcinoma. *American Journal of Clinical Oncology, 32,* 296–303. doi:10.1097/COC.0b013e318187132a

DeLaney, T. (2008). *Proton and charged particle radiotherapy.* In T.F. DeLaney & H.M. Kooy (Eds.), Clinical issues in proton radiotherapy (pp. 108–114). Philadelphia, PA: Lippincott Williams & Wilkins.

DeLaney, T.F., & Kirsch, D.G. (2008). Bone and soft tissue. In T.F. DeLaney & H.M. Kooy (Eds.), *Proton and charged particle radiotherapy* (pp. 172–185). Philadelphia, PA: Lippincott Williams & Wilkins.

Durante, M., & Loeffler, J.S. (2010). Charged particles in radiation oncology. *Nature Reviews Clinical Oncology, 7,* 37–43. doi:10.1038/nrclinonc.2009.183

Feng, M., & Eisbruch, A. (2007). Future issues in highly conformal radiotherapy for head and neck cancer. *Journal of Clinical Oncology, 25,* 1009–1013. doi:10.1200/JCO.2006.10.4638

Georg, D., Hillbrand, M., Stock, M., Dieckmann, K., & Pötter, R. (2008). Can protons improve SBRT for lung lesions? Dosimetric considerations. *Radiotherapy and Oncology, 88,* 368–375. doi:10.1016/j.radonc.2008.03.007

Gottschalk, B. (2008). Treatment delivery systems: Passive beam scattering. In T.F. DeLaney & H.M. Kooy (Eds.), *Proton and charged particle radiotherapy* (pp. 33–40). Philadelphia, PA: Lippincott Williams & Wilkins.

Hall, E. (2009). Protons for radiotherapy: A 1946 proposal. *Lancet Oncology, 10,* 196. doi:10.1016/S1470-2045(09)70022-1

Halperin, E.C. (2006). Particle therapy and treatment of cancer. *Lancet Oncology, 7,* 676–685. doi:10.1016/S1470-2045(06)70795-1

Hillbrand, M., Georg, D., Gadner, H., Pötter, R., & Dieckmann, K. (2008). Abdominal cancer during early childhood: A dosimetric comparison of proton beams to standard and advanced photon radiotherapy. *Radiotherapy and Oncology, 89,* 141–149. doi:10.1016/j.radonc.2008.06.012

Krengli, M., Hug, E.B., Adams, J.A., Smith, A.R., Tarbell, N.J., & Munzenrider, J.E. (2005). Proton radiation therapy for retinoblastoma: Comparison of various intraocular tumor locations and beam arrangements. *International Journal of Radiation Oncology, Biology, Physics, 61,* 583–593. doi:10.1016/j.ijrobp.2004.06.003

Lee, C.T., Bilton, S.D., Famiglietti, R.M., Riley, B.A., Mahajan, A., Chang, E.L., ... Smith, A.R. (2005). Treatment planning with protons for pediatric retinoblastoma, medulloblastoma, and pelvic sarcoma: How do protons compare with other conformal techniques? *International Journal of Radiation Oncology, Biology, Physics, 63,* 362–372. doi:10.1016/j.ijrobp.2005.01.060

Levin, W.P., Kooy, H., Loeffler, J.S., & DeLaney, T.F. (2005). Proton beam therapy. *British Journal of Cancer, 93,* 849–854. doi:10.1038/sj.bjc.6602754

MacDonald, S.M., Safai, S., Trofimov, A., Wolfgang, J., Fullerton, B., Yeap, B.Y., ... Yock, T. (2008). Proton radiotherapy for childhood ependymoma: Initial clinical outcomes and dose comparisons. *International Journal of Radiation Oncology, Biology, Physics, 71,* 979–986. doi:10.1016/j.ijrobp.2007.11.065

Merchant, T.E., Mulhern, R.K., Krasin, M.J., Kun, L.E., Williams, T., Li, C., ... Sanford, R.A. (2004). Preliminary results from a phase II trial of conformal radiation therapy and evaluation of radiation-related CNS effects for pediatric patients with localized ependymoma. *Journal of Clinical Oncology, 22,* 3156–3162. doi:10.1200/JCO.2004.11.142

Nguyen, P.L., Trofimov, A., & Zietman, A.L. (2008). Proton-beam vs. intensity-modulated radiation therapy: Which is best for treating prostate cancer? *Oncology, 22,* 748–754.

Patel, S., & DeLaney, T.F. (2008). Advanced-technology radiation therapy for bone sarcomas. *Cancer Control, 15,* 21–37.

Schulz-Ertner, D., Jäkel, O., & Schlegel, W. (2006). Radiation therapy with charged particles. *Seminars in Radiation Oncology, 16,* 249–259. doi:10.1016/j.semradonc.2006.04.008

Shih, H.A., Chapman, P.H., Bussière, M.R., Chen, C.C., & Loeffler, J.S. (2008). Central nervous system. In T.F. DeLaney & H.M. Kooy (Eds.), *Proton and charged particle radiotherapy* (pp. 140–150). Philadelphia, PA: Lippincott Williams & Wilkins.

Smith, A.R. (2009). Vision 20/20: Proton therapy. *Medical Physics, 36,* 556–568. doi:10.1118/1.3058485

Trofimov, A., Nguyen, P.L., Coen, J.J., Doppke, K.P., Schneider, R.J., Adams, J.A., ... Shipley, W.U. (2007). Radiotherapy treatment of early-stage prostate cancer with IMRT and protons: A treatment planning comparison. *International Journal of Radiation Oncology, Biology, Physics, 69,* 444–453. doi:10.1016/j.ijrobp.2007.03.018

Vargas, C., Fryer, A., Mahajan, C., Indelicato, D., Horne, D., Chellini, A., ... Keole, S. (2008). Dose-volume comparison of proton therapy and intensity-modulated radiotherapy for prostate cancer. *International Journal of Radiation Oncology, Biology, Physics, 70,* 744–751. doi:10.1016/j.ijrobp.2007.07.2335

Yock, T., DeLaney, T.F., Esty, B., & Tarbell, N.J. (2008). Pediatric tumors. In T.F. DeLaney & H.M. Kooy (Eds.), *Proton and charged particle radiotherapy* (pp. 125–139). Philadelphia, PA: Lippincott Williams & Wilkins.

Yock, T., Schneider, R., Friedmann, A., Adams, J., Fullerton, B., & Tarbell, N. (2005). Proton radiotherapy for orbital rhabdomyosarcoma: Clinical outcome and a dosimetric comparison with photons. *International Journal of Radiation Oncology, Biology, Physics, 63,* 1161–1168. doi:10.1016/j.ijrobp.2005.03.052

Yock, T.I., & Tarbell, N.J. (2004). Technology insight: Proton beam radiotherapy for treatment in pediatric brain tumors. *Nature Clinical Practice Oncology, 1,* 97–103. doi:10.1038/ncponc0090

IX. Special populations

A. Pediatric radiation oncology
   1. Pediatric cancer incidence
      - a) In the United States in 2011, approximately 11,210 children younger than 15 years old were diagnosed with cancer.
      - b) Cancer is the leading cause of death from disease in children younger than 15 years old and is surpassed only by accidents in all causes of death in children. In 2011, it was projected that 1,320 children would die from cancer (ACS, 2011).
   2. Specific differences between pediatric and adult cancers
      - a) Childhood cancer is not one disease entity but a spectrum of different malignancies. They vary by type of histology, site of disease origin, race, sex, and age. The common cancers seen in children are leukemias, brain and other CNS tumors, bone cancers, lymphomas, soft tissue sarcomas, kidney cancers, and eye tumors (see Figure 28). In contrast, the common cancers in adults are skin, prostate, breast, lung, and colorectal (ACS, 2010).
      - b) Childhood cancers tend to respond better to treatment with chemotherapy and radiation, and children tend to tolerate treatment better than adults. Multimodality treatment has become the standard, and a significant proportion of children with cancer will receive RT as part of their clinical course. The caveat to this, however, is that children will require follow-up for the rest of their lives. Many will need medical interventions as a result of the long-term side effects of radiation and chemotherapy.
      - c) Most children with cancer are best treated at a medical center that is a member of the Children's Oncology Group. These centers often are associated with a university or a children's hospital. The treatment at these centers is coordinated by a team of experts who specialize in the diagnosis and treatment of pediatric cancers (ACS, 2010). Not all facilities have the capability to deliver specialized treatments such as proton beam RT; therefore, some families may need to relocate during the time of the child's treatment.
      - d) In contrast to adults with cancer, most children with cancer will be cured of their disease (Stegmaier & Sellers, 2009)
   3. Patient- and family-centered care (Branowicki, Houlahan, & Conley, 2009)
      - a) Commonly practiced in pediatric oncology settings, patient- and family-centered care is based on the understanding of the following.
         - (1) The child's main source of support and strength is family.
         - (2) Clinical decision making requires an understanding of the perspectives and information provided by the parents and the child or young adult.
         - (3) Consideration must be given to the psychosocial and cultural needs of the family and the child throughout the course of the disease.
         - (4) The goal is to help the parents develop confidence in their ability to care for their child throughout the course of the illness.
      - b) Pediatric oncology nurses collaborate with members of the oncology team to reduce the burden that cancer has placed on the family by ensuring that their needs are met through
         - (1) Providing compassionate, developmentally appropriate care
         - (2) Nurturing the support systems already established in the family
         - (3) Fostering normalcy
         - (4) Educating the child and family about the cancer diagnosis, its treatment, and management of side effects.
   4. Radiation treatment and planning
      - a) Goal of RT is to increase disease-free survival while limiting normal tissue morbidity. If achieving disease-free survival is not possible, then the attempt is to offer a better quality of life (Bussière & Adams, 2003).

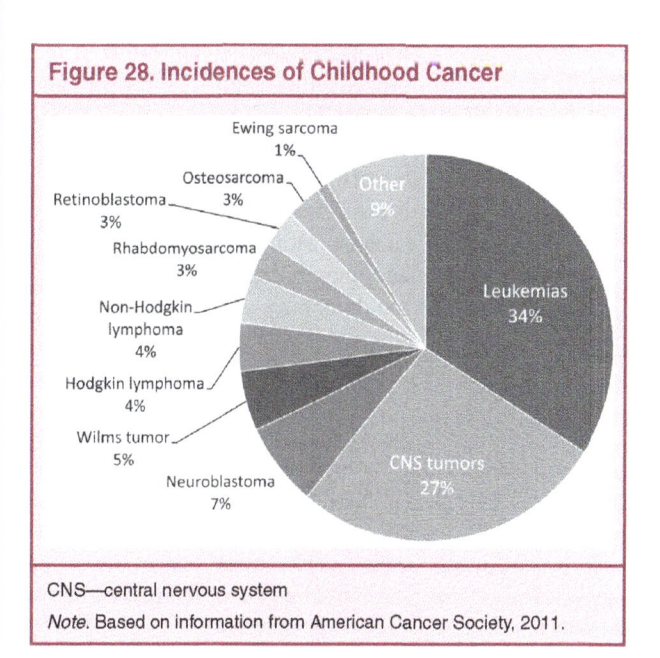

Figure 28. Incidences of Childhood Cancer

- Ewing sarcoma 1%
- Osteosarcoma 3%
- Retinoblastoma 3%
- Rhabdomyosarcoma 3%
- Non-Hodgkin lymphoma 4%
- Hodgkin lymphoma 4%
- Wilms tumor 5%
- Neuroblastoma 7%
- Other 9%
- CNS tumors 27%
- Leukemias 34%

CNS—central nervous system

Note. Based on information from American Cancer Society, 2011.

RT also provides excellent palliation of troublesome symptoms.

b) Evaluation for treatment eligibility begins at a tumor board meeting. The data reviewed includes

(1) The goal of therapy: Cure or palliation

(2) Pertinent facts about the tumor: Size, location, type, and grade

(3) Relative volume of necrotic or poorly vascularized tissue within the treatment field as assessed by imaging studies: Tissue oxygenation influences the response of tumors to radiation

(4) Clinical condition

(5) The age of the child

(6) The requirement of anesthesia or sedation (Lew, 1997; Marcus & Haas-Kogan, 2009).

c) Purpose of treatment planning is to delineate target volumes and the critical anatomic structures obtained from the imaging studies (CT and MRI) in order to shape the beam to precisely match the tumor (Bussière & Adams, 2003).

(1) Immobilization devices: With proper immobilization, treatment setup errors will be reduced, which results in improved tumor control probability and reduces normal tissue complications (Light & Halperin, 2011). The delivery of the precise treatment prescribed is possible through the use of devices such as customized masks, bite blocks, and immobilization systems or body molds; or the placement of permanent skin marks or tattoos at specific locations on the child's body (Cullen, Derrickson, & Potter, 2002).

(a) Goals that must be met regardless of the device used (Light & Halperin, 2011)

i. The child should feel comfortable and secure.

ii. The patient setup must be reproducible.

iii. The setup should be quick and easy.

iv. Construction of the device should be relatively quick.

v. The device must not interfere with the establishment of a secure airway and monitoring devices when anesthesia is required for young children.

d) Sedation/anesthesia

(1) The malignancies treated with RT require a specific location of the beam to spare or limit normal tissue morbidity. Any movement, no matter how small, could undermine the techniques employed to spare normal tissue and thus diminish the efficacy of the treatment (Chalabi & Patel, 2009). Determination of the need for anesthesia often is made at the initial consultation when the child and family are seen by the anesthesiologist, the radiation oncologist, and other members of the team. These members include the radiation oncology nurse, social worker, child life specialist, and psychiatrist. All play a vital role in decreasing child and family anxiety. It is crucial that a good rapport is established with the child and family at this initial contact, as it sets the tone for subsequent treatments (Chalabi & Patel, 2009).

(2) Several demographic, medical, child, and parental psychosocial variables are influential in making the decision. It is typically high child anxiety, high expectations of distress, and high parent anxiety in combination with the child's age that determines the need for sedation or anesthesia (Klosky et al., 2007).

(a) A behavioral program that teaches children how to cooperate with their radiation treatment without anesthesia or sedation, either through distraction or rehearsal, may be successful. If these techniques fail to achieve the child's cooperation, anesthesia or sedation must be used. For very young children, those less than three years, anesthesia is almost always needed. After five years of age, however, anesthesia is rarely needed (Schulman, Frederick, & Halperin, 2011). The following are some pharmaceutical and psychological measures employed to ensure accurate delivery.

  i. Administration of a mild sedative such as lorazepam or diazepam one hour before treatment (Cullen et al., 2002)

  ii. Distraction therapy or behavioral rehearsal to address the separation anxiety experienced by this age group. The parents may accompany the child to the treatment room, but they must leave once the child is positioned. The child must remain in the room alone during the treatment (Buehrer, Immoos, Frei, Timmermann, & Weiss, 2007; Chalabi & Patel, 2009; Krauss & Green, 2006). The expertise of a child life specialist is invaluable in making a child more at ease in the treatment area. With their knowledge of the various techniques of play, the child's anxiety may be reduced, and perhaps the need for sedation or anesthesia may be prevented (Light & Halperin, 2011).

(b) Other deciding factors include the following.

  i. The location of the malignancy—Retinoblastoma requires absolute immobility of the eye and prevention of disconjugate gaze during the treatment.

  ii. The length of the therapy

  iii. The position required for treatment—Certain brain tumors (medulloblastoma, germ-cell tumors, and CNS leukemia) require prone positioning with a flexed head for cranial spinal irradiation. This treatment is an hour long and is difficult to maintain without anesthesia for most children younger than 11 years. Occasionally, stabilization of the airway is required by either intubation, placement of a nasal trumpet, or laryngeal mask airway (Chalabi & Patel, 2009).

(3) Anesthetic considerations

(a) Pediatric anesthesiologists have knowledge of pediatric malignancies and appropriate anesthetic agents and can intervene in the event of complications.

(b) The desired elements of pediatric anesthesia include

  i. Assurance of the child's immobility

  ii. Rapid onset and reliable sedation

  iii. Short recovery period

  iv. Early hospital discharge

  v. No development of tolerance to the anesthetic

  vi. Assurance of patent airway despite treatment position (Krauss & Green, 2006).

(c) Anesthesia may be delivered with IV agents (ketamine, midazolam, propofol) or with inhalation agents (sevoflurane, isoflurane) (Schulman et al., 2011).

  i. Propofol is the drug of choice for RT because it provides reliable sedation with lower incidence of nausea and vomiting and only rare occurrences of emergence delirium.

  ii. Ketamine is contraindicated in children with brain tumors because it increases intracranial pressure and in children with disease in the head and neck area because it causes nystagmus, which could interfere with precision of RT delivery. It increases recovery time more than 20 times of that seen with propofol.

  iii. Sevoflurane is excellent in children without venous access because it is delivered by nasal insufflations, but it causes excessive emergence delirium and rapid recovery. It does pollute the environment in the radiation treatment rooms where air conditioning may be unlike that seen in operating room suites. For this reason, no pregnant staff should be in the room when it is being delivered (Anghelescu et al., 2008; Buehrer et al., 2007; Gottschling et al., 2005; Krauss & Green, 2006).

(d) Although adhering to fasting guidelines is important, children

who are receiving concurrent chemotherapy and daily treatments can become dehydrated and nutritionally depleted. Ideally, early morning treatments will limit the child's distress (Chalabi & Patel, 2009; Branowicki et al., 2009).

(e) Consent is obtained by the anesthesiologist at the initial consult. This will encompass all planning procedures (MRI and CT) as well as the daily treatments.

(f) Parents must be instructed on the fasting guidelines recommended by the treating institution. Generally, instructions specify no solid food or milk products after midnight and no clear liquids two hours prior to the treatment. Exceptions can be made by the anesthesiologist for children whose treatment will be later in the day. Not following the guidelines could possibly result in the cancellation of the child's treatment for that particular day.

(g) An RN with pediatric advanced life support certification should be available to assist the anesthesiologist. Short of that, a nurse certified in cardiopulmonary resuscitation and with recovery room experience or proficiency in airway management should be available.

(h) An emergency response policy/procedure should be in place. The child must be monitored with closed-circuit television monitors clearly visible to the anesthesiologist while outside the RT room. These monitors will display electrocardiogram, pulse oximeter, blood pressure, and end-tidal carbon dioxide measurements. All emergency equipment, including oxygen source, suction equipment, and a pediatric code cart, must be readily available. These should be checked daily (Schulman et al., 2011).

(i) Continuous monitoring during the recovery period is performed until the child is fully awake and vital signs are stable.

5. Supportive care initiatives

a) Psychosocial care of children and families: Distress in cancer is defined as "a multifactorial unpleasant emotional experience of a psychological (cognitive, behavioral, emotional), social, and/or spiritual nature that may interfere with the ability to cope effectively with cancer, its physical symptoms and its treatment" (NCCN, 2010b, p. DIS-2)

(1) The diagnosis of cancer in a child is the most stressful and difficult experience a family will ever face. The majority will be able to make adequate adjustments, with support and information, although confronting the diagnosis and coping with the multiple challenges is a demanding process. They may exhibit signs of acute distress necessitating additional services and interventions, or the level of distress may escalate and behavioral or psychological intervention is required. Clearly, in pediatric oncology, the families have to be a target of attention as much as the children. Good communication results in better care outcomes (Recklitis, Casey, & Zeltzer, 2009).

(2) Clinical assessment of the child and the family should be performed at the initial visit and as clinically indicated, especially with a change in the disease state (remission, recurrence, or progression) (NCCN, 2010b).

(3) Certain factors will influence how parents, children, and siblings experience the disease (Recklitis et al., 2009).

(a) Status of marital relationship
(b) Socioeconomic status
(c) Disrupted routine
(d) Fear and uncertainty
(e) Emotional state
(f) Poor relationships
(g) School performance
(h) Peer relations
(i) Self-confidence
(j) Adjustment

(4) How children react to the environment will have an influence on both their emotions and their behavior. The strongest predictor of increased anticipatory distress is the age of the child, specifically those between the ages of two to seven years (Klosky et al., 2007). In addition, the parent's stress level has an impact on the child's stress level and behavior (Krauss & Green, 2006; Recklitis et al., 2009).

(5) Licensed mental health professionals and chaplains should be readily available (NCCN, 2010b).

(6) Children undergoing RT frequently experience distress despite the fact that the treatment is painless and noninvasive (Cullen et al., 2002). Their reactions result from their fear of the unknown, the unfamiliar conditions under which the treatment will be given, the unfamiliar staff, their previous experiences with medical procedures, and the separation from their parents during the treatment (Cullen et al., 2002; Kreitler et al., 2011).

(7) The ability to help these children through their course of treatment lies in understanding that:

   (a) No single individual can meet all the needs of the children and their families.

   (b) Knowledge of the stages of child development—infancy, toddler, preschool, school age, and adolescence—and the developmental tasks associated with each is crucial to providing the appropriate care, support, and communication to these children (Recklitis et al., 2009) (see Table 18).

   (c) Honesty can help children grow to trust that adults will not withhold information from them (Recklitis et al., 2009). Educate parents about the impact that withholding information has on increasing children's anxieties and fears about their illness.

   (d) Children will be noncompliant at some interval during their treatment. Behavioral interventions should not be implemented until there has been a discussion with the family and they have expressed a willingness to accept and use the approach (Recklitis et al., 2009).

(8) Siblings—The challenges that siblings face can be extremely stressful as they, too, undergo a tremendous change in their lives. How they deal with them will depend on their developmental level and the support they receive. They may ask, "What about me?" as their parents tend to the needs of the ill sibling. The sibling's adjustment to the diagnosis can have both positive and negative out-

Table 18. Developmental Considerations of Children Undergoing Radiation Therapy

Needs	Interventions
Infants (birth–12 months): Trust versus mistrust	
Trust	Provide consistent caregivers. Keep the parent within the infant's line of sight. Allow parents to assist with assessment procedures, if desired. Cuddle the infant.
Sensorimotor	Provide a soothing environment. Have parent hold the infant during induction of anesthesia, stroking the skin and speaking softly. Provide soft, cuddly toys.
Nutrition	Provide adequate fluids, both IV and oral.
Object permanence	Encourage parents to accompany the child to the treatment room. Assess parental ability to provide comfort and care. Place a familiar object with the infant, such as a stuffed animal, special blanket, or pacifier.
Toddlers (12–36 months): Autonomy versus shame and doubt	
Autonomy	Allow choices when possible. Allow the child to participate in care when possible (e.g., flushing the catheter, removing pulse oximeter probe or blood pressure cuff, cleaning injection port of IV tubing).
Limited reasoning	Explain sensory aspects of procedure. Prepare the child prior to procedures, using simple words that are used by the child and family. Use distraction techniques (blowing bubbles, reading or telling stories, singing songs). Have a nonthreatening item in the treatment room as a focus of attention (e.g., animated stuffed animal that the child can manipulate), thus steering attention from threatening equipment. Inform the child that it is acceptable to cry or yell to express discomfort or fear. Use positive reinforcement: offer verbal praise, stickers, or a trip to the toy box. Role play.
Security	Allow the child to have a familiar object, such as a favorite blanket, stuffed animal, or pacifier. Provide a consistent caregiver. Encourage parents to accompany the child to the treatment room. Assess parental ability to provide comfort and care.
Body integrity	Allow the child to wear own clothes. Protect dressings, bandages, or catheters.

(Continued on next page)

Table 18. Developmental Considerations of Children Undergoing Radiation Therapy *(Continued)*

Needs	Interventions
Preschool (3–6 years): Initiative versus guilt	
Initiative	Allow participation in care (e.g., flushing the catheter, assisting with assessment procedures). Provide choices, but avoid excessive delays. Offer positive reinforcement (e.g., verbal praise, stickers, a trip to the toy box).
Fear of the unknown	Provide simple explanations using nonthreatening words. Ask for the child's thoughts about why the treatment or procedure is needed. Explain sensory aspects of the procedure and how it will affect the child. Consider a behavioral rehearsal the day before the initial treatment. This is beneficial when it is uncertain whether the child will require anesthesia, especially with a child 5 years old or older. Encourage parents to view an instructional video on radiation treatment, specific to the institution, if available.
Imitative	Observe another child's treatment preparation.
Security	Encourage parental presence. Bring a favorite toy, security object, or favorite music or audiobook. Provide a consistent caregiver.
Body integrity	Allow the child to wear own clothes.
Magical thinking	Employ play therapy, imagery, and fantasy as distraction techniques.
School-aged (6–12 years): Industry versus inferiority	
Industry	Include the child in decision making. Encourage active participation. Discuss the behavioral expectations and ways of maintaining control. Provide opportunity for behavioral rehearsal or encourage the child to be a mentor for another child. Remain with the child during treatment to provide support and information. This may be needed until the child becomes comfortable with setup. Offer praise and encouragement.
Increase language skills/interest in learning	Assess the child's level of understanding. Explain the procedure using correct medical and scientific terminology and provide them with an instructional video. Allow time for questions and discussion. Explain the function of equipment.
Body image	Discuss the temporary side effects and the interventions to help minimize them. Explore feelings about body image changes. Respect the need for privacy.
Independence	Encourage involvement in self-care activities. Promote participation in school and social activities. Encourage the family to set a daily routine and maintain normal limit-setting. Normalize activities as much as possible.
Security	Provide consistent caregivers. Provide the child with the chance to express feelings or concerns through art, play, or music. Refer to additional counseling as needed.
Adolescent (12–18 years): Identity versus role confusion	
Identity	Promote continued participation in school and social activities. Arrange schedule to accommodate academic needs. Introduce the adolescent to other adolescents receiving radiation treatment. Explain the rationale for treatment, behavioral expectations, and side effects. Encourage responsibility for self-care. Be available to facilitate an open and positive adolescent-parent communication.
Independence	Involve the child in decision making. Realize that the adolescent may be noncompliant. Empathize with the child's plight of feeling pushed around. Learn from the teen the preferences for receiving information (e.g., advance preparation for procedures or information delivered the day before).
Body image	Provide a supportive relationship. Discuss how appearance may change as a result of the radiation treatment (e.g., erythema, hair loss at treatment field). Refer to additional counseling if needed.
Self-concept	Promote a support network among other teens. Provide privacy, confidentiality, and opportunity to discuss feelings.

Note. Based on information from Recklitis et al., 2009; Wilson & Hockenberry, 2008.

comes. Any interventions should follow the sibling throughout the entire treatment, not simply at certain phases of treatment. The nonprofit organization SuperSibs! (www.supersibs.org) provides siblings with opportunities to share with others through activities and services. Institutions caring for children with cancer should ensure opportunities to praise and support the healthy sibling (Recklitis et al., 2009; Sidhu, Passmore, & Baker, 2005; Woodgate, 2006).

b) Nutritional status—At the time of diagnosis, incidence of malnutrition is 6%–50% and is dependent on the histology, stage, and location of the disease (Ladas et al., 2005). For this reason, nutritional support should be initiated as soon as the diagnosis is made (Ladas et al., 2005). This requires a multidisciplinary approach.

  (1) Children's nutritional needs must meet their requirements for growth and development, as well as what is needed to support them throughout their treatment (Ladas et al., 2005).

  (2) Nursing assessment should include a medical and surgical history, the anticipated treatments, anthropometric measurements, biochemical parameters, clinical observations, and dietary history, including the use of herbs, supplements, and other complementary alternative therapies (the use of which may require additional discussion with the radiation oncologist). The registered dietitian completes the assessment and determines the nutrient requirements.

  (3) Children who must fast daily for delivery of anesthesia for RT are at high risk for malnutrition. They could very quickly lose greater than 5% of their pre-illness weight, which is the point at which nutritional interventions should be implemented (Cullen et al., 2002). These can include encouraging nutrient-dense foods and beverages, enteral tube feedings, or TPN.

  (4) Side effects from RT may result in malnutrition. These include mucositis, esophagitis, nausea, vomiting, constipation, and xerostomia.

  (5) Nutrition may become a control issue between the parents, the child, and the healthcare providers. In all other aspects of care, the child feels a lack of control. The psychosocial team can work with the child and the family to identify ways that can relieve the tension around food (Ladas et al., 2005).

c) Radiation somnolence syndrome: This is a side effect of cranial irradiation.

  (1) The supposition is that irradiation results in either the dysfunction of myelin or the destruction of microvasculature leading to interruption of cell integrity. This affects the oligodendroglia (Ryan, 2000; Vern & Salvi, 2009).

  (2) The symptoms of this syndrome are theorized to occur when the synthesis of myelin is most acute, and the recovery phase represents a resumption of the myelin synthesis. The symptoms appear approximately four to six weeks after the completion of RT and may last 3–14 days until resolution. In children with acute lymphocytic leukemia, it has been observed in 60%–79% of those who received treatment to 2,400 cGy and in 13%–58% of those who received treatment to 1,800 cGy (Vern & Salvi, 2009).

  (3) Symptoms include excessive sleepiness (sometimes sleeping up to 20 hours a day), headache, anorexia, irritability, nausea, vomiting, ataxia, and low-grade fever.

  (4) The most important intervention is anticipatory guidance and preparation. For many parents, the symptoms of somnolence syndrome mimic the similar signs and symptoms that initially alerted the parents prior to the diagnosis. The parents should be reassured that the syndrome is self-limiting and has no known long-term consequences. Children in whom the symptoms persist and are severe may benefit from a course of steroids (Ryan, 2000; Vern & Salvi, 2009).

d) Fatigue: Cancer-related fatigue is defined by NCCN as a "distressing persistent, subjective sense of physical, emotional, and/or cognitive tiredness or exhaustion related to cancer or cancer treatment that is not proportional to recent activity and interferes with usual functioning" (NCCN, 2010a, p. FT-1). It has been found to be one of the most distressing symptoms experienced by children receiving cancer treatment (Hockenberry, 2004). It is the only factor associated with poor health-related quality of life in pediatric cancer survivors. Some of the factors considered to be associated with fatigue can be divided into physical and psychosocial factors (Ullrich, Berde, & Billett, 2009). They include

(1) Destruction of cells by RT
(2) Poor nutritional status
(3) Anemia
(4) Delivery of concurrent chemotherapy
(5) Medications used for symptom management
(6) Pain
(7) Psychological distress
(8) Sleep impairment.

e) Cerebellar mutism syndrome, also known as posterior fossa syndrome, is a unique postoperative complication.

(1) Incidence and risk factors: It has been recognized for the past 30 years in children who have undergone surgical resections for posterior fossa tumors (Souweidane, 2010). Its incidence varies, although it has been reported to be nearly 40% (Souweidane, 2010).

(2) Presentation: The syndrome typically presents 24–48 hours after resection with diminishing of speech patterns leading to mutism, emotional lability, ataxia, and hypotonia. These symptoms may persist from weeks to months (Turgut, 2008).

(3) Sequelae: Of those children affected, approximately 50% will have significant sequelae one year after surgery (Packer, MacDonald, & Vezina, 2010). These include balance difficulties, neurocognitive challenges, and speech impairments (Keiran et al., 2009; Packer et al., 2010).

(4) Prevention: It is known that surgical intervention is contributory; however, limited tumor removal is not a justifiable option unless it is known that the tumor is invading the brain stem. It is a well-supported fact that significant residual tumor is a negative prognostic indicator (Packer et al., 2010; Souweidane, 2010).

6. Childhood cancer survivorship

a) Innovations in cancer treatment have resulted in a decrease in morbidity and mortality in childhood pediatric oncology. Children are surviving, some into their second and third decades. The ability to decrease the RT field, thus sparing dose to normal tissues, has provided further hopes for decreasing sequelae, which is especially crucial in children diagnosed with brain tumors (Eshelman-Kent, Gilger, & Galla-

gher, 2009). The overall five-year survival rate for childhood cancer has improved from 58% for patients diagnosed between 1975 and 1977 to 82% for those diagnosed between 1999 and 2005 (Jemal, Siegel, Xu, & Ward, 2010). This translates into almost 300,000 childhood cancer survivors (Ruccione, 2009).

b) There must be a delicate balance between effective therapy and acceptable toxicity. A cure may be achievable at the cost of increasing morbidity. In contrast, adhering to therapeutic regimens to minimize toxicities may increase the chance of relapse, progression, metastasis, or death (Askins & Moore, 2008). Regardless of the course chosen, there will be untoward late effects, increasing the rate of mortality of adult survivors of childhood cancer or impairing survivors' quality of life (see Table 19). Of the adults who survived childhood cancer, 60%–70% will develop at least one health-related complication as a result of their treatment. Of these complications, the most emotionally and physically devastating are secondary cancers (Bhatia & Constine, 2011).

c) Risk factors for developing late effects (Kenney & Diller, 2009)

(1) Modality, site, dose, and intensity of treatment: Larger doses of chemotherapy or radiation generally have worse outcomes.

(2) Concurrent treatments: Exposure to more than one modality with related toxicities

(3) Age, sex, and genetic predisposition

(4) Health behaviors and comorbidities

d) Follow-up: There is a growing need for comprehensive, specialized follow-up care for childhood cancer survivors. Developing long-term follow-up clinics (survivorship clinics) can provide these survivors the advantage of a multidisciplinary team of experts and survivor education programs (Kenney & Diller, 2009). The Children's Oncology Group has developed a comprehensive set of guidelines to assist both healthcare providers and survivors in understanding the health issues that are specific to the type of cancer and the treatment received. These guidelines can be found at www.survivorshipguidelines.org (Kurt et al., 2008).

7. Ethical considerations and clinical trials

a) Most children with cancer are enrolled in clinical trials. The knowledge acquired

Table 19. Late Effects by Organ System	
Organ System	**Late Effects**
Central nervous system	Leukoencephalopathy Myelopathy Necrosis Neurocognitive deficits Psychosocial distress
Neuroendocrine	Gonadotropin deficiencies Growth hormone deficiencies Hyperthyroidism Hypothyroidism Panhypopituitarism Precocious puberty Thyroid cancer
Bone	Avascular necrosis Bone growth retardation Fractures Kyphosis Osteopenia Scoliosis
Cardiac	Cardiomyopathy Coronary artery disease Pericarditis Valvular disease
Lung	Fibrosis Lung cancer
Ovary	Impaired development of secondary sexual characteristics Menstrual irregularities: amenorrhea, early menopause Sterilization Suppressed hormone production
Testes	Infertility Sterility Testicular failure
Kidney	Fibrosis Hypoplastic kidney Nephropathy
Gastrointestinal	Adhesions Cirrhosis Diabetes mellitus Enteritis
Eyes	Cataracts Glaucoma Lacrimal duct stenosis Retinopathy
Hearing	Chondritis Chronic otitis media Sensorineural hearing loss
Teeth and saliva	Dental abnormalities Xerostomia

* Any organ exposed to radiation therapy is at risk for secondary cancers.

Note. Based on information from Bhatia & Constine, 2011; Friedman & Constine, 2011.

from evaluating the interventions is one reason for the dramatic improvement in survival over the past 30 years (Barfield & Kodish, 2009). The ethical issues are more complex because a child is the recipient, and the person making the decision (the parent, parents, or advocate) is not the person who will be facing the risks or benefits. It becomes more difficult as children become adolescents. The ethics of assent are a difficult issue. Questions include when should it be required, and whether it is binding.

(1) Theoretically, any child able to maturely evaluate the risks and benefits of the clinical trial should assent to participate (Klimaszewski, 2008). The child should understand what the clinical trial entails (goals, objectives, procedures, and risks) and any alternatives before assenting. This brings the child's maturity into question, and with that, guidance from the institution's institutional review board (IRB) is required.

(2) The IRB has tremendous responsibility regarding a child's assent (45 CFR 46.408) (U.S. Department of Health and Human Services Office for Human Research Protections, 2009).

   (a) The IRB can determine whether a child is able to provide assent, taking the child's age, level of maturity, and psychological state into consideration. At the IRB's discretion, this determination can be made for one child or for all children to be enrolled in a specific clinical trial.

   (b) The IRB may determine that assent is not a necessary condition for proceeding with the clinical trial. Even if the children are capable of assenting, the IRB may determine assent unnecessary.

   (c) An institution's IRB may determine that adolescents do not need parental consent if asked to participate in a low-risk study.

   (d) When the IRB determines that a child's assent is required, it must stipulate whether and how that assent will be documented.

(3) More ethical questions surface if the child or adolescent is pregnant.

(4) Much remains to be learned.

b) Principles governing the participation of children in research
  (1) Children are individuals, and their developing autonomy in decisions needs to be respected.
  (2) The parent's wisdom in assessing what is in the best interest of the child and in guiding the child's moral development should be respected.
  (3) Policies regarding assent should be amenable to the medical and psychological circumstances often seen in pediatric oncology.
c) Two questions that must be asked when discussing advances in pediatric cancer therapies are "What can be done next?" and "What should be done next?" Good clinical trials require ethical decisions made at every level, both scientific and philosophical (Barfield & Kodish, 2009).

References

American Cancer Society. (2011). Cancer facts and figures 2011. Retrieved from http://www.cancer.org/Research/CancerFactsFigures/CancerFactsFigures/cancer-facts-figures-2011

Anghelescu, D.L., Burgoyne, L.L., Liu, W., Hankins, G.M., Cheng, C., Beckham, P.A., … Bikhazi, G.B. (2008). Safe anesthesia for radiotherapy in pediatric oncology: St. Jude Children's Research Hospital Experience, 2004–2006. *International Journal of Radiation Oncology, Biology, Physics, 71*, 491–497. doi:10.1016/j.ijrobp.2007.09.044

Askins, M.A., & Moore, B.D., III. (2008). Preventing neurocognitive late effects in childhood cancer survivors. *Journal of Child Neurology, 23*, 1160–1171. doi:10.1177/0883073808321065

Barfield, R.C., & Kodish, E. (2009). Ethical considerations in pediatric oncology clinical trials. In S.H. Orkin, D.E. Fisher, A.T. Look, S. Lux, D. Ginsburg, & D.G. Nathan (Eds.), *Oncology of infancy and childhood* (pp. 1319–1336). Philadelphia, PA: Elsevier Saunders.

Bhatia, S., & Constine, L.S. (2011). Second primary cancers. In E.C. Halperin, L.S. Constine, N.J. Tarbell, & L.E. Kun (Eds.), *Pediatric radiation oncology* (5th ed., pp. 397–413). Philadelphia, PA: Lippincott Williams & Wilkins.

Branowicki, P.A., Houlahan, K.E., & Conley, S.B. (2009). Nursing care of patients with childhood cancer. In S.H. Orkin, D.E. Fisher, A.T. Look, S. Lux, D. Ginsburg, & D.G. Nathan (Eds.), *Oncology of infancy and childhood* (pp. 1145–1175). Philadelphia, PA: Elsevier Saunders.

Buehrer, S., Immoos, S., Frei, M., Timmermann, B., & Weiss, M. (2007). Evaluation of propofol for repeated prolonged deep sedation in children undergoing proton radiation therapy. *British Journal of Anaesthesia, 99*, 556–560. doi:10.1093/bja/aem207

Bussière, M.R., & Adams, J.A. (2003). Treatment planning for conformal proton radiation therapy. *Technology in Cancer Research and Treatment, 2*, 389–399.

Chalabi, J., & Patel, S. (2009). Radiation therapy in children. *International Anesthesiology Clinics, 47*, 45–53. doi:10.1097/AIA.0b013e3181a4698a

Cullen, P.M., Derrickson, J.D., & Potter, J.A. (2002). Radiation therapy. In C.R. Baggott, K.P. Kelly, D. Fochtman, & G.V. Foley (Eds.), *Nursing care of children and adolescents with cancer* (3rd ed., pp. 116–132). Philadelphia, PA: Saunders.

Eshelman-Kent, D., Gilger, E., & Gallagher, M. (2009). Transitioning survivors of central nervous system tumors: Challenges for patients, families, and health care providers. *Journal of Pediatric Oncology Nursing, 26*, 280–294. doi:10.1177/1043454209343209

Friedman, D.L., & Constine, L.S. (2011). Late effects of cancer treatment. In E.C. Halperin, L.S. Constine, N.J. Tarbell, & L.E. Kun (Eds.), *Pediatric radiation oncology* (5th ed., pp. 353–396). Philadelphia, PA: Lippincott Williams & Wilkins.

Gottschling, S., Meyer, S., Krenn, T., Reinhard, H., Lothschuetz, D., Nunold, H., & Graf, N. (2005). Propofol versus midazolam/ketamine for procedural sedation in pediatric oncology. *Journal of Pediatric Hematology/Oncology, 27*, 471–476.

Hockenberry, M. (2004). Symptom management research in children with cancer. *Journal of Pediatric Oncology Nursing, 21*, 132–136. doi:10.1177/1043454204264387

Keiran, M., Chi, S., Samuel, D., Lechpammer, M., Blackman, S., Prabhu, S., … Segal, R. (2009). Tumors of the brain and spinal cord. In S.H. Orkin, D.E. Fisher, A.T. Look, S. Lux, D. Ginsburg, & D.G. Nathan (Eds.), *Oncology of infancy and childhood* (pp. 601–720). Philadelphia, PA: Elsevier Saunders.

Kenney, L.B., & Diller, L. (2009). Childhood cancer survivorship. In S.H. Orkin, D.E. Fisher, A.T. Look, S. Lux, D. Ginsburg, & D.G. Nathan (Eds.), *Oncology of infancy and childhood* (pp. 1255–1289). Philadelphia, PA: Elsevier Saunders.

Klimaszewski, A. (2008). Informed consent. In A.D. Klimaszewski, M. Bacon, H.E. Deininger, B.A. Ford, & J.G. Westendorp (Eds.), *Manual for clinical trials nursing* (2nd ed., pp. 97–105). Pittsburgh, PA: Oncology Nursing Society.

Klosky, J.L., Tyc, V.L., Tong, X., Srivastava, D.K., Kronenberg, M., de Armendi, A.J., & Merchant, T.E. (2007). Predicting pediatric distress during radiation therapy procedures: The role of medical, psychosocial, and demographic factors. *Pediatrics, 119*, e1159–e1166. doi:10.1542/peds.2005-1514

Krauss, B., & Green, S.M. (2006). Procedural sedation and analgesia in children. *Lancet, 367*, 766–780. doi:10.1016/S0140-6736(06)68230-5

Kreitler, S., Arush, M., Krivoy, E., Golan, H., Kreitler, M., & Toren, A. (2011). Psychosocial aspects of radiotherapy for the child and family with cancer. In E.C. Halperin, L.S. Constine, N.J. Tarbell, & L.E. Kun (Eds.), *Pediatric radiation oncology* (5th ed., pp. 447–455). Philadelphia, PA: Lippincott Williams & Wilkins.

Kurt, B.A., Armstrong, G.T., Cash, D.K., Krasin, M.J., Morris, E.B., Spunt, S.L., … Hudson, M.M. (2008). Primary care management of the childhood cancer survivor. *Journal of Pediatrics, 152*, 458–466. doi:10.1016/j.jpeds.2007.10.002

Ladas, E.J., Sacks, N., Meacham, L., Henry, D., Enriquez, L., Lowry, G., … Rogers, P. (2005). A multidisciplinary review of nutrition considerations in the pediatric oncology population: A perspective from Children's Oncology Group. *Nutrition in Clinical Practice, 20*, 377–393. doi:10.1177/0115426505020004377

Lew, C. (1997). Pediatric cancers—The special needs of children receiving radiation therapy. In K.H. Dow, J.D. Bucholtz, R. Iwamoto, V. Fieler, & L. Hilderley (Eds.), *Nursing care in radiation oncology* (2nd ed., pp. 316–354). Philadelphia, PA: Saunders.

Light, K.L., & Halperin, E.C. (2011). Stabilization and immobilization devices. In E.C. Halperin, L.S. Constine, N.J. Tarbell, & L.E. Kun (Eds.), *Pediatric radiation oncology* (5th ed., pp. 425–428). Philadelphia, PA: Lippincott Williams & Wilkins.

Marcus, K.M., & Haas-Kogan, D. (2009). Pediatric radiation oncology. In S.H. Orkin, D.E. Fisher, A.T. Look, S. Lux, D. Ginsburg, & D.G. Nathan (Eds.), *Oncology of infancy and childhood* (pp. 241–255). Philadelphia, PA: Elsevier Saunders.

National Comprehensive Cancer Network. (2010a). *NCCN Clinical Practice Guidelines in Oncology: Cancer-related fatigue* [v.1.2011]. Retrieved from http://www.nccn.org/professionals/physician_gls/PDF/fatigue.pdf

National Comprehensive Cancer Network. (2010b). *NCCN Clinical Practice Guidelines in Oncology: Distress management* [v.1.2011]. Retrieved from http://www.nccn.org/professionals/physician_gls/PDF/distress.pdf

Packer, R.J., MacDonald, T., & Vezina, G. (2010). Central nervous system tumors. *Hematology/Oncology Clinics of North America, 24,* 87–108. doi:10.1016/j.hoc.2009.11.012

Recklitis, C.J., Casey, R.L., & Zeltzer, L. (2009). Psychosocial care of children and families. In S.H. Orkin, D.E. Fisher, A.T. Look, S. Lux, D. Ginsburg, & D.G. Nathan (Eds.), *Oncology of infancy and childhood* (pp. 1291–1317). Philadelphia, PA: Elsevier Saunders.

Ruccione, K. (2009). The legacy of pediatric oncology nursing in advancing survivorship research and clinical care. *Journal of Pediatric Oncology Nursing, 26,* 255–265. doi:10.1177/1043454209343179

Ryan, J. (2000). Radiation somnolence syndrome. *Journal of Pediatric Oncology Nursing, 17,* 50–53. doi:10.1177/104345420001700107

Schulman, S.R., Frederick, H., & Halperin, E.C. (2011). Anesthesia for external beam radiotherapy. In E.C. Halperin, L.S. Constine, N.J. Tarbell, & L.E. Kun (Eds.), *Pediatric radiation oncology* (5th ed., pp. 414–424). Philadelphia, PA: Lippincott Williams & Wilkins.

Sidhu, R., Passmore, A., & Baker, D. (2005). An investigation into parent perceptions of the needs of siblings of children with cancer. *Journal of Pediatric Oncology Nursing, 22,* 276–287. doi:10.1177/1043454205278480

Siegel, R., Ward, E., Brawley, O., & Jemal, A. (2011). Cancer statistics, 2011. *CA: A Cancer Journal for Clinicians, 61,* 212–236. doi:10.3322/caac.20121

Souweidane, M.M. (2010). Posterior fossa syndrome [Editorial]. *Journal of Neurosurgery Pediatrics, 5,* 325–328. doi:10.3171/2009.11.PEDS09369

Stegmaier, K., & Sellers, W.R. (2009). Targeted approaches to drug development. In S.H. Orkin, D.E. Fisher, A.T. Look, S. Lux, D. Ginsburg, & D.G. Nathan (Eds.), *Oncology of infancy and childhood* (pp. 57–98). Philadelphia, PA: Elsevier Saunders.

Turgut, M. (2008). Cerebellar mutism [Letter to the editor]. *Journal of Neurosurgery Pediatrics, 1,* 262. doi:10.3171/PED/2008/1/3/262

Ullrich, C.K., Berde, C.B., & Billett, A.L. (2009). Symptom management in children with cancer. In S.H. Orkin, D.E. Fisher, A.T. Look, S. Lux, D. Ginsburg, & D.G. Nathan (Eds.), *Oncology of infancy and childhood* (pp. 1203–1253). Philadelphia, PA: Elsevier Saunders.

U.S. Department of Health and Human Services Office for Human Research Protections. (2009, January). Title 25, part 46: Protection of human subjects. In *Code of federal regulations.* Retrieved from http://www.hhs.gov/ohrp/humansubjects/guidance/45cfr46.html#46.408

Vern, T.Z., & Salvi, S. (2009). Somnolence syndrome and fever in pediatric patients with cranial irradiation. *Journal of Pediatric Hematology/Oncology, 31,* 118–120. doi:10.1097/MPH.0b013e31818cd698

Wilson, D., & Hockenberry, M.J. (2008). *Wong's clinical manual of pediatric nursing* (7th ed.). St. Louis, MO: Elsevier Mosby.

Woodgate, R.L. (2006). Siblings' experiences with childhood cancer: A different way of being in the family. *Cancer Nursing, 29,* 406–414.

B. Geriatric radiation oncology
  1. Because of significant heterogeneity among older oncology patients, the practice of "geriatric oncology" is not defined by a specific age cutoff but rather "when the health status of a patient population begins to interfere with the oncologic decision-making guidelines" (Extermann, 2000).
  2. Approximately 50% of all cancers diagnosed and 70% of cancer deaths occur in patients age 65 and older (Ries et al., 2003). Increased cancer prevalence among older patients is multifactorial and may be related to (Taylor & Kuchel, 2009)
      a) Increased length of exposure to carcinogens
      b) Age-related decline in immune function
      c) Cumulative genetic defects such as defects in tumor suppressor genes.
  3. Older adult patients may be underrepresented in clinical trials that set the standards for oncology practice (Yee, Pater, Pho, Zee, & Siu, 2003), particularly patients older than 80 (Cyr, Gillanders, Aft, Eberlein, & Margenthaler, 2011). As little data exist to describe the benefits and risks of treatment in older adult patients, optimal therapy recommendations generally are not clearly defined. More research is needed to evaluate the response of older adults to aggressive cancer therapies.
      a) Historically, many perceived that treatment in older adult patients was more toxic or less effective. This may not be true. Jantunen et al. (2011) used data from the European Group for Blood and Marrow Transplantation to retrospectively compare 655 patients older than 65 years of age to 79 patients age 65 and younger. All patients had mantle cell lymphoma with similar characteristics treated with autologous stem cell transplantation. No significant difference existed in the number of CD34+ cells transfused, the use of granulocyte colony-stimulating factor, the cumulative incidence of neutrophil engraftment, or the time to an unsupported platelet count of greater than 20×10^9/L. Both groups had similar relapse rates at two and five years (older group was 28.4% versus 24.5% in the younger group), and progression-free survival did not differ significantly at five years (28.6% in the older group versus 39.9% in the younger group). Overall survival did not differ significantly at five years between older and younger patients (60.7% versus 67.4%, respectively, p = 0.15).

b) Greater prevalence of comorbidities or declining functional status in older patients may limit treatment options (Extermann, 2007).

c) Patients may choose not to pursue aggressive therapies because of personal conditions or values (NCCN, 2011).

4. Significant heterogeneity exists among older adult patients in terms of life expectancy, functional status, comorbidities, and social support.

   a) In a systematic review of 345 cooperative clinical trials, no evidence of worse survival or treatment-related mortality was found among patients older than 65 receiving experimental cancer therapy compared with younger patients (Kumar, Soares, Balducci, & Djulbegovic, 2007).

   b) Generalizability of these findings is limited, as study inclusion criteria limited patients to those without a history of prior malignancies, evidence of organ dysfunction, or poor performance status. Therefore, although this sample represented only the very healthiest older patients, it offered compelling support that in well-selected older patients with good performance status and adequate supportive care, age alone does not indicate worse treatment tolerance than younger patients.

5. Treatment decisions in older adult patients should be tailored to the individual circumstances and desires of the patient.

   a) Specific differences between geriatric and adult cancers

      (1) Age-related tumor changes

         (a) Cancers associated with a more aggressive course in older adults

            i. Acute myeloid leukemia is often associated with an unfavorable cytogenetic profile in older adults (Balducci & Behge, 2001).

            ii. NHL (large cell and follicular lymphoma) is associated with shorter remission duration (Balducci & Behge, 2001).

            iii. Gliomas (Peschel et al., 1993)

         (b) Cancers often associated with a more indolent course in older adults (Balducci & Behge, 2001)

            i. Prostate

            ii. Breast

            iii. Lung

      (2) Age-related treatment changes

         (a) Some tumors may be less responsive to chemotherapy in older patients (Balducci & Behge, 2001).

            i. Acute myeloid leukemia

            ii. Ovarian cancer

         (b) Cancers associated with worse treatment tolerance in older adults

            i. Colon cancer (adjuvant 5-FU–based therapy) (Sargent et al., 2001)

            ii. NSCLC (concurrent chemoradiation)

      (3) Changes in physiologic reserve

         (a) Declining physiologic reserve may affect the tolerance of treatment stress. Commonly occurring functional changes that may affect treatment tolerance include

            i. Bone marrow/immune function

            ii. Renal function

            iii. Cardiac function

            iv. Neurologic function

         (b) Healing of mucosal tissue damage in response to radiation treatment appears to occur at the same rate in both older and younger patients (Horiot, 2007).

   b) Issues associated with treatment of older adults with cancer

      (1) Physiologic changes

         (a) The potential for age-related decline in organ function should be considered.

         (b) RT can exacerbate underlying system compromise related to the intended treatment field.

            i. Neurologic

               • Underlying sensory deficits (neuropathy, hearing loss)

               • Alteration in cerebral blood flow

            ii. Cardiac: Greater prevalence of occult heart disease (coronary artery disease, reduced ejection fraction) (Sawhney, Sehl, & Naeim, 2005)

iii. Pulmonary: Consider baseline pulmonary function tests prior to treating significant lung volume.

iv. GI
- Prior history of colitis, surgery, ulcers, or bleeding
- Mucosal atrophy may be more prevalent
- Age-related decline in liver function (decreased liver size and blood flow) (Sawhney et al., 2005; Sehl, Sawhney, & Naeim, 2005)
  - Greater caution with chemotherapy agents that are metabolized in the liver
  - Generally does not require dose modification unless significant hepatic insufficiency (due to chronic liver disease or liver metastasis)

v. Renal
- Age-related decline in glomerular filtration rate (less than 60 ml/min per 1.73 m^2)
- Particular caution with chemotherapy or medications that are cleared by the kidneys

vi. Bone marrow function
- Incidence of early/severe neutropenia is increased among older adult patients receiving chemotherapy (Lyman, Kuderer, Agboola, & Balducci, 2003; Sehl et al., 2005).
- Severe neutropenia is associated with increased risk of infections, sepsis, and hospitalizations (Lyman et al., 2003; Sehl et al., 2005).
- Radiation treatment to the pelvis, spine, sternum, ribs, long bones, and skull may contribute to bone marrow suppression, prompting greater consideration for complete blood count monitoring (Haas, 2004).

(2) Comorbidities
  (a) Number of comorbidities does not correlate with functional status (Extermann, Overcash, Lyman, Parr, & Balducci, 1998).

  (b) Impact of comorbid disease in relation to the treatment plan (such as the potential for additive toxicity or exacerbation of underlying disease)
    i. Do comorbidities make the treatment plan more risky?
    ii. Does the severity of comorbidities limit the benefit likely to occur from radiation treatment?

(3) Functional reserve
  (a) Poor baseline functional status may adversely affect treatment tolerance and outcome.
  (b) Frail patients are generally at greater risk. Frailty may exist without significant identified comorbid conditions and is manifested by the following (Fried et al., 2001).
    i. Weight loss
    ii. Fatigue
    iii. Generalized weakness
    iv. Impaired mobility or decline in physical activity

c) Assessment
  (1) Estimating life expectancy (Walter & Covinsky, 2001): A reasonable estimation of life expectancy influences treatment goals and approach (i.e., curative, control, or palliative) and should include consideration of the following.
    (a) Chronologic age
      i. Neither age nor comorbidities are absolute contraindications to radiation treatment unless they indicate a much shorter life expectancy than the evolution of the cancer to be treated.
      ii. Determining the average estimated life expectancy based on age and general health condition, however, can provide useful information about potential for longevity (Walter & Covinsky, 2001).
    (b) Functional status
      i. Performance status (e.g., Karnofsky scale, Zubrod, Eastern Cooperative Oncology Group performance status scales)
      ii. ADL: Ability to perform basic tasks of daily living, including feeding, bathing, and toileting.
      iii. Instrumental ADL: Skills necessary to live independently,

including ability to grocery shop, prepare meals, pay bills, manage the household (i.e., maintenance and housekeeping), and take medications independently (NCCN, 2011).

- Instrumental ADL are a more sensitive predictor of mortality among patients with cancer (Malone et al., 2005).
- Performance status scores often underestimate actual functional ability. Independence with ADL/instrumental ADL activities may be more reliable indicators of functional status (Repetto et al., 2002).

(c) Comorbidities

i. Identify comorbidities contributing to life expectancy estimation.

ii. Optimize treatment of comorbidities that are unrecognized or poorly controlled before beginning treatment.

(2) Estimated morbidity from cancer diagnosis

(a) Stage of disease

(b) Likelihood of recurrence or progression

(c) Disease behavior (indolent versus aggressive)

(3) Significant risk of cancer-related mortality or morbidity leads to further assessment of functional status and comorbidities to determine suitability for treatment (curative or control intent). Low risk of morbidity/mortality or limited life expectancy may prompt consideration of best supportive care approach (NCCN, 2011).

(a) If good performance status and no contraindicated comorbidities, the patient may be a candidate for curative therapy.

(b) If the patient has marginal performance status, consider modified therapy or identify interventions that may improve condition to allow for curative therapy (e.g., improve comorbidity management, nutritional intervention, physical therapy).

(c) If the patient has poor performance status or declines therapy, offer best supportive care.

(4) The Comprehensive Geriatric Assessment is recommended as an important aspect of the treatment decision-making process (Extermann et al., 2005). It is a useful tool to better support the needs of the geriatric patients with cancer, including

(a) Predicting treatment tolerance or side effects

(b) Tailoring treatment to predicted survival benefit (overall and cancer related)

(c) Identifying and managing subclinical problems potentially affecting treatment tolerance or outcomes

(d) Improving symptom management (pain, physical and psychosocial functioning).

(5) The Comprehensive Geriatric Assessment includes evaluation of the following domains.

(a) Functional status (ADL and instrumental ADL performance)

(b) Comorbid medical conditions

i. Presence of comorbid conditions that affect life expectancy

ii. Recognition of both clinical and subclinical comorbidities that might impede treatment

- Obtain baseline audiology examination if the ear is in the treatment field (NCCN, 2011).
- Perform pulmonary function testing prior to treating significant lung volume.
- For patients with implanted cardiac devices (such as a pacemaker or defibrillator), consider need for beam modification (Mell & Mundt, 2005) and post-treatment device interrogation.

iii. Identification of the potential impact of comorbidities on treatment tolerance

iv. State of comorbid conditions (e.g., controlled, poorly controlled, end-organ compromise): Evidence of poorly controlled or undiagnosed comorbidities should be identified and corrected, particularly if they interfere with optimal treatment delivery or tolerance risk.

(c) Cognitive status

    i. Ability of the patient to understand/comply with treatment instructions
- Complying with daily treatment
- Positioning on treatment table/immobilization, breath holding
- Taking medication as instructed
- Participating in self-care activities

    ii. Predictor of survival (dementia portends poor survival risk)

(d) Psychological state

    i. Depression prevalence is estimated to be 3%–25% among older adult patients with cancer (Kua, 2005).

    ii. Unrecognized psychological disturbance (distress, anxiety, depression) may negatively affect patient well-being.

(e) Social support

    i. Loss of independence and poor social support among older adults can contribute to isolation and psychological distress (Hurria et al., 2009).

    ii. Many patients benefit from social services assessment and supportive care interventions or referrals.

(f) Nutritional status

    i. Malnutrition or weight loss may be attributable to underlying disease process, poor intake, or both.

    ii. Weight loss 5% or greater is associated with increased mortality risk in the older general population (Newman et al., 2001).

    iii. Poor nutritional status may negatively affect expected treatment tolerance and response (Nitenberg & Raynard, 2000).

(g) Medication list review

    i. Medication use increases with advancing age.

    ii. Limit potential for drug interactions or polypharmacy, and discontinue or decrease unnecessary medications.

(h) Geriatric syndromes

    i. Polypharmacy

    ii. Sensory deficit

    iii. Malnutrition

    iv. Limited social support

    v. Depression

    vi. Dementia

    vii. Fall risk

(6) Comprehensive Geriatric Assessment delivery

(a) Patient administered

    i. Completion of mailed/e-mailed assessment tool

    ii. In-office completion of form

(b) Provider-administered: Interview

(c) Combination of both

(7) Other related screening tools

(a) Mini-Mental State Examination (Crum, Anthony, Bassett, & Folstein, 1993; Tombaugh & McIntyre, 1992)

(b) Geriatric Depression Scale (Jongenelis et al., 2005)

(c) NCCN distress thermometer (Mitchell, 2007; NCCN, 2010)

(d) Mini Nutritional Assessment (Guigoz, Lauque, & Vellas, 2002; Vellas et al., 1999)

(8) Patient decision making

(a) Assess the patient's cognitive ability to make decisions.

(b) Assess the patient's and family's treatment goals and values.

d) Reducing treatment toxicity in older adults

(1) Conformal, IMRT, and stereotactic treatment modalities limit toxicity to healthy tissues and have significantly improved tolerance of radiation in older adult patients (Horiot, 2007).

(2) Hypofractionated treatment may be offered for convenience when treatment is for palliative or symptom management intent or if tolerance of full treatment course is an issue (Donato, Valeriani, & Zurlo, 2003).

(3) Caution with concurrent chemoradiation

(a) Consider less toxic agents when possible.

(b) Consider dose reduction if necessary, especially if palliation is the intent of treatment.

(c) Colony-stimulating factor support should be offered if neutropenia is expected with chemotherapy (Doorduijn et al., 2003).

(d) Consider use of radioprotectants (e.g., amifostine in head and neck cancer) (NCCN, 2011).

(4) Early identification and correction of toxicity

(a) Monitor for symptoms/provide adequate symptom management.
  i. Radiation-induced nausea and vomiting is less common in older than younger patients, but when it occurs, it may be more serious (Horiot, 2007).
  ii. Older patients may be less likely to report signs or symptoms of dehydration.
  iii. The risk of fatigue, pain, and depression may be increased during and after radiation among older adult patients (Rao & Harvey, 2004).
(b) Early management of nutrition deficit/fluid depletion
  i. Early and aggressive rehydration/electrolyte correction if needed
  ii. Nutritional support, supplements, and education
(5) A multidisciplinary approach to prevention and management of symptoms may be needed (Horiot, 2007).
  (a) Dietitian
  (b) Pain specialist
  (c) Physical or occupational therapist
  (d) Speech pathologist
  (e) Psycho-oncologist
  (f) Social worker
  (g) Oncology nurse
e) Psychosocial issues: Emotional and social support
  (1) Caregiver needs and availability
  (2) Assistance with meals and ADL
  (3) Transportation burden to treatment facility
  (4) Visiting nurse and homecare services/hospice services
f) Transportation and positioning issues: Daily transportation to the radiation oncology facility may be burdensome for some patients.
  (1) Problems
    (a) Distance to treatment facility
    (b) Access to transportation
    (c) Dependence on others
    (d) Fatigue or other treatment side effects
  (2) Interventions
    (a) Availability of local temporary housing
    (b) Hospitalization during treatment
    (c) Hypofractionated approach, if appropriate
g) Common cancers in older adults

(1) Prostate
  (a) Seventy percent of prostate cancers occur in men older than 65 (Horiot, 2007).
  (b) RT is generally preferable to surgery in men older than 70 or in younger men with comorbidities portending high surgical risk.
  (c) Given the more indolent course of prostate cancer in older adults, treatment is generally offered to patients with estimated life expectancy of more than 10 years, unless the patient is symptomatic.
(2) Breast
  (a) Half of all breast cancers occur in women 65 or older, with more than 60% presenting with localized disease (Jemal, Siegel, Xu, & Ward, 2010).
  (b) Older adult women more commonly undergo mastectomy as compared to breast-conservation surgery with radiation (Bouchardy et al., 2003).
  (c) In women receiving breast irradiation, the local control benefit of the boost is less significant in women older than 60 and may reasonably be omitted in selected patients (Bartelink et al., 2001).
  (d) Partial breast irradiation, brachytherapy, or hypofractionated RT techniques may offer reasonable alternatives in the future to protracted radiation courses for eligible older women with breast cancer (Ortholan, Hannoun-Lévi, Ferrero, Largillier, & Courdi, 2005).
(3) Lung
  (a) More than half of all lung cancers are diagnosed in patients older than 65 (Ries et al., 2003). Patients older than 80 are less likely to receive local therapy and have reduced survival compared to younger patients (Ries et al., 2003).
  (b) For early-stage disease, radiation alone may be considered if patient is not a surgical candidate.
    i. Smaller than 5 cm tumor: Hypofractionated stereotactic radiation
    ii. Larger than 5 cm tumor: Definitive conventional RT

iii. Radiation alone is well tolerated in older people, with a high percentage of patients completing treatment and low rates of grade 3 or 4 toxicities (Zachariah et al., 1997).
- Acute risks: Fatigue, esophagitis, pneumonitis
- Late toxicity: Decline in pulmonary function, pulmonary fibrosis

(4) Caution with combined-modality chemoradiation in older patients is required because of the increased incidence of treatment toxicity (Schild et al., 2007).

h) Survivorship issues in older patients with cancer

(1) According to Rowland et al. (2004), 61% of cancer survivors are older than 65, representing approximately 6.5 million older adult survivors.

(2) Older cancer survivors report greater functional impairment and may be at greater risk of comorbidities than age-matched noncancer populations (Hewitt, Rowland, & Yancik, 2003).

(3) Uptake of recommended primary care and preventive care services among cancer survivors is less consistent than patients without a cancer history, despite evidence indicating a greater risk of other significant health impact (Snyder et al., 2009).

(4) Attention to physical and psychosocial impact of cancer treatment is important to maintaining health and optimizing quality of life among older cancer survivors.

i) Resources

(1) Cancer Supportive Survivorship Care, Geriatric Oncology: http://www.cancersupportivecare.com/Geriatric/geriatric.html

(2) Cope, D.G., & Reb, A.M. (Eds.). (2006). *An evidence-based approach to the treatment and care of the older adult with cancer.* Pittsburgh, PA: Oncology Nursing Society.

(3) National Gerontological Nursing Association: www.ngna.org

(4) NCCN (2011) guidelines for senior adult oncology: www.nccn.org

(5) ONS and the Geriatric Oncology Consortium Joint Position on Cancer Care in the Older Adult: www.ons.org/Publications/Positions/Geriatric

References

Balducci, L., & Behge, C. (2001). Cancer and age in the USA. *Critical Reviews in Oncology/Hematology, 37,* 137–145. doi:10.1016/S1040-8428(00)00109-8

Bartelink, H., Horiot, J.C., Poortmans, P., Struikmans, H., Van den Bogaert, W., Barillot, I., ... Pierart, M. (2001). Recurrence rates after treatment of breast cancer with standard radiotherapy with or without additional radiation. *New England Journal of Medicine, 345,* 1378–1387. doi:10.1056/NEJMoa010874

Bouchardy, C., Rapiti, E., Fioretta, G., Laissue, P., Neyroud-Casper, I., Schäfer, P., ... Vlastos, G. (2003). Undertreatment strongly decreases prognosis of breast cancer in elderly women. *Journal of Clinical Oncology, 21,* 3580–3587. doi:10.1200/JCO.2003.02.046

Crum, R.M., Anthony, J.C., Bassett, S.S., & Folstein, M.F. (1993). Population-based norms for the Mini-Mental State Examination by age and educational level. *JAMA, 269,* 2368–2391. doi:10.1001/jama.1993.03500180078038

Cyr, A., Gillanders, W.E., Aft, R.L., Eberlein, T.J., & Margenthaler, J.A. (2011). Breast cancer in elderly women (≥ 80 years): Variation in standard of care? *Journal of Surgical Oncology, 103,* 201–206. doi:10.1002/jso.21799

Donato, V., Valeriani, M., & Zurlo, A. (2003). Short course radiation therapy for elderly cancer patients. Evidences from the literature review. *Critical Reviews in Oncology/Hematology, 45,* 305–311. doi:10.1016/S1040-8428(02)00082-3

Doorduijn, J.K., van der Holt, B., van Imhoff, G.W., van der Hem, K.G., Kramer, M.H., van Oers, M.H., ... Sonneveld, P. (2003). CHOP compared with CHOP plus granulocyte colony-stimulating factor in elderly patients with aggressive non-Hodgkin's lymphoma. *Journal of Clinical Oncology, 21,* 3041–3050. doi:10.1200/JCO.2003.01.076

Extermann, M. (2000). Measuring comorbidity in older cancer patients. *European Journal of Cancer, 36,* 453–471. doi:10.1016/S0959-8049(99)00319-6

Extermann, M. (2007). Interaction between comorbidity and cancer. *Cancer Control, 14,* 13–22.

Extermann, M., Aapro, M., Bernabei, R., Cohen, H.J., Droz, J.P., Lichtman, S., ... Topinkova, E. (2005). Use of comprehensive geriatric assessment in older cancer patients: Recommendations from the task force on CGA of the International Society of Geriatric Oncology (SIOG). *Critical Reviews in Oncology/Hematology, 55,* 241–252. doi:10.1016/j.critrevonc.2005.06.003

Extermann, M., Overcash, J., Lyman, G.H., Parr, J., & Balducci, L. (1998). Comorbidity and functional status are independent in older cancer patients. *Journal of Clinical Oncology, 16,* 1582–1587.

Fried, L.P., Tangen, C.M., Walston, J., Newman, A.B., Hirsch, C., Gottdiener, J., ... McBurnie, M.A. (2001). Frailty in older adults: Evidence for a phenotype. *Journals of Gerontology, Series A: Biological Sciences and Medical Sciences, 56,* M146–M156.

Guigoz, Y., Lauque, S., & Vellas, B.J. (2002). Identifying the elderly at risk for malnutrition. The Mini Nutritional Assessment. *Clinics in Geriatric Medicine, 18,* 737–757.

Haas, M.L. (2004). Utilizing geriatric skills in radiation oncology. *Geriatric Nursing, 25,* 355–360. doi:10.1016/j.gerinurse.2004.09.001

Hewitt, M., Rowland, J.H., & Yancik, R. (2003). Cancer survivors in the United States: Age, health, and disability. *Journals of Gerontology. Series A: Biological Sciences and Medical Sciences, 58,* 82–91.

Horiot, J.C. (2007). Radiation therapy and the geriatric oncology patient. *Journal of Clinical Oncology, 25,* 1930–1935. doi:10.1200/JCO.2006.10.5312

Hurria, A., Li, D., Hansen, K., Patil, S., Gupta, R., Nelson, C., ... Kelly, E. (2009). Distress in older patients with cancer.

Journal of Clinical Oncology, 27, 4346–4351. doi:10.1200/JCO.2008.19.9463

Jantunen, E., Canals, C., Attal, M., Thomson, K., Milpied, N., Buzyn, A., … Sureda, A. (2011). Autologous stem-cell transplantation in patients with mantle cell lymphoma beyond 65 years of age: A study from the European Group for Blood and Marrow Transplantation (EBMT). *Annals of Oncology.* Advance online publication. doi:10.1093/annonc/mdr035

Jemal, A., Siegel, R., Xu, J., & Ward, E. (2010). Cancer statistics, 2010. *CA: A Cancer Journal for Clinicians, 60,* 277–300. doi:10.3322/caac.20073

Jongenelis, K., Pot, A.M., Eisses, A.M., Gerritsen, D.L., Derksen, M., Beekman, A.T., … Ribbe, M.W. (2005). Diagnostic accuracy of the original 30-item and shortened versions of the Geriatric Depression Scale in nursing home patients. *International Journal of Geriatric Psychiatry, 20,* 1067–1074. doi:10.1002/gps.1398

Kua, J. (2005). The prevalence of psychological and psychiatric sequelae of cancer in the elderly—How much do we know? *Annals of the Academy of Medicine, Singapore, 34,* 250–256.

Kumar, A., Soares, H.P., Balducci, L., & Djulbegovic, B. (2007). Treatment tolerance and efficacy in geriatric oncology: A systematic review of phase III randomized trials conducted by five National Cancer Institute-sponsored cooperative groups. *Journal of Clinical Oncology, 25,* 1272–1276. doi:10.1200/JCO.2006.09.2759

Lyman, G.H., Kuderer, N., Agboola, O., & Balducci, L. (2003). Evidence-based use of colony-stimulating factors in elderly cancer patients. *Cancer Control, 10,* 487–499.

Malone, P., Perrone, F., Gallo, C., Manzione, L., Piantedosi, F., Barbera, S., … Cazzaniga, M. (2005). Pretreatment quality of life and functional status assessment significantly predict survival of elderly patients with advanced non-small-cell lung cancer receiving chemotherapy: A prognostic analysis of the multicenter Italian lung cancer in the elderly study. *Journal of Clinical Oncology, 23,* 6865–6872. doi:10.1200/JCO.2005.02.527

Mell, L.K., & Mundt, A.J. (2005). Radiation therapy in the elderly. *Cancer Journal, 11,* 495–505.

Mitchell, A.J. (2007). Pooled results from 38 analyses of the accuracy of distress thermometer and other ultra-short methods of detecting cancer-related mood disorders. *Journal of Clinical Oncology, 25,* 4670–4681. doi:10.1200/JCO.2006.10.0438

National Comprehensive Cancer Network. (2010). *NCCN Clinical Practice Guidelines in Oncology: Distress management* [v.1.2011]. Retrieved from http://www.nccn.org/professionals/physician_gls/pdf/distress.pdf

National Comprehensive Cancer Network. (2011). *NCCN Clinical Practice Guidelines in Oncology: Senior adult oncology* [v.2.2011]. Retrieved from http://www.nccn.org/professionals/physician_gls/pdf/senior.pdf

Newman, A.B., Yanez, D., Harris, T., Duxbury, A., Enright, P.L., & Fried, L.P. (2001). Weight change in old age and its association with mortality. *Journal of the American Geriatrics Society, 49,* 1309–1318. doi:10.1046/j.1532-5415.2001.49258.x

Nitenberg, G., & Raynard, B. (2000). Nutritional support of the cancer patient: Issues and dilemmas. *Critical Reviews in Oncology/Hematology, 34,* 137–168. doi:10.1016/S1040-8428(00)00048-2

Ortholan, C., Hannoun-Lévi, J.M., Ferrero, J.M., Largillier, R., & Courdi, A. (2005). Long-term results of adjuvant hypofractionated radiotherapy for breast cancer in elderly patients. *International Journal of Radiation Oncology, Biology, Physics, 61,* 154–162. doi:10.1016/j.ijrobp.2004.04.059

Peschel, R.E., Wilson, L., Haffty, B., Papadopoulos, D., Rosenzweig, K., & Feltes, M. (1993). The effect of advanced age on the efficacy of radiation therapy for early breast cancer, local prostate cancer and grade III–IV gliomas. *International Journal of Radiation Oncology, Biology, Physics, 26,* 539–544. doi:10.1016/0360-3016(93)90973-Y

Rao, A., & Harvey, H.J. (2004). Symptom management in the elderly cancer patient: Fatigue pain and depression. *Journal of the National Cancer Institute Monographs, 2004,* 150–157. doi:10.1093/jncimonographs/lgh031

Repetto, L., Fratino, L., Audisio, R.A., Venturino, A., Gianni, W., Vercelli, M., … Zagonel, V. (2002). Comprehensive geriatric assessment adds information to Eastern Cooperative Oncology Group performance status in elderly cancer patients: An Italian Group for Geriatric Oncology Study. *Journal of Clinical Oncology, 20,* 494–502. doi:10.1200/JCO.20.2.494

Ries, L.A.G., Eisner, M.P., Kosary, C.L., Hankey, B.F., Miller, B.A., Clegg, L., … Edwards, B.K. (Eds.). (2003). *SEER cancer statistics review, 1975–2000.* Bethesda, MD: National Cancer Institute.

Rowland, J., Mariotto, A., Aziz, N., Tesauro, G., Feuer, E.J., Blackman, D., … Pollack, L.A. (2004). Cancer survivorship—United States, 1971-2001. *Morbidity and Mortality Weekly Report, 53,* 526–529.

Sargent, D.J., Goldberg, R.M., Jacobson, S.D., Macdonald, J.S., Labianca, R., Haller, D.G., … Francini, G. (2001). A pooled analysis of adjuvant chemotherapy for resected colon cancer in elderly patients. *New England Journal of Medicine, 345,* 1091–1097. doi:10.1056/NEJMoa010957

Sawhney, R., Sehl, M., & Naeim, A. (2005). Physiologic aspects of aging: Impact on cancer management and decision making, part I. *Cancer Journal, 11,* 449–460.

Schild, S.E.., Mandrekar, S.J., Jatoi, A., McGinnis, W.L., Stella, P.J., Deming, R.L., … Adjei, A.A. (2007). The value of combined-modality therapy in elderly patients with stage III nonsmall cell lung cancer. *Cancer, 15,* 363–368. doi:10.1002/cncr.22780

Sehl, M., Sawhney, R., & Naeim, A. (2005). Physiologic aspects of aging: Impact on cancer management and decision making, part II. *Cancer Journal, 11,* 461–473.

Snyder, C.F., Frick, K.D., Kantsiper, M.E., Pearis, K.S., Herbert, R.J., Blackford, A.L., … Earle, C.C. (2009). Prevention, screening, and surveillance care for breast cancer survivors compared with controls: Changes from 1998 to 2002. *Journal of Clinical Oncology, 27,* 1054–1061. doi:10.1200/JCO.2008.18.0950

Taylor, J.A., III, & Kuchel, G.A. (2009). Bladder cancer in the elderly: Clinical outcomes, basic mechanisms, and future research direction. *Nature Clinical Practice Urology, 6,* 135–144. doi:10.1038/ncpuro1315

Tombaugh, R.N., & McIntyre, N.J. (1992). The mini-mental state examination: A comprehensive review. *Journal of the American Geriatrics Society, 40,* 922–935.

Vellas, B., Guigoz, Y., Garry, P.J., Nourhashemi, F., Bennahum, D., Lauque, S., & Albarede, J.L. (1999). The Mini Nutritional Assessment (MNA) and its use in grading the nutritional state of elderly patients. *Nutrition, 15,* 116–122. doi:10.1016/S0899-9007(98)00171-3

Walter, L.C., & Covinsky, K.E. (2001). Cancer screening in elderly patients: A framework for individualized decision making. *JAMA, 285,* 2750–2756.

Yee, K.W., Pater, J.L., Pho, L., Zee, B., & Siu, L.L. (2003). Enrollment of older patients in cancer treatment trials in Canada: Why is age a barrier? *Journal of Clinical Oncology, 21,* 1618–1623. doi:10.1200/JCO.2003.12.044

Zachariah, B., Balducci, L., Venkattaramanabalaji, G.V., Casey, L., Greenberg, H.M., & DelRegato, J.A. (1997). Radiotherapy for cancer patients aged 80 and older: A study of effectiveness and side effects. *International Journal of Radiation Oncology, Biology, Physics, 39,* 1125–1129. doi:10.1016/S0360-3016(97)00552-X

C. Radiation therapy for people with special needs
  1. Definition: *Special needs* is defined in a variety of ways, depending on the country or geographic region or the context within which special needs are addressed, such as education, health care, or government. In North America, the term is often linked to diagnostic or functional development and refers to individuals with medical, physical, and psychological or mental disabilities, including those requiring additional support beyond what is required by the general group or population.
  2. In the context of RT, *special needs* relates to comorbidities and/or disabilities affecting the delivery or side effects of treatment, psychosocial and functional concerns of patients undergoing RT, and special populations (e.g., pediatric, geriatric) or unique concerns of populations of patients receiving RT.
    a) Medical comorbidities
      (1) Defined as ailments other than the primary oncologic diagnosis that can influence the outcome of treatment (Geraci, Escalante, Freeman, & Goodwin, 2005).
      (2) Medical comorbidities represent a major prognostic factor in the long-term survival of patients with cancer (Geraci et al., 2005).
      (3) Survival rates decrease for patients with cancer based on the overall number and severity of comorbid illnesses (Geraci et al., 2005).
      (4) Various challenges exist in assessing the actual consequences of comorbidities in the oncology population (Geraci et al., 2005), including the cancer diagnosis and available treatment options. The range of severity of comorbidities affects the patient's trajectory of care and the influence of confounding medical issues, age, sex, ethnicity, and socioeconomic status.
    b) Treatment side effects
      (1) Magnan and Wood (2003) conducted a descriptive, correlation study of 384 patients with cancer treated with RT to differing primary cancer sites. The research revealed that patients with higher functional quality of life and hemoglobin levels prior to treatment initiation tended to experience delayed onset, shorter duration, and lower levels of fatigue. Patients with higher pretreatment mood disturbances or global symptom distress were associated with earlier onset, longer duration, and worsened severity of fatigue.
      (2) Nourissat et al. (2010) researched predictors of greater weight loss during RT for patients with head and neck cancer as a part of a phase III chemoprevention trial. They found that preexisting factors for increased weight loss during RT included all head and neck cancer sites other than the glottic larynx, higher pre-RT body weight, stage II disease, dysphagia and/or odynophagia before RT, and a lower Karnofsky performance score.
      (3) Practice implications: Pretreatment screening and risk assessment of patients is necessary to identify comorbidities that may affect the onset, duration, and intensity of experienced side effects from the planned RT (Magnan & Wood, 2003). Coordination with other specialties in managing comorbidities is important.
    c) Physical disability
      (1) WHO (n.d.) defined *disabilities* as "an umbrella term, covering impairments, activity limitations, and participation restrictions. An impairment is a problem in body function or structure; an activity limitation is a difficulty encountered by an individual in executing a task or action; while a participation restriction is a problem experienced by an individual regarding involvement in life situations. Thus, disability is a complex phenomenon, reflecting an interaction between features of a person's body and features of the society in which he or she lives."
      (2) Pretreatment practice implications
        (a) Patients may require assistance with transportation arrangements for daily RT appointments.
        (b) Consideration of disability transportation schedules may influence the timing of RT appointments.

(c) RT staff will need to educate staff and provide appropriate equipment to facilitate safe transfers.

(d) The patient and staff must anticipate increased time for RT and physical examinations on treatment visits.

(3) Treatment practice implications: Goal is to maintain functional independence of patient during and after treatment by staff anticipating and reducing the occurrence of secondary conditions.

(4) Post-treatment practice implications: Oncology rehabilitation is an appropriate option and takes into consideration both disease progression and individualized goals. It can be an appropriate option for most patients with cancer with loss of independent mobility and self-care (Cheville, 2005).

d) Obesity

(1) *Obesity* is defined by the Centers for Disease Control and Prevention (2010) as a BMI greater than 30, more than what is healthy for the given height of an individual, and increasing the risk for diabetes, hypertension, and cardiovascular diseases. *Morbid obesity* is a BMI greater than 40.

(2) Practice implications

(a) Appropriate supplies and equipment should be accessible to facilitate patient care (extra-large hospital gowns, a scale, Hoyer lift with a weight capacity beyond 300 pounds, and large blood pressure cuffs).

(b) CT planning and the use of daily cone beam imaging may provide challenges with morbidly obese patients because of the small size of the CT machine opening (bore) and difficulty moving equipment around the patient when using cone beam imaging.

(c) Provide assistance as required on and off the radiation table. Always treat the patient with dignity and respect.

e) Visual impairment/blindness

(1) Preexisting visual impairment/blindness: Patients with visual impairments or blindness can encounter unique challenges that can hinder their ability to obtain oncology care that is safe, efficient, and patient centered. Potential barriers that these patients may ex-

perience throughout their trajectory of care include lack of basic respect, poor communication, limited physical access, and inadequate information (O'Day, Killeen, & Iezzoni, 2004).

(2) Practice implications: Vision Australia (2007) recommended the following interventions for healthcare providers to improve the overall cancer treatment experience.

(a) Communication

i. All RT team members participating in the patient interaction should introduce themselves.

ii. Team members should address the patient by name so that he or she is cognizant that the healthcare professionals are conversing with the patient.

iii. Speak to the patient in a normal tone of voice.

iv. Ensure that the patient is aware when the radiation therapist is exiting the treatment room and will be monitoring the patient by intercom and camera.

v. Explain all procedures to the patient and always inform the patient prior to commencement of any physical contact.

(b) Respect

i. The patient must be central in all discussions about the cancer diagnosis and planned RT. Visual impairment does not hinder the patient's ability to fully participate in healthcare decision making.

ii. Ask the patient what assistance, if any, is required.

iii. Guide dogs are permitted in patient areas. Do not touch or play with guide dogs when they are wearing a working harness.

(c) Physical access and mobility

i. Orient the patient to the examination room or radiation suite by utilizing a central point.

ii. Accompany the patient when orienting the individual to new clinical areas, which will aid the patient in deciphering both spatial and sensory cues.

iii. The clinician should invite the patient to take his or her arm for guiding purposes.

(d) Access to information: Whenever possible, provide information regarding cancer diagnosis and RT in Braille, large print, or audio formats (tape, CD, MP3).

(3) Treatment-related visual impairment

(a) Patients whose RT fields encompass critical eye structures may lose their vision immediately or over time as a result of treatment (e.g., patients with brain or nasopharyngeal cancers where treatment margins are close to or involve the optic nerve or optic chiasm).

(b) Practice implications: Provide education, supportive counseling, and referral to resources for patients who will lose their vision immediately or over time as a result of RT.

f) Hearing impairment

(1) Preexisting hearing impairment: Impairment can affect understanding of one's cancer diagnosis and proposed treatment options as well as medication adherence (Iezzoni, O'Day, Killeen, & Harker, 2004).

(2) Practice implications: Iezzoni et al. (2004) described interventions for the hearing impaired.

(a) Ask the patient about preferred methods of communication. Make appropriate accommodations as needed, such as the usage of interpreters, e-mails, and faxes.

(b) Minimize background noise during interactions.

(c) Assessment rooms should have appropriate lighting to facilitate communication (e.g., lip reading).

(d) Ask the patient if the current communication style is effective, and if not, what measures could be employed to rectify unsatisfactory circumstances.

(e) Always look at and speak directly to the patient.

(f) Be mindful not to speak loudly in public places when speaking with the patient due to privacy issues.

(g) Prior to touching the patient, always inform the individual immediately before doing so.

(h) Describe all physical maneuvers before proceeding.

(i) Request that the patient summarize provided information in order to assess understanding.

(j) When possible, provide patient information on written handouts.

(3) Treatment-related hearing impairment—Practice implications

(a) Provide referrals for routine and follow-up hearing testing for patients who are at risk of hearing loss as a result of radiation or combined modality treatment (e.g., IMRT plus cisplatin chemotherapy for head and neck cancers).

(b) Advocate for funding of hearing aids or devices.

3. Psychosocial issues/coping/mental health (see section IV.E—Distress/coping)

a) Overview: A cancer diagnosis can result in an emotional upheaval for the involved person and the family or caregivers. The array of emotions experienced and the support required can vary throughout the patient's trajectory of care.

b) Susceptible patients: NCCN (2010) guidelines identified the following preexisting patient factors that place an individual with a cancer diagnosis at increased risk for emotional distress throughout the care experience.

(1) History of depression or suicide attempt

(2) Uncontrolled symptoms

(3) Substance abuse

(4) Diminished cognitive functioning

(5) Multiple medical comorbidities

(6) Spiritual or religious conflicts

(7) Limited support network

(8) Family or caregiver discord

(9) Financial concerns

(10) Living alone

(11) Dependent child or children

(12) Younger age; female

(13) Communication issues (language, literacy, speech/hearing problems)

(14) Past abuse (physical and/or sexual)

(15) Psychiatric disorder

c) Pretreatment: Planning phase prior to the initiation of RT involves periods of waiting, multiple consultations, and various medical investigations—all of which can produce emotional suffering for a patient with cancer (NCCN, 2010).

d) During treatment: Larsson, Hedelin, and Athlin (2007) conducted a qualitative study examining the experience of daily life for patients with head and neck cancer undergoing RT and reported that the actual treatment phase of radiation results in a major upheaval of the patient's life and, in turn, emotional turmoil. Although many patients found the regular contact with healthcare professionals to be a source of comfort throughout treatment, the following have been reported as potential sources of emotional discord during this time.

   (1) The travel back and forth for daily RT treatment

   (2) Separation from family because of the need to stay at a patient hotel or lodging as a result of the patient's residence being too distant from the treating facility

   (3) The development of various treatment-related side effects and physical impairment

e) Post-treatment: Larsson et al. (2007) found that the conclusion of RT can produce a vast array of emotions, including accomplishment and relief, for patients with head and neck cancer; some experience anxiety and worry as they struggle with side effects and await the outcome regarding treatment response. Others have a sense of feeling alone or abandoned as they attempt to address problems at home away from the support of their oncology team.

f) Treatment implications/recommended interventions: Anticipate stressful situations and recognize patients who are vulnerable to experience emotional discord. Interventions for those requiring emotional support during any aspect of their oncology trajectory of care is both situational and patient dependent. Regardless, NCCN (2010) recommended the following options to improve patients' overall emotional status.

   (1) Symptom management

   (2) Timely education and information

   (3) Pharmacology options

   (4) Referral to the mental health team

   (5) Support groups

   (6) Individual or family counseling

   (7) Relaxation, meditation, and music therapy

   (8) Exercise

   (9) Referral to spiritual care

g) Anxiety: Feelings of nervousness, apprehension, irritability, unease, or dread. Physical symptoms of anxiety include nausea, tachycardia, shortness of breath, light-headedness, insomnia, tremors, and diaphoresis. Patients with cancer have increased levels of anxiety compared to the general population. Moreover, anxiety has been found to worsen as cancer progresses or physical functioning deteriorates (Roth & Massie, 2007).

   (1) Pretreatment: A systematic review of 45 studies examined the psychological status of patients with cancer before, during, and after completion of RT. Prior to the initiation of RT, anxiety was the more commonly reported psychological reaction. Specifically, 10%–20% of patients with cancer experienced anxiety before treatment (Stiegelis, Ranchor, & Sanderman, 2004).

   (2) During treatment: Anxiety levels tend to peak during the first week of RT with 21%–54% of patients experiencing this emotion (Stiegelis et al., 2004).

   (3) Post-treatment: Reports of anxiety following RT were inconsistent. However, longitudinal studies have indicated general improvement with patients with cancer and psychological functioning (Stiegelis et al., 2004).

     (a) Anxiety levels increase as the patient awaits medical follow-up or the results of diagnostic tests for disease surveillance (NCCN, 2010).

     (b) Anxiety increases in patients who have tumor progression and a decline in physical status (Roth & Massie, 2007).

   (4) Treatment implications/recommended interventions for anxiety: Recognition of anxiety in radiation oncology patients is necessary to provide patient-centered care and manage patients' needs effectively. Screening tools are an efficient and reliable means of identifying anxiety in this patient population (NCCN, 2010). The oncology team should be aware of circumstances that may

heighten anxiety and offer the patient specific interventions, which may include any of the following (NCCN, 2010).

(a) Rule out or appropriately address potential contributing factors such as medications, medical states, and substance withdrawal.

(b) Emotional support (i.e., referral to community resources)

(c) Education (i.e., problem solving)

(d) Referral to psychiatry/psychology for interventions such as cognitive-behavioral therapy, supportive psychotherapy, or individual, couples, or family counseling

(e) Pharmacologic interventions

(f) Spiritual counseling when appropriate

(f) Wellness activities—Yoga, Reiki, meditation

h) Claustrophobia: An intense fear of enclosed spaces; specifically, the individual's trepidation centers on being physically constrained and potentially suffocating (McIsaac, Thordarson, Shafran, Rachman, & Poole, 1998). Claustrophobia is considered an anxiety disorder that can produce significant feelings of both dread and panic (Thorpe, Salkovskis, & Dittner, 2008).

(1) Pretreatment and during treatment: Unfortunately, patients who suffer from claustrophobia will encounter situations throughout their oncology trajectory of care that will undoubtedly trigger this disorder. The diagnosis and staging of cancer requires various investigations to be performed, many of which can be distressing for the claustrophobic patient. In particular, these patients find MRI almost impossible to endure. As a result, some patients may simply refuse to have the test performed. However, for those with claustrophobia who do undergo an MRI, approximately 15% of patients report experiencing some type of claustrophobic reaction during the imaging (Norton & Price, 2008). This reaction not only affects the individual negatively on both physical and psychological levels but also can result in less-than-ideal images because of early termination of the test (Norton & Price, 2008).

(a) Thorpe et al. (2008) studied the role of cognitive factors in the occurrence of a claustrophobic reaction during MRI. The researchers reported that claustrophobic patients frequently experienced thoughts of suffocation, harm triggered by the machine itself, and lack of perceived control.

(b) Recommendations from the study were to provide identified claustrophobic patients detailed information before the MRI pertaining to airflow and descriptions of the physical and safety aspects of the MRI machine.

(2) The planning phase of RT and the treatment itself can be unbearable for claustrophobic patients. Those with this phobia will unquestionably encounter extreme difficulties with the required immobilization of the body part being treated. The panic experienced may be heightened for patients with head and neck cancer who require a hard, plastic, mesh mask placed over their face and shoulders to secure them onto to the radiation table to minimize movement.

(3) Kim et al. (2009) investigated alternative immobilization devices for patients with head and neck cancer receiving IMRT. The efficacy of the standard thermoplastic mask was compared to that of a Vac Fix mold used specifically for claustrophobic patients at the University of Florida. This mold requires the placement of one to two straps wrapped around the patient's head. Setup and monitoring for isocenter movement necessitate the usage of an infrared camera system and a customized bite plate. Three patients were studied with the Vac Fix mold with the accompanying camera system. Of these patients, one was identified as being claustrophobic and the remaining two simply could not tolerate the standard mask. The comparison group consisted of five patients immobilized with a thermomask. The Vac Fix with camera was found to be as effective as the thermomask, with mean displacements being very close between the two systems. However, the Vac Fix patients required more beam interruptions for the purpose of repo-

sitioning; specifically, this occurred 7.7 times versus 1.8 times for those with the thermomask over the span of 20 treatments.

(4) Norton and Price (2008) conducted a meta-analysis to examine cognitive-behavioral treatment outcomes for adults with various anxiety problems. The reviewers cited that cognitive-behavioral treatment had a tendency to generate positive effects from pre- to post-testing across all types of anxiety disorders.

(5) Practice implications: The oncology team needs to identify patients with claustrophobia early in the care process to enable timely referrals and prevent delays with diagnosis and treatment. Treatment will depend on the patient and severity of the claustrophobic disorder and may include the following.

  (a) Referral to psychology, psychiatry, social work, or pastoral care for cognitive-behavioral therapy

  (b) Use of previously listed interventions for anxiety disorders including sedatives (see section IV.E—Distress/coping)

  (c) Detailed information on the particular test or radiation immobilization device

  (d) The Vac Fix may be a future option for patients with head and neck cancer and claustrophobia; however, more research is required in this area.

i) Depression: Is underdiagnosed despite its high prevalence. The rate of depression within the oncology population is 3%–38% (Snyderman & Wynn, 2009). It is common for patients with cancer to experience an array of emotions upon diagnosis, including sadness, shock, anger, and fear; however, these feelings tend to dissipate within two weeks as patients adjust to their circumstances and focus on the required treatment

(Snyderman & Wynn, 2009). According to the *Diagnostic and Statistical Manual of Mental Disorders*, a patient must have five or more symptoms for over a two-week period to be diagnosed with a major depressive disorder (Snyderman & Wynn, 2009). Screening tools are an efficient and reliable means of identifying depression in the oncology population (NCCN, 2010).

(1) Pretreatment: According to a systematic review of 45 studies examining the psychological status of patients with cancer during various aspects of their trajectory of care, psychological distress prior to treatment commencement primarily consisted of anxiety, whereas depression tended to only be experienced in 1.5%–8% of patients (Stiegelis et al., 2004).

(2) During treatment: During RT, depression tends to increase and occurs in 12%–31% of patients, with a peak occurring during the final week of treatment as physical side effects worsen (Stiegelis et al., 2004).

(3) Post-treatment: Post-treatment depression occurs in 8%–21.5% of patients (Stiegelis et al., 2004).

(4) Treatment implications/interventions for depression: The oncology team must be knowledgeable regarding the prevalence of depression among patients and specific periods during treatment where symptoms can worsen in order to best anticipate and manage this illness. Potential contributing factors of depressive symptoms must be assessed and include medications, disease- and treatment-related symptoms, medical conditions, and withdrawal states. Furthermore, patients' safety, suicide, and/or self-harm potential must be assessed. Potential treatments for a depressed patient should be individualized and can include any of the following (NCCN, 2010).

  (a) Pharmacologic interventions: Appropriate referral to psychiatry or family physician

  (b) Psychosocial interventions such as cognitive-behavioral therapy, supportive psychotherapy, and individual, couples, or family counseling and referral to other team members such as social work, psychology, or pastoral care

j) Cognitive impairment

(1) Overview
  (a) Definition: *Cognitive function* is the mental capacity to perceive, respond to, and comprehend ideas ("Cognitive Function," 2009).
  (b) Dysfunction with intellectual processes can cause impairment in one or more of the following cognitive subdomains: Awareness, language, intelligence, personality, disposition, behavior, perception, visuospatial abilities, and executive function (Fox, Mitchell, & Booth-Jones, 2006).
  (c) Cognitive impairment in a patient with cancer can be the result of multiple conditions, some of which may be preexisting, including dementia, delirium, brain tumors, mental illness, developmental delays, learning disabilities, medication side effects, and medical comorbidities, to name a few.
(2) Treatment considerations: Patients with cognitive impairment may not be able to provide informed consent because of their inability to reason or to comprehend the risks versus benefits of various therapeutic options, long-term consequences of the disease process, and treatment implications (Fox et al., 2006).
(3) The patient's ability to be compliant during treatment must be considered, such as the ability to attend daily treatments and be immobilized for therapy.
(4) Cognitive impairment can be worsened by the oncology disease process, side effects experienced by the treatment, and medications prescribed. The impact on the patient's ability to perform ADL must be considered.
(5) Cognitive screening is recommended for patients with impaired intellectual functioning at the initial visit and subsequent follow-ups (Fox et al., 2006). Time is limited during clinic visits; therefore, a short, reliable, and sensitive instrument should be used, such as the Mini-Mental State Examination or Modified Mini-Mental State Examination (Fox et al., 2006). This will provide a baseline assessment of the patient in order to anticipate and manage challenges during the treatment process (Fox et al.,

2006). Screening will help to identify support, education, and guidance that may be required to assist with the coping of the patient and the patient's caregivers (Fox et al., 2006).
(6) Practice implications: The healthcare team should recognize the need for appropriate consultations such as psychiatry, neuropsychology, and patient advocacy groups.
  (a) If decision-making capacity is impeded, involvement of the substitute decision maker or medical power of attorney will be required.
  (b) The patient and family may benefit from attendance of support groups.
  (c) Assist the caregiver in creating a list of things that friends or family can help with in order to ease the caregiver's burden (Fox et al., 2006).
  (d) Provide information about the trajectory of care and illness so that the patient and family can anticipate needs, communicate concerns, accomplish short-term goals, and perform end-of-life planning as needed (Fox et al., 2006).
  (e) Facilitate maintenance of the patient's roles and functioning by making appropriate referrals to social work, physiotherapy, or occupational therapy (Fox et al., 2006).
  (f) Whenever possible, maintain patient participation and dignity regardless of impediments (Fox et al., 2006).
4. Social support and family burden of care: A diagnosis of cancer and its treatment can result in disruption of both the individual's and family members' lives. The patient's routine must now accommodate daily RT, new medication regimens, and a number of self-care measures. As treatment progresses and side effects worsen, the patient may find it difficult to cope with the expectations of the new schedules, especially those patients with limited support networks. Furthermore, the patient may continue to struggle during the initial periods after treatment as he or she recovers and tries to reestablish old routines. Often, family members are the ones who assist the patient with these functional aspects.
  a) An Australian study investigated the impact of such additional responsibilities on

caregivers. Many reported feeling a dual burden of care. Specifically, they were organizing and assisting the patient with his or her needs while also having to take on more household and financial responsibilities (Clavarino, Lowe, Carmont, & Balanda, 2002).

    b) Practice implications: The healthcare team must make appropriate and timely referrals (social work, home care, and meal delivery services).

5. Financial: A diagnosis of cancer and its sequelae can have a devastating impact on one's financial circumstances because of the inability to work and the overall cost of oncologic care.

    a) Inability to work; benefit claims: A synthesis of British-based qualitative studies demonstrated a lack of accessible information regarding financial concerns at initial diagnosis and treatment. The oncology team's deficiency in providing appropriate and timely financial counseling early within the trajectory of care can result in general hardship for the patient and potentially financial ruin. Patients who require submission of benefit claims, whether it be via their employer or the government, can find the process complicated, lengthy, and often frustrating. To avoid exacerbation of the patient's already tenuous monetary status, late applications and the loss of benefits must be avoided (Wilson & Amir, 2008).

        (1) Practice implications: It is necessary that the oncology team discuss potential financial issues prior to treatment initiation and make referrals as needed to the social worker, who can both explain and expedite claim form completion (Wilson & Amir, 2008).

    b) Insurance: Approximately 16% of Americans lacked health coverage in 2005 (Meropol & Schulman, 2007). The uninsured tend to be overly represented from low-income households. This vulnerable population has no financial means for health care despite being a group most in need. Furthermore, those with insurance may encounter financial hardships because of copayments and/or coinsurance programs (Meropol & Schulman, 2007). The cost of cancer treatment can be financially devastating to some patients. Braud et al. (2003) conducted a retrospective study to determine the average cost of hospital-based oncology care in France for patients with recurrent lung cancer from the time of diagnosis to death. The researchers found the average cost per patient to be approximately 12,500 euros. In the United States, this price tag increased to a staggering $48,000 (USD) (Braud et al., 2003). Unfortunately, uninsured people or individuals burdened with high copayments may be required to make difficult decisions regarding their oncology care and corresponding treatment (Meropol & Schulman, 2007).

        (1) Practice implications: The healthcare team needs to have a discussion with the patient early in the delivery of care and make referrals as appropriate.

    c) Drug coverage: Radiation oncology patients with partial or a lack of drug coverage are confronted with additional and often overwhelming expenditures. Patients with cancer require medications to manage both disease symptoms and side effects from the RT. For some, their recommended treatment regimen includes either concurrent or adjuvant chemotherapy. This will undoubtedly result in significant financial hardship for many patients, as cytotoxic and biologic agents are among the costliest drugs within the medical system. As the price tag for one's oncology care increases, the patient may be more apt to ration medications or not purchase them at all (Meropol & Schulman, 2007).

        (1) Practice implications: Referral to the social worker is necessary for assessment regarding qualification and, if appropriate, assistance with applications to various government or compassionate drug plans.

        (2) Supplies are an additional expense that often is not covered by insurance plans. These include medical items such as dressings and wound or ostomy care supplies.

    d) Transportation

        (1) The vast majority of patients receive RT on an outpatient basis. This requires individuals to travel back and forth to the treating facility for their daily therapy. The encumbrance of daily travel on patients can include the following.

           (a) Travel time (Meden, St. John-Larkin, Hermes, & Sommerschield, 2002)

           (b) Travel expenses (Meden et al., 2002)

           (c) Driving during hazardous weather conditions (Meden et al., 2002)

           (d) Reliance on family or friends for rides

(e) Fatigue or exhaustion upon arrival to the treatment facility or on return home (Hjörleifsdóttir, Hallberg, Bolmsjö, & Gunnarsdóttir, 2007)

(f) Difficulty in performing necessary aspects of care

(2) Practice implications: The oncology team may refer the patient to organizations that provide transportation through volunteers. The use of volunteer drivers can decrease the burden on the patient and family. However, such volunteer services often transport more than one patient, resulting in individuals waiting for extended periods of time for others to complete their treatments and appointments.

e) Accommodation: Patients who live far from the treating facility or find the daily travel unmanageable may opt to stay at lodgings closer to the hospital, such as a patient hotel. These hotels typically offer accommodations and various support services for independent patients and their spouse for a reasonable cost.

(1) Research is inconsistent regarding the impact on individuals who temporarily reside at patient hotels during their RT. Larsson et al. (2007) reported that many patients with head and neck cancer who utilized such lodgings found the separation from their families and friends to be emotionally difficult. Conversely, no significant disparity in psychological distress was noted between Icelandic patients with cancer who had their RT close to home in comparison to those who lived significant distances away and were required to stay at an alternative residence during treatment (Hjörleifsdóttir et al., 2007). These differences may be accounted for by the fact that for a number of patients, their partner resides at the hotel with them, whereas others must stay alone because of various circumstances. Furthermore, some may take comfort in the shared experience and camaraderie with other patient guests residing at the hotel.

(2) Although patient hotels tend to offer discounted fees for patients and their spouse or partner, this cost can still represent an added expense and financial burden.

(3) Practice implications: Referral to social work may help with financial assistance or the waiving of patient hotel fees for those with limited household income.

(4) Discuss the potential of a loved one staying with the patient at the hotel during treatment.

(5) Recommend that patients who find it difficult being away from family or friends return home on weekends.

f) Distance: Patients who live at a distance from the treating facility can experience difficulties with daily transportation, and alternative accommodations may be required as discussed previously. More significantly, distance also can affect the treatment decisions of patients, especially with older adults (Punglia, Weeks, Neville, & Earle, 2006).

(1) Patients with early-stage breast cancer who lived greater distances from radiation treatment facilities were more likely to undergo a mastectomy instead of the equally efficacious treatment of breast-conserving therapy, which involves a wide excision followed by RT (Meden et al., 2002). The incidence of breast-conserving therapy was only 24.2% for the women from rural, northern Michigan, which is almost half the U.S. average (Meden et al., 2002).

(2) Punglia et al. (2006) investigated the impact of distance to the treating hospital on the obtainment of postmastectomy RT in older adult women. In the analysis, increasing distance to the radiation treatment facility was independently associated with a reduced likelihood of the individual receiving postmastectomy RT (overall risk = 0.996 per additional mile, p = 0.01). Furthermore, the decreased use of postmastectomy RT occurred at distances greater than 25 miles and was statistically significant for patients living 75 miles from the closest radiation facility (Punglia et al., 2006). Lastly, this consequence of distance on postmastectomy RT was increasingly evident in patients older than 75 (Punglia et al., 2006).

(3) Practice implications: The oncology team must be mindful of this fact when discussing potential therapeutic options (Punglia et al., 2006).

g) Access to care: Urban centers tend to have elite oncology programs or cancer-focused hospitals that appeal to high concentrations of oncology medical professionals; however, these hospital services are not disseminated equally to inner-city neighborhoods or urban populations. Blumenthal and Kagen (2002) outlined various factors for such inequity in healthcare access, including

(1) A shortage of primary care physicians to perform screening, assessments, required diagnostics, and in turn make appropriate referrals to oncology specialists

(2) Rural communities' tendency to have limited hospital resources per capita in comparison to cities

(3) Cultural barriers

(4) Lack of insurance

(5) Unawareness of obtainable health care by residents

(6) Transportation to treating facilities

(7) Treatment adherence.

6. Treatment adherence: WHO (2003) defined *treatment adherence* as "the extent to which a person's behavior—taking medication, following a diet, and/or executing lifestyle changes—corresponds with agreed recommendations from a healthcare provider" (p. 3). Adherence can become a predicament at any aspect of the radiation oncology patient's trajectory of care (Edmonds & McGuire, 2007).

a) Edmonds and McGuire (2007) detailed potential barriers to treatment adherence for patients with head and neck cancer who were undergoing RT; however, many of these described obstacles could be applicable to other radiation oncology populations.

(1) The patient's ability to effectively cope with symptoms from the disease and resulting side effects from the RT can negatively affect not only one's quality of life but also one's capacity to endure further treatment.

(2) The patient's inability to fully appreciate and comprehend the diagnosis and potential outcomes of treatment can affect adherence. This lack of understanding can be the result of multiple and often coexisting patient factors including cultural background, educational and literacy levels, socioeconomic status, age, and gender.

(3) Potential physical barriers that can impede patient attendance to daily RT include transportation issues and distance from the treatment center.

(4) Lack of health insurance coverage may influence adherence.

(5) Another indentified barrier was the inability to take time off from work because of financial obligations or inflexible work schedules.

(6) The patient may be emotionally overwhelmed by life circumstances such that he or she can no longer manage the demands of daily treatment.

b) Practice implications and interventions for adherence: The oncology team needs to anticipate patient-specific concerns and make efforts to address them in a timely fashion to reduce episodes of missed radiation treatments. Edmonds and McGuire (2007) outlined the following strategies to improve patient adherence.

(1) Cultivate a relationship with the patient that is both mutually respectful and trusting.

(2) Be cognizant of patient limitations, and provide tailored education to meet the patient's individual needs.

(3) Assess and ensure involvement of the patient's support system.

(4) Discuss financial and work-related issues.

(5) Whenever possible, make appropriate referrals on the patient's behalf.

c) Language barriers can negatively affect access to oncology services, quality of care, provider effectiveness, patient satisfaction, and treatment outcomes (Health Canada, 2001).

(1) Utilizing family members or friends as interpreters during healthcare visits is the most common response to encountered language barriers (Health Canada, 2001). However, this reliance on untrained interpreters throughout the patient's trajectory of care is unacceptable, as it can result in potential problems and risks for the patient. Specifically, the information communicated about the diagnosis, prognosis, and treatment may not be accurate for the following reasons.

(a) The interpreter may purposely conceal aspects of the information from the patient to protect the individual.

(b) The interpreter may not comprehend what is being communicated by the healthcare team.

(c) The interpreter may not correctly translate medical terminology.

(d) The interpreter may be placed in an unfair position translating emotional discussions to the patient.

(2) For precise translation to occur, a healthcare interpreter must be utilized. Such appropriate interpretation services can include

(a) A healthcare team member who is bilingual

(b) Hospital-employed interpreters

(c) Language lines (e.g., telephone service, interpretation phone lines)

(d) Outside agencies with interpreters

(e) Patient education material in languages of common populations in the area, whenever possible.

d) Health care in North America is primarily based upon Western values and beliefs. Specifically, scientific evidence and technology is the cornerstone of the medical system (Rose, 2007). However, the increasing diversity of North America's population can present challenges to healthcare professionals who are having more frequent encounters with patients from multiple cultures and ethnic backgrounds.

(1) To provide optimal care, the healthcare community must be cognizant of the differing needs of patients from various cultures while not stereotyping individuals (Rose, 2007). Rose (2007) performed a literature review regarding the special needs of patients with cancer who were from transcultural backgrounds. In particular, the author highlighted the following areas that the oncology team must consider when caring for such patients.

(a) The importance of extended family in treatment decisions and providing care to the patient is much more prevalent in non-Western cultures. Under such circumstances, the oncology team should provide, whenever possible, a family-focused care approach.

(b) Styles of communication vary among cultures. Some patients may avoid eye contact or physical touch. Others may feel it is undignified to complain, ask questions, speak about the cancer diagnosis, or show emotions. Healthcare professionals must be aware of these communication styles in order to participate in dialogue that is sensitive to the patient and his or her needs.

(c) The Western philosophy regarding healthcare management is to trust in modern medicine. However, non-Western cultures may have strong beliefs that religion or faith will intervene on behalf of the individual. This may result in a lack of adherence to treatment plans. It is important that the oncology team work with the patient to incorporate conventional therapies in a manner that is respectful of the individual and his or her personal beliefs.

(d) Diet has significance in each culture in regard to general well-being, treatment of illness, and socially, as it represents a means to comfort the individual. During RT, the patient often is advised to avoid certain food selections. Adherence to this advice may be difficult depending on the person's background and food preferences. Some patients will ingest foods only at room temperature; others are vegetarians; and some will fast for periods at a time. It is best to seek the assistance of the dietitian, who can make appropriate and culturally based recommendations.

(e) Sexuality may be a topic considered inappropriate for discussion by patients of certain cultures. Healthcare professionals need to have knowledge of sexual concerns and be sensitive to individual and cultural norms.

e) Literacy: Patients with inadequate general literacy have decreased capacity to attain and comprehend information regarding their oncology diagnosis and the risks versus benefits of proposed treatment options (Davis, Williams, Marin, Parker, & Glass, 2002).

(1) Patients often hide illiteracy because it can be a source of embarrassment and shame for them. Such patients are not easily identifiable; however, they are more likely to have multiple medical comorbidities, have lower levels of education, be elderly, and live in poverty. The healthcare team may suspect a patient to have limited reading skills if, on a consistent basis, forms are not completed or are completed by family or the patient requests a healthcare member to read the questions and fill in the answers because of forgotten glasses (Davis et al., 2002).

(2) Whenever possible, provide verbal information regarding the cancer diagnosis and treatment to patients with reading deficits (Davis et al., 2002).

(3) Davis et al. (2002) recommended the following practical guidelines for oncology team members when interacting with patients who have low literacy levels.

   (a) Use simple language and avoid medical terminology.
   (b) Slow the conversation down.
   (c) Avoid information overload.
   (d) Repeat instructions.
   (e) Use pictures and stories to facilitate the patient's comprehension.
   (f) Do not ask if the patient understands. Rather, obtain a sense of information appreciation by using teach-back methods.
   (g) Always be courteous and sensitive to the patient.
   (h) Written patient education materials should be at a grade 4–8 reading level.
   (i) Videos and interactive computer programs may be beneficial to this patient population; however, assistance may be required with use and setup of the technology (Davis et al., 2002).

7. Return to work: Out of financial necessity, some patients with cancer manage to continue working throughout RT, whereas others return to employment shortly after treatment (Canadian Cancer Society, 2010). However, many patients require a longer post-treatment recovery period (Canadian Cancer Society, 2010). The length of recuperation and one's ability to regain employment depend on patient characteristics, the job itself, the cancer diagnosis, and corresponding treatment. Return

to work for many cancer survivors symbolizes a complete recovery and the reclaiming of a sense of normalcy to their lives (de Boer et al., 2008). On the contrary, the inability to work can negatively affect cancer survivors' quality of life, self-esteem, and financial well-being (Tamminga, de Boer, Verbeek, Taskila, & Frings-Dresen, 2010).

a) Four separate studies have reported that approximately 60% of patients with cancer resume employment within one to two years of diagnosis (de Boer et al., 2008). However, a meta-analysis examining cancer survivors and their resumption of work demonstrated a 37% higher probability of unemployment for the oncology population in comparison to healthy controls (de Boer, Taskila, Ojajärvi, van Dijk, & Verbeek, 2009).

b) Limited research exists examining the impact of cancer and the corresponding treatment on the individual's capacity to resume work functions (de Boer et al., 2008).

c) de Boer et al. (2008) investigated the degree to which self-reported work ability can predict the return to employment in patients with cancer. The researchers found that patients treated with chemotherapy alone or in conjunction with another modality, such as radiation or surgery, consistently exhibited lower work ability scores (de Boer et al., 2008). Furthermore, these patients' risk of not returning to work was 2.4 times higher than those treated with surgery alone (de Boer et al., 2008).

d) Cancer survivors of prostate, testicular, or breast malignancies who had resumed employment two to six years after initial diagnosis demonstrated no difference in hours worked compared to controls. However, they did report significantly worse physical and mental workplace abilities (Gudbergsson, Fosså, Borgeraas, & Dahl, 2006).

e) Hoving, Broekhuizen, and Frings-Dresen (2009) performed a systematic review on breast cancer survivors and return-to-work interventions. The authors reported a lack of methodologically sound research pertaining to this topic. However, they did find studies pertaining to cancer and other diseases in the occupational health literature. Specifically, some evidence suggests that provisions made by employers, such as flexibility with hours, ease the transition of cancer survivors back to their work environment. Moreover, rehabilitation that focuses on graded activity may be a necessary option for patients to address issues of fatigue, endurance, physical work aptitude, and psychosocial performance. Lastly, the authors recommended that both timely and open communication with employers regarding these necessary accommodations should occur (Hoving et al., 2008).

f) ACS (2011) outlined practical work modifications that may assist cancer survivors.

(1) The availability of modified devices and equipment

(2) Reorganization or reassignment of work-related duties

(3) Tailored work schedules and reduced hours as needed

g) Practice implications: It is the healthcare team's responsibility to assist the patient in identifying accommodations required to facilitate a smooth and successful transition back into the workplace. Moreover, support should be provided to the patient in both making appropriate arrangements and with completing necessary work-related forms.

8. Special populations

a) Rare cancers: More than 200 types of cancer are considered rare diseases, which in the United States are defined as conditions with an incidence of fewer than 200,000 cases per year (Orphan Drug Act, 1983).

(1) Access to specialized centers: Those diagnosed with rare cancers often have challenges in finding a doctor with the expertise to diagnose, treat, or refer to a radiation facility.

(2) Although RT often can be available closer to the patient's home, referral to radiation centers with more experience in the management of rare cancers, infrastructures to provide access to combined-modality treatment including clinical trials, and a multidisciplinary team to support the patient should be considered. Patients may need to be referred to centers with specialized equipment including IMRT or proton therapy to manage specific cases.

(3) A recent Cancer Care Ontario guideline for the management of head and neck cancer recommended that patients with rare tumors or other uncommon histologies "be referred to a multidisciplinary team at a center seeing at least 100 head and neck cases annually, to develop a treatment plan that may be executed in whole or in part closer to home in collaboration with the referring center" (Gilbert et al., 2009, p. 33).

b) Pediatric cancers (see section IX.A—Pediatric radiation oncology)

(1) Conscious sedation for procedures/treatment

(a) Depending on the developmental age of the child, the number of fractions and the time required for daily treatment, the level of the child's anxiety, and the need for the child to be motionless during treatment, conscious or deep sedation or general anesthesia may be required.

(b) Sedation is used to reduce fear and anxiety in children and parents, achieve immobilization, and ensure pain control and overall safety of the child being treated (Gozal & Gozal, 2008).

(c) A team of well-trained personnel is required to safely manage the sedation and recovery.

(2) Distress: Children younger than 10 years of age often experience procedural distress.

(a) Younger age, observed behavioral distress, and treatment in the prone position may be predictors of RT-related distress (Klosky et al., 2007).

(b) Cognitive-behavioral and psychological strategies have been useful in reducing distress and motion in children undergoing invasive procedures, but up to 60% of children may still require sedation (Schiff, Holtz, Peterson, & Rakusan, 2001; Slifer, Bucholtz, & Cataldo, 1994).

(c) With the addition of in-room multimedia/multisensory distractions, even younger children may be able to tolerate procedures without sedation (Slifer, 1996).

(d) Children with less distress during MRI procedures and RT simulation may be weaned off sedation over the course of the treatment (Klosky et al., 2004).

(3) Transition to adult centers

(a) The age at which children transition to receiving care in an adult facility may vary depending on the center, the program, and the location of the treating/follow-up center.

(b) Preparation for the transition, understanding of the differences and expectations of receiving care in an adult facility, and introduction of team members prior to the transfer of care can ease the transition (Henderson, Friedman, & Meadows, 2010).

(c) Young adults between the ages of 16 and 24 have been identified as a vulnerable group with unmet needs.

(d) Long-term follow-up and monitoring of late effects and secondary cancers are needed (Eshelman-Kent, Gilger, & Gallagher, 2009; Hobbie & Ogle, 2001).

c) Long-term follow-up: Assessment of late effects

(1) Up to 60% of young adults have chronic health problems following pediatric cancer treatment, and up to 20% may have more than three chronic health issues (Skinner, Wallace, & Levitt, 2007).

(2) It is important to identify high-risk patients based on the site and volume of radiation treatment as well as when the treatment was delivered (i.e., prior to modern technologies, when larger volumes to critical tissues were treated).

(3) Late effects by treatment field

(a) Cardiovascular effects

i. Adults who received radiation as children are at increased risk for stroke and myocardial infarction five or more years following treatment as a result of radiation-induced arterial damage (Dickerman, 2007).

ii. Cardiovascular effects can include valve abnormalities, arrhythmias, autonomic dysfunction, abnormal stress tests, pericardial disease, carotid disease, stroke, fatigue, and shortness of breath (Carver et al., 2007; Greving & Santacroce, 2005).

iii. Radiation-induced cardiac disease accounts for 25% of the deaths not attributable to the cancer in patients with HL who had received a greater than 40 Gy dose of radiation (Carver et al., 2007).

(b) Pulmonary effects

i. Thoracic irradiation is associated with an increased risk of pulmonary fibrosis and abnormal pulmonary function, both dependent upon dose and fractionation (Marina, Sharis, & Tarbell, 2004).

ii. The risk of fibrosis increases when patients are younger at the time of radiation treatment and when RT is delivered in combination with bleomycin chemotherapy, even with lower radiation doses (Marina et al., 2004; Weiner, Maity, Carlson, & Ginsberg, 2006).

iii. A cumulative incidence of lung fibrosis has been reported at 3.5% 20 years following diagnosis and treatment (Mertens et al., 2002). The incidence of pulmonary fibrosis has been reported as 5%–15%, lower in patients with HL and breast cancer and higher in patients with lung cancer (Carver et al., 2007).

iv. A yearly history and physical should be performed, along with pulmonary function tests every one to two years depending on results. A chest CT should be ordered for any abnormal pulmonary function tests.

(c) Cranial irradiation

i. Growth hormone abnormalities resulting in abnormal bone growth can occur and have been associated with obesity (dose greater than 20 Gy, females treated at younger than four years of age) (Dickerman, 2007).

ii. Cognitive challenges can include difficulties in reading, spelling, visual auditory learning, adaptive behavior, communication, and academic achievement (Dickerman, 2007).

iii. Children treated with conformal RT for low-grade glioma at five years of age or younger experienced the greatest decline in cognition, with age being more influential than radiation dose (Merchant, Conklin, Wu, Lustig, & Xiong, 2009). In children with ependymoma, reading abilities seem to be affected more so than other academic or intellectual functions (Conklin, Lim, Xiong, Ogg, & Merchant, 2008).

iv. The use of conformal RT or delay of RT needs to be considered when treating young children. Patients should be followed with a yearly history and physical and specific testing related to the risk of late effects.

v. Cognitive screening and referral to a neuropsychologist should be considered in both children and adults treated with CNS irradiation for brain tumors (Fox et al., 2006).

(d) GI and genitourinary late effects may include asplenia with lifelong risk of sepsis, GI obstruction secondary to fibrosis, nephropathy, and bladder damage. Routine monitoring should involve an annual history and physical.

(e) Thyroid—Hypothyroidism has been associated with thoracic, cranial, and neck irradiation.

i. The relative risk of hypothyroidism in a group of patients treated for HL was 17.1. An increased risk has been linked to doses greater than 4.5 Gy, age older than 15 years, female sex, and time since radiation treatment of less than five years (Sklar et al., 2000).

ii. Other studies have reported the incidence of hypothyroidism

to be 25%–43% within a median of three years following treatment and up to 50% at 20 years following RT (Metzger et al., 2006; Sklar et al., 2000).

iii. An annual history and physical including thyroid levels should be performed.

(f) Gonadal impairment resulting from radiation to the testes or ovaries or the hypothalamic-pituitary axis is related to dose, fractionation schedule, and age (Dickerman, 2007).

i. Doses greater than 20 Gy in girls usually result in ovarian failure or reduced follicular development at puberty (Oeffinger & Hudson, 2004).

ii. In boys, doses greater than 3 Gy usually result in azoospermia (Oeffinger & Hudson, 2004). Fertility preservation options should be considered.

iii. Routine history and physical including hormone levels should be conducted.

(g) Secondary cancers—Childhood cancer survivors may have an increased lifetime risk, 15–20 times that of the general population with a latency period of up to 15 years (Oeffinger & Hudson, 2004).

i. Risk factors include age, total dose, and number of fractions of RT. Secondary cancers may develop in any tissue within the original treatment field and may include bone tumors and thyroid, breast, lung, and colon cancers (Ruble & Kelly, 1999).

ii. Young women receiving thoracic irradiation during puberty for HL were found to have up to a 35% cumulative probability of developing breast cancer by age 40, with a mean age at breast cancer diagnosis of 31.5 years (Bhatia et al., 2003; Kenney et al., 2004). Focus groups held with young women who had received RT for HL between the ages of 16 and 26 identified motivating factors for learning about and participating in a breast health program to promote health practices (Crom, Hinds, Gattuso, Tyc, & Hudson, 2005). The need for a positive learning environment, the sharing of experiences, and the use of multiple formats of education are important.

    iii. An annual history and physical with an initial mammogram at age 25 has been recommended (Smith, 2002).

d) Geriatric/older adults: 60% of cancers occur in older adults, with a similar number receiving RT for their disease.

    (1) Chronologic age should not be the determining factor for offering RT. Physical and cognitive changes associated with aging do need to be taken into account when assessing a patient undergoing RT, but with the advent of advanced techniques (e.g., IMRT) that spare more normal tissue, many older adult patients with good performance status tolerate treatment as well as younger patients do, with good response and survival rates (Zachariah & Balducci, 2000; Zachariah et al., 1997).

    (2) Comorbidities—RT is beneficial to older adult patients with comorbidities who may not be eligible for chemotherapy or surgery. Most of the studies identifying toxicities of treatment in older adults are based on conformal or older treatment techniques. Additionally, many older adult patients were not included in clinical trials in the past, a trend that is changing (Horiot, 2007).

    (3) Assessment—Use of a tool such as the Comprehensive Geriatric Assessment is important to identify symptoms and changes related to aging versus radiation-induced symptoms (Haas, 2004; Rao, Seo, & Cohen, 2004).

    (4) A thorough assessment will identify social, functional, and economic factors that may play a larger role in older adult patients' toleration of treatment. For example, the long duration of treatment may increase the risk of fatigue, induce challenges with daily transportation to and from treatment, alter the time required to continue with ADL including making meals and maintaining nutrition and hydra-

tion, and add burden to the usual management of existing comorbidities.

    (5) Frail older adults—The definition of *frailty* varies by author but includes factors that increase the individual's susceptibility to minor stresses, further affecting preexisting functional dependence, comorbidities, and geriatric syndromes (e.g., dementia, delirium, falls, incontinence) (Balducci & Stanta, 2000). More research is needed to better understand how this group of older adults will tolerate and respond to RT.

e) Sexual orientation and gender: Most clinical assessment tools are heterocentric with questions related to social support, marriage, or partner relationships and identify gender only as male or female. There is a need to address sexual orientation and gender identification to best meet the needs of patients and support them through RT and other treatments.

    (1) Studies addressing the needs of gay or lesbian individuals tend to be focused on traditional sites of disease such as breast, gynecologic, or prostate cancer but need to be broadened to address side effects, late effects, sexuality, and body image concerns related to other types of cancers treated with RT (e.g., colon cancer, anal cancer, head and neck cancer).

    (2) Prostate cancer in a transgender woman is rare but has been diagnosed in patients 12–41 years following male-to-female reassignment surgery. Treatment has included RT (72 Gy in 1.8 cGy fractions) (Miksad et al., 2006). There is a lack of understanding about the experience and needs of transgender individuals with cancer undergoing RT.

References

American Cancer Society. (2011). *Returning to work after cancer treatment.* Retrieved from http://www.cancer.org/Treatment/SurvivorshipDuringandAfterTreatment/StayingActive/WorkingDuringandAfterTreatment/returning-to-work-after-cancer-treatment

Balducci, L., & Stanta, G. (2000). Cancer in the frail patient: A coming epidemic. *Hematology/Oncology Clinics of North America, 14,* 235–250.

Bhatia, S., Yasui, Y., Robison, L.L., Birch, J.M., Bogue, M.K., Diller, L., ... Meadows, A.T. (2003). High risk of subsequent neoplasms continues with extended follow-up of childhood Hodgkin's disease: Report from the Late Effects Study Group. *Journal of Clinical Oncology, 21,* 4386–4394. doi:10.1200/JCO.2003.11.059

Blumenthal, S.J., & Kagen, J. (2002). The effects of socioeconomic status on health in rural and urban America. *JAMA, 287,* 109. doi:10.1001/jama.287.1.109

Braud, A.C., Lévy-Piedbois, C., Piedbois, P., Piedbois, Y., Livartovski, A., Le Vu, B., ... Durand-Zaleski, I. (2003). Direct treatment costs for patients with lung cancer from first recurrence to death in France. *PharmacoEconomics, 21,* 671–679.

Canadian Cancer Society. (2010). *Work and cancer.* Retrieved from http://www.cancer.ca/Canada-wide/About%20cancer/Coping%20 with%20cancer/Life%20after%20cancer/Work%20and%20cancer .aspx?sc_lang=en

Carver, J.R., Shapiro, C.L., Ng, A., Jacobs, L., Schwartz, C., Virgo, K.S., ... Vaughn, D.J. (2007). American Society of Clinical Oncology clinical evidence review on the ongoing care of adult survivors: Cardiac and pulmonary late effects. *Journal of Clinical Oncology, 25,* 3991–4008. doi:10.1200/JCO.2007.10.9777

Centers for Disease Control and Prevention. (2010, June 21). Overweight and obesity. Retrieved from http://www.cdc.gov/obesity/ defining.html

Cheville, A.L. (2005). Cancer rehabilitation. *Seminars in Oncology, 32,* 219–224. doi:10.1053/j.seminoncol.2004.11.009

Clavarino, A.M., Lowe, J.B., Carmont, S.A., & Balanda, K. (2002). The needs of cancer patients and their families from rural and remote areas of Queensland. *Australian Journal of Rural Health, 10,* 188–195. doi:10.1046/j.1440-1584.2002.00436.x

Cognitive function. (2009). In *Mosby's medical dictionary* (8th ed.). Retrieved from http://medical-dictionary.thefreedictionary.com/ cognitive+function

Conklin, H.M., Lim, C., Xiong, X., Ogg, R.J., & Merchant, T.E. (2008). Predicting change in academic abilities after conformal radiation therapy for localized ependymoma. *Journal of Clinical Oncology, 26,* 3965–3970. doi:10.1200/JCO.2007.15.9970

Crom, D.B., Hinds, P.S., Gattuso, J.S., Tyc, V., & Hudson, M.M. (2005). Creating the basis for a breast health program for female survivors of Hodgkin disease using a participatory research approach. *Oncology Nursing Forum, 32,* 1131–1141. doi:10.1188/05. ONF.1131-1141

Davis, T.C., Williams, M.V., Marin, E., Parker, R.M., & Glass, J. (2002). Health literacy and cancer communication. *CA: A Cancer Journal for Clinicians, 52,* 134–149. doi:10.3322/canjclin.52.3.134

de Boer, A.G., Taskila, T., Ojajärvi, A., van Dijk, F.J., & Verbeek, J.H. (2009). Cancer survivors and unemployment: A meta-analysis and meta-regression. *JAMA, 301,* 753–762. doi:10.1001/ jama.2009.187

de Boer, A.G., Verbeek, J.H., Spelten, E.R., Uitterhoeve, A.L.J., Ansink, A.C., de Reijke, T.M., ... van Dijk, F.J. (2008). Work ability and return-to-work in cancer patients. *British Journal of Cancer, 98,* 1342–1347. doi:10.1038/sj.bjc.6604302

Dickerman, J.D. (2007). The late effects of childhood cancer therapy. *Pediatrics, 119,* 554–568. doi:10.1542/peds.2006-2826

Edmonds, M.F., & McGuire, D.B. (2007). Treatment adherence in head and neck cancer patients undergoing radiation therapy: Challenges for nursing. *Journal of Radiology Nursing, 26,* 87–92. doi:10.1016/j.jradnu.2007.04.003

Eshelman-Kent, D., Gilger, E., & Gallagher, M. (2009). Transitioning survivors of central nervous system tumors: Challenges for patients, families, and health care providers. *Journal of Pediatric Oncology Nursing, 26,* 280–294. doi:10.1177/1043454209343209

Fox, S.W., Mitchell, S.A., & Booth-Jones, M. (2006). Cognitive impairment in patients with brain tumors: Assessment and intervention in the clinic setting. *Clinical Journal of Oncology Nursing, 10,* 169–176. doi:10.1188/06.CJON.169-176

Geraci, J.M., Escalante, C.P., Freeman, J.L., & Goodwin, J.S. (2005). Comorbid disease and cancer: The need for more relevant conceptual models in health services research. *Journal of Clinical Oncology, 23,* 7399–7404. doi:10.1200/JCO.2004.00.9753

Gilbert, R., Devries-Aboud, M., Winquist, E., Waldron, J., McQuestion, M., & Head and Neck Disease Site Group. (2009). *The management of head and neck cancer in Ontario: Organizational and clinical practice guideline recommendations. A quality initiative of the Program in Evidence-Based Care (PEBC), Cancer Care Ontario (CCO)* (Evidence-based Series #5-3). Retrieved from http://www.cancercare.on.ca/common/pages/UserFile .aspx?fileId=58592

Gozal, D., & Gozal, Y. (2008). Pediatric sedation/anesthesia outside the operating room. *Current Opinion in Anaesthesiology, 21,* 494–498. doi:10.1097/ACO.0b013e3283079b6c

Greving, D.M., & Santacroce, S.J. (2005). Cardiovascular late effects. *Journal of Pediatric Oncology Nursing, 22,* 38–47. doi:10.1177/1043454204272531

Gudbergsson, S.B., Fosså, S.D., Borgeraas, E., & Dahl, A.A. (2006). A comparative study of living conditions in cancer patients who have returned to work after curative treatment. *Supportive Care in Cancer, 14,* 1020–1029. doi:10.1007/s00520-006-0042-9

Haas, M.L. (2004). Utilizing geriatric skills in radiation oncology. *Geriatric Nursing, 25,* 355–360. doi:10.1016/j.gerinurse.2004.09.001

Health Canada. (2001). Language barriers in access to health care. Retrieved from http://www.hc-sc.gc.ca/hcs-sss/alt_formats/hpb-dgps/ pdf/pubs/2001-lang-acces/2001-lang-acces-eng.pdf

Henderson, T.O., Friedman, D.L., & Meadows, A.T. (2010). Childhood cancer survivors: Transition to adult-focused risk-based care. *Pediatrics, 126,* 129–136. doi:10.1542/peds.2009-2802

Hjörleifsdóttir, E., Hallberg, I.R., Bolmsjö, I.A., & Gunnarsdóttir, E.D. (2007). Icelandic cancer patients receiving chemotherapy or radiotherapy: Does distance from treatment center influence distress and coping? *Cancer Nursing, 30*(6), E1–E10. doi:10.1097/01. NCC.0000300161.06016.a9

Hobbie, W.L., & Ogle, S. (2001). Transitional care for young adult survivors of childhood cancer. *Seminars in Oncology Nursing, 17,* 268–273. doi:10.1053/sonu.2001.27922

Horiot, J.C. (2007). Radiation therapy and the geriatric oncology patient. *Journal of Clinical Oncology, 25,* 1930–1935. doi:10.1200/ JCO.2006.10.5312

Hoving, J.L., Broekhuizen, M.L.A., & Frings-Dresen, M.H.W. (2009). Return to work of breast cancer survivors: A systematic review of intervention studies. *BMC Cancer, 9,* 117. doi:10.1186/1471 -2407-9-117

Iezzoni, L.I., O'Day, B.L., Killeen, M., & Harker, H. (2004). Communicating about health care: Observations from persons who are deaf or hard of hearing. *Annals of Internal Medicine, 140,* 356–362.

Kenney, L.B., Yasui, Y., Inskip, P.D., Hammond, S., Neglia, J.P., Mertens, A.C., ... Diller, L. (2004). Breast cancer after childhood cancer: A report from the Childhood Cancer Survivor Study. *Annals of Internal Medicine, 141,* 590–597.

Kim, E., Jahan, T., Aouizerat, B.E., Dodd, M.J., Cooper, B.A., Paul, S.M., ... Miaskowski, C. (2009). Differences in symptom clusters identified using occurrence rates versus symptom severity ratings in patients at the end of radiation therapy. *Cancer Nursing, 32,* 429–436. doi:10.1097/NCC.0b013e3181b046ad

Klosky, J.L., Tyc, V.L., Srivastava, D.K., Tong, X., Kronenberg, M., Booker, Z.J., ... Merchant, T.E. (2004). Brief report: Evaluation of an interactive intervention designed to reduce pediatric distress during radiation therapy procedures. *Journal of Pediatric Psychology, 29,* 621–626. doi:10.1093/jpepsy/jsh064

Klosky, J.L., Tyc, V.L., Tong, X., Srivastava, D.K., Kronenberg, M., de Armendi, A.J., & Merchant, T.E. (2007). Predicting pediatric distress during radiation therapy procedures: The role of medical, psychosocial, and demographic factors. *Pediatrics, 119,* e1159–e1166. doi:10.1542/peds.2005-1514

Larsson, M., Hedelin, B., & Athlin, E. (2007). Needing a hand to hold: Lived experiences during the trajectory of care for patients with head and neck cancer treated with radiotherapy. *Cancer Nursing, 30,* 324–332. doi:10.1097/01.NCC.0000281722.56996.07

Magnan, M.A., & Wood, D.W. (2003). The effects of health state, hemoglobin, global symptom distress, mood disturbance, and treatment site on fatigue onset, duration, and distress in patients receiving radiation therapy [Online exclusive]. *Oncology Nursing Forum, 30,* E33–E39. doi:10.1188/03.ONF.E33-E39

Marina, N., Sharis, C., & Tarbell, N. (2004). Respiratory complications. In W.H. Wallace & D.M. Green (Eds.), *Late effects of childhood cancer* (pp. 114–122). London, England: Arnold.

McIsaac, H.K., Thordarson, D.S., Shafran, R., Rachman, S., & Poole, G. (1998). Claustrophobia and the magnetic resonance imaging procedure. *Journal of Behavioral Medicine, 21,* 255–268. doi:10.1023/A:1018717016680

Meden, T., St. John-Larkin, C., Hermes, D., & Sommerschield, S. (2002). Relationship between travel distance and utilization of breast cancer treatment in rural northern Michigan. *JAMA, 287,* 111. doi:10.1001/jama.287.1.111

Merchant, T.E., Conklin, H.M., Wu, S., Lustig, R.H., & Xiong, X. (2009). Late effects of conformal radiation therapy for pediatric patients with low-grade glioma: Prospective evaluation of cognitive, endocrine, and hearing deficits. *Journal of Clinical Oncology, 27,* 3691–3697. doi:10.1200/JCO.2008.21.2738

Meropol, N.J., & Schulman, K.A. (2007). Cost of cancer care: Issues and implications. *Journal of Clinical Oncology, 25,* 180–186. doi:10.1200/JCO.2006.09.6081

Mertens, A.C., Yasui, Y., Liu, Y., Stovall, M., Hutchinson, R., Ginsberg, J., ... Robison, L.L. (2002). Pulmonary complications in survivors of childhood and adolescent cancer: A report from the Childhood Cancer Survivor Study. *Cancer, 95,* 2431–2441. doi:10.1002/cncr.10978

Metzger, M.L., Hudson, M.M., Somes, G.W., Shorr, R.I., Li, C.S., Krasin, M.J., ... Howard, S.C. (2006). White race as a risk factor for hypothyroidism after treatment for pediatric Hodgkin's lymphoma. *Journal of Clinical Oncology, 24,* 1516–1521. doi:10.1200/JCO.2005.05.0195

Miksad, R.A., Bubley, G., Church, P., Sanda, M., Rofsky, N., Kaplan, I., & Cooper, A. (2006). Prostate cancer in a transgender woman 41 years after initiation of feminization. *JAMA, 296,* 2316–2317. doi:10.1001/jama.296.19.2316

National Comprehensive Cancer Network. (2010). *NCCN Clinical Practice Guidelines in Oncology: Distress management* [v.1.2011]. Retrieved from http://www.nccn.org/professionals/physician_gls/PDF/distress.pdf

Norton, P.J., & Price, E.C. (2008). A meta-analytic review of adult cognitive-behavioral treatment outcome across the anxiety disorders. *Journal of Nervous and Mental Disease, 195,* 521–531. doi:10.1097/01.nmd.0000253843.70149.9a

Nourissat, A., Bairati, I., Samson, E., Fortin, A., Gélinas, M., Nabid, A., ... Meyer, F. (2010). Predictors of weight loss during radiotherapy in patients with stage I or II head and neck cancer. *Cancer, 116,* 2275–2283. doi:10.1002/cncr.25041

O'Day, B.L., Killeen, M., & Iezzoni, L.I. (2004). Improving health care experiences of persons who are blind or have low vision: Suggestions from focus groups. *American Journal of Medical Quality, 19,* 193–200. doi:10.1177/106286060401900503

Oeffinger, K.C., & Hudson, M.M. (2004). Long-term complications following childhood and adolescent cancer: Foundations for providing risk-based health care for survivors. *CA: A Cancer Journal for Clinicians, 54,* 208–236. doi:10.3322/canjclin.54.4.208

Orphan Drug Act, 21 U.S.C. § 316 *et seq.* (1983). Retrieved from http://ecfr.gpoaccess.gov

Punglia, R.S., Weeks, J.C., Neville, B.A., & Earle, C.C. (2006). Effect of distance to radiation treatment facility on use of radiation therapy after mastectomy in elderly women. *International Journal of Radiation Oncology, Biology, Physics, 66,* 56–63. doi:10.1016/j.ijrobp.2006.03.059

Rao, A.V., Seo, P.H., & Cohen, H.J. (2004). Geriatric assessment and comorbidity. *Seminars in Oncology Nursing, 31,* 149–159. doi:10.1053/j.seminoncol.2003.12.026

Rose, T.A. (2007). The special needs of adult trans-cultural cancer patients. *Canadian Journal of Medical Radiation Technology, 38*(2), 10–16. doi:10.1016/S0820-5930(09)60244-9

Roth, A.J., & Massie, M.J. (2007). Anxiety and its management in advanced cancer. *Current Opinion in Supportive and Palliative Care, 1,* 50–56. doi:10.1097/SPC.0b013e32813aeb23

Ruble, K., & Kelly, K.P. (1999). Radiation therapy in childhood cancer. *Seminars in Oncology Nursing, 15,* 292–302. doi:10.1016/S0749-2081(99)80058-8

Schiff, W.B., Holtz, K.D., Peterson, N., & Rakusan, T. (2001). Effect of an intervention to reduce procedural pain and distress for children with HIV infection. *Journal of Pediatric Psychology, 26,* 417–427. doi:10.1093/jpepsy/26.7.417

Skinner, R., Wallace, W.H.B., & Levitt, G. (2007). Long-term follow-up of children treated for cancer: Why is it necessary, by whom, where and how? *Archives of Disease in Childhood, 92,* 257–260. doi:10.1136/adc.2006.095513

Sklar, C., Whitton, J., Mertens, A., Stovall, M., Green, D., Marina, N., ... Robison, L. (2000). Abnormalities of the thyroid in survivors of Hodgkin's disease: Data from the Childhood Cancer Survivor Study. *Journal of Clinical Endocrinology and Metabolism, 85,* 3227–3232. doi:10.1210/jc.85.9.3227

Slifer, K.J. (1996). A video system to help children cooperate with motion control for radiation treatment without sedation. *Journal of Pediatric Oncology Nursing, 13,* 91–97. doi:10.1177/104345429601300208

Slifer, K.J., Bucholtz, J.D., & Cataldo, M.D. (1994). Behavioral training of motion control in young children undergoing radiation treatment without sedation. *Journal of Pediatric Oncology Nursing, 11,* 55–63. doi:10.1177/104345429401100204

Smith, P.C.K. (2002). The role of the primary care advanced practice nurse in evaluating and monitoring childhood cancer survivors for a second malignant neoplasm. *Journal of Pediatric Oncology Nursing, 19,* 84–96. doi:10.1053/jpon.2002.123450

Snyderman, D., & Wynn, D. (2009). Depression in cancer patients. *Primary Care, 36,* 703–719. doi:10.1016/j.pop.2009.07.008

Stiegelis, H.E., Ranchor, A.V., & Sanderman, R. (2004). Psychological functioning in cancer patients treated with radiotherapy. *Patient Education and Counseling, 52,* 131–141. doi:10.1016/S0738-3991(03)00021-1

Tamminga, S.J., de Boer, A.G., Verbeek, J.H., Taskila, T., & Frings-Dresen, M.H. (2010). Enhancing return-to-work in cancer patients, development of an intervention and design of a randomized controlled trial. *BMC Cancer, 10,* 345. doi:10.1186/1471-2407-10-345

Thorpe, S., Salkovskis, P.M., & Dittner, A. (2008). Claustrophobia in MRI: The role of cognitions. *Magnetic Resonance Imaging, 26,* 1081–1088. doi:10.1016/j.mri.2008.01.022

Vision Australia. (2007, February 20). Fact sheet: Caring for patients who are blind or have low vision. Retrieved from http://www.visionaustralia.org.au/info.aspx?page=644

Weiner, D.J., Maity, A., Carlson, C.A., & Ginsberg, J.P. (2006). Pulmonary function abnormalities in children treated with whole lung irradiation. *Pediatric Blood and Cancer, 46*, 222–227. doi:10.1002/pbc.20457

Wilson, K., & Amir, Z. (2008). Cancer and disability benefits: A synthesis of qualitative findings on advice and support. *Psycho-Oncology, 17*, 421–429. doi:10.1002/pon.1265

World Health Organization. (2003). *Adherence to long-term therapies: Evidence for action.* Retrieved from http://www.who.int/chp/knowledge/publications/adherence_report/en/index.html

World Health Organization. (n.d.). Disability. Retrieved from http://www.who.int/topics/disabilities/en

Zachariah, B., & Balducci, L. (2000). Radiation therapy of the older patient. *Hematology/Oncology Clinics of North America, 14,* 131–167. doi:10.1016/S0889-8588(05)70282-3

Zachariah, B., Balducci, L., Venkattaramanabalaji, G.V., Casey, L., Greenberg, H.M., & DelRegato, J.A. (1997). Radiotherapy for cancer patients aged 80 and older: A study of effectiveness an side effects. *International Journal of Radiation Oncology, Biology, Physics, 39,* 1125–1129. doi:10.1016/S0360-3016(97)00552-X

X. Chemical modifiers of cancer treatment

A. Radioprotectors
1. Definition: *Radioprotectors* (also called *radioprotectants*) are drugs designed to protect normal cells from damage resulting from RT by promoting cellular repair (NCI, 2010).
2. *Cytoprotectants* are defined as chemical modifiers designed to minimize normal tissue damage resulting from chemotherapy administration without compromising tumor control (Kouvaris, Kouloulias, & Vlaho, 2007; MedImmune, LLC, 2010; Rosenthal, 2006; Rosenthal &Trotti, 2009; Samuels, 2004). The term is also used for amifostine administration for both chemotherapy and radiation protection.
    a) Amifostine—The active thiol metabolite binds to and detoxifies the reactive metabolites of cisplatin (MedImmune, LLC, 2010; Schuchter, Hensley, Meropol, & Winer, 2002).
    b) Mesna—Cytoprotectant used to decrease the incidence of ifosfamide-associated bladder/urethral toxicity (Schuchter et al., 2002).
    c) Dexrazoxane—Cardioprotectant used to reduce the incidence and severity of cardiomyopathy in women with metastatic breast cancer who have received more than 300 mg/m^2 of doxorubicin in the metastatic setting and who will continue doxorubicin-containing therapy to control their disease. It is not recommended for use when doxorubicin therapy is initiated (Pfizer Inc., 2011; Schuchter et al., 2002). Increased nausea and vomiting are noted with use of this therapy.
3. Protection of normal tissue against adverse effects from RT and chemotherapy may permit dose escalation, increased patient survival, and better quality of life for patients requiring cancer treatments (Citrin et al., 2010; Samuels, 2004; Wasserman et al., 2000).
4. An organic thiophosphate cytoprotective agent with FDA approval: Amifostine (Ethyol®, MedImmune, LLC). It is a prodrug that is dephosphorylated by alkaline phosphatase in tissues to pharmacologically active free thiol metabolite. The active free thiol metabolite is believed to be responsible for the reduction of the toxic effects of radiation on normal oral tissues (MedImmune, LLC, 2010; Schuchter et al., 2002).
    a) It is FDA approved as a cytoprotectant to reduce the cumulative renal toxicity associated with repeated administration of cisplatin with advanced ovarian cancer (MedImmune, LLC, 2010).
    b) It also is FDA approved as a radioprotectant to reduce the incidence of moderate to severe xerostomia in patients undergoing postoperative RT for head and neck cancer where the RT field includes a substantial portion of the parotid gland (Brizel et al., 2000; Kouvaris et al., 2007; MedImmune, LLC, 2010).
    c) For the previous indications, the clinical data do not suggest that amifostine alters the effectiveness of cisplatin or RT (MedImmune, LLC, 2010).
    d) Numerous clinical trials have examined the safety and efficacy of amifostine in the prevention of mucositis in radiation-induced and combined-modality therapy–induced mucositis in three major areas: head and neck cancer, NSCLC, and pelvic cancer (Antonadou et al., 2001; Büntzel, Küttner, Fröhlich, & Glatzel, 1998; Koukourakis et al., 2000).
    e) Based on extensive data available, additions were made to the amifostine U.S. Pharmacopeia drug information monograph for off-label use in mucosal RT or RT combined with chemotherapy (U.S. Pharmacopeia, 2002).
5. The use of a radioprotectant such as amifostine needs to be considered even with the advantages of IMRT in an attempt to decrease the acute and chronic toxicity of RT (Thorstad, Chao, & Haughey, 2004).
6. Head and neck cancer (Logan, 2009; Ribeiro, Kowalski, & Latorre, 2000; Trotti, 2000)
    a) Significant toxicities from head and neck irradiation
        (1) Acute mucositis
        (2) Acute and chronic xerostomia
        (3) Acute esophagitis
        (4) Candidiasis
        (5) Skin reactions
    b) Results of significant toxicities caused by radiation to the head and neck region include
        (1) Weight loss
        (2) Taste alterations

(3) Oral complications and pain
(4) Extreme fatigue
(5) Dehydration
(6) Dental complications
(7) Treatment interruptions
(8) Dose limitations
(9) Discontinuation of treatment
(10) Hospitalizations
(11) Ultimately poor outcomes.

c) Combined-modality treatment with chemotherapy and RT increases the toxicities of xerostomia, mucositis, and esophagitis. IMRT has enabled increased delivery of therapeutic doses of radiation to tumors while limiting exposure to normal tissue, thereby reducing the incidence, duration, and severity of xerostomia in patients with head and neck cancer (Kam et al., 2007; Samuels, 2004; Thorstad et al., 2004; Vissink, Jansma, Spijkervet, Burlage, & Coppes, 2003).

d) Amifostine as a radioprotector in head and neck cancer
(1) Clinical trials have suggested that amifostine protects against radiation-induced toxicity in both patients receiving RT alone and those receiving radiochemotherapy (Anné & Curran, 2002; Brizel et al., 2000; Büntzel, Glatzel, Mücke, Micke, & Bruns, 2007; Büntzel et al., 1998).
(2) In a phase III randomized trial with amifostine as a radioprotector in squamous cell cancer of the head and neck, amifostine reduced acute and chronic xerostomia while preserving antitumor efficacy and reducing the overall incidence of grade 2 or higher xerostomia from 78% to 51% (p < 0.0001) (Brizel et al., 2000). The median time to onset of grade 2 or higher acute xerostomia was longer in the amifostine plus RT group (45 days) compared to the control group (30 days, p = 0.0001). In addition, patients pretreated with amifostine were able to tolerate larger doses of radiation (60 Gy) compared to the RT-alone group (42 Gy, p = 0.0001). The radiation dose necessary to cause grade 2 or higher acute xerostomia was 40% higher in the amifostine plus RT group (Brizel et al., 2000).
(3) Clinical benefit was measured by the use of an eight-item validated patient benefit questionnaire during and up to 11 months after RT. Amifostine-treated patients consistently reported better scores on the questionnaire beginning at week 4 of radiation (p < 0.05), which was indicative of improved oral toxicity–related outcomes and improved clinical benefit (Wasserman et al., 2000).
(4) Additionally, 18- and 24-month follow-up data obtained from a pivotal phase III study (Brizel et al., 2000) further established the selective cytoprotection and lack of tumor protection with the use of amifostine. At 18 and 24 months, no statistically significant difference existed in locoregional control (p = 0.610; p = 0.535, respectively), progression-free survival (p = 0.958; p = 0.982, respectively), and overall survival rate (p = 0.184; p = 0.184, respectively) between patients receiving amifostine and those in the control group, confirming that amifostine did not compromise antitumor efficacy of RT (Brizel et al., 2000).
(5) The use of amifostine has not been embraced as fully as other strategies to reduce toxic effects of RT or chemotherapy. Some radiation oncologists remain hesitant to adopt cytoprotective agents because of their limited use of and experience with injectable medications, lack of appreciation of symptom burden (e.g., nausea/vomiting, hypotension, rash), and the clinical impact of mucositis and xerostomia (Samuels, 2004).
(6) Some radiation and medical oncologists have questions about the risk-benefit profiles of cytoprotective agents, including the potential for tumor protection and the belief that IMRT eliminates the need for cytoprotective agents (Rosenthal, 2006; Samuels, 2004).
(7) Cytoprotection can be used to prevent unnecessary delays in RT treatments for postoperative patients with head and neck cancer where the radiation port will include a large part of the parotid glands.

e) Targeted therapy with cetuximab may be combined with radiation in initial treatment or used alone to treat recurrent head and neck cancer. With the use of targeted therapy, patients with head and neck cancer receiving radiation experience increased skin reaction toxicities in the treatment field; therefore, amifostine (which can cause a skin reaction) is NOT used with targeted therapies (Koukourakis et al., 2010). Patients treated with cetuximab develop temporary acneform skin reaction (rash) on the face and body that usually disappears after treatment. The presence and intensity of the rash from the targeted therapies have been associated with better survival in patients treated with cetuximab (Koukourakis et al., 2010).

7. NSCLC

    a) Toxicities from lung irradiation for NSCLC (Antonadou et al., 2000; Gopal et al., 2003; Komaki et al., 2002)

        (1) Dysphagia

        (2) Esophagitis

        (3) Dyspnea

        (4) Cough

        (5) Pneumonitis

        (6) Fibrosis

    b) Amifostine has shown a reduction in the incidence of both radiation-induced toxicities, such as esophagitis and pneumonitis, and chemotherapy-related toxicities, including nephrotoxicity, hematologic toxicity, and possibly neurotoxicity (Antonadou et al., 2000, 2001; Antonadou, Pepelassi, Synodinou, Puglisi, & Throuvalas, 2002; Komaki et al., 2002; Leong et al., 2001; Movsas et al., 2005; Werner-Wasik et al., 2001).

    c) Multiple trials have demonstrated a reduction in acute and late lung toxicity without affecting antitumor efficacy of RT in advanced lung cancer. In a study of 73 patients with advanced-stage lung cancer, the incidence of esophagitis grade 2 or higher during week 4 of treatment with daily fraction of 2 Gy/ five days/week was 42% (31/73) in the radiation-alone group compared to 4% (3/73) in the group that also received amifostine (p < 0.001). Amifostine was administered daily at 340 mg/m². Two months following therapy, 73 patients were evaluated for the incidence of pneumonitis. Forty-three percent (23/53) of patients in the radiation arm and 9% (4/44) in the amifostine plus radiation arm demonstrated changes representative of grade 2 or greater lung damage (p < 0.001). Fibrosis was present in 53% (19/36) of patients receiving RT alone versus 28% (9/32) of those receiving radiation plus amifostine (Antonadou et al., 2001).

    d) In a study of 26 patients treated with thoracic irradiation for lung cancer, 11 patients received concurrent hyperfractionated radiation with chemotherapy (cisplatin, etoposide) and amifostine (Gopal et al., 2003). The cytoprotective benefit of amifostine in this report was illustrated with an increase in

the threshold for local diffusion capacity in the lung (DL_{CO}) loss from 13 to 36 Gy. Amifostine has previously been found to reduce the decrease in DL_{CO} from 42% to 24% in patients with NSCLC treated with chemoradiation (Antonadou et al., 2001). The authors emphasized the importance of evaluating the relationship between local radiation dose and the loss of DL_{CO} (Gopal et al., 2003). The utilization of this information in combination with a DVH allows for the prediction of the expected loss of whole lung diffusion capacity associated with a treatment plan. Clinically, this is relevant because the DL_{CO} should not decrease much more than 50% than predicted if patients are to maintain a reasonable quality of life (Antonadou et al., 2001; Gopal et al., 2007).

    e) Data from preclinical studies support the hypothesis that cytoprotection in the RT clinical setting appears to be most effective when the drug is given in a specific time frame before daily radiation treatments and the flat dose of 500 mg of amifostine (Bachy, Fazenbaker, Kifle, & Cassatt, 2003; Cassatt, Fazenbaker, Kifle, & Bachy, 2002; Fazenbaker, Bachy, Kifle, & Cassatt, 2003).

    f) Several large clinical trials have demonstrated significant cytoprotection with the use of amifostine as a single injection prior to each standard fraction of radiation treatment five days each week for six to seven weeks (Antonadou et al., 2000, 2001, 2002; Brizel et al., 2000).

8. Dosing and administration of amifostine

    a) The recommended dose of amifostine in patients with head and neck cancer is 200 mg/m² administered once daily as a three-minute IV push starting 15–30 minutes prior to RT (MedImmune, LLC, 2010) for reduction of moderate to severe xerostomia.

    b) Several clinical trials have provided evidence that amifostine at 300–340 mg/m² can provide mucosal protection and reduction of mucositis associated with RT or radiochemotherapy (Antonadou et al., 2001, 2002; Büntzel et al., 1998).

    c) Although not FDA approved, rapid IV push as a 10-second push may reduce the occurrence of nausea, vomiting, and hypotension associated with amifostine versus a slower IV push while still maintaining the effectiveness and antitumor efficacy of RT or chemotherapy (Boccia, 2002; Wagner, Radmard, & Schönekaes, 1999).

d) Other research and preliminary data suggest subcutaneous administration at a 500 mg flat dose mixed in 2.5 ml of normal saline, given in one to two injections daily, 20–60 minutes prior to daily radiation, demonstrates a reduction in xerostomia and mucositis (Anné & Curran, 2002; Koukourakis et al., 2000).

e) Adverse effects of amifostine as a radioprotector
  (1) Nausea and vomiting
  (2) Hypotension
  (3) Cutaneous reactions (local skin irritation/localized rash at the injection site, generalized rash, erythema multiforme, Stevens-Johnson syndrome, toxic epidermal necrolysis, exfoliative dermatitis) (MedImmune, LLC, 2010)
  (4) Fever, chills
  (5) Asthenia (Anné & Curran, 2002; Boccia, 2002; Koukourakis et al., 2000)

9. Specific nursing care and instructions for patients
  a) Premedicate with an oral antiemetic 90–120 minutes before amifostine daily.
    (1) Prochlorperazine 10 mg orally may be effective for some patients who cannot afford a 5-HT$_3$ antagonist, but MedImmune recommends a 5-HT$_3$ antagonist as the frontline antiemetic to be used (MedImmune, LLC, 2010).
    (2) Assess the patient's nausea profile and recommend a 5-HT$_3$ antagonist if the patient has risk factors for increased nausea and vomiting. Keep in mind the patient's full treatment regimen when assessing the need for antiemetics.
  b) Hydration is key for patients receiving amifostine to prevent hypotension.
    (1) Encourage the patient to drink two to three 8 oz glasses of water or sports drink prior to amifostine administration.
    (2) If the patient has a gastrostomy tube or percutaneous endoscopic gastrostomy tube, have the patient take 250 ml of fluid (water or sports drink) prior to amifostine administration.
    (3) Encourage the patient to drink an additional liter throughout the day.
    (4) Assess for symptoms of dehydration daily before giving amifostine.
      (a) Dizziness
      (b) Light-headedness
      (c) Hypotension
      (d) Tachycardia
      (e) Concentrated urine
      (f) Change in weight
    (5) Hold treatment if the patient is dehydrated or hypotensive.
    (6) Give IV hydration if needed.
    (7) Monitor blood pressure daily with a baseline and every 5–15 minutes or until stable or as clinically indicated (Daly, Holloway, & Ameen, 2003; Wagner et al., 1999).
  c) Cutaneous reaction with or without a fever
    (1) Local cutaneous reaction at the injection site can be treated with injection site rotation, local steroidal cream, and an oral antihistamine one hour before daily amifostine administration (Daly et al., 2003; Wang, Kagan, & Tome, 2003).
    (2) If a systemic rash occurs, which is defined as a rash outside the RT portal or local injection site, amifostine should be discontinued. Rash can be treated with comfort measures.
    (3) Discontinue if a fever occurs, and rule out other possible etiologies before continuing use (Boccia et al., 2003).
  d) Other important information to know before administering amifostine: Nausea and vomiting may be increased when patients are also receiving chemotherapy with RT, leading to uncertainty as to the cause of nausea and vomiting and whether discontinuation of the amifostine is needed. Reevaluation of antinausea medications and the patient's hydration status should be done first (Samuels, 2004).

10. A variety of radioprotective or cytoprotective agents are currently being investigated and include the following (Jatoi & Thomas, 2002; Kushi et al., 2006).
  a) Gene therapy: Intratumor injection of manganese superoxide dismutase-plasmid/liposome
  b) Transforming growth factor-beta
  c) Keratinocyte growth factor
  d) Glutamine
  e) Interleukin-15
  f) Melatonin
  g) Omega-3 fatty acids

References

Anné, P.R., & Curran, W.J., Jr. (2002). A phase II trial of subcutaneous amifostine and radiation therapy in patients with head and neck cancer. *Seminars in Radiation Oncology, 12*(1, Suppl. 1), 18–19. doi:10.1053/srao.2002.31358

Antonadou, D., Coliarakis, N., Synodinou, M., Athanassiou, H., Kouveli, A., Verigos, C., ... Clinical Radiation Oncology Hellenic Group. (2001). Randomized phase III trial of radiation treatment ± amifostine in patients with advanced-stage lung cancer. *International Journal of Radiation Oncology, Biology, Physics, 51*, 915–922. doi:10.1016/S0360-3016(01)01713-8

Antonadou, D., Pepelassi, M., Synodinou, M., Puglisi, M., & Throuvalas, N. (2002). Prophylactic use of amifostine to prevent radiochemotherapy-induced mucositis and xerostomia in head-and-neck cancer. *International Journal of Radiation Oncology, Biology, Physics, 52*, 739–747. doi:10.1016/S0360-3016(01)02683-9

Antonadou, D., Synodinou, M., Boufi, M., Sagriotis, A., Paloudis, S., & Throuvalas, N. (2000). Amifostine reduces acute toxicity during radiochemotherapy in patients with localized advanced stage non small cell lung cancer [Abstract 1960]. *Proceedings of the American Society of Clinical Oncology, 19*. Retrieved from http://www.asco.org/ASCOv2/Meetings/Abstracts?&vmview=abst_detail_view&confID=2&abstractID=201307

Bachy, C.M., Fazenbaker, C.A., Kifle, G., & Cassatt, D.R. (2003). Daily dosing with amifostine is necessary for full protection against oral mucositis caused by fractionated radiation in rats: Protection and pharmacokinetics [Abstract 2081]. *Proceedings of the American Society of Clinical Oncology, 22*. Retrieved from http://www.asco.org/ASCOv2/Meetings/Abstracts?&vmview=abst_detail_view&confID=23&abstractID=102840

Boccia, R.V. (2002). Improved tolerability of amifostine with rapid infusion and optimal patient preparation. *Seminars in Oncology, 29*(6, Suppl. 19), 9–13. doi:10.1053/sonc.2002.37358

Boccia, R.V., Bourhis, D., Brizel, D., Daly, C., Holloway, N., Hymes, S., ... Wasserman, T. (2003). Management of cutaneous reactions associated with amifostine: Findings of an independent panel [Abstract 3175]. *Proceedings of the American Society of Clinical Oncology, 22*. Retrieved from http://www.asco.org/ASCOv2/Meetings/Abstracts?&vmview=abst_detail_view&confID=23&abstractID=103868

Brizel, D.M., Wasserman, T.H., Henke, M., Strnad, V., Rudat, V., Monnier, A., ... Sauer, R. (2000). Phase III randomized trial of amifostine as a radioprotector in head and neck cancer. *Journal of Clinical Oncology, 18*, 3339–3345.

Büntzel, J., Glatzel, M., Mücke, N., Micke, O., & Bruns, F. (2007). Influence of amifostine on late radiation-toxicity in head and neck cancer—A follow-up study. *Anticancer Research, 27*, 1953–1956.

Büntzel, J., Küttner, K., Fröhlich, D., & Glatzel, M. (1998). Selective cytoprotection with amifostine in concurrent radiochemotherapy for head and neck cancer. *Annals of Oncology, 9*, 505–509.

Cassatt, D.R., Fazenbaker, C.A., Kifle, G., & Bachy, C.M. (2002). Preclinical studies on the radioprotective efficacy and pharmacokinetics of subcutaneously administered amifostine. *Seminars in Oncology, 29*(6, Suppl. 19), 2–8. doi:10.1016/S0093-7754(02)70002-X

Citrin, D., Cotrim, A.P., Hyodo, F., Baum, B.J., Krishna, M.C., & Mitchell, J.B. (2010). Radioprotectors and mitigators of radiation-induced normal tissue injury. *Oncologist, 15*, 360–371. doi:10.1634/theoncologist.2009-S104

Daly, C., Holloway, D., & Ameen, D. (2003). Subcutaneous administration of amifostine during radiotherapy: A clinical perspective [Abstract 3154]. *Proceedings of the American Society of Clinical Oncology, 22*. Retrieved from http://www.asco.org/ASCOv2/Meetings/Abstracts?&vmview=abst_detail_view&confID=23&abstractID=103144

Fazenbaker, C.A., Bachy, C.M., Kifle, G., & Cassatt, D.R. (2003). Dose and schedule dependency of amifostine protection against hyperfractionated radiotherapy in a rat model [Abstract 2083]. *Proceedings of the American Society of Clinical Oncology, 22*. Retrieved from http://www.asco.org/ASCOv2/Meetings/Abstracts?&vmview=abst_detail_view&confID=23&abstractID=102979

Gopal, R., Tucker, S.L., Komaki, R., Liao, Z., Forster, K.M., Stevens, C., ... Starkschall, G. (2003). The relationship between local dose and loss of function for irradiated lung. *International Journal of Radiation Oncology, Biology, Physics, 56*, 106–113. doi:10.1016/S0360-3016(03)00094-4

Jatoi, A., & Thomas, C.R., Jr. (2002). Esophageal cancer and the esophagus: Challenges and potential strategies for selective cytoprotection of the tumor-bearing organ during cancer treatment. *Seminars in Radiation Oncology, 12*(1, Suppl. 1), 62–67. doi:10.1053/srao.2002.31376

Kam, M.K., Leung, S.F., Zee, B., Chau, R.M., Suen, J.J., Mo, F., ... Chan, A.T. (2007). Prospective randomized study of intensity-modulated radiotherapy on salivary gland function in early-stage nasopharyngeal carcinoma patients. *Journal of Clinical Oncology, 25*, 4873–4879. doi:10.1200/JCO.2007.11.5501

Komaki, R., Lee, J.S., Kaplan, B., Allen, P., Kelly, J.F., Liao, Z., ... Cox, J.D. (2002). Randomized phase III study of chemoradiation with or without amifostine for patients with favorable performance status inoperable stage II–III non-small cell lung cancer: Preliminary results. *Seminars in Radiation Oncology, 12*(Suppl. 1), 46–49. doi:10.1053/srao.2002.31363

Koukourakis, M.I., Kyrias, G., Kakolyris, S., Kouroussis, C., Frangiadaki, C., Giatromanolaki, A., ... Georgoulias, V. (2000). Subcutaneous administration of amifostine during fractionated radiotherapy: A randomized phase II study. *Journal of Clinical Oncology, 18*, 2226–2233.

Koukourakis, M.I., Tsoutsou, P.G., Karpouzis, A., Tsiarkatsi, M., Karapantzos, I., Daniilidis, V., & Kouskoukis, C. (2010). Radiochemotherapy with cetuximab, cisplatin, and amifostine for locally advanced head and neck cancer: A feasibility study. *International Journal of Radiation Oncology, Biology, Physics, 77*, 9–15. doi:10.1016/j.ijrobp.2009.04.060

Kouvaris, J.R., Kouloulias, V.E., & Vlahos, L.J. (2007). Amifostine: The first selective-target and broad-spectrum radioprotector. *Oncologist, 12*, 738–747. doi:10.1634/theoncologist.12-6-738

Kushi, L.H., Byers, T., Doyle, C., Bandera, E.V., McCullough, M., McTiernan, A., ... Thun, M.J. (2006). American Cancer Society Guidelines on Nutrition and Physical Activity for cancer prevention: Reducing the risk of cancer with healthy food choices and physical activity. *CA: A Cancer Journal for Clinicians, 56*, 254–281. doi:10.3322/canjclin.56.5.254

Leong, S.S., Tan, E.H., Fong, K.W., Ong, Y.K., Ang, P.T., Wilder-Smith, E., & Lim, S.H. (2001). Randomized double-blind study of combined modality treatment with or without amifostine in unresectable stage III non-small cell lung cancer (NSCLC) [Abstract 1310]. *Proceedings of the American Society of Clinical Oncology, 20*. Retrieved from http://www.asco.org/ASCOv2/Meetings/Abstracts?&vmview=abst_detail_view&confID=10&abstractID=1310

Logan, R.M. (2009). Advances in understanding of toxicities in treatment for head and neck cancer. *Oral Oncology, 45*, 844–848. doi:10.1016/j.oraloncology.2009.03.018

MedImmune, LLC. (2010). *Ethyol®* [Package insert]. Retrieved from http://www.ethyol.com/resources/pdf/Ethyol-PI.pdf

Movsas, B., Scott, C., Langer, C., Werner-Wasik, M., Nicolaou, N., Komaki, R., ... Byhardt, R. (2005). Randomized trial of amifostine in locally advanced non-small-cell lung cancer patients receiving chemotherapy and hyperfractionated radiation: Radiation Therapy Oncology Group 98-01. *Journal of Clinical Oncology, 23,* 2145–2154. doi:10.1200/JCO.2005.07.167

National Cancer Institute. (2010, June 3). Fact sheet: Radiation therapy for cancer. Retrieved from http://www.cancer.gov/cancertopics/factsheet/Therapy/radiation

Pfizer Inc. (2011). *Zinecard®* [Package insert]. New York, NY: Author.

Ribeiro, K.C., Kowalski, L.P., & Latorre, M.R. (2000). Impact of comorbidity, symptoms, and patients' characteristics on the prognosis of oral carcinomas. *Archives of Otolaryngology—Head and Neck Surgery, 126,* 1079–1085.

Rosenthal, D.I. (2006). Established and emerging uses of cytoprotection in head and neck cancer [Editorial]. *Archives of Otolaryngology—Head Neck Surgery, 132,* 129–130.

Rosenthal, D.I., & Trotti, A. (2009). Strategies for managing radiation-induced mucositis in head and neck cancer. *Seminars in Radiation Oncology, 19,* 29–34. doi:10.1016/j.semradonc.2008.09.006

Samuels, M.A. (2004). Cytoprotection in head and neck cancer: Issues in oral care. *Journal of Supportive Oncology, 2*(6, Suppl. 3), 9–12.

Schuchter, L.M., Hensley, M.L., Meropol, N.J., & Winer, E.P. (2002). 2002 update of recommendations for the use of chemotherapy and radiotherapy protectants: Clinical practice guidelines of the American Society of Clinical Oncology. *Journal of Clinical Oncology, 20,* 2895–2903. doi:10.1200/JCO.2002.04.178

Thorstad, W.L., Chao, K.S.C., & Haughey, B. (2004). Toxicity and compliance of subcutaneous amifostine in patients undergoing postoperative intensity-modulated radiation therapy for head and neck cancer. *Seminars in Oncology, 31*(Suppl. 18), 8–12.

Trotti, A. (2000). Toxicity in head and neck cancer: A review of trends and issues. *International Journal of Radiation Oncology, Biology, Physics, 47,* 1–12. doi:10.1016/S0360-3016(99)00558-1

U.S. Pharmacopeia. (2002). *Amifostine, finalized drug information.* Rockville, MD: Author.

Vissink, A., Jansma, J., Spijkervet, F.K.L., Burlage, F.R., & Coppes, R.P. (2003). Oral sequelae of head and neck radiotherapy. *Critical Reviews in Oral Biology and Medicine, 14,* 199–212. doi:10.1177/154411130301400305

Wagner, W., Radmard, A., & Schönekaes, K.G. (1999). A new administration schedule for amifostine as a radioprotector in cancer therapy. *Anticancer Research, 19,* 2281–2283.

Wang, R., Kagan, R.A., & Tome, M.A. (2003). Subcutaneous (SQ) amifostine (A) is safe and effective in the treatment of head and neck cancers [Abstract 2065]. *Proceedings of the American Society of Clinical Oncology, 22.* Retrieved from http://www.asco.org/ASCOv2/Meetings/Abstracts?&vmview=abst_detail_view&confID=23&abstractID=100174

Wasserman, T., Mackowiak, J.I., Brizel, D.M., Oster, W., Zhang, J., Peeples, P.J., & Sauer, R. (2000). Effect of amifostine on patient assessed clinical benefit in irradiated head and neck cancer. *International Journal of Radiation Oncology, Biology, Physics, 48,* 1035–1039. doi:10.1016/S0360-3016(00)00735-5

Werner-Wasik, M., Axelrod, R.S., Friedland, D.P., Hauck, W., Rose, L.J., Chapman, A.E., ... Curran, W.J. (2001). Preliminary report on reduction of esophagitis by amifostine in patients with non–small-cell lung cancer treated with chemoradiotherapy. *Clinical Lung Cancer, 2,* 284–289. doi:10.3816/CLC.2001.n.011

B. Radiosensitizers and concurrent chemotherapy and biotherapy
   1. Radiosensitizers
      a) Definition: *Radiosensitizers* are chemical or pharmacologic agents that increase radiation damage to sensitive cells when given concurrently with radiation (Wilkes & Barton-Burke, 2011).
      b) Rationale: To enhance damage to tumor cells while minimizing normal tissue toxicity (Bryer, 2001)
      c) Types of radiosensitizers
         (1) Hypoxic cell sensitizers, such as nitroimidazoles, misonidazole, etanidazole, and nimorazole, can make hypoxic cells sensitive to damage from radiation by acting like oxygen in the chemical reactions occurring after RT treatment (Wilkes & Barton-Burke, 2011).
         (2) Nonhypoxic cell sensitizers, such as bromodeoxyuridine and iododeoxyuridine, are incorporated into the DNA of rapidly dividing tumor cells, thus increasing sensitivity to RT (Bryer, 2001; Wilkes & Barton-Burke, 2011).
         (3) Chemotherapy agents, such as fluoropyrimidines (5-FU), taxanes (docetaxel, paclitaxel), platinum agents (such as carboplatin, cisplatin), etoposide (VP-16), gemcitabine hydrochloride, and bleomycin sulfate, are capable of radiosensitization and can be given either before RT or concurrently (Wilkes & Barton-Burke, 2011). Topoisomerase inhibitors, such as irinotecan hydrochloride and topotecan hydrochloride, have been used as radiosensitizing agents.
         (4) Molecular-targeted therapy agents are the newest compounds to be used as radiosensitizer agents, increasing the effectiveness of RT. EGFR agents such as cetuximab, oral EGFR agents, cyclooxygenase-2 inhibitor agents, and antiangiogenic agents have been studied in combination with RT in an effort to increase cell kill (Herrera, Vidal, Oza, Milosevic, & Fyles, 2008; Shannon & Williams, 2008).
   2. Concurrent chemotherapy
      a) Definition: Chemotherapy is given at the same time as RT, which provides more activity on tumor cells than either agent alone and with acceptable toxicity (Mierzwa, Nyati, Morgan, & Lawrence, 2010). Concurrent chemotherapy improves clinical results

compared to induction or adjuvant chemotherapy and RT (Mierzwa et al., 2010).

b) Rationale: To take advantage of the radiosensitizing effects of chemotherapy agents (Zaidi, Huddart, & Harrington, 2009) and improve locoregional tumor control with the goal of decreasing the possibility for distant metastases (Brizel & Esclamado, 2006; Gérard et al., 2003). Combined-modality therapy increases the effectiveness of RT or chemotherapy alone at tissue and cellular levels (Mierzwa et al., 2010). Radiation can affect vascular permeability, allowing enhanced drug delivery and increased drug concentration at the tissue level. At the cellular level, systemic therapies increase the sensitivity of RT by interfering with DNA repair mechanisms (Mierzwa et al., 2010).

c) Generally used for locally advanced or unresectable solid tumors and preoperatively (neoadjuvant) to reduce tumor size and make surgical resection possible (Mierzwa et al., 2010). Specific chemotherapy agents improve the effectiveness of RT in destruction of tumor cells while demonstrating nonoverlapping toxicities (Mierzwa et al., 2010). The most commonly treated cancers with this modality include the following.

(1) Head and neck cancer (platinum agents; taxanes)

(a) A retrospective study examined the results of 146 patients with nasopharyngeal cancer receiving concurrent chemoradiation with cisplatin. Although retrospective, the results demonstrated a markedly improved overall survival and progression-free survival (Kim et al., 2008). The results of concurrent chemoradiation compared to RT alone in nasopharyngeal cancer showed significant improvement in local control and survival with the combined-therapy approach in 190 consecutive patients receiving cisplatin and 5-FU (Venkitaraman, Ramanan, Vasanthan, & Sagar, 2009).

(b) Common regimens for chemotherapy combined with RT for head and neck cancer include doses of cisplatin of 100 mg/m^2 on days 1, 22, and 43 of RT or lower doses given in different schedules. The use of low-dose cisplatin has been studied and found to be feasible with lower acute and chronic toxicity (Wolff et al., 2009).

(2) Lung cancer (platinum agents)

(a) NSCLC: Several trials have validated the effectiveness of chemoradiation in patients with NSCLC using various agents, although cisplatin is the most commonly used agent (Curran et al., 2003; Fournel et al., 2005; Furuse et al., 1999). The American College of Clinical Pharmacy evidence-based clinical practice guidelines call for chemoradiation for selected patients with stage IIIB disease but not for patients with stage IIIB NSCLC as a result of N3 disease (Jett, Schild, Keith, & Kesler, 2007). Patients with significant comorbidities and of older age often are not eligible for concurrent chemoradiation. De Ruysscher et al. (2009) determined that less toxic alternatives are needed for this group of patients, as in one study, more than half of patients with stage III lung cancer were ineligible for the combined treatment.

(b) SCLC: The current recommended therapy for patients with limited-stage disease includes cisplatin and etoposide plus thoracic RT. Response rates of 70%–90% have been noted in this group of patients (NCCN, 2011c). RT is usually started on chemotherapy cycle 1 or 2, with concurrent chemoradiation preferred compared to sequential (in patients fit to receive therapy) (NCCN, 2011c).

(3) GI cancers—esophagus, gastric, colorectal (gemcitabine, platinum agents, 5-FU, oxaliplatin)

(a) Rectal cancer: Standard therapy for select patients with rectal cancer includes 5-FU–based chemotherapy delivered concurrently with RT

(Glynne-Jones & Harrison, 2007; NCCN, 2011b).

(b) Newer studies are exploring additional agents such as oxaliplatin and capecitabine in patients with rectal cancer with intriguing results (Gérard et al., 2010).

(4) Cervical cancer (platinum agents): In one recent trial, 57 patients with locally advanced cervical cancer who received concurrent chemoradiation with 5-FU and cisplatin were followed for 53 months; the overall response rate was 91.5% with a five-year overall survival and three-year progression-free survival of 69.4% and 74.9%, respectively (Choi et al., 2008). The treatment was effective and well tolerated. This treatment is considered standard therapy for appropriate patients with cervical cancer.

(5) Pancreatic cancer (5-FU, gemcitabine)

(a) Chemoradiation is considered an option for the management of unresectable locoregional pancreatic cancer (NCCN, 2011a). The use of 5-FU with split-course RT was found to be more effective than RT alone (Moertel et al., 1981), with an early twofold increase in median survival (42.2 weeks versus 22.9 weeks) (Boz et al., 2006).

(b) The current recommendation for combined-modality therapy for this tumor type is upfront fluoropyrimidine (continuous infusion 5-FU or capecitabine)–based chemoradiation for locally advanced disease in select patients followed by additional maintenance chemotherapy in some patients. Recommended adjuvant therapy should be upfront fluoropyrimidine (bolus 5-FU or capecitabine)–based or gemcitabine-based chemoradiation followed by maintenance therapy or gemcitabine or continuous infusion 5-FU followed by continuous infusion 5-FU/RT followed by maintenance therapy. Additional options may include chemotherapy alone or RT alone (for palliative therapy) (NCCN, 2011a). For patients able to receive neoadjuvant therapy, a combination of upfront fluoropyrimidine (continuous infusion 5-FU or capecitabine)–

based chemoradiation or upfront gemcitabine-based chemoradiation may be considered (NCCN, 2011a).

(6) High-grade glioma, brain metastases (temozolomide): Stupp et al. (2005) demonstrated the benefit of temozolomide added to RT for newly diagnosed glioblastoma in a trial of 573 patients randomized to combined therapy or RT alone. The two-year survival rate for the combined therapy was 26.5% versus 10.4% for RT alone.

3. Concurrent biotherapy

a) Definition: Biotherapy agents are given at the same time as RT, increasing the effectiveness of RT versus RT alone, with acceptable toxicity and with the goal of improving control of locoregional disease and improving survival (Bonner et al., 2006).

(1) Epidermal growth factor receptor inhibitor (EGFRI) agents are now approved in the combined-modality treatment of head and neck cancers and are being studied in other tumor types.

(a) Mechanism of action: EGFR is abnormally activated in epithelial cancers, and almost all cells of these neoplasms (including head and neck) have high levels of the receptor, with tumors displaying poor outcomes (Bonner et al., 2006). Radiation treatment increases EGFR expression (Bonner et al., 2006). This increased expression of EGFR is thought to increase the radioresistance of cancer cells; therefore, using an EGFRI agent can block the EGFR signaling, enhancing the radiosensitivity of the cells (Bonner et al., 2006; Karar & Maity, 2009).

i. Based on the pivotal trial by Bonner et al. (2006), the FDA approved the EGFR agent cetuximab in 2006. In this randomized phase III trial of 211 patients receiving the combined therapy compared to 213 patients receiving RT alone, the combined-therapy group had a median duration of locoregional control of 24.4 months versus 14.9 months for the RT-alone patients (Bonner et al., 2006). Patients receiving the combined therapy had a significantly reduced mortality as well; common toxic effects associated with RT to the head and neck were not increased.

ii. Phase II studies in NSCLC have shown that cetuximab with concurrent RT can be safe without leading to higher rates of acute treatment toxicities (Mierzwa et al., 2010). Ongoing research in this area should further define the role of cetuximab and RT in this tumor type.

iii. Research with cetuximab, gemcitabine, and RT in the treatment of pancreatic cancer has been published; results did not show a significant difference in patient survival, which may be because RAS (part of the cell signaling pathway involved in EGFR signaling) is mutated in more than 90% of patients with pancreatic cancer (Mierzwa et al., 2010).

(b) Small-molecule tyrosine kinase inhibitor agents inhibit unregulated EGFR and have been studied in combination with chemotherapy and RT. Results with gefitinib have been variable and appear to be dependent on the schedule of administration (Mierzwa et al., 2010).

i. In head and neck cancer, adding gefitinib in combination with RT and docetaxel (after induction therapy with carboplatin, docetaxel, and 5-FU) produced a moderate increase in toxicity and similar efficacy to other chemoradiation trials (Hainsworth et al., 2009).

ii. Reports exist from phase I and II trials of gefitinib and erlotinib in combination with RT and other chemotherapy agents in the treatment of NSCLC, gliomas, and esophageal and pancreatic cancer. Further research is needed to refine the role of oral tyrosine kinase inhibitor agents in the treatment of these and other solid tumor types (Mierzwa et al., 2010).

(2) Antiangiogenesis agents offer another treatment strategy for several tumor types, including colorectal and breast cancer.

(a) Mechanism of action: Antiangiogenesis agents are important in the prevention of the formation of new blood vessels critical to continued tumor growth and metastasis (Wilkes & Barton-Burke, 2011). Tumors expressing vascular endothelial growth factor tend to be more aggressive and more likely to metastasize and thus present an intriguing target for cancer therapy (Wilkes & Barton-Burke, 2011).

(b) Combining these therapies with radiation has been a target of research over several years. It has been theorized that an angiogenesis inhibitor would affect the efficacy of ionizing radiation by inducing tumor hypoxia (O'Reilly, 2007). Vascular endothelial growth factor and platelet-derived growth factor inhibition reduces cell signaling integral to tumor growth; adding radiation enhances the effect (Timke et al., 2008).

i. Early-phase studies with bevacizumab and temozolomide with concurrent RT in the treatment of patients with glioblastoma have shown that the regimen is tolerated well and does not produce significantly higher toxicity rates (Kirkpatrick, Desjardins, Reardon, & Vredenburgh, 2008).

ii. Phase I and II studies of bevacizumab in combination with capecitabine followed by maintenance chemotherapy and bevacizumab have been published with similar survival results to other combined-modality studies in pancreatic cancer (Crane et al., 2009).

iii. Additional tumor types under study with antiangiogenesis agents include colon and rectal cancers, NSCLC, prostate cancer, cervical cancer, and sarcoma (Zaidi et al., 2009). These ongoing studies will continue to explore various angiogenesis inhibitor drugs in combination with RT. Further research will help to define the combined-modality approach with these agents.

(3) Immunotherapy agents act to enhance the immune system's ability to kill tumor cells (Stevens, 2003).

(a) Immunotherapy agents include vaccines made from the tumor cells of patients, which improve the ability of the immune system to identify, target, and destroy similar tumor cells (Stevens, 2003).

(b) Radiation may help to alter tumor cell environment, making the cells more susceptible to immune-mediated killing (Ferrara, Hodge, & Gulley, 2009).

(4) Nursing considerations: Radiation nurses face increasing responsibilities in caring for patients receiving concurrent therapies. Although the nurses may not be primarily responsible for the administration of some of these additional chemotherapy and biotherapy treatments, the enhanced side effects in these patients can be challenging.

(a) Incorporating new information into clinical practice related to new RT techniques, new agents, and genetic and molecular therapies

(b) Serving as a resource for RT staff regarding concurrent therapies, schedules, and patient assessment

(c) Serving as a liaison to medical oncology and collaborating with nuclear medicine and other departments or offices regarding treatment schedules, laboratory work, side effect management, and follow-up to ensure that patients receive follow-up care as appropriate

(d) Monitoring patients receiving concurrent therapy: Although most chemotherapy agents are given in lower systemic doses than if given alone, concomitant side effects can be severe and may necessitate treatment interruptions (Mierzwa et al., 2010; Wilkes & Barton-Burke, 2011).

i. Bone marrow suppression: Almost all chemotherapy agents, especially taxanes, gemcitabine, carboplatin, and mitomycin

ii. GI effects (nausea and vomiting, diarrhea, anorexia): Taxanes, platinum compounds

iii. Stomatitis: Taxanes, fluorouracil

iv. Peripheral neuropathies: Platinum compounds, taxanes

v. Esophagitis: Cisplatin with etoposide and RT

vi. Dermatologic: Cetuximab, as an EGFRI agent, interferes with normal growth and differentiation of skin cells (keratinocytes), causing a characteristic EGFRI rash (Wilkes & Barton-Burke, 2011).

• With patients with head and neck cancer who are receiving concurrent RT and EGFRI therapy, rash occurs in most patients (Viale, Haas, & Lacouture, 2010).

• Initial reports from the pivotal clinical trials noted the presence of the EGFRI rash but no significant increase in radiation dermatitis. Subsequent reports have demonstrated enhanced skin toxicity in select patients with combined-modality treatment. Data showed that the summary incidence of high-grade radiation dermatitis in patients receiving combined-modality treatment was 31.3%, with rash in 16.1% and mucositis in 52.7% (Tejwani et al., 2009).

• Suggested management strategies include topical moisturizers, antibiotics, and steroids for in-field dermatitis, consideration of systemic doxycycline, and, for patients with grade 3–4 toxicity, interruption of therapy or possibly discontinuing the EGFRI agent (Viale et al., 2010). Patients should be given the same information and cautions as those receiving chemotherapy or RT alone.

References

Bonner, J.A., Harari, P.M., Giralt, J., Azarnia, N., Shin, D.M., Cohen, R.B., ... Ang, K.K. (2006). Radiotherapy plus cetuximab for squamous-cell carcinoma of the head and neck. *New England Journal of Medicine, 354*, 567–578. doi:10.1056/NEJMoa053422

Boz, G., De Paoli, A., Innocente, R., Rossi, C., Tosolini, G.C., Bassi, C., ... Trovò, M.G. (2006). Radiotherapy and chemotherapy in pancreatic cancer. Topical issues and future perspectives. *Journal of the Pancreas, 7*, 122–130.

Brizel, D.M., & Esclamado, R. (2006). Concurrent chemoradiotherapy for locally advanced, nonmetastatic, squamous carcinoma of the head and neck: Consensus, controversy, and conundrum. *Journal of Clinical Oncology, 24*, 2612–2617. doi:10.1200/JCO.2005.05.2829

Bryer, M.P. (2001). Combined modality therapy. In M.C. Perry (Ed.), *The chemotherapy source book* (3rd ed., pp. 73–81). Philadelphia, PA: Lippincott Williams & Wilkins.

Choi, I.J., Cha, M.S., Park, E.S., Han, M.S., Choi, Y., Je, G.H., & Kim, H.H. (2008). The efficacy of concurrent cisplatin and 5-flurouracil chemotherapy and radiation therapy for locally advanced cancer of the uterine cervix. *Journal of Gynecologic Oncology, 19*, 129–134. doi:10.3802/jgo.2008.19.2.129

Crane, C.H., Winter, K., Regine, W.F., Safran, H., Rich, T.A., Curran, W., ... Willet, C.G. (2009). Phase II study of bevacizumab with concurrent capecitabine and radiation followed by maintenance gemcitabine and bevacizumab for locally advanced pancreatic cancer: Radiation Therapy Oncology Group RTOG 0411. *Journal of Clinical Oncology, 27*, 4096–4102. doi:10.1200/JCO.2009.21.8529

Curran, W.J., Scott, C.B., Langer, C.J., Komaki, R., Lee, J.S., Hauser, S., ... Cox, J.D. (2003). Long-term benefit is observed in a phase III comparison of sequential vs concurrent chemo-radiation for patients with unresected stage III NSCLC: RTOG 9410 [Abstract 2499]. *Proceedings of the American Society of Clinical Oncology, 22*, 621.

De Ruysscher, D., Botterweck, A., Dirx, M., Pijls-Johannesma, M., Wanders, R., Hochstenbag, M., ... Lambin, P. (2009). Eligibility for concurrent chemotherapy and radiotherapy of locally advanced lung cancer patients: A prospective, population-based study. *Annals of Oncology, 20*, 98–102. doi:10.1093/annonc/mdn559

Ferrara, T.A., Hodge, J.W., & Gulley, J.L. (2009). Combining radiation and immunotherapy for synergistic antitumor therapy. *Current Opinion in Molecular Therapeutics, 11*, 37–42.

Fournel, P., Robinet, G., Thomas, P., Souquet, P.-J., Léna, H., Vergnenégre, A., ... Pérol, M. (2005). Randomized phase III trial of sequential chemoradiotherapy compared with concurrent chemoradiotherapy in locally advanced non–small-cell lung cancer: Groupe

Lyon-Saint-Etienne d'Oncologie Thoracique–Groupe Français de Pneumo-Cancérologie NPC 95-01 Study. *Journal of Clinical Oncology, 23*, 5910–5917. doi:10.1200/JCO.2005.03.070

Furuse, K., Fukuoka, M., Kawahara, M., Nishikawa, H., Takada, Y., Kudoh, S., ... Ariyoshi, Y. (1999). Phase III study of concurrent versus sequential thoracic radiotherapy in combination with mitomycin, vindesine, and cisplatin in unresectable stage III non–small cell lung cancer. *Journal of Clinical Oncology, 17*, 2692–2699.

Gérard, J.P., Azria, D., Gourgou-Bourgade, S., Martel-Laffay, I., Hennequin, C., Etienne, P.L., ... Conroy, T. (2010). Comparison of two neoadjuvant regimens for locally advanced rectal cancer: Results of the phase III trial ACCORD 12/0405-Prodige 2. *Journal of Clinical Oncology, 28*, 1638–1644. doi:10.1200/JCO.2009.25.8376

Gérard, J.P., Chapet, O., Nemoz, C., Romestaing, P., Mornex, F., Coquard, R., ... Freyer, G. (2003). Preoperative concurrent chemoradiotherapy in locally advanced rectal cancer with high-dose radiation and oxaliplatin-containing regimen: The Lyon R0-04 phase II trial. *Journal of Clinical Oncology, 21*, 1119–1124. doi:10.1200/JCO.2003.10.045

Glynne-Jones, R., & Harrison, M. (2007). Locally advanced rectal cancer: What is the evidence for induction chemoradiation? *Oncologist, 12*, 1309–1318. doi:10.1634/theoncologist.12-11-1309

Hainsworth, J.D., Spigel, D.R., Burris, H.A., III, Markus, T.M., Shipley, D., Kuzur, M., ... Greco, F.A. (2009). Neoadjuvant chemotherapy/gefitinib followed by concurrent chemotherapy/radiation therapy/gefitinib for patients with locally advanced squamous carcinoma of the head and neck. *Cancer, 115*, 2138–2146. doi:10.1002/cncr.24265

Herrera, F.G., Vidal, L., Oza, A., Milosevic, M., & Fyles, A. (2008). Molecular targeted agents combined with chemo-radiation in the treatment of locally advanced cervical cancer. *Reviews on Recent Clinical Trials, 3*, 111–120.

Jett, J.R., Schild, S.E., Keith, R.L., & Kesler, K.A. (2007). Treatment of non-small cell lung cancer, stage IIIB: ACCP evidence-based clinical practice guidelines (2nd edition). *Chest, 132*(Suppl. 3), 266S–276S. doi:10.1378/chest.07-1380

Karar, J., & Maity, A. (2009). Modulating the tumor microenvironment to increase radiation responsiveness. *Cancer Biology and Therapy, 8*, 1994–2001. doi:10.4161/cbt.8.21.9988

Kim, Y.-S., Kim, B.-S., Jung, S.-L., Lee, Y.-S., Kim, M.-S., Sun, D.-I., ... Kang, J.-H. (2008). Radiation therapy combined with (or without) cisplatin-based chemotherapy for patients with nasopharyngeal cancer: 15-years experience of a single institution in Korea. *Cancer Research and Treatment, 40*, 155–163. doi:10.4143/crt.2008.40.4.155

Kirkpatrick, J.P., Desjardins, A., Reardon, D.A., & Vredenburgh, J.J. (2008). Radiotherapy, temozolomide, and bevacizumab followed by irinotecan, temozolomide, and bevacizumab in newly diagnosed glioblastoma multiforme: Preliminary results from an ongoing phase II trial [Abstract 2089]. *International Journal of Radiation Oncology, Biology, Physics, 72*(1, Suppl. 1), S209. doi:10.1016/j.ijrobp.2008.06.1537

Mierzwa, M.L., Nyati, M.K., Morgan, M.A., & Lawrence, T.S. (2010). Recent advances in combined modality therapy. *Oncologist, 15*, 372–381. doi:10.1634/theoncologist.2009-S105

Moertel, C.G., Frytak, S., Hahn, R.G., O'Connell, M.J., Reitemeier, R.J., Rubin, J., ... Novak, J.W. (1981). Therapy of locally unresectable pancreatic carcinoma: A randomized comparison of high dose (6000 rads) radiation alone, moderate dose radiation

(4000 rads + 5-fluorouracil), and high dose radiation + 5-fluo-rouracil. The Gastrointestinal Tumor Study Group. *Cancer, 48,* 1705–1710. doi:10.1002/1097-0142(19811015)48:8<1705::AID -CNCR2820480803>3.0.CO;2-4

National Comprehensive Cancer Network. (2011a). *NCCN Clinical Practice Guidelines in Oncology: Pancreatic adenocarcinoma* [v.2.2011]. Retrieved from http://www.nccn.org/professionals/ physician_gls/PDF/pancreatic.pdf

National Comprehensive Cancer Network. (2011b). *NCCN Clinical Practice Guidelines in Oncology: Rectal cancer* [v.4.2011]. Retrieved from http://www.nccn.org/professionals/physician_ gls/pdf/rectal.pdf

National Comprehensive Cancer Network. (2011c). *NCCN Clinical Practice Guidelines in Oncology: Small cell lung cancer* [v.2.2011]. Retrieved from http://www.nccn.org/professionals/ physician_gls/PDF/sclc.pdf

O'Reilly, M.S. (2007). Antiangiogenesis and vascular endothelial growth factor/vascular endothelial growth factor receptor tar-geting as part of a combined-modality approach to the treat-ment of cancer. *International Journal of Radiation Oncology, Biology, Physics, 69*(2, Suppl. 1), S64–S66. doi:10.1016/j. ijrobp.2007.04.093

Shannon, A.M., & Williams, K.J. (2008). Antiangiogenics and ra-diotherapy. *Journal of Pharmacy and Pharmacology, 60,* 1029–1036. doi:10.1211/jpp.60.8.0009

Stevens, C.W. (2003). Clinical applications of new modalities. In J.D. Cox & K.K. Ang (Eds.), *Radiation oncology: Rationale, tech-nique, results* (8th ed., pp. 987–1002). St. Louis, MO: Mosby.

Stupp, R., Mason, W.P., van den Bent, M.J., Weller, M., Fisher, B., Taphoorn, M.J.B., ... Mirimanoff, R.O. (2005). Radiotherapy plus concomitant and adjuvant temozolomide for glioblastoma. *New England Journal of Medicine, 352,* 987–996. doi:10.1056/ NEJMoa043330

Tejwani, A., Wu, S., Jia, Y., Agulnik, M., Millender, L., & Lacouture, M.E. (2009). Increased risk of high-grade dermatologic toxici-ties with radiation plus epidermal growth factor receptor inhib-itor therapy. *Cancer, 115,* 1286–1299. doi:10.1002/cncr.24120

Timke, C., Zieher, H., Roth, A., Hauser, K., Lipson, K.E., Weber, K.J., ... Huber, P.E. (2008). Combination of vascular endothe-lial growth factor receptor/platelet-derived growth factor re-ceptor inhibition markedly improves radiation tumor therapy. *Clinical Cancer Research, 14,* 2210–2219. doi:10.1158/1078 -0432.CCR-07-1893

Venkitaraman, R., Ramanan, S.G., Vasanthan, A., & Sagar, T.G. (2009). Results of combined modality treatment for nasopha-ryngeal cancer. *Journal of Cancer Research and Therapeutics, 5,* 102–106. doi:10.4103/0973-1482.52798

Viale, P.H., Haas, M.L., & Lacouture, M.E. (2010). Epidermal growth factor receptor inhibitors and radiation therapy in head and neck cancer: Potential management strategies for skin reactions. *Journal of the Advanced Practitioner in Oncology, 1,* 75–86.

Wilkes, G.M., & Barton-Burke, M. (2011). *2010 oncology nursing drug handbook.* Sudbury, MA: Jones and Bartlett.

Wolff, H.A., Overbeck, T., Roedel, R.M., Hermann, R.M., Herrmann, M.K.A., Kertesz, T., ... Christiansen, H. (2009). Toxicity of daily low dose cisplatin in radiochemotherapy for locally advanced head and neck cancer. *Journal of Cancer Research and Clinical Oncology, 135,* 961–967. doi:10.1007/ s00432-008-0532-x

Zaidi, S.H., Huddart, R.A., & Harrington, K.J. (2009). Novel target-ed radiosensitisers in cancer treatment. *Current Drug Discovery Technologies, 6,* 103–134.

C. Radioimmunotherapy and radiopharmaceuticals
   1. Radioimmunotherapy (radioimmunoconjugate treatment)
      a) Definition: *Radioimmunotherapy* is the administration of radionuclides chemical-ly conjugated to antibodies. The antibod-ies can recognize and bind to antigens on tumor cells and serve as carriers of the ra-dionuclide to the tumor cells (Robinson, Borghaei, Adams, & Weiner, 2008). These products are also called *radiopharmaceu-ticals* (Temple, 2007).
      b) Rationale
         (1) *Chimeric* monoclonal antibodies are mouse-human hybrids synthesized in laboratories by humanizing *murine* antibodies (derived from mouse ami-no acid) with normal human immuno-globulin genes. The hybridization of these antibodies seeks to prevent the induction of antiglobulin human anti-mouse antibody (HAMA) response of the host immune system that had neu-tralized the therapeutic monoclonal an-tibodies. Chimeric, or humanized, an-tibodies also have a prolonged half-life in vivo and therefore increased potency as cytotoxic therapy (Dearden, 2007).
         (2) The chimeric monoclonal antibody is then bound (conjugated) to a radioac-tive isotope by a strong linking agent called a *chelator* (for example, in ibri-tumomab treatment, the chelator is tiuxetan) to deliver therapeutic radio-isotopes to produce tumor kill by a single cell mechanism. The therapeu-tic monoclonal antibody activates the host effector mechanisms on tumor-specific antigens, whereas the radio-isotope is able to deliver a cytotox-ic dose to the adjacent negative an-tigen cells (Dearden, 2007). This ad-ditional cytotoxicity is referred to as "crossfire" or "bystander" effect and has been shown to decrease toxicity to nontumor cells, therefore lessen-ing side effects of therapy (Dearden, 2007; Schaefer-Cutillo, Friedberg, & Fisher, 2007) (see Figure 29).
         (3) Cells adjacent to the antibody-binding cell will also be affected by the radi-ation that emits from the radiolabeled antibody (Hagenbeek & Lewington, 2005).
         (4) Radioimmunotherapy is used in com-bination with chemotherapy to enhance targeting of tumor cells and direct cell

Figure 29. The "Crossfire" Effect

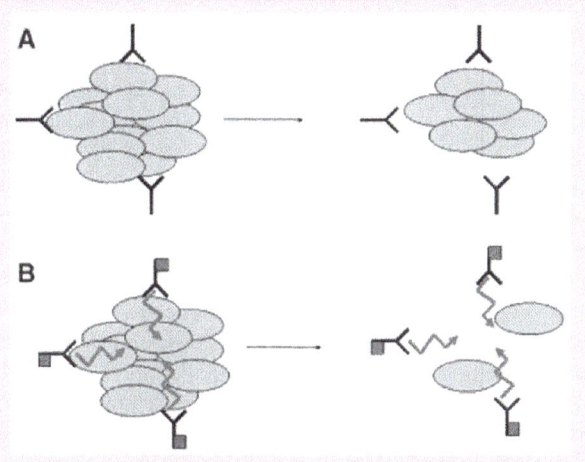

(A) Monoclonal antibody binding to cells on periphery of tumor with antibody-mediated cell death. (B) Antibody plus radioimmunotherapy: Red squares indicate radioimmunoconjugate. Antibody binds to periphery, with additional cytotoxicity mediated by radiotherapy-unbound cells via a "crossfire" (or "bystander") effect.

Note. From "Novel Concepts in Radioimmunotherapy for Non-Hodgkin's Lymphoma," by J. Schaefer-Cutillo, J.W. Friedberg, and R.I. Fisher, 2007, *Oncology, 21*, p. 204. Copyright 2007 by UBM Medica, LLC. Reprinted with permission.

kill with cross-reactivity (Dearden, 2007; Schaefer-Cutillo et al., 2007) (see Figure 29).

c) Contraindications
   (1) Patients should not receive the regimens if they have more than 25% marrow involvement with lymphoma or impaired bone marrow reserve because of the increased potential for hematologic toxicities (Spectrum Pharmaceuticals, Inc., 2010).
   (2) Dosing modifications must be made per manufacturer inserts if platelet counts are less than or equal to 150,000/mm³; platelets must be greater than 100,000/mm³.
   (3) Type I sensitivity is the production of HAMA to murine components of the monoclonal antibody. The number of patients who develop HAMA has been very low (1.3%, 6/446 in 8 studies reported with ibritumomab tiuxetan therapy), and the development of antibody after treatment was most often transient and did not increase with time (Spectrum Pharmaceuticals, Inc., 2010).

d) Pretreatment tests (GlaxoSmithKline, 2005; Spectrum Pharmaceuticals, Inc., 2010)
   (1) Bilateral bone marrow biopsy and aspiration to determine the extent of lymphoma present in the bone marrow
   (2) Complete blood count with platelets
   (3) Hepatitis B surface antigen and hepatitis B core antibody testing in all patients prior to rituximab therapy (NCCN, 2011)

e) Treatment regimen for radioimmunotherapy: Dosing guidelines are based on the patient's weight and platelet count (GlaxoSmithKline, 2005; Spectrum Pharmaceuticals, Inc., 2010).

f) Types: Two radionuclides used for radioimmunotherapy regimens are ^{131}I and ^{90}Y (Kersten, 2011).
   (1) ^{90}Y has a long path length, high-energy beta emissions, lack of volatility, and ease and safety with its conjugation to antibodies and patient administration (Robinson et al., 2008).
      (a) Ibritumomab tiuxetan (Zevalin®, Spectrum Pharmaceuticals, Inc.) is indicated for patients with previously untreated follicular NHL who achieve a partial or complete response to first-line chemotherapy and relapsed or refractory, low-grade or follicular B-cell NHL (Spectrum Pharmaceuticals, Inc., 2010).
      (b) Ibritumomab is a murine monoclonal antibody that specifically targets the CD20 antigen found on 95% of B-cell lymphomas (Spectrum Pharmaceuticals, Inc., 2010). It forms a covalent bond to tiuxetan, which is a high-affinity chelator (binder) to the radioactive isotopes ^{90}Y and ^{111}In (Spectrum Pharmaceuticals, Inc., 2010). The radioisotope used in the Zevalin therapeutic dose is ^{90}Y, and ^{111}In, a gamma emitter, is the radioisotope used in the biodistribution imaging dose of the Zevalin regimen. The compounds used in the Zevalin therapeutic regimen are known as ^{90}Y-radiolabeled Zevalin (^{90}Y-Zevalin) and ^{111}In-radiolabeled Zevalin (^{111}In-Zevalin) (Spectrum Pharmaceuticals, Inc., 2010).
      (c) The ibritumomab tiuxetan (Zevalin) therapeutic regimen has three main parts administered over seven to nine days on an outpatient basis (Spectrum Pharmaceuticals, Inc., 2010).

i. Imaging dose: Premedication plus rituximab plus ^{111}In-Zevalin

ii. Indium scan: Gamma camera scan to assess ^{111}In-Zevalin biodistribution in the body

iii. Therapeutic dose: Premedication plus rituximab plus ^{90}Y-Zevalin

(d) Administration (Spectrum Pharmaceuticals, Inc., 2010)

i. **Day 1:** Premedicate with acetaminophen 650 mg orally and diphenhydramine 50 mg orally prior to rituximab infusion.

ii. Rituximab 250 mg/m[2] IV at 50 mg/hr. Do not mix or dilute rituximab with other drugs. **Never administer by IV push or bolus.**

iii. If no reactions, increase by 50 mg/hr every 30 minutes to a maximum of 400 mg/hr.

iv. Temporarily slow or interrupt the rituximab infusion for less severe infusion reactions. If symptoms improve, continue the infusion at one-half the previous rate.

v. Administer 5 mCi ^{111}In-Zevalin calibrated and prepared by nuclear medicine/radiation physicist over 10 minutes as an IV injection within four hours following the rituximab infusion. Use a 0.22 micron low-protein-binding in-line filter between the syringe and the infusion port. After injection, flush the line with at least 10 ml of normal saline.

vi. **Indium scan:** First whole body camera image is taken 2–24 hours after the first dose was given to assess ^{111}In-Zevalin biodistribution in the body.

vii. Second whole body camera image is taken 48–72 hours later (optional).

viii. **Day 7, 8, or 9:** Premedicate with acetaminophen 650 mg orally and diphenhydramine 50 mg orally prior to rituximab infusion.

ix. Infuse rituximab 250 mg/m[2] IV at 100 mg/hr. Increase rate by 100 mg/hr increments every 30 minutes to a maximum rate of 400 mg/hr as tolerated. If the patient experienced a reaction to rituximab on day 1, administer at an initial rate of 50 mg/hr and escalate the infusion rate in 50 mg/hr increments every 30 minutes to a maximum of 400 mg/hr.

x. Within four hours of completion of rituximab infusion, the patient receives the ^{90}Y-Zevalin injection through a free-flowing IV line by a physician. Use a 0.22 micron low-protein-binding in-line filter between the syringe and the infusion port. After injection, flush the line with at least 10 ml of normal saline. Monitor the patient closely for signs of extravasation of ^{90}Y-Zevalin. If extravasation occurs, stop infusion immediately and restart in another limb.

xi. **Never administer more than 32 mCi ^{90}Y-Zevalin regardless of the patient's body weight.**

xii. See full prescribing information in package insert for dose determinations based on the patient's platelet count.

xiii. Acrylic shielding blocks beta emissions; absorbent pads are placed under infusion sites (Hendrix, 2004).

(e) Patient and family education (Spectrum Pharmaceuticals, Inc., 2010)

i. The patient should contact the doctor if signs or symptoms of reactions related to rituximab infusion develop within the first 24 hours. These would be the same as any allergic reaction, such as breathing difficulties, chest pain, and cardiac symptoms (Spectrum Pharmaceuticals, Inc., 2010).

ii. The patient should have weekly blood counts and contact the doctor if signs or symptoms of cytopenias develop, such as bleeding, easy bruising, pallor, petechiae (small red or purple spots) or pur-

pura (purple-colored patches), weakness, or fatigue (Spectrum Pharmaceuticals, Inc., 2010).

iii. The patient should avoid medications that interfere with platelet function such as aspirin and NSAIDs, except as the physician directs (Spectrum Pharmaceuticals, Inc., 2010).

iv. The patient should go to the emergency department if a diffuse rash, bullae (blisters greater than 5 mm in diameter containing clear fluid), or desquamation (peeling) of the skin or oral mucosa develops (Spectrum Pharmaceuticals, Inc., 2010).

v. The patient should immediately contact the doctor if signs or symptoms of infection develop, such as fever with cough or problems with urination. The patient may experience flu-like symptoms 12–24 hours after the infusion of ibritumomab tiuxetan (Spectrum Pharmaceuticals, Inc., 2010).

vi. No limits on activity are needed because radiation is low dose.

vii. The patient may have family contact.

viii. Family members and caregivers should avoid exposure to the patient's body fluids (vomit, urine, and stool) for 3 days (72 hours) after treatment. Contaminated materials used for cleaning should be flushed down the toilet or put in a plastic bag before being placed in household garbage (Spectrum Pharmaceuticals, Inc., 2010).

ix. The patient should use a condom during sexual relations for one week after treatment and should avoid pregnancy for 12 months after treatment with ibritumomab tiuxetan. Teratogenic effects (effects on a fetus) are not known (Spectrum Pharmaceuticals, Inc., 2010).

x. Nursing mothers should discontinue breast-feeding during and after treatment with ibritumomab tiuxetan. The effect of exposure to ibritumomab tiuxetan in infants is not known (Spectrum Pharmaceuticals, Inc., 2010).

xi. The patient should not receive a live viral vaccine within 12 months of ibritumomab tiuxetan treatment (Spectrum Pharmaceuticals, Inc., 2010).

(2) ^{131}I, a beta- and gamma-emitting radionuclide, has a relatively short average path length and enables both patient dose optimization and tumor cell kill with a single agent (Srinivasan & Mukherji, 2011).

(a) Tositumomab is indicated for the treatment of patients with CD20 antigen–expressing relapsed or refractory, low-grade, follicular, or transformed NHL, including patients with rituximab-refractory NHL.

(b) Tositumomab is a murine monoclonal antibody that is radiolabeled with ^{131}I. This antibody targets the CD20 antigen on the surface of mature B cells and B-cell tumors.

(c) Dosing (GlaxoSmithKline, 2005)

i. ^{131}I tositumomab requires thyroid blockage with potassium iodide taken orally to prevent uptake of radioactive iodine in the thyroid at least 24 hours prior to the dosimetric dose and for at least two weeks following the therapeutic dose (GlaxoSmithKline, 2005).

ii. Unlabeled tositumomab is given prior to the dosimetric labeled dose to protect the more easily accessible spleen and blood cells that share the same antigen as the tumor cells. The tumor cells are more difficult to access; therefore, theoretically, the labeled tositumomab will have an improved chance to attach and destroy the antigen-bearing tumor cells once the unlabeled has attached to the more easily accessed cells (Wahl, 2005).

iii. Three whole body gamma scans are performed to determine biodistribution and dosimetry of the radiation in the labeled dose.

(d) Administration (GlaxoSmith-Kline, 2005)

i. Oral potassium iodide supplements are administered beginning day 1 for 14 days after the infusion of the therapeutic ^{131}I dose.

ii. Patients are premedicated with acetaminophen and diphenhydramine.

iii. Tositumomab (unlabeled) 450 mg is given on day 0 over 60 minutes.

iv. A 5 mCi dosimetric dose of ^{131}I tositumomab (35 mg) is administered over 20 minutes.

v. The whole body gamma scan is completed on day 0.

vi. The patient usually returns for two subsequent whole body scans on days 2, 3, or 4 and 6 or 7.

vii. If the biodistribution (uptake and clearance of the labeled test dose) is acceptable as calculated by the scans and whole body dosimetries, the patient's therapeutic dose is calculated. If the platelets are between 100,000 and 150,000/mm^3, the dose is lowered. If the biodistribution is not acceptable, there is no administration of the therapeutic dose of [131]I.

viii. Between days 7 and 14, the patient will be given the therapeutic dose calculated on the patient-specific activity of [131]I.
- Patients are premedicated with acetaminophen and diphenhydramine.

- Tositumomab (unlabeled) 450 mg is given over 60 minutes.
- The prescribed therapeutic dose of ^{131}I tositumomab is administered over 20 minutes.

(e) Patient and family education are the same as those for any radiolabeled iodine treatment (Wahl, 2005). No national safety standards currently exist for using [131]I. Therefore, the American Thyroid Association has proposed the following recommendations when treating with [131]I (Sisson et al., 2011).

i. The patient should drive himself/herself to the treatment site in a private car.
- If the patient must be driven by another person, time and distance rules apply to minimize exposure to the nontreated person.
- If the person driving the patient is a member of the patient's household, the time in the car will limit the time at home with the patient after the procedure.
- The minimum distance separating the patient from the driver must be greater than three feet. It is advised that a large vehicle such as a passenger van or minivan is used for transportation of patients with longer drives.
- The patient should use the bathroom prior to leaving the facility and then frequently to prevent the accumulation of radiation in the bladder.

ii. The patient should wear scrubs during isolation to prevent risk of contamination of personal clothing going home. Personal care items should be disposable or disposed prior to discharge (Al-Shakhrah, 2008).

iii. The treatment room should be private and either lead lined or of thick concrete walls in a corner to minimize radiation exposure in the hallway or to adjacent rooms. The room should have a private bathroom attached (Al-Shakhrah, 2008).

iv. No visitors should be present during the infusion of ^{131}I, and visitors should be highly discouraged during the immediate time after the patient has been treated (Al-Shakhrah, 2008; Sisson et al., 2011).

v. The discharge of the patient after administration of labeled tositumomab must be carried out with specific guidelines, including patient-specific radiation safety instructions.

- The patient must be able to provide self-care for two weeks after the therapeutic infusion, or he or she may not be an appropriate candidate for tositumomab therapy.
- Radiation exposure of family members and caregivers who are close to the patient must be ALARA and within NRC limits.
- The following recommendations are of average durations and vary according to the clearance calculations of ^{131}I based on the scans of the patient (Al-Shakhrah, 2008; Sisson et al., 2011).
- Encourage the patient to drink fluids to assist in clearing ^{131}I from the urinary system.
- The patient should not take long trips (car, bus, plane, or train) sitting near others for at least four months after treatment with [131]I.
- The patient should limit contact closer than six feet with individuals and maximize distance from other individuals for a minimum of eight days.
- The patient must sleep in a separate bed with at least six feet of separation from the next person for 3–11

days (this recommendation is dose and clearance rate dependent).

- The patient must avoid sexual intercourse for one to five days after treatment (this recommendation is dose and clearance rate dependent).
- The patient should avoid contact with pregnant women, nursing mothers, infants, and young children for one to five days (Al-Shakhrah, 2008; Rao, Akabani, & Rizzieri, 2005; Sisson et al., 2011).

vi. Nursing mothers should cease breast-feeding or pumping breast milk six weeks prior to treatment with ^{131}I and delay resuming breast-feeding until three months after treatment to limit radiation to both the infant's thyroid and the patient's breast. If breast milk continues to be produced, ^{131}I treatment should be delayed (Sisson et al., 2011).

vii. For seven days after treatment

- Patients should wash hands frequently and should have sole use of a bathroom if possible. Towels, toothbrushes, and washcloths should be separate from other family or household members' items. The patient's home toothbrush should be discarded in a separate bag two weeks after the tositumomab infusion (Sisson et al., 2011).
- The patient should urinate only while sitting down to avoid splashing urine outside of the toilet. The toilet should be flushed two times with the lid down after use (Rao et al., 2005; Sisson et al., 2011).
- Clothing and linen should be kept in a separate bag for one week before laundering because of the presence of ^{131}I in the patient's sweat (Sisson et al., 2011).

- Washable food utensils are advised because disposable utensils will require special discard procedures. The dishware can be washed with those of the family/household (Rao et al., 2005; Sisson et al., 2011).
- Patients are advised to use personal cell phones to avoid the need for special cleaning of shared telephones (Sisson et al., 2011).

(3) Toxicities of radioimmunotherapy
- (a) Hematologic (GlaxoSmithKline, 2005; Spectrum Pharmaceuticals, Inc., 2010)
  - i. Bone marrow suppression
    - Thrombocytopenia
    - Neutropenia
    - Anemia
    - Asthenia
  - ii. Hematologic toxicity is the most common acute side effect. The median time to nadir is seven to nine weeks (Wahl, 2005) and it can last for as long as 12 weeks (Spectrum Pharmaceuticals, Inc., 2010).
- (b) Nonhematologic (GlaxoSmithKline, 2005; Spectrum Pharmaceuticals, Inc., 2010)
  - i. Rash
  - ii. Fever
  - iii. Chills
  - iv. Myalgia
  - v. Diaphoresis
  - vi. Pruritus
  - vii. Nausea and vomiting
  - viii. Diarrhea
  - ix. Nasal congestion
  - x. Hypotension
- (c) Other toxicities
  - i. Rigors
  - ii. Bronchospasm

- iii. Laryngeal edema
- (d) Postmarketing toxicities
  - i. Ibritumomab (Spectrum Pharmaceuticals, Inc., 2010)
    - Erythema multiforme, Stevens-Johnson syndrome, toxic epidermal necrolysis, bullous dermatitis, and exfoliative dermatitis
    - Radiation injury in tissues near areas of lymphomatous involvement within a month of ibritumomab administration
    - Infusion-site erythema and ulceration following extravasation
  - ii. Tositumomab: Postmarketing data are not available (FDA, 2011).

g) Documentation (Catlin-Huth, Haas, & Pollock, 2002)
- (1) Monitoring: Injury potential, bleeding, infection
- (2) Complete blood count with differential; weekly until levels recover

h) Collaborative management
- (1) Treatment with radioimmunotherapy involves the coordinated efforts of hematologists, oncologists, nurses, pharmacists, nuclear medicine personnel, radiation physicists and dosimetrists, and radiation oncologists.
- (2) Nurses must adhere to strict guidelines for radiation safety and protection (see section III—Radiation protection and safety).
- (3) All personnel involved in the administration of tositumomab and ^{131}I should follow radiation safety precautions for standard radioactive iodine.
- (4) Guidelines for outpatient care for patients treated with radioimmunotherapy for NHL have been reported in the literature (Wahl, 2005).
- (5) Patient education is crucial to facilitate early recognition of symptoms of infusion side effects within the first 24 hours of the infusion.
- (6) Review with the patient the importance of premedications, such as acetaminophen and diphenhydramine, as well as steroids, antihistamines, oxygen, and pain medications.

i) Related Web sites
- (1) Lymphoma Research Foundation: www.lymphoma.org

(2) Patients Against Lymphoma: www .lymphomation.org. Site includes a nationwide one-to-one support program where patients with lymphoma and their caregivers can share their experiences and find emotional support.

2. Radionuclide therapy (Temple, 2007)

a) Definition: Systemic radionuclide therapy is brachytherapy that is administered using unsealed radioactive sources in a liquid, capsule, or colloidal suspension that is ingested, injected, or instilled directly into the body.

b) Rationale: Radionuclide therapy is very effective in treating specific tumors and has relatively few side effects (Wahl, 2005).

c) Types and uses in specific cancers

(1) ^{131}I (referred to as MIBG—iodine-131-meta-iodobenzylguanidine): Used mainly for thyroid cancer and other neuroendocrine tumors; localizes within well-differentiated thyroid cancer cells (Al-Shakhrah, 2008; Carling & Udelsman, 2008)

(a) Administration: Given by mouth, either in capsules or liquid form

(b) Nursing care (Al-Shakhrah, 2008)

i. Dose
   • Less than 33 mCi: Treated as outpatient
   • Greater than 33 mCi: Hospitalization required

ii. Follow radiation precautions (see section III—Radiation protection and safety).

iii. Encourage oral intake of fluids to facilitate disbursement/absorption of ^{131}I.

iv. Follow body fluid precautions (blood, saliva, urine, stool, and perspiration).

v. Do not have carpeting or rugs in the room. Use plastic covering on pillows, mattresses, and anything the patient touches while in the hospital (e.g., telephone, television, sink handles, bedside table, toilet, bedside commode).

vi. Have the patient use washable eating utensils to avoid special procedures for discard.

(c) Patient and family education (see Patient and Family Education for ^{131}I tositumomab)

i. Educate regarding the previous nursing care considerations.

ii. Offer emotional support. The experience can be very distressing to the patient (Al-Shakhrah, 2008).

iii. Offer suggestions for passing time and reducing anxiety (e.g., reading, watching television, listening to music on MP3 players, talking on the telephone, doing crossword puzzles, using tablet computers, using programs such as Skype to communicate with friends and family and discouraging visitors).

(d) Inpatient staff education (Al-Shakhrah, 2008; Wahl, 2005)

i. Provide in-service education regarding brachytherapy/^{131}I and radiation safety.

ii. Provide written instructions, protocols, and references.

iii. Be available for consultation or questions in person or by telephone.

(2) ^{89}Sr (Metastron™, GE Healthcare): Used mainly for the treatment of painful bone metastasis. Localizes in the mineral content of the bone by combining with calcium (Chow, Finkelstein, & Coleman, 2008; GE Healthcare, 2006).

(a) Administration

i. Outpatient procedure

ii. Administered by radiation oncologist or nuclear medicine physician (Temple, 2007)

iii. IV administration: The manufacturer recommended dose is 148 MBq, 4 mCi given slowly (1–2 minutes) IV. There is also an alternative dose based on weight (GE Healthcare, 2006).

(b) Nursing care

i. Establish IV access.

ii. Provide education regarding rationale and side effects.

iii. Obtain baseline blood counts (platelets can be affected).

iv. Obtain orders for blood counts within one week of therapy and then every two weeks (for 12 weeks for hematologic recovery). Hematologic toxicity is related to the extent of bony metastasis (Temple, 2007; Williams & Burrows, 2007).

(c) Patient and family education: For first week

  i. Wipe up urine spills, and flush the toilet after each use.

  ii. Wash hands after each use of the toilet.

  iii. Wash linens separately when they are exposed to body fluids.

(d) Other education

  i. Educate about pain flare, which can occur up to 72 hours after administration; treat with analgesics (acetaminophen or stronger). Flare may last up to one week (Temple, 2007; Williams & Burrows, 2007). The use of glucocorticosteroids has been beneficial to minimize this reaction.

  ii. Inform about laboratory appointments for frequent monitoring of blood counts (^{89}Sr has known bone marrow toxicity), the importance of follow-up, and thrombocytopenia precautions, if necessary (GE Healthcare, 2006).

(3) ^{153}Sm (Quadramet®, EUSA Pharma [USA], Inc.): Is neutron irradiation with isotopically enriched samarium oxide (^{152}Sm). It emits both medium-energy beta particles and a gamma photon (EUSA Pharma [USA], Inc., 2008). Samarium is indicated for use in patients with osteoblastic metastatic bone lesions (Temple, 2007).

(a) Administration (EUSA Pharma [USA], Inc., 2008)

  i. Outpatient procedure

  ii. Given intravenously undiluted over one minute followed by IV saline flush

  iii. Dosage: 1 mCi/kg of patient's body weight

  iv. Administered by radiation oncologist or nuclear medicine physician

(b) Nursing care (EUSA Pharma [USA], Inc., 2008; Temple, 2007)

  i. Obtain baseline complete blood count, platelet count, and creatinine.

  ii. No fasting is necessary.

  iii. Establish IV access.

  iv. Infuse 500 ml normal saline prior to samarium administration or have the patient drink two quarts of water before arriving.

  v. Provide a shielded syringe for physician.

  vi. The patient cannot be discharged until radioactivity levels and exposure rates comply with federal and local regulations. Levels are calculated using clearance activity measured in urine. In study, clearance activity is greatest in the first 6 hours after administration but continues to be significant for up to 12 hours.

(c) Patient and family education (EUSA Pharma [USA], Inc., 2008; Temple, 2007; Williams & Burrows, 2007)

  i. Educate the patient that mild and transient flare of pain may occur within 72 hours of injection.

  ii. Instruct the patient to follow up with repeat blood counts weekly for eight weeks starting two weeks after injection. Hematologic events are the most common adverse events and usually are reversible.

  iii. Precautions need to be taken for at least 12 hours after administration (EUSA Pharma [USA], Inc., 2008).

    • Flush the toilet at least two times after each use. Spilled urine or blood should be immediately cleaned up with flushable toilet paper and disposed via the toilet, or the nonflushable paper or cloths placed in separate bag for storage and disposal outside the home.

    • Wash hands thoroughly with soap and water after using the toilet.

  iv. Clothing or linens should be immediately washed separately from other items, or stored in a bag for one to two weeks prior to washing to allow for radioactive decay prior to mingling.

(4) ^{32}P: A pure beta emitter radionuclide. It is used for the treatment of chronic my-

eloproliferative disorders such as primary proliferative polycythemia in patients older than 70 years of age who have not responded to other standard therapies (Balan & Critchley, 1997), and, rarely, to treat malignant ascites associated with ovarian cancer (Saul et al., 1996).

(a) Primary proliferative polycythemia: An unnatural proliferation of one or more elements of the hematopoietic system (Balan & Critchley, 1997; Perkins, 2005)

　i. The radionuclide targets the nucleic acids of rapidly proliferating cells (Perkins, 2005).

　ii. Without therapy, complications of panmyelosis, splenomegaly, and a predisposition to venous or arterial thrombosis, myelofibrosis, and acute leukemia have been reported (Streiff, Smith, & Spivak, 2002).

　iii. The rationale for its use is to reduce the patient's hematocrit level, maintain a normal platelet count, and prevent complications of cerebral thrombosis, thrombophlebitis, or myocardial infarction (Balan & Critchley, 1997).

　iv. Administration: A radiation oncologist or nuclear medicine physician administers it by IV injection. ^{32}P is mixed in an isotonic solution of sodium orthophosphate and calibrated by a radiation oncology physicist (Balan & Critchley, 1997)

　v. Patients with polycythemia vera are at risk for the following side effects after use of ^{32}P: 5.5% risk of myelofibrosis, 7.6% risk of acute leukemia, and 8% risk of developing other cancers (Balan & Critchley, 1997; Parmentier, 2003).

(b) Nursing care

　i. Perform baseline clinical laboratory evaluation for measurement of red cell volume to establish diagnosis of primary proliferative polycythemia.

　ii. ^{32}P is administered in the outpatient/clinic setting.

　iii. Establish IV access.

　iv. Acrylic shielding blocks beta emissions; place absorbent pads under infusion sites.

　v. Follow universal precautions to prevent contact with bodily fluids.

(c) Patient and family education

　i. Reinforce universal precautions when handling bodily fluids, soiled linens, or clothing.

　ii. Stress importance of follow-up.

(d) The use of intraperitoneal ^{32}P in the treatment of epithelial ovarian cancer is rarely done (Saul et al., 1996). However, intraperitoneal ^{32}P may be used for management of malignant ascites.

　i. Because of the high rate of late bowel complications, including chronic abdominal cramping and small bowel obstruction, it has been recommended that intraperitoneal cisplatin be used as standard adjuvant treatment for ovarian cancer rather than ^{32}P (Class, Jost, Mose, Weber, & Brady, 2008; Vergote et al., 1992).

　ii. ^{32}P has been shown to lack efficacy in intraperitoneal administration for stage III ovarian cancer after a negative second-look laparotomy (Class et al., 2008).

　iii. A radiation oncologist or nuclear medicine physician administers ^{32}P through an intraperitoneal catheter.

　iv. It is often instilled as an outpatient procedure.

　v. Nursing care—Precautions are the same as when given for polycythemia vera. Wound dressing should be observed for drainage, discarded in a doubled plastic bag, and disposed of in the trash (Balan & Critchley, 1997; Parmentier, 2003).

　vi. Patient and family education (Balan & Critchley, 1997; Parmentier, 2003)

　　• Once the ^{32}P is instilled into the patient's peritoneal cavity, no special radiation precautions are necessary because abdominal tissues provide adequate shielding of the radiation.

- For 12 hours after the infusion of ^{32}P, instruct the patient on the following.
  - Wash hands thoroughly with soap and water after using the toilet.
  - Drink extra fluids to speed elimination of the isotope via the urine.
  - Do not have sexual intercourse or contact with partner.

(5) Related Web sites

(a) ACR-ASTRO Practice Guideline for the Performance of Therapy With Unsealed Radiopharmaceutical Sources (revised 2010): www.acr.org/SecondaryMainMenuCategories/quality_safety/guidelines/nuc_med/unsealed_radiopharmaceuticals.aspx

(b) NCCN: www.nccn.org

(c) NCI What You Need to Know About™ Thyroid Cancer: www.cancer.gov/cancertopics/wyntk/thyroid

(d) State Government of Victoria (Australia) Department of Human Services, Radiation Safety Program's Guidelines for the Therapeutic Administration of Strontium-89: www.health.vic.gov.au/environment/downloads/guidelines_strontium.pdf

(e) World Nuclear Association: www.world-nuclear.org

References

Al-Shakhrah, I.A. (2008). Radioprotection using iodine-131 for thyroid cancer and hyperthyroidism: A review. *Clinical Journal of Oncology Nursing, 12,* 905–912. doi:10.1188/08.CJON.905-912

Balan, K.K., & Critchley, M. (1997). Outcome of 259 patients with primary proliferative polycythaemia (PPP) and idiopathic thrombocythaemia (IT) treated in a regional nuclear medicine department with phosphorus-32—A 15 year review. *British Journal of Radiology, 70,* 1169–1173.

Carling, T., & Udelsman, R. (2008). Thyroid tumors. In V.T. DeVita Jr., T.S. Lawrence, & S.A. Rosenberg (Eds.), *Cancer: Principles and practice of oncology* (8th ed., pp. 1663–1681). Philadelphia, PA: Lippincott Williams & Wilkins.

Catlin-Huth, C., Haas, M., & Pollock, V. (Eds.). (2002). *Radiation therapy patient care record: A tool for documenting nursing care.* Pittsburgh, PA: Oncology Nursing Society.

Chow, E., Finkelstein, J.A., & Coleman, R.E. (2008). Metastatic cancer to the bone. In V.T. DeVita Jr., T.S. Lawrence, & S.A. Rosenberg (Eds.), *Cancer: Principles and practice of oncology* (8th ed., pp. 2510–2522). Philadelphia, PA: Lippincott Williams & Wilkins.

Class, R., Jost, M., Mose, S., Weber, H., & Brady, L.W. (2008). Radioimmunoglobulins and nonsealed radionuclide therapy. In E.C. Halperin, C.A. Perez, & L.W. Brady (Eds.), *Perez and Brady's principles and practice of radiation oncology* (5th ed., pp. 583–598). Philadelphia, PA: Lippincott Williams & Wilkins.

Dearden, C.E. (2007). Role of antibody therapy in lymphoid malignancies. *British Medical Bulletin, 83,* 275–290. doi:10.1093/bmb/ldm025

EUSA Pharma (USA), Inc. (2008). *Quadramet®* [Package insert]. Retrieved from http://www.quadramet-us.com/assets/pdf/QuadrametPI.pdf

GE Healthcare. (2006). *Metastron™* [Prescribing information]. Retrieved from http://md.gehealthcare.com/shared/pdfs/pi/Metastron.pdf

GlaxoSmithKline. (2005). *Bexxar®* [Package insert]. Research Triangle Park, NC: Author.

Hagenbeek, A., & Lewington, V. (2005). Report of a European consensus workshop to develop recommendations for the optimal use of (90)Y-ibritumomab tiuxetan (Zevalin) in lymphoma. *Annals of Oncology, 16,* 786–792. doi:10.1093/annonc/mdi148

Hendrix, C. (2004). Radiation safety guidelines for radioimmunotherapy with yttrium 90 ibritumomab tiuxetan. *Clinical Journal of Oncology Nursing, 8,* 31–34. doi:10.1188/04.CJON.31-34

Kersten, M.J. (2011). Radioimmunotherapy in follicular lymphoma: Some like it hot…. *Transfusion and Apheresis Science, 44,* 173–178. doi:10.1016/j.transci.2011.01.015

National Comprehensive Cancer Network. (2011). *NCCN Clinical Practice Guidelines in Oncology: Non-Hodgkin's lymphomas* [v.3.2011]. Retrieved from http://www.nccn.org/professionals/physician_gls/pdf/nhl.pdf

Parmentier, C. (2003). Use and risks of phosphorus-32 in the treatment of polycythemia vera. *European Journal of Nuclear Medicine and Molecular Imaging, 30,* 1413–1417. doi:10.1007/s00259-003-1270-6

Perkins, A. (2005). In vivo molecular targeted radiotherapy. *Biomedical Imaging and Intervention Journal, 1*(2), e9. doi:10.2349/biij.1.2.e9

Rao, A.V., Akabani, G., & Rizzieri, D.A. (2005). Radioimmunotherapy for non-Hodgkin's lymphoma. *Clinical Medicine and Research, 3,* 157–165. doi:10.3121/cmr.3.3.157

Robinson, M.K., Borghaei, H., Adams, G.P., & Weiner, L.M. (2008). Monoclonal antibodies. In V.T. DeVita Jr., T.S. Lawrence, & S.A. Rosenberg (Eds.), *Cancer: Principles and practice of oncology* (8th ed., pp. 537–547). Philadelphia, PA: Lippincott Williams & Wilkins.

Saul, H.M., Sedlacek, T.V., Heller, P.B., Glassburn, J.R., Riva, J., Bertoli, R., … Lin, J.K. (1996). Intracavitary use of radioactive colloidal phosphorus 32 in the treatment of epithelial ovarian cancer. *Journal of the American Osteopathic Association, 96,* 727–732.

Schaefer-Cutillo, J., Friedberg, J.W., & Fisher, R.I. (2007). Novel concepts in radioimmunotherapy for non-Hodgkin's lymphoma. *Oncology, 21,* 203–212.

Sisson, J.C., Freitas, J., McDougall, I.R., Dauer, L.T., Hurley, J.R., Brierley, J.D., … Greenlee, C. (2011). Radiation safety in the treatment of patients with thyroid diseases by radioiodine ^{131}I: Practice recommendations of the American Thyroid Association. *Thyroid, 21,* 335–346. doi:10.1089/thy.2010.0403

Spectrum Pharmaceuticals, Inc. (2010). *Zevalin®* [Package insert]. Irvine, CA: Author.

Srinivasan, A., & Mukherji, S.K. (2011). Tositumomab and iodine I 131 tositumomab (Bexaar). *American Journal of Neuroradiology, 32,* 637–638. doi:10.3174/ajnr.A2593

Streiff, M.B., Smith, B., & Spivak, J.L. (2002). The diagnosis and management of polycythemia vera in the era since the Polycythemia Vera Study Group: A survey of American Society of Hematology members' practice patterns. *Blood, 99,* 1144–1149. doi:10.1182/blood.V99.4.1144

Temple, S.V. (2007). Radiopharmaceuticals. In M.L. Haas, W.P. Hogle, G.J. Moore-Higgs, & T.K. Gosselin-Acomb (Eds.), *Radiation therapy: A guide to patient care* (pp. 399–412). St. Louis, MO: Elsevier Mosby.

U.S. Food and Drug Administration. (2011). Summary minutes of the Oncologic Drugs Advisory Committee Meeting February 8, 2011. Retrieved from http://www.fda.gov/downloads/Advisory Committees/CommitteesMeetingMaterials/Drugs/Oncologic DrugsAdvisoryCommittee/UCM250472.pdf

Vergote, I.B., Vergote-De Vos, L.N., Abeler, V.M., Aas, M., Lindegaard, M.W., Kjørstad, K.E., & Tropé, C.G. (1992). Randomized trial comparing cisplatin with radioactive phosphorus or whole-abdomen irradiation as adjuvant treatment of ovarian cancer. *Cancer, 69,* 741–749. doi:10.1002/1097-0142(19920201)69:3<741::AID -CNCR2820690322>3.0.CO;2-G

Wahl, R.L. (2005). Tositumomab and ^{131}I therapy in non-Hodgkin's lymphoma. *Journal of Nuclear Medicine, 46*(Suppl. 1), 128S–140S.

Williams, D., & Burrows, K. (2007). Spinal cord and bone metastases. In M.L. Haas, W.P. Hogle, G.J. Moore-Higgs, & T.K. Gosselin-Acomb (Eds.), *Radiation therapy: A guide to patient care* (pp. 267–280). St. Louis, MO: Elsevier Mosby.

XI. General radiation oncology issues

A. Survivorship
 1. Cancer survivorship has been an essential part of cancer care since 1986.
   a) The National Coalition for Cancer Survivorship (n.d.) (www.canceradvocacy.org) began in 1986.
   b) NCI's Cancer Survivorship Research Department established the Office of Cancer Survivorship in 1996. A *cancer survivor* is anyone who has been diagnosed with cancer, including the person's family members, friends, and caregivers, from the time of diagnosis through the balance of his or her life (NCI Office of Cancer Survivorship, 2010). Individual settings may define the area of survivorship they will focus on depending on their activities and expertise (NCI Office of Cancer Survivorship, n.d.).
   c) The Lance Armstrong Foundation (www.livestrong.org) was established in 1997 (LIVESTRONG, n.d.).
   d) The Institute of Medicine published a report in 2006 titled *From Cancer Patient to Cancer Survivor: Lost in Transition* (Hewitt, Greenfield, & Stovall, 2006).
   e) Components of survivorship care include four major areas (see Figure 30).
     (1) Prevention and detection
     (2) Surveillance
     (3) Interventions for symptoms associated with cancer and its treatment
     (4) Coordination of care and information among oncologists, primary care physicians, patients, and consultants
   f) Promotion of treatment summary and survivorship care plans: Goal is to promote communication and healthy choices to improve quality of life. Journey Forward (www.journeyforward.org) and LIVESTRONG and OncoLink (www.livestrongcareplan.org) offer survivorship care plan builders.
 2. The number of survivors continues to rise; 20 million survivors are expected by 2020 (ACS, 2010).
   a) According to Radiological Society of North America and ACR (n.d.), 50%–60% of patients receive radiation as part of their cancer treatment.
   b) Focus on long-term care of survivors is based on changes in survivors' physical, psychological, social, and spiritual response to cancer and its treatments (Ferrell, Dow, & Grant, 1995).
   c) Sixty percent of cancer survivors are age 65 or older (Ries et al., 2006).

 3. Risk factors that lead to long-term and late effects for cancer survivors are related to intensity of their treatments and comorbidities they have that are complicated by their disease or treatment (Aziz, 2007; Hurria et al., 2008).
   a) Older adults and young children may tolerate treatments differently related to organ development or aging results (Aziz, 2007; Bhatia, Landier, & Robison, 2002; Hurria et al., 2008).
   b) Late effects of treatment may not occur for months to years and are caused by damage to organs during active treatment (Aziz & Rowland, 2003; Ganz, 2006; Paice, 2011).
 4. Survivorship issues related to surgery
   a) Depend on site of surgery, such as lymphedema from breast surgery
   b) Long-term and late effects associated with surgical sites can include changes in physical functioning, circulatory changes, pain, neuropathy, and lymphedema. Physical changes may include ostomies and limb amputations, which result in body image changes and have psychosocial implications. Risk for multiple painful symptoms are related to nerve entrapment, plexopathies, or fistula formation (Paice, 2011). Impairment in motor sensory function, impaired immune function, and elimination problems are associated with cancer surgery (Hewitt et al., 2006).

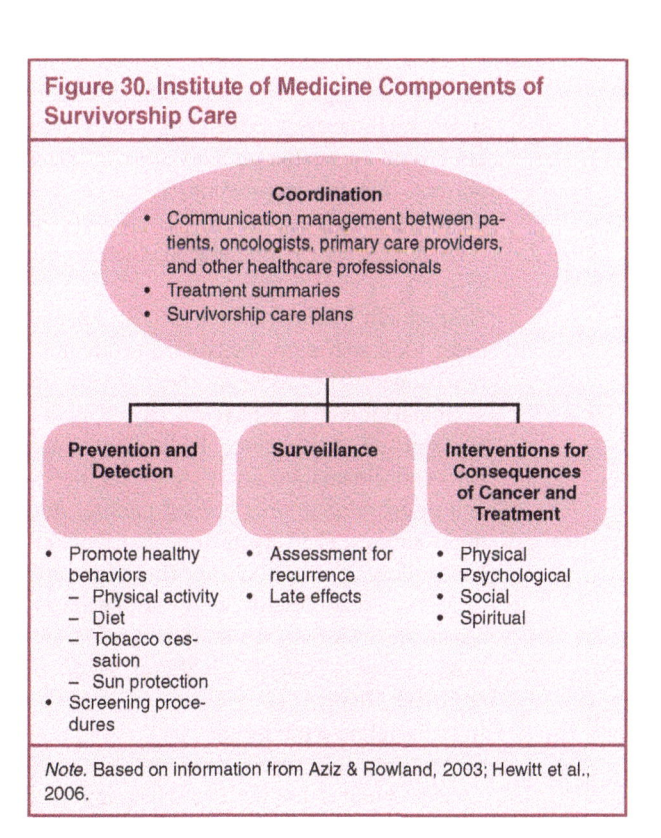

Figure 30. Institute of Medicine Components of Survivorship Care

Coordination
- Communication management between patients, oncologists, primary care providers, and other healthcare professionals
- Treatment summaries
- Survivorship care plans

Prevention and Detection
- Promote healthy behaviors
  - Physical activity
  - Diet
  - Tobacco cessation
  - Sun protection
- Screening procedures

Surveillance
- Assessment for recurrence
- Late effects

Interventions for Consequences of Cancer and Treatment
- Physical
- Psychological
- Social
- Spiritual

Note. Based on information from Aziz & Rowland, 2003; Hewitt et al., 2006.

5. Survivorship issues related to chemotherapy
   a) Initial responses include nausea and vomiting, hematologic effects, pain, neuropathy, and fatigue (Aziz, 2007; Badin, Iqbal, Sikder, & Chang, 2008; Camp-Sorrell, 2008; Ganz, 2007; Lockwood-Rayermann, 2006).
   b) Long-term effects are related to the type of chemotherapy, such as anthracycline and cardiovascular disease, infertility issues, sexuality issues, neuropathy, cognitive dysfunction, and pulmonary or endocrine-related late effects (Adams et al., 2003; Camp-Sorrell, 2008; Correa & Ahles, 2008; Deimling, Kahana, Bowman, & Schaefer, 2002; Fosså, Vassilopoulou-Sellin, & Dahl, 2008; Ganz, 2007; Lipshultz et al., 1991; Miller & Triano, 2008; Paice, 2011; Pinder, Duan, Goodwin, Hortobagyi, & Giordano, 2007).
   c) Second malignancies (Bhatia et al., 1996; van Leeuwen et al., 2000)
6. Survivorship issues related to RT: Systemic effects are related to the site and dose of radiation. Although RT is responsible for many successes in cancer survivorship, multiple late effects are associated with RT such as osteoporosis, immune suppression, hormone deficiencies, arthralgias, and risks for second cancers (Aziz, 2007; Economou & Grant, 2010; Miller & Triano, 2008).
7. Assessment of survivorship needs: Assessment tools can help focus care to areas of most concern for cancer survivors. Needs assessment tools include physical, psychosocial, and spiritual components. Focused care can help coordinate care around patients' needs and improve quality of life for patients and their families. The City of Hope Pain and Palliative Care Resource Center (http://prc.coh.org) has a section with samples of needs assessment tools that can be downloaded and used to assess patients (Schlairet, Heddon, & Griffis, 2010).
8. Interdisciplinary models of care
   a) Multiple disciplines work together to provide support for the ever-changing care needs of cancer survivors (Asher, 2010; Ganz, 2009; Grant & Economou, 2007; Landier, 2009; McCabe & Jacobs, 2008).
   b) Over the course of care from diagnosis to death, cancer survivors may need interventions from multiple specialists. These include oncologists, primary care physicians, APNs, nurses, social workers, dietitians, and rehabilitation specialists (Asher, 2010).
   c) Models of care include pediatric long-term follow-up programs, which care for pediatric patients from diagnosis until transition into an adult-focused program; community-based shared-care models, which coordinate care between caregivers and settings; disease-specific cancer survivor programs, which are built around specific diseases (e.g., breast cancer, prostate cancer, lung cancer); and comprehensive survivor programs, which usually are part of large academic centers where all specialties are available at one site. Patients may see psychosocial specialists as well as rehabilitation and palliative care specialists as needed (McCabe & Jacobs, 2008; Oeffinger & McCabe, 2006).
9. Communicating survivorship patient needs
   a) Treatment summaries and survivorship care plans help document the care received and the individualized follow-up plan for patients according to their diagnosis and treatment summary (Institute of Medicine, 2007; Morgan, 2009) (see www.journeyforward.org and www.livestrongcareplan.org).
   b) RT patients should receive a summary of areas of their body that were irradiated, how much radiation (total dose in Gy) was received, and a documentation of any severe side effects experienced. Toxicities related to radiation affect the musculoskeletal system and bones and may cause muscle atrophy. Additional effects include changes in organ function, as well as pain, neuropathy, and skin changes or fibrosis (Aziz, 2007; Paice, 2011; Polomano & Farrar, 2006). Survivorship care plans for survivors who have received radiation must include screening information that is site specific and detection recommendations to diagnose secondary cancers in the radiation site early (Mayer et al., 2007). This information can help oncologists and primary care physicians anticipate and prepare the patient for future healthcare issues and needs.
10. See Table 20 for key survivorship resources for patients and families.

Table 20. Key Survivorship Resources for Patients and Families

Organization	Web Address
American Cancer Society	www.cancer.org
American Cancer Society Cancer Survivors Network	http://csn.cancer.org
American Society of Clinical Oncology's Cancer.Net	www.cancer.net
Cancer Support Community	www.cancersupportcommunity.org
CancerCare	www.cancercare.org
Centers for Disease Control and Prevention	www.cdc.gov
City of Hope Pain and Palliative Care Resource Center	http://prc.coh.org
Fertile Hope	www.fertilehope.org
Lance Armstrong Foundation	http://livestrong.org
National Cancer Institute Office of Cancer Survivorship	http://survivorship.cancer.gov
National Coalition for Cancer Survivorship	www.canceradvocacy.org
Oncology Nursing Society's Cancer Journey	http://www.thecancerjourney.org/survivor
Planet Cancer (young adults with cancer)	www.planetcancer.org

Note. Based on information from Economou & Grant, 2010.

References

Adams, M.J., Lipshultz, S.E., Schwartz, C., Fajardo, L.F., Coen, V., & Constine, L.S. (2003). Radiation-associated cardiovascular disease: Manifestations and management. *Seminars in Radiation Oncology, 13,* 346–356. doi:10.1016/S1053-4296(03)00026-2

American Cancer Society. (2010, June 3). National Cancer Survivors Day®: A milestone for survivors and the American Cancer Society Hope Lodge [Press release]. Retrieved from http://pressroom.cancer.org/index.php?s=43&item=247

Asher, A. (2010). Cancer rehabilitation and survivorship: Cedars-Sinai Medical Center experience. *Oncology Nurse-APN/PA, 3*(6), 1, 18–21.

Aziz, N.M. (2007). Late effects of cancer treatments. In P.A. Ganz (Ed.), *Cancer survivorship: Today and tomorrow* (pp. 54–76). New York, NY: Springer.

Aziz, N.M., & Rowland, J.H. (2003). Trends and advances in cancer survivorship research: Challenge and opportunity. *Seminars in Radiation Oncology, 13,* 248–266. doi:10.1016/S1053-4296(03)00024-9

Badin, S., Iqbal, A., Sikder, M., & Chang, V.T. (2008). Persistent pain in anal cancer survivors. *Journal of Cancer Survivorship, 2,* 79–83. doi:10.1007/s11764-008-0051-4

Bhatia, S., Landier, W., & Robison, L.L. (2002). Late effects of childhood cancer therapy. In V.T. DeVita Jr., S. Hellman, & S.A. Rosenberg (Eds.), *Progress in oncology 2002* (pp. 171–213). Sudbury, MA: Jones and Bartlett.

Bhatia, S., Robison, L.L., Oberlin, O., Greenberg, M., Bunin, G., Fossati-Bellani, F., & Meadows, A.T. (1996). Breast cancer and other second neoplasms after childhood Hodgkin's disease. *New England Journal of Medicine, 334,* 745–751. doi:10.1056/NEJM199603213341201

Camp-Sorrell, D. (2008). Cardiovascular late effects. *Oncology, 22*(Suppl. 2, Nurse Ed.), 42–44.

Correa, D.D., & Ahles, T.A. (2008). Neurocognitive changes in cancer survivors. *Cancer Journal, 14,* 396–400. doi:10.1097/PPO.0b013e31818d8769

Deimling, G.T., Kahana, B., Bowman, K.F., & Schaefer, M.L. (2002). Cancer survivorship and psychological distress in later life. *Psycho-Oncology, 11,* 479–494. doi:10.1002/pon.614

Economou, D., & Grant, M. (2010). Late and long-term physical effects in cancer survivors. *Oncology Nurse-APN/PA, 3*(6), 1, 12, 34.

Ferrell, B.R., Dow, K.H., & Grant, M. (1995). Measurement of the quality of life in cancer survivors. *Quality of Life Research, 4,* 523–531.

Fosså, S.D., Vassilopoulou-Sellin, R., & Dahl, A.A. (2008). Long term physical sequelae after adult-onset cancer. *Journal of Cancer Survivorship, 2,* 3–11. doi:10.1007/s11764-007-0039-5

Ganz, P.A. (2006). Monitoring the physical health of cancer survivors: A survivorship-focused medical history. *Journal of Clinical Oncology, 24,* 5105–5111. doi:10.1200/JCO.2006.06.0541

Ganz, P.A. (2007). Cancer survivors: Issues in symptom management. *Journal of Supportive Oncology, 5,* 73.

Ganz, P.A. (2009). Quality of care and cancer survivorship: The challenge of implementing the Institute of Medicine recommendations. *Journal of Oncology Practice, 5,* 101–105. doi:10.1200/JOP.0934402

Grant, M., & Economou, D.D. (2007, July/August). Survivorship education for quality cancer care. *Oncology Issues, 22*(4), 24–29.

Hewitt, M., Greenfield, S., & Stovall, E. (Eds.). (2006). *From cancer patient to cancer survivor: Lost in transition* (Institute of Medicine report). Washington, DC: National Academies Press.

Hurria, A., Wong, F.L., Villaluna, D., Bhatia, S., Chung, C.T., Mortimer, J., ... Naeim, A. (2008). Role of age and health in treatment recommendations for older adults with breast cancer: The perspective of oncologists and primary care providers. *Journal of Clinical Oncology, 26,* 5386–5392. doi:10.1200/JCO.2008.17.6891

Institute of Medicine. (2007). *Implementing cancer survivorship care planning—Workshop summary.* Washington, DC: National Academies Press.

Landier, W. (2009). Survivorship care: Essential components and models of delivery. *Oncology, 23*(Suppl. 4, Nurse Ed.), 46–53.

Lipshultz, S.E., Colan, S.D., Gelber, R.D., Perez-Atayde, A.R., Sallan, S.E., & Sanders, S.P. (1991). Late cardiac effects of doxorubicin therapy for acute lymphoblastic leukemia in childhood. *New England Journal of Medicine, 324,* 808–815. doi:10.1056/NEJM199103213241205

LIVESTRONG. (n.d.). Who we are. Retrieved from http://www.livestrong.org/Who-We-Are/Our-History

Lockwood-Rayermann, S. (2006). Survivorship issues in ovarian cancer: A review. *Oncology Nursing Forum, 33,* 553–662. doi:10.1188/06.ONF.553-562

Mayer, D.K., Terrin, N.C., Menon, U., Kreps, G.L., McCance, K., Parsons, S.K., & Mooney, K.H. (2007). Screening practices in cancer survivors. *Journal of Cancer Survivorship, 1,* 17–26. doi:10.1007/s11764-007-0007-0

McCabe, M.S., & Jacobs, L. (2008). Survivorship care: Models and programs. *Seminars in Oncology Nursing, 24,* 202–207. doi:10.1016/j.soncn.2008.05.008

Miller, K.D., & Triano, L.R. (2008). Medical issues in cancer survivors—A review. *Cancer Journal, 14,* 375–387. doi:10.1097/PPO.0b013e31818ee3dc

Morgan, M.A. (2009). Cancer survivorship: History, quality-of-life issues, and the evolving multidisciplinary approach to implementation of cancer survivorship care plans. *Oncology Nursing Forum, 36,* 429–436. doi:10.1188/09.ONF.429-436

National Cancer Institute Office of Cancer Survivorship. (2010, June). Fact sheet (public). Retrieved from http://cancercontrol.cancer.gov/ocs/ocs_factsheet.pdf

National Cancer Institute Office of Cancer Survivorship. (n.d.). Office of Cancer Survivorship key initiatives. Retrieved from http://cancercontrol.cancer.gov/ocs/key.html

National Coalition for Cancer Survivorship. (n.d.). About us: The organization. Retrieved from http://www.canceradvocacy.org/about/org/

Oeffinger, K.C., & McCabe, M.S. (2006). Models for delivering survivorship care. *Journal of Clinical Oncology, 24,* 5117–5124. doi:10.1200/JCO.2006.07.0474

Paice, J.A. (2011). Chronic treatment-related pain in cancer survivors. *Pain, 152*(Suppl. 3), S84–S89. doi:10.1016/j.pain.2010.10.010

Pinder, M.C., Duan, Z., Goodwin, J.S., Hortobagyi, G.N., & Giordano, S.H. (2007). Congestive heart failure in older women treated with adjuvant anthracycline chemotherapy for breast cancer. *Journal of Clinical Oncology, 25,* 3808–3815. doi:10.1200/JCO.2006.10.4976

Polomano, R.C., & Farrar, J.T. (2006). Pain and neuropathy in cancer survivors. Surgery, radiation, and chemotherapy can cause pain; research could improve its detection and treatment. *American Journal of Nursing, 106*(Suppl. 3), 39–47.

Radiological Society of North America & American College of Radiology. (n.d.). Introduction to cancer therapy (radiation oncology). Retrieved from http://www.radiologyinfo.org/en/info.cfm?pg=intro_onco

Ries, L.A.G., Melbert, D., Krapcho, M., Mariotto, A., Miller, B.A., Feuer, E.J., ... Edwards, B.K. (2006). *SEER cancer statistics review 1975–2004.* Bethesda, MD: National Cancer Institute.

Schlairet, M., Heddon, M.A., & Griffis, M. (2010). Piloting a needs assessment to guide development of a survivorship program for a community cancer center. *Oncology Nursing Forum, 37,* 501–508. doi:10.1188/10.ONF.501-508

van Leeuwen, F.E., Klokman, W.J., Veer, M.B., Hagenbeek, A., Krol, A.D., Vetter, U.A., ... Aleman, B.M. (2000). Long-term risk of second malignancy in survivors of Hodgkin's disease treated during adolescence or young adulthood. *Journal of Clinical Oncology, 18,* 487–497.

B. Palliative care
    1. RT and palliative care
        a) In radiation oncology, an estimated 30%–50% of therapy undertaken is for palliation (van Oorschot, Rades, Schulze, Beckmann, & Feyer, 2011).
        b) It is important that palliation be achieved with as efficient a fractionation schedule as possible in patients with limited life expec-

tancy and with as few side effects as possible (Lutz et al., 2011).
        c) Other issues such as symptom management, homecare status, and factors affecting quality of life are relevant for patients and families receiving palliative care.
    2. Definition of palliative care: An approach that improves the quality of life of patients and their families facing the problems associated with life-threatening illness through the prevention and relief of suffering by means of early identification and impeccable assessment and treatment of pain and other problems, such as physical, psychosocial, and spiritual. The general criteria for acceptance into a palliative care program is a diagnosis of an illness that is life threatening and not curable. The components that make up palliative care (WHO, n.d.) are listed in Figure 31.
    3. Benefits of palliative care
        a) Higginson et al. (2002) looked at whether palliative care teams within hospitals improved care at the end of life for patients and families. A systematic literature review identified nine hospital-based populations where the impact of the palliative care team was reported. Only one of these studies was controlled. The conclusion in this paper suggested that palliative care teams provided some benefit to patients that resulted in shorter hospital stays. The patients were hospitalized and at the end of life. The remainder of the studies were observational or retrospective.

Figure 31. The Essentials of Palliative Care

- Provides relief from pain and other distressing symptoms
- Affirms life and regards dying as a normal process
- Intends neither to hasten nor postpone death
- Integrates the psychological and spiritual aspects of patient care
- Offers a support system to help patients live as actively as possible until death
- Offers a support system to help the family cope during the patient's illness and in their own bereavement
- Uses a team approach to address the needs of patients and their families, including bereavement counseling, if indicated
- Will enhance quality of life and also may positively influence the course of illness
- Is applicable early in the course of illness, in conjunction with other therapies that are intended to prolong life, such as chemotherapy or radiation therapy, and includes those investigations needed to better understand and manage distressing clinical complications

Note. From "WHO Definition of Palliative Care," by World Health Organization, n.d. Retrieved from http://www.who.int/cancer/palliative/definition/en/. Copyright 2011 by World Health Organization. Reprinted with permission.

b) In 2003, Higginson et al. undertook a systematic review and meta-analysis of 19 relevant studies of patients who were in the hospital or hospice or at home related to the impact of palliative care teams on the experience of patients and caregivers at the end of life. Two patient outcomes, namely pain and "other symptoms," indicated a small significant benefit (by chi square testing) in favor of the palliative care team. There was also a trend toward improved satisfaction and therapeutic interventions with the palliative care team, but this did not reach significance using the random effects model.

c) In a study involving 151 patients with metastatic NSCLC, patients who received early palliative care as opposed to standard oncologic care had significant improvements in both quality of life and mood (p = 0.02). In addition, patients who received early palliative care received less aggressive care (*aggressive care* being defined as chemotherapy within 14 days of death, no hospice care or admission to hospice, to hospice within three days of death) at the end of life but had longer survival (11.6 versus 8.9 months; p = 0.02) (Temel et al., 2010).

4. Misunderstandings about the use of RT in palliative care

 a) Palliative RT may be underutilized because of several possible misconceptions among healthcare professionals.

  (1) A perception may exist that insurance does not pay for RT while the patient is in hospice (in jurisdictions where this might be an issue).

  (2) Patients need not travel repeatedly when they are very ill and in pain, as studies show that one fraction of 6–8 Gy (delivered in a single visit) can have a major positive impact on pain control and be just as effective as longer treatment schedules lasting one to two weeks (Hartsell et al., 2003).

  (3) A mistaken perception may exist that short RT courses were more damaging to normal tissues, especially in older adults, and therefore many patients would have side effects (Lutz et al., 2011).

   (a) One comprehensive study comparing a single treatment with 8 Gy versus 30 Gy over 10 treatments showed that the acute tox-icity rates were almost identical (p < 0.0001). In the single-fraction arm (n = 432), 9% of patients experienced grade 2–3 acute toxicity and less than 1% experienced grade 4 toxicity (Hartsell et al., 2003).

   (b) A study by Campos et al. (2010) (N = 558) showed that patients of all ages should be referred for palliative RT, as older patients received equal benefit compared with their younger counterparts without increased toxicity.

  (4) Indications for urgent palliative RT may include the following.

   (a) Oncologic emergencies
    i. SCC (Kaplan, 2006)
    ii. Superior vena cava obstruction (Kaplan, 2006)
    iii. Symptomatic bronchial obstruction (Wan & Bezjak, 2010)
    iv. Orbital nerve compression

   (b) Skeletal metastasis, including pathologic fracturing

   (c) Brain metastasis and raised intracranial pressure

   (d) Control of bleeding (e.g., hemoptysis, vaginal and rectal bleeding)

   (e) Control of fungating or ulcerating tumor

5. Components of palliative care

 a) Palliative care assessment

  (1) Comprehensive holistic assessment is undertaken at the initial visit.

  (2) Nursing assessment is ongoing during and after RT for a period of one to two weeks as the acute tissue reactions diminish (Lutz et al., 2011). Patients rarely experience late side effects from palliative RT because of the low doses administered (Lutz et al., 2011). Using Ferrell's (1995) quality-of-life framework, the assessment focuses on

   (a) Physical well-being
   (b) Psychological well-being
   (c) Social well-being
   (d) Spiritual well-being (Ferrell, 1995; Glass, Cluxton, & Rancour, 2001).

 b) Plan of care: Develop a plan of care, and evaluate and adjust it as required on an ongoing basis, with the patient and family setting mutual goals (Registered Nurses' Association of Ontario, 2006).

  (1) Assist the patient in understanding the diagnosis and prognosis, and promote informed choice.

     (2) Respect the patient's values, goals, and priorities.

     (3) Honor preferences of the patient and family.

     (4) Respect the patient's cultural and spiritual perspective.

     (5) Attempt to meet the patient's preferences related to living situations, care settings, and services.

     (6) Encourage the patient and family to address advance care planning and directives (i.e., living will, do-not-resuscitate order, preference regarding end-of-life care, such as hospice).

     (7) Identify potential areas of conflict between the patient, family, financial institutions, and care providers, and develop a plan to bring about a resolution.

  c) Acknowledge and address caregiver needs (NCCN, 2011b).

     (1) Appreciate the considerable demands and responsibilities that caregivers face (emotional, financial, and physical) while caring for the person at home and attempting to meet their own needs.

     (2) Ensure supportive services are available to caregivers (e.g., telephone support, respite care, help with personal care for the patient, counseling following bereavement).

     (3) Recognize that certain caregivers are at high risk for fatigue and physical and emotional illnesses or distress. Address these needs when implementing services.

     (4) Recognize and initiate conversation about possible financial concerns that caregivers may face (e.g., loss of income) while looking after a person at home.

  d) Pain and symptom management

     (1) Providing relief of pain and other symptoms experienced by patients with cancer can contribute significantly to their quality of life (Kirou-Mauro et al., 2009).

     (2) Pain and symptom management strategies should be the first priority of care and implemented, assessed, and adjusted accordingly during and after treatment (NCCN, 2011a).

  e) Interdisciplinary approach to care: Use an interdisciplinary approach (i.e., nurses, physicians, social workers, dietitians, pastoral caregivers, pharmacists, psychologists, family, and volunteers) to deal with the multifaceted needs of care (American College of Surgeons Commission on Cancer, 2011).

     (1) Ensure facilitation of smooth communication and continuity of care among members of the interdisciplinary team within healthcare settings/institutions, particularly as illness progresses (American College of Surgeons Commission on Cancer, 2011).

     (2) Ensure open, ongoing, and consistent communication among the patient, family members, and the interdisciplinary team (Registered Nurses' Association of Ontario, 2006).

  f) Perform ongoing documentation of symptoms, assessment, plan of care, and evaluation.

6. Related Web sites

  a) American Academy of Hospice and Palliative Medicine: www.aahpm.org

  b) American Association of Colleges of Nursing End-of-Life-Care: www.aacn.nche.edu/elnec

  c) Canadian Hospice Palliative Care Association: www.chpca.net

  d) Center to Advance Palliative Care: www.capc.org

  e) Edmonton Regional Palliative Care Program (Canada): www.palliative.org

  f) End of Life/Palliative Education Resource Center: www.eperc.mcw.edu

  g) Hospice and Palliative Nurses Association: www.hpna.org

  h) Hospice Foundation of America: www.hospicefoundation.org

  i) National Hospice and Palliative Care Organization: www.nhpco.org

  j) NCCN: www.nccn.org

  k) ONS Home Care and Palliative Care Special Interest Group: http://hcpc.vc.ons.org/page/4918

  l) Palliative Drugs.com (United Kingdom): www.palliativedrugs.com

References

American College of Surgeons Commission on Cancer. (2011, February). Cancer program standards 2012: Ensuring patient-centered care. Working draft. Retrieved from http://www.facs.org/cancer/coc/cps2012draft.pdf

Campos, S., Presutti, R., Zhang, L., Salvo, N., Hird, A., Tsao, M., ... Chow, E. (2010). Elderly patients with painful bone metastases should be offered palliative radiotherapy. *International Journal Radiation Oncology, Biology, Physics, 76*, 1500–1506. doi:10.1016/j.ijrobp.2009.03.019

Ferrell, B.R. (1995). The impact of pain on quality of life: A decade of research. *Nursing Clinics of North America, 30*, 609–624.

Glass, E., Cluxton, D., & Rancour, P. (2001). Principles of patient and family assessment. In B.R. Ferrell & N. Coyle (Eds.), *Textbook of palliative nursing* (pp. 37–50). New York, NY: Oxford University Press.

Hartsell, W.F., Scott, C., Bruner, D.W., Scarantino, C.W., Ivker, R., Roach, M., ... Konski, A. (2003). Phase III randomized trial of 8 Gy in 1 fraction vs. 30 Gy in 10 fractions for palliation of painful bone metastases: Preliminary results of RTOG 97-14 (Plenary abstract presentation at the 45th Annual Meeting of American Society of Therapeutic Radiology and Oncology, Salt Lake City, UT, October 19–23). *International Journal of Radiation Oncology, Biology, Physics, 57*(2, Suppl. 1), S124. doi:10.1016/S0360-3016(03)00823-X

Higginson, I.J., Finlay, I., Goodwin, D.M., Cook, A.M., Hood, K., Edwards, A.G.K., ... Normand, C.E. (2002). Do hospital-based palliative teams improve care for patients or families at the end of life? *Journal of Pain and Symptom Management, 23*, 96–106. doi:10.1016/S0885-3924(01)00406-7

Higginson, I.J., Finlay, I.G., Goodwin, D.M., Hood, K., Edwards, A.G.K., Cook, A., ... Normand, C.E. (2003). Is there evidence that palliative care teams alter end-of-life experiences of patients and their caregivers? *Journal of Pain and Symptom Management, 25*, 150–168. doi:10.1016/S0885-3924(02)00599-7

Kaplan, M. (Ed.). (2006). *Understanding and managing oncologic emergencies: A resource for nurses.* Pittsburgh, PA: Oncology Nursing Society.

Kirou-Mauro, A.M., Hird, A., Wong, J., Sinclair, E., Barnes, E.A., Tsao, M., ... Chow, E. (2009). Has pain management in cancer patients with bone metastases improved? A seven-year review at an outpatient palliative radiotherapy clinic. *Journal of Pain and Symptom Management, 37*, 77–84. doi:10.1016/j.jpainsymman.2007.12.014

Lutz, S., Berk, L., Chang, E., Chow, E., Hahn, C., Hoskin, P., ... Hartsell, W. (2011). Palliative radiation therapy for bone metastasis: An ASTRO evidence-based guideline. *International Journal of Radiation Oncology, Biology, Physics, 79*, 965–976. doi:10.1016/j.ijrobp.2010.11.026

National Comprehensive Cancer Network. (2011a). *NCCN Clinical Practice Guidelines in Oncology: Adult cancer pain* [v.1.2011]. Retrieved from http://www.nccn.org/professionals/physician_gls/pdf/pain.pdf

National Comprehensive Cancer Network. (2011b). *NCCN Clinical Practice Guidelines in Oncology: Palliative care* [v.2.2011]. Retrieved from http://www.nccn.org/professionals/physician_gls/pdf/palliative.pdf

Registered Nurses' Association of Ontario. (2006, March). *Supporting and strengthening families through expected and unexpected life events* (Rev. ed.). Toronto, Ontario, Canada: Author.

Temel, J.S., Greer, J.A., Muzikansky, A., Gallagher, E.R., Admane, S., Jackson, V.A., ... Lynch, T.J. (2010). Early palliative care for patients with metastatic non–small-cell lung cancer. *New England Journal of Medicine, 363*, 733–742. doi:10.1056/NEJMoa1000678

van Oorschot, B., Rades, D., Schulze, W., Beckmann, G., & Feyer, P. (2011). Palliative radiotherapy—New approaches. *Seminars in Oncology, 38*, 443–449. doi:10.1053/j.seminoncol.2011.03.015

Wan, J.F., & Bezjak, A. (2010). Superior vena cava syndrome. *Hematology/Oncology Clinics of North America, 24*, 501–513. doi:10.1016/j.hoc.2010.03.003

World Health Organization. (n.d.). WHO definition of palliative care. Retrieved from http://www.who.int/cancer/palliative/definition/en/

C. Cancer clinical trials
 1. Definition: Research studies involving people that answer scientific questions in order to find improved ways to prevent, detect, diagnose, and treat cancer (NCI, 2010)
 2. Purpose
  a) Evaluation of the safety and efficacy of novel treatments
  b) Assessment of the safety and efficacy of new combinations and indications for existing FDA-approved treatments
  c) Advancement of cancer therapy in participants with cancer: Although still inconclusive, some research suggests that participation in clinical trials may have a positive effect on participant outcomes (Braunholtz, Edwards, & Lilford, 2001; Kandzari et al., 2005).
 3. Phases (NCI, 2010)
  a) Phase I—Determination of the route, frequency, dose, and preliminary safety information for a new treatment
  b) Phase II—Assessment of the effectiveness and continued appraisal of safety for a new treatment
  c) Phase III—Evaluation of the effectiveness of a new treatment or combination of treatments compared to standard treatment
  d) Phase IV—Appraisal of a treatment after it has been FDA-approved and marketed to further assess treatment effectiveness and safety over a longer period of time
 4. Types of trials (NCI, 2010)
  a) Treatment—Determination of the safety and effectiveness of a new treatment, including new drugs, new combinations of treatments, new radiation or surgical techniques, and new therapeutic approaches such as gene therapy
  b) Prevention—Assessment of the effectiveness and safety of various treatments for people at risk for developing cancer, those at risk for a cancer recurrence, and those who have had cancer and are at risk for developing a new cancer

c) Screening—Appraisal of the safety and effectiveness of new methods for detecting cancer at earlier stages

d) Quality-of-life/supportive care trials—Evaluation of interventions to reduce side effects from treatment and increase the quality of life of patients with cancer and cancer survivors

5. The role of the clinical trials nurse

a) Recruitment of study participants (ONS, 2010)

(1) Have knowledge of current clinical trials and resources for obtaining information for current trial availability. RT clinical trials can be found on the RTOG Web site (www.rtog.org) and the ACR Imaging Network Web site (www.acrin.org).

(2) Understanding barriers to accrual: Less than 5% of all adult patients newly diagnosed with cancer participate in NCI clinical trials (NCI, 2005). Additionally, women, racial and ethnic minorities, and older adults are significantly underrepresented in clinical trials compared to non-Hispanic White men (Ford et al., 2008; Lewis et al., 2003; Murthy, Krumholz, & Gross, 2004).

(a) Healthcare provider–level barriers

i. Lack of time; conflict between role of clinician and researcher (Ford et al., 2008; NCI, 2005)

ii. Administrative burden associated with trial participation (NCI, 2005)

iii. Lack of awareness of available trials (Ford et al., 2008; NCI, 2005)

iv. Failure to explicitly offer clinical trial participation; difficulty with communication (Albrecht et al., 2008)

(b) Patient-level barriers (Ford et al., 2008; Mills et al., 2006)

i. Lack of insurance/direct and indirect costs of study participation

ii. Preference for a specific treatment

iii. Interference with everyday life; frequency of tests/procedures

iv. Issues with transportation; distance from treatment center

v. Dislike of randomization

vi. Fear of potential side effects

vii. Lack of information on cancer, treatment options, and overall health literacy

viii. Fears of exploitation or being treated as a "guinea pig"

ix. Uncertainty of benefits

(c) Organization-level barriers

i. Lack of infrastructure to support clinical trials (Hudson, Momperousse, & Leventhal, 2005; Joseph & Dohan, 2009; Murray et al., 2010; Somkin et al., 2005, 2008)

ii. Delayed clinical trial activation time (Dilts & Sandler, 2006; Dilts et al., 2006, 2008, 2009)

iii. Organizational culture not conducive to clinical trial participation (Joseph & Dohan, 2009; Somkin et al., 2008)

iv. Study design barriers (Ford et al., 2008)

• Stringent inclusion/exclusion criteria

• Women, racial and ethnic minorities, and older adults are significantly underrepresented in clinical trials (Ford et al., 2008; Lewis et al., 2003; Murthy et al., 2004).

(3) Understanding facilitators to clinical trial accrual (Chang, Hendricks, Slawsky, & Locastro, 2004; Nurgat et al., 2005; Wright et al., 2004)

(a) Patient-level facilitators

i. Being insured

ii. Higher socioeconomic status

iii. Perceived personal benefit from participation

iv. Altruism

v. Receiving state-of-the-art treatment

vi. Closer monitoring and follow-up on trial

vii. Monetary compensation

viii. Certain characteristics of the recruiter

(b) Provider-level facilitators

i. Recommendation from a trusted health professional

ii. Provision of incentives (Holland, 2008)

• Increased funding for grants

• Per-patient reimbursement

• Professional and public recognition

(c) Organization-level facilitators (Sateren et al., 2002)
   i. Presence of approved cancer program
   ii. Number of oncology specialists

b) Participation in the informed consent process
   (1) The Belmont Report (U.S. Department of Health, Education & Welfare, 1979) guides the informed consent process in the United States.
   (2) Basis of the informed consent process is the principle of respect for persons: Recognizing a subject's personal dignity and autonomy, or the right of subjects to act in their best interest, as well as recognizing that subjects with diminished autonomy (e.g., children, older adults) require additional protection.
   (3) Elements of informed consent process
      (a) Information: Individuals, knowing that the procedure is neither necessary for their care nor perhaps fully understood, can decide whether they wish to participate in the furthering of knowledge. Even when some direct benefit to them is anticipated, the subjects should understand clearly the range of risk and the voluntary nature of participation.
      (b) Comprehension: Because the subject's ability to understand is a function of intelligence, rationality, maturity, and language, it is necessary to adapt the presentation of the information to the subject's capacities. Investigators are responsible for ascertaining whether the subject has comprehended the information. Although there is always an obligation to ascertain that the information about risk to subjects is complete and adequately comprehended, when the risks are more serious, that obligation increases. On occasion, it may be suitable to give some oral or written tests of comprehension.
      (c) Voluntariness: An agreement to participate in research constitutes a valid consent only if it has been voluntarily given—free of coercion and undue influence. *Coercion* is when an overt threat of harm is intentionally presented by one person to another to obtain compliance. *Undue influence* is an offer of an excessive, unwarranted, inappropriate, or improper reward or other overture to obtain compliance.
   (4) Definition (National Institutes of Health, 2007): *Informed consent* is the process of learning the key facts about a clinical trial before deciding whether to participate. It is a continuing process throughout the study to provide information for participants.
      (a) The research team explains the details of the study.
      (b) Translation assistance is provided for non-English-speaking patients.
      (c) An informed consent document is given to the patient, which includes the study's purpose, duration, required procedures, risks and benefits, and key contacts.
      (d) The participant has adequate time to review the document and then decide whether to sign it.
      (e) Informed consent is not a contract, and the participant may withdraw from the trial at any time.
   (5) Steps in the informed consent process using various communication techniques such as video, interactive computer programs, and discussions, and supplemental materials such as written materials (Klimaszewski, 2008)
      (a) Initial meeting
      (b) Time to read and consider participation
      (c) Assessment of understanding
      (d) Questions
      (e) Signing of informed consent document
      (f) New information is provided throughout study, and if required, an updated informed consent document is presented to the patient for signature.

c) Health Insurance Portability and Accountability Act (HIPAA): Privacy rule governing the use and disclosure of protected health information that is transmitted or maintained in any form (Holt, 2003). See the following Web resources for further details.
   (1) American Medical Association: www.ama-assn.org

(2) U.S. Department of Health and Human Services: www.hhs.gov/ocr/privacy

d) The nurse's role in the informed consent process

(1) Provide the patient or patient advocate with information at his or her level of understanding to allow autonomous decision making.

(2) Ensure that content of consent is complete and includes the following (U.S. Department of Health and Human Services Office for Human Research Protections, 2009).

   (a) Study purpose, including an explanation of study procedures and whether any procedures are experimental

   (b) Alternative therapeutic options

   (c) Risks, including side effects of treatment, and benefits

   (d) Emphasis that participation is voluntary, the participant may discontinue participation at any time without penalty or loss of benefits to which the participant is otherwise entitled, and that refusal to participate will involve no penalty or loss of benefits

   (e) The name and contact information of the principal investigator and whom to contact in the event of a research-related injury

   (f) The extent to which confidentiality of records identifying the participant will be maintained

   (g) If the study involves more than minimal risk, an explanation about whether any compensation and medical treatments are available if injury occurs, what they entail, and where more information is available

   (h) Current IRB stamp of approval

(3) Ensure that content of informed consent includes the six essential elements to comply with the HIPAA privacy rule (Holt, 2003).

   (a) A description of information to be disclosed

   (b) Notice of the patient's right to revoke the authorization

   (c) To whom information will be disclosed

   (d) The purpose for which it will be disclosed

   (e) The expiration date for transferring protected health information

   (f) A patient's dated signature

(4) Assess the patient's decision-making capacity.

(5) Clarify and expand on information given by physicians.

(6) Provide and assist the patient in gathering additional relevant sources of information.

(7) Allow sufficient time for the patient to read the consent form, ask questions, and decide whether to participate

(8) Verify understanding of content by summarizing and asking open-ended questions (Jefford & Moore, 2008).

(9) Assess informed consent for appropriate reading level (Coyne et al., 2003), language (Roberts, 2001), and font size (for the visually impaired).

(10) Outline the progression of the protocol and what the participant can expect at each stage, as well as his or her responsibilities as a trial participant.

(11) Explain the patient's rights as a research participant (Joshi & Ehrenberger, 2001; NCI, 2002).

(12) Utilize various modes of communication to improve comprehension (Cohn & Larson, 2007).

(13) Validate the patient's consent at each visit before each clinical trial treatment (Klimaszewski, 2008).

6. The nurse's role in clinical trial patient management (ONS, 2010)

a) Verify that the potential participant meets study eligibility criteria.

b) Assess the participant for adverse events and assist in the management of side effects.

c) Provide contact numbers and educate patients regarding how and when to report changes in health status.

d) Coordinate protocol-related tests and appointments.

e) Perform timely identification, documentation, and communication of serious or unexpected side effects.

f) Determine whether a dose-limiting toxicity has occurred or if a dose modification is necessary based on adverse event assessments, and communicate this to the study team.

g) Ensure compliance with the protocol (ONS, 2010).

(1) Assess the patient's ability to adhere to protocol requirements (e.g., com-

pletion of diaries, keeping treatment schedule).

(2) Ensure that protocol guidelines, processes, and procedures are followed.

(3) Maintain participant confidentiality by securing research data and patient health information.

(4) Ensure accurate and timely completion of research data.

(5) Prepare for monitor and auditor reviews.

h) Facilitate clinical trial–related communication (ONS, 2010).

(1) Act as a liaison among the patient, physician, study team, IRB, and study sponsor.

(2) Provide clinical trial information to health professionals within the organization and develop relationships with referring departments and organizations to promote accrual and improve protocol compliance.

(3) Coordinate site initiation visits with the study sponsor and study team members.

(4) Provide community education and outreach regarding clinical trials.

i) Ensure appropriate clinical trial–related documentation (ONS, 2010).

(1) Follow protocol, institutional, and IRB requirements related to appropriate documentation in source data.

(2) Educate study team members regarding the protocol, institutional, and IRB requirements for documentation in source data.

(3) Confirm that all data can be verified within source documents.

j) Ensure ethical practice in the conduct of clinical trials (ONS, 2010).

(1) Adhere to ethical principles, including informed consent, patient autonomy, justice, and beneficence.

(2) Identify and protect the rights of vulnerable patient populations participating in clinical trials.

(3) Report scientific misconduct according to institutional guidelines.

k) Practice financial stewardship in the conduct of clinical trials (ONS, 2010).

(1) Guide participants in verifying healthcare coverage.

(2) Identify routine care costs versus research-related costs and the impact on the research participant.

(3) Identify financial factors that may influence the cost of trial conduct.

l) For a more in-depth description of the role of the clinical trials nurse, refer to ONS's *Oncology Clinical Trials Nurse Competencies* (2010).

7. Additional resources

a) Related Web sites

(1) National Institutes of Health: www .clinicaltrials.gov

(2) NCI: www.cancer.gov

(3) NCI's Center for Cancer Research: http://ccr.nci.nih.gov

(4) NCI Dictionary of Cancer Terms: www.cancer.gov/dictionary

(5) NCI Drug Dictionary: www.cancer .gov/drugdictionary

(6) ONS: www.ons.org

(7) U.S. Department of Health and Human Services Office for Human Research Protections: www.hhs.gov/ohrp

(8) U.S. Department of Health and Human Services Office for Human Research Protections, *Code of Federal Regulations* title 25, part 46: Protection of human subjects: www.hhs.gov/ohrp/ humansubjects/guidance/45cfr46 .html

b) Book: Klimaszewski, A.D., Bacon, M., Deininger, H.E., Ford, B.A., & Westendorp, J.G. (Eds.). (2008). *Manual for clinical trials nursing* (2nd ed.). Pittsburgh, PA: Oncology Nursing Society.

c) Journal: *Applied Clinical Trials*: www .actmagazine.com

References

Albrecht, T.L., Eggly, S.S., Gleason, M.E.J., Harper, F.W.K., Foster, T.S., Peterson, A.M., ... Ruckdeschel, J.C. (2008). Influence of clinical communication on patients' decision making on participation in clinical trials. *Journal of Clinical Oncology, 26,* 2666–2673. doi:10.1200/JCO.2007.14.8114

Braunholtz, D.A., Edwards, S.J.L., & Lilford, R.J. (2001). Are randomized clinical trials good for us (in the short term)? Evidence for a "trial effect." *Journal of Clinical Epidemiology, 54,* 217–224. doi:10.1016/S0895-4356(00)00305-X

Chang, B.-H., Hendricks, A.M., Slawsky, M.T., & Locastro, J.S. (2004). Patient recruitment to a randomized clinical trial of behavioral therapy for chronic heart failure. *BMC Medical Research Methodology, 4,* 8. doi:10.1186/1471-2288-4-8

Cohn, E., & Larson, E. (2007). Improving participant comprehension in the informed consent process. *Journal of Nursing Scholarship, 39,* 273–280. doi:10.1111/j.1547-5069.2007.00180.x

Coyne, C.A., Xu, R., Raich, P., Plomer, K., Dignan, M., Wenzel, L.B., ... Cella, D. (2003). Randomized, controlled trial of an easy-to-read informed consent statement for clinical trial participation: A study of the Eastern Cooperative Oncology Group. *Journal of Clinical Oncology, 21,* 836–842. doi:10.1200/JCO.2003.07 .022

Dilts, D.M., & Sandler, A.B. (2006). Invisible barriers to clinical trials: The impact of structural, infrastructural, and procedural barriers to opening oncology clinical trials. *Journal of*

Clinical Oncology, 24, 4545–4552. doi:10.1200/JCO.2005.05 .0104

Dilts, D.M., Sandler, A.B., Baker, M., Cheng, S.K., George, S.L., Karas, K.S., … Schilsky, R.L. (2006). Process to activate phase III clinical trials in a Cooperative Oncology Group: The case of Cancer and Leukemia Group B. *Journal of Clinical Oncology, 24,* 4553–4557. doi:10.1200/JCO.2006.06.7819

Dilts, D.M., Sandler, A.B., Cheng, S., Crites, J.S., Ferranti, L., Wu, A., … Comis, R. (2008). Development of clinical trials in a cooperative group setting: The Eastern Cooperative Oncology Group. *Clinical Cancer Research, 14,* 3427–3433. doi:10.1158/1078 -0432.CCR-07-5060

Dilts, D.M., Sandler, A.B., Cheng, S.K., Crites, J.S., Ferranti, L.B., Wu, A.Y., … Abrams, J. (2009). Steps and time to process clinical trials at the Cancer Therapy Evaluation Program. *Journal of Clinical Oncology, 27,* 1761–1766. doi:10.1200/JCO.2008.19 .9133

Ford, J.G., Howerton, M.W., Lai, G.Y., Gary, T.L., Bolen, S., Gibbons, M.C., … Bass, E.B. (2008). Barriers to recruiting underrepresented populations to cancer clinical trials: A systematic review. *Cancer, 112,* 228–242. doi:10.1002/cncr.23157

Holland, J. (2008). Recruitment and promotion strategies for clinical trials. In A.D. Klimaszewski, M. Bacon, H. Deininger, B.A. Ford, & J.G. Westendorp (Eds.), *Manual for clinical trials nursing* (2nd ed., pp. 147–150). Pittsburgh, PA: Oncology Nursing Society.

Holt, E. (2003). The HIPAA privacy rule, research, and IRBs. *Applied Clinical Trials, 12*(6), 48–66.

Hudson, S.V., Momperousse, D., & Leventhal, H. (2005). Physician perspectives on cancer clinical trials and barriers to minority recruitment. *Cancer Control, 12*(Suppl. 2), 93–96.

Jefford, M., & Moore, R. (2008). Improvement of informed consent and the quality of consent documents. *Lancet Oncology, 9,* 485–493. doi:10.1016/S1470-2045(08)70128-1

Joseph, G., & Dohan, D. (2009). Recruiting minorities where they receive care: Institutional barriers to cancer clinical trials recruitment in a safety-net hospital. *Contemporary Clinical Trials, 30,* 552–559. doi:10.1016/j.cct.2009.06.009

Joshi, T.G., & Ehrenberger, H.E. (2001). Cancer clinical trials in the new millennium: Novel challenges and opportunities for oncology nursing. *Clinical Journal of Oncology Nursing, 5,* 147–152.

Kandzari, D.E., Roe, M.T., Chen, A.Y., Lytle, B.L., Pollack, C.V., Jr., Harrington, R.A., … Peterson, E.D. (2005). Influence of clinical trial enrollment on the quality of care and outcomes for patients with non-ST-segment elevation acute coronary syndromes. *American Heart Journal, 149,* 474–481. doi:10.1016/j.ahj.2004.11 .014

Klimaszewski, A.D. (2008). Informed consent. In A.D. Klimaszewski, M. Bacon, H.E. Deininger, B.A. Ford, & J.G. Westendorp (Eds.), *Manual for clinical trials nursing* (2nd ed., pp. 97–105). Pittsburgh, PA: Oncology Nursing Society.

Lewis, J.H., Kilgore, M.L., Goldman, D.P., Trimble, E.L., Kaplan, R., Montello, M.J., … Escarce, J.J. (2003). Participation of patients 65 years of age or older in cancer clinical trials. *Journal of Clinical Oncology, 21,* 1383–1389. doi:10.1200/JCO.2003.08 .010

Mills, E.J., Seely, D., Rachlis, B., Griffith, L., Wu, P., Wilson, K., … Wright, J.R. (2006). Barriers to participation in clinical trials of cancer: A meta-analysis and systematic review of patient-reported factors. *Lancet Oncology, 7,* 141–148. doi:10.1016/ S1470-2045(06)70576-9

Murray, P., Kerridge, I., Tiley, C., Catanzariti, A., Welberry, H., Lean, C., … Bradstock, K. (2010). Enrollment of patients to clinical trials in haematological cancer in New South Wales: Current status, perceived barriers and opportunities for improvement. *Internal Medicine Journal, 40,* 133–138. doi:10.1111/j.1445-5994.2009 .01911.x

Murthy, V.H., Krumholz, H.M., & Gross, C.P. (2004). Participation in cancer clinical trials: Race-, sex-, and age-based disparities. *JAMA, 291,* 2720–2726. doi:10.1001/jama.291.22.2720

National Cancer Institute. (2002, September 26). Cancer clinical trials: The in-depth program. Retrieved from http://www .cancer.gov/clinicaltrials/resources/in-depth-program

National Cancer Institute. (2005, January 19). Doctors, patients face different barriers to clinical trials. Retrieved from http:// www.cancer.gov/clinicaltrials/conducting/developments/ doctors-barriers0401

National Cancer Institute. (2010). Factsheet: Cancer clinical trials. Retrieved from http://www.cancer.gov/cancertopics/factsheet/ Information/clinical-trials

National Institutes of Health. (2007, September 20). Understanding clinical trials. Retrieved from http://www.clinicaltrials.gov/ ct2/info/understand

Nurgat, Z.A., Craig, W., Campbell, N.C., Bissett, J.D., Cassidy, J., & Nicolson, M.C. (2005). Patient motivations surrounding participation in phase I and phase II clinical trials of cancer chemotherapy. *British Journal of Cancer, 92,* 1001–1005. doi:10.1038/ sj.bjc.6602423

Oncology Nursing Society. (2010). *Oncology clinical trials nurse competencies.* Retrieved from http://www.ons.org/media/ons/ docs/publications/ctncompetencies.pdf

Roberts, D.M. (2001). Meeting the needs of patients with limited English proficiency. *Journal of Medical Practice Management, 17,* 71–75.

Sateren, W.B., Trimble, E.L., Abrams, J., Brawley, O., Breen, N., Ford, L., … Christian, M.C. (2002). How sociodemographics, presence of oncology specialists, and hospital cancer programs affect accrual to cancer treatment trials. *Journal of Clinical Oncology, 20,* 2109–2117. doi:10.1200/JCO.2002.08 .056

Somkin, C.P., Altschuler, A., Ackerson, L., Geiger, A.M., Greene, S.M., Mouchawar, J., … Wagner, E. (2005). Organizational barriers to physician participation in cancer clinical trials. *American Journal of Managed Care, 11,* 413–421.

Somkin, C.P., Altschuler, A., Ackerson, L., Tolsma, D., Rolnick, S.J., Yood, R., … Go, A.S. (2008). Cardiology clinical trial participation in community-based healthcare systems: Obstacles and opportunities. *Contemporary Clinical Trials, 29,* 646–653. doi:10.1016/j.cct.2008.02.003

U.S. Department of Health and Human Services Office for Human Research Protections. (2009, January). Title 25, part 46: Protection of human subjects. In *Code of federal regulations.* Retrieved from http://www.hhs.gov/ohrp/humansubjects/guidance/45cfr46. html

U.S. Department of Health, Education, and Welfare. (1979). The Belmont report. *Federal Register, 44,* 23192–23197. Retrieved from http://www.hhs.gov/ohrp/archive/documents/19790418 .pdf

Wright, J.R., Whelan, T.J., Schiff, S., Dubois, S., Crooks, D., Haines, P.T., … Levine, M.N. (2004). Why cancer patients enter randomized clinical trials: Exploring the factors that influence their decision. *Journal of Clinical Oncology, 22,* 4312–4318. doi:10.1200/ JCO.2004.01.187

D. Nursing management in radiation oncology
  1. Definition: *Nursing management* is the process of planning, organizing, staffing, directing, and controlling a nursing unit or service (Clark, 2009). *Nursing leadership* is the process whereby nurse managers empower themselves and others to achieve organizational goals. The goal of the manager is to create an environment that attracts and retains outstanding nurses.
  2. Managing staff
    a) Staffing
      (1) Evaluate the needs of the practice.
        (a) Setting (e.g., academic, specialty hospital, hospital-based clinic, freestanding clinic, private practice)
        (b) Patient population (e.g., case mix, acuity index, age-specific needs, percentage of curative and palliative patients, percentage of pediatric and older adult patients, socioeconomic status, survivorship needs, and cultural diversity of patients)
        (c) Treatments (e.g., EBRT, brachytherapy, hypofractionated treatments, protocols, clinical trials)
        (d) Physician expectations, referral base
        (e) Hours of operation (e.g., flexible scheduling, early morning and late-night treatments, weekend operations)
        (f) Reimbursement practices (based on third-party payer policies, contracts, and state regulations)
      (2) Determine staffing patterns.
        (a) RN, bachelor's-prepared
          i. Oncology nursing certification
          ii. RN role in radiation oncology includes patient assessment, education, support, counseling, physical care, research, coordination, and leadership activities (Gosselin-Acomb, 2006; Moore-Higgs et al., 2003a; Smith, Arslanian-Carlin, & Cartwright-Alcarese, 2011).
        (b) Clinical nurse specialist (CNS), master's-prepared, advanced oncology certified clinical nurse specialist (AOCNS®). CNS role includes clinician, educator, mentor, consultant, and researcher (ONS, 2008).
        (c) Nurse practitioner (NP), master's-prepared, advanced oncology certified nurse practitioner (AOCNP®). NP role, in collaboration with a radiation oncologist, involves the care of the physiologic and psychological needs of patients with cancer, including cancer prevention and detection, cancer diagnosis and treatment, rehabilitation, survivorship, and end-of-life care (Carper & Haas, 2006). ONS (2007) has established oncology NP competencies that reflect the work of a multiorganizational national panel and can serve as minimum standard for role development with a radiation oncology department.
      (3) Determine the number of nursing staff.
        (a) The American College of Radiation Oncology has published guidelines for accreditation (Cotter & Parsai, 2009) recommending 1 RN per 200–300 new patients annually, based on an eight-hour/five-day workweek.
        (b) Current models need to include not only direct patient care hours but time spent on other ancillary responsibilities. These include answering telephones, scheduling appointments or tests, performing clinical trial activities, obtaining test results, cleaning equipment, and developing patient education materials
      (4) Establish the model of practice.
        (a) Collaborative practice model: The nurse and physician collaboratively care for a specific patient practice.
        (b) Clinical model primary: The RN follows the patient during consultation, treatment, and follow-up (Gosselin-Acomb, 2006).

(5) Write the position descriptions. The American Academy of Ambulatory Care Nursing (2006) *Core Curriculum for Ambulatory Care Nursing* includes a comprehensive discussion of the scope of ambulatory care nursing and includes the American Academy of Ambulatory Care Nursing Administrative and Practice Standards. A conceptual framework for ambulatory practice is provided that may be helpful in developing a position description. Moore-Higgs et al. (2003b) applied this framework to radiation oncology practice.

    (a) Accountability (scope of responsibilities)

    (b) Reporting structure

    (c) Requirements (educational, experience, knowledge, skills, and abilities)

    (d) Responsibilities (clinical, quality, professional)

    (e) Coordination/leadership

    (f) Education/development

(6) Under the Americans with Disabilities Act of 1990 (see www.ada.gov/pubs/ada.htm), if an employee can perform essential job functions, the employer has to make reasonable accommodations (e.g., modifying work schedule, reassigning nonessential functions, modifying equipment).

3. Hiring

    a) Recruit eligible candidates (e.g., nurse recruitment department, Web sites, multimedia advertising campaigns, professional conferences, individual referrals, social networks, local job fairs).

    b) Screen applicants.

    c) Review curriculum vitae/résumé.

    d) Certification within the specialty (such as ONS's Certified Breast Care Nurse [CBCN™]) validates the RN's specialized knowledge, indicates a level of clinical competence, and enhances professional credibility (American Nurses Credentialing Center, 2010).

    e) Interview applicants. Goal of interview is to judge the applicant's dependability, willingness to assume responsibility for the job, willingness and ability to work with others, interest in the job, and adaptability, and the consistency of the applicant's goals with available opportunities (Tomey, 2009).

    f) Prepare for the interview by structuring questions to (Tomey, 2009)

    (1) Obtain information

    (2) Give information

    (3) Determine if the applicant meets the requirements of the position.

    (4) Formulate open-ended questions that reveal candidate's strengths and weaknesses (e.g., "Tell me about how you handled a difficult conflict with a colleague," or "What would your coworkers say is a strength of yours? What would they say you are challenged by?"

    (5) Avoid discriminatory questions (e.g., national origin, race, color, religion, marital status, parental status, age).

    (6) Describe position responsibilities, hours, and working conditions framed around the needs of the patient population and the department.

    (7) Encourage questions.

    g) Schedule the interview.

    (1) Conduct the interview: State the purpose of the interview is to give and receive information to determine if there is a mutual fit. Review and clarify items on the curriculum vitae. Ensure a quiet, uninterrupted interview.

        (a) One-on-one interviews with leadership

        (b) Panel interview consisting of all levels of nursing staff

        (c) Panel interview consisting of multidisciplinary team members

    (2) Check references (usually conducted by nurse recruitment). Review credentialing process for APNs.

4. Education—Programs should emphasize teamwork, conflict resolution, and the use of informatics to promote collaboration in patient care, planning, and implementation (Studer, 2003; Wakefield & O'Grady, 2000).

    a) Staff development

    (1) Malcolm Knowles' assumptions regarding adult learning (Abruzzese, 1996; Knowles, Holton, & Swanson, 2005) remain relevant. Adults are self-directed and need to know the reason for why they should learn something. They are ready to learn when they perceive the need to learn and when the information is immediately applicable.

    (2) Orientation to unit and organization, mandatory annual and continuing education

        (a) Unit-based educational offerings for ongoing clinical and staff development (e.g., radiation safety,

in-services on equipment, supplies, procedures, and regulatory requirements)

(b) Competency-based orientation program with preceptor support

(c) Continuing education to maintain and enhance knowledge (e.g., unit-based, conferences, journal club)

(d) Mandatory annual: Web-based, drills (e.g., The Joint Commission)

(e) Certification requirements

(f) Professional development opportunities: As mentor/mentee

(3) Plan and implement educational programs.

(a) Assess staff learning needs. Identify knowledge, skills, and attitudes required.

(b) Establish learning objectives that are observable and measurable (begin with action verbs).

(c) Develop an outline of the content needed to ensure achievement of objectives.

(d) Determine the method of presenting content. Use various methodologies (e.g., readings, didactic presentations, audiovisuals, interactive media, clinical rotations with preceptors). Consider strategies to make educational programs meaningful to the learner (Marquis & Huston, 2009; Sullivan & Decker, 2008).

(e) Develop a tool to evaluate if objectives were met.

i. Post-test for didactic information

ii. Competency checklist for skills

b) Performance appraisal: Key points outlined by Sullivan and Decker (2008, Chapter 18, p. 241) and Marquis and Huston (2009, Chapter 14, pp. 423–451) include the following.

(1) Performance appraisal is the systematic evaluation of the quality of the employee's performance based on defined standards.

(a) It is a tool to integrate, facilitate, and coordinate the work of employees in alignment with the goals of the organization and department.

(b) It is an opportunity to establish mutual goals with clear objectives.

(c) It establishes a motivational climate for professional develop-

ment, role-modeling, mentoring, coaching, and disciplining, when needed.

(d) It is results-oriented; goals are concrete, quantifiable, objective, and easily measured with an established time frame.

(2) Rating scale: Notes performance (outcomes and behavior) at a point on a continuum. The following example illustrates use of a rating scale (Marquis & Huston, 2009).

(a) 5—Significantly exceeds expectations (significant contributions to the department's effectiveness).

(b) 4—Exceeds expectations (performance above average; at times exceeds some job expectations and requirements).

(c) 3—Meets expectations (performance consistently meets the normal job expectations and requirements).

(d) 2—Needs improvement (performance occasionally fails to meet some job expectations and requirements; improvement is expected in order to meet all job expectations).

(e) 1—Fails to meet performance standards (performance does not meet the critical job expectations and requirements. Successful completion of a performance improvement plan is essential for continued employment in the position).

(3) Sullivan and Decker (2008) and Marquis and Huston (2009) described the RN's role in performance appraisal.

(a) Self-evaluation is an expectation of Magnet® nurses (American Nurses Credentialing Center, 2010). The RN completes and reviews with supervisor for feedback and revisions.

(b) Group evaluation can be incorporated into performance evaluation. Several managers are asked to rank employee performance based on job descriptions and performance standards.

(c) Peer review provides valuable feedback. RNs assess and judge the performance of professional peers against predetermined standards.

(4) Sullivan and Decker (2008) and Marquis and Huston (2009) listed key elements of an appraisal.

(a) State the purpose of the appraisal interview.

(b) Review each rating with the employee, and discuss discrepancies, if appropriate.

(c) Include anecdotal notes/critical notes that record timely observations of performance; seek input from other sources if work not directly observed.

(d) Reinforce strengths and confidence in the employee.

(5) Factors that influence errors in performance evaluation (Marquis & Huston, 2009; Sullivan & Decker, 2008)

(a) Leniency error: Evaluator overrates staff's performance.

(b) Recency error: A recent mistake or accomplishment is used to frame the entire evaluation period.

(c) Halo error: Evaluator rates high across all categories.

(d) Horns effect: The evaluator is hypercritical.

(e) Bias: A person who does not complain is likely to have higher ratings than a person who does; a person on a successful team is likely to have higher ratings than a person on less successful team.

c) Coaching: The day-to-day process of helping employees improve their performance (Sullivan & Decker, 2008). Coaching consists of

(1) Needs analysis

(2) Decision making

(3) Problem solving

(4) Analytical thinking, active listening, and motivation.

d) Team building: Essentials to optimal team building (Marquis & Huston, 2009; Smith et al., 2011; Sullivan & Decker, 2008)

(1) A high-performance team works cooperatively with a leader on clearly defined objectives and tasks; roles are well defined.

(a) Maintain a positive work group climate.

(b) Communicate openly, candidly, and clearly with one another about procedures, expectations, and plans.

(c) Mutual respect is a requisite; suggestions and critiques are encouraged from all members of the team.

(d) Decision-making model is clear (e.g., the rational model uses deliberate actions to select the best solutions; the collegial model facilitates decisions by a group of peers) (Sullivan & Decker, 2008).

(e) Decisions support the needs of the department and patient population.

(f) Provide and seek feedback from all team members to plan and to understand outcomes from action plans implemented and to learn and apply to future solutions.

(2) Housekeeping items

(a) Develop an agenda with clear objectives.

(b) Start and end each meeting on time.

(c) Include membership that reflects needed expertise and scope.

(d) Set expectations for attendance and commitment.

(e) Provide adequate time for each member to complete duties.

(3) Team-building concepts specific to radiation oncology (Smith et al., 2011)

(a) The RT team is a matrix of personnel within the department and within the organization or cancer center.

(b) The planning and delivery of RT is a team effort that requires collaboration and coordination among radiation, medical, and surgical staff that includes the radiation oncologist, medical physicist, dosimetrist, radiation therapist, radiation oncology nurse, and ideally, a dedicated supportive care team (e.g., social work, nutritionist) and clerical staff.

5. Managing operations

a) Collaboration

(1) Defined as mutual attention to the problem in which the talents of all parties are used. Focus is on solving the problem (Sullivan & Decker, 2008).

It is an essential element in providing quality health care.

(2) The manager is a role model for staff collaboration when interacting with colleagues in leadership roles. This will help enhance team building within the collaborative practice model.

(3) An important element is role delineation that clearly defines who has oversight and who is responsible for the day-to-day operations of the department, the budget, new equipment needs, development, staffing, quality performance improvement, and standards of care (Smith et al., 2011).

(4) Promote intradepartmental collaboration. This includes physicians, therapists, physicists, administration, and ancillary parties involved within the department.

(5) Promote interdepartmental collaboration (e.g., medical oncology, radiology, surgery, social work, dietary services).

(6) Strategies to promote collaboration
  (a) Five concepts: Sharing, partnership, power, interdependency, and process (D'Amour, Ferrada-Videla, Rodriguez, & Beaulieu, 2005)
  (b) Education—Programs should emphasize teamwork, conflict resolution, and the use of informatics to promote collaboration in patient care, planning, and implementation (Wakefield & O'Grady, 2000).

b) Information technology
  (1) The Institute of Medicine Committee on Quality of Health Care in America (2001) supported the use of information regarding patient encounters that should focus on safety, EBP, and patient satisfaction. The use of electronic medical records is further supported by HIPAA, the American Recovery and Reinvestment Act of 2009, and the Health Information Technology for Economic and Clinical Health Act of 2009.
  (2) All staff must have a basic knowledge of computers. RNs are in a pivotal role to access and retrieve electronic data. Patients may have a *personal health record*, or PHR, or an *electronic health record*, or EHR. Communications may occur via e-mail, social networking Web sites, or online teaching modules.

(3) The nurse manager should have knowledge of electronic systems to support care within the department and to assist in the selection of the system.
(4) Using the Internet to support EBP

c) Finance: Key points (Marquis & Huston, 2009; Perez & Halperin, 2004; Smith et al., 2011; Sullivan & Decker, 2008)
  (1) A *budget* is a detailed, written plan for the allocation of resources and a control for ensuring that results reflect the plans.
    (a) Direct costs: Expenses that directly affect patient care and hands-on nursing, including but not limited to salaries, benefits, and supplies
    (b) Indirect costs: Necessary expenses but not hands-on nursing, including but not limited to maintenance personnel, receptionists, nurse managers, or overhead costs (e.g., depreciation)
  (2) The budget is generated from the radiation oncology department's strategic plan (Perez & Halperin, 2004).
    (a) Aligned with well-defined goals and objectives
    (b) Determines resource needs: Proactive fiscal planning
    (c) Projects both controllable and noncontrollable expenses (e.g., depreciation of RT equipment is noncontrollable)
    (d) Analyzes and budgets for all levels of tasks associated with delivery of RT (e.g., activity-based cost system)
        i. Staff: Radiation oncologists, physicists, therapists, dosimetrists, nurses, and receptionists
        ii. Physical resources: Space, equipment, and machines
        iii. Supplies: X-ray films and office supplies
        iv. Support services: Administration and information technology
  (3) Budget control: Analyze expenses, and anticipate, recognize, and proactively address budgetary challenges.
    (a) Review variance when above or below expectations (e.g., 5% positive or negative variance) (Marquis & Huston, 2009; Perez & Halperin, 2004).
    (b) Transparent budget: Staff understand how the resources are

being used; engage team to find innovative ways to be more cost-effective.

(c) Accountability: Organization charts and job descriptions are available and are aligned with the department's goals and objectives.

(d) Communication: The team understands the relationships among goals, expenses, and revenues.

(4) Types of budgets

(a) Operating budget (annual budget coincides with fiscal year): Projects the planned activities and operations for the upcoming year

(b) Revenue budget: Represents the patient care revenues expected for the budget period based on volume and mix of patients, rates, and discounts

(c) Zero-based budget: Justifies every expense item based on current fiscal environment and department/organization strategic plan

(d) Incremental budget: Lists expenses "line by line" by salary and nonsalary items

(e) Fixed budgets: Set; do not consider making changes (e.g., volume).

(f) Variable budgets: Set; do make adjustments based on changes (e.g., volume).

(g) Expense budget: Reflects patient care objectives and activity parameter established; represents the expenses expected for the budget period.

(h) Personnel (salary) budget: Estimates the cost of direct labor necessary to meet the department's goals and objectives

(5) Overview of financial/budgetary considerations relevant to RT (Perez & Halperin, 2004; Smith et al., 2011; Sullivan & Decker, 2008)

(a) RT is primarily a fixed-cost business.

(b) Primary goal is to increase patient volumes while managing the use of resources.

(c) Advancements and changes in expensive technology increase direct and nondirect costs.

d) Managing quality patient care: Key points for developing and maintaining quality patient care (Marquis & Huston, 2009; Smith et al., 2011; Sullivan & Decker, 2008)

(1) Radiation oncology nursing role: Using an evidence-based model of practice, the radiation oncology nurse provides assessment, diagnosis, outcome identification, planning, implementation, and evaluation, focusing on the continuum of care to support patients who are receiving RT and their families and caregivers (Smith et al., 2011).

(2) Standards, policies, and procedures

(a) *Standards* define the level of care by which quality can be evaluated. The scope and standards of nursing care provide the foundation for quality care (Eaton & Tipton, 2009a). The *Statement on the Scope and Standards of Oncology Nursing Practice* (Brant & Wickham, 2004) provides a comprehensive discussion of the scope and standards of oncology nursing practice, standards of care, and professional performance.

(b) *Structure standards* are defined as the rules and regulations or policies of varying levels of the organization (describe the environment, staffing plan, and physical resources).

(c) *Process standards* define the actions and behaviors of giving care as well as what constitutes that care (e.g., assessments, patient education, interventions).

  i. Policies: Define who can do what under what circumstances.

  ii. Procedures: Specify the psychomotor skills involved in the actions of carrying out a task.

  iii. Protocols: Dependent, interdependent, and independent service structure standards are developed to be consistent with departmental or interdisciplinary standards and apply to the role of each professional because of the nature of the care provided or the setting in which it is provided. iv. Guidelines: Document care or personnel actions.

(d) Outcome standards: Delineate the expected results of nursing care (e.g., health status, functioning, knowledge, behavior). *Nursing care plans* and *interdisciplinary clinical pathways* document defined outcomes.

(e) Use best current evidence to develop policies, procedures, and standards.

i. Standards, policies, and procedures developed using ONS Putting Evidence Into Practice resources (Eaton & Tipton, 2009a, 2009b; Eaton, Tipton, & Irwin, 2011) and nationally recognized organizations by specialty (e.g., ACR).

ii. Many Internet resources are available for searching for evidence, although at some sites, full-text articles are available only to members or subscribers (see Figure 32).

(3) Continuous performance improvement projects are important to improving and evaluating the quality of care.

(a) "The measurement of outcomes may translate into more cost-effective care, improved patient satisfaction, recognition of a professional approach to care, increased collaboration with physicians and other healthcare professionals, and optimal patient outcomes" (Gobel & Tipton, 2009, p. 1).

(b) Healthcare quality indicators are used to measure and improve the quality, effectiveness, and efficiency of patients with cancer.

(c) The Agency for Healthcare Research and Quality (www.ahrq .gov) provides clinical EBP guidelines and outcomes, some of which are relevant in the radiation oncology setting (e.g., pain management for patients with cancer; breast cancer screening schedule).

(d) See section XII—Accreditation and quality improvement.

6. Documentation: Documentation of nursing assessment, nursing interventions, and evaluation of patient outcomes is included in the patient's treatment record and is essential for provision and evaluation of quality care and for regulatory and financial assessments. The *Radiation Therapy Patient Care Record: A Tool for Documenting Nursing Care* (Catlin-Huth,

Haas, & Pollock, 2002) provides instructions and tools to standardize the documentation of nursing care provided to patients receiving RT.

Figure 32. Useful Internet Sites for Nursing Management in Radiation Oncology

Searching within a specific database
- CINAHL®: Members-only search: www.cinahl.com
- U.S. National Library of Medicine, PubMed database (includes MEDLINE®): www.ncbi.nlm.nih.gov/entrez/query.fcgi

Searching for systematic reviews from multiple resources/sites
- SUMSearch 2: http://sumsearch.org
- TRIP Database: www.tripdatabase.com

Searching for systematic reviews within particular sites (nursing)
- *Evidence-Based Nursing*: Select "Topic Collections" to browse or use the search box to look for a specific topic: http://ebn.bmj.com
- Joanna Briggs Institute (Australia): www.joannabriggs.edu .au
- National Institute of Nursing Research: www.ninr.nih.gov/ NewsAndInformation/NINRPublications

Searching for systematic reviews within particular sites (general)
- Agency for Healthcare Research and Quality: www.ahrq .gov/clinic/epcix.htm
- Bandolier (United Kingdom): Summarizes systematic reviews, includes focus on pain: www.medicine.ox.ac.uk/ bandolier
- Clinical Evidence: http://clinicalevidence.bmj.com/ceweb/ index.jsp
- Cochrane Library: www.thecochranelibrary.com/view/0/ index.html
- *Evidence-Based Medicine*: http://ebm.bmj.com
- National Health Service (United Kingdom) Centre for Reviews and Dissemination: www.york.ac.uk/inst/crd/welcome .htm

Searching for practice guidelines
- Agency for Healthcare Research and Quality, National Guideline Clearinghouse: www.ngc.gov
- American Association of Critical-Care Nurses: www.aacn .org
- American College of Radiology: www.acr.org
- American Hospital Association: www.aha.org
- American Medical Association: www.ama-assn.org
- American Nurses Association: www.nursingworld.org
- American Society of Clinical Oncology: www.asco.org
- American Society of periAnesthesia Nurses: www.aspan .org
- Association of Pediatric Hematology/Oncology Nurses: www.aphon.org
- Dermatology Nurses' Association: www.dnanurse.org
- National Comprehensive Cancer Network: www.nccn.org
- Oncology Nursing Society: www.ons.org
- Society of Gynecologic Nurse Oncologists: www.sgno.org
- Society of Gastroenterology Nurses and Associates: www .sgna.org

7. Patient education
   a) Identify existing printed resources that nursing staff can distribute to patients.
      (1) ACS: www.cancer.org
      (2) Cancer Information Network: www.thecancer.net
      (3) LIVESTRONG: www.livestrong.org
      (4) NCCN: www.nccn.org
      (5) NCI: www.cancer.gov
      (6) OncoLink: www.oncolink.com
      (7) ONS's Cancer Journey: www.thecancerjourney.org
   b) Develop department- and practice-specific information.
   c) Patient education committee—Develop practice-specific or site-specific patient education materials based on the best evidence available. Membership collaborates with and seeks expert critique from the interdisciplinary team and optimally includes the patient.
      (1) Printed material (available in multiple languages)
      (2) Audiovisual material (e.g., CDs, podcasts)
   d) Patient education in radiation oncology is focused on self-care to prevent, minimize, and delay treatment-related side effects (Smith et al., 2011). Patient outcomes associated with optimal self-care and side effect management include treatment interruption (dose delay), dose reduction, decrease in inpatient length of stay, decrease in emergency department visits, fewer hospitalizations, and increased functional status and quality of life.
8. Research
   a) It is essential that the care of patients with cancer be evidence based and that research be conducted in areas where this is lacking (e.g., quality of life, symptom experience, late effects of cancer, survivorship).
      (1) Read and critique relevant nursing research articles and application of research findings to practice; participate in journal clubs.
      (2) Join ONS special interest groups (SIGs) to engage with other radiation department teams to discuss concepts, literature, and other issues. Visit the Radiation SIG Virtual Community at www.radiation.vc.ons.org.
      (3) Participate in organization's nursing research or professional development committee; propose beginning one if not in place.
   b) The nurse's role in clinical trials (see section XI.C—Cancer clinical trials)
      (1) Depending upon the setting, the radiation oncology nurse's role and the research nurse's role are separate.
      (2) For diseases/programs that have the majority of patients enrolled in clinical trials, an integrated role is ideal.
      (3) The level of integration of research and clinical practice into the radiation oncology nurse's role varies based on the number of patients enrolled in clinical trials.
      (4) Because treatment for patients with cancer is based on the outcome of clinical trials, it is important that radiation oncology nurses remain current in clinical trials and research.
9. Leadership
   a) Characteristics of leaders (Hesselbein, Goldsmith, & Somerville, 2002; Koestenbaum, 2002; Studer, 2003)
      (1) Develop trust by being honest and fair
      (2) Facilitate two-way communication
      (3) Inspire high performance
      (4) Inspire the dream/vision of others
      (5) Communicate effectively
      (6) Create cohesive teams that work toward the vision and stay focused
      (7) Cultivate a culture of innovation
      (8) Promote motivation and growth through coaching and role modeling
   b) Review leadership models: Hesselbein et al. (2002) and Studer (2003) described leadership models. Following is an example of the leadership diamond (Studer, 2003).
      (1) Leadership diamond: Distinguishes four interdependent leadership imperatives
         (a) Ethics: Be of service (e.g., act with integrity and in accordance with one's principles).
         (b) Vision: Think big and new (e.g., exercise abstract visioning).
         (c) Reality: Have no illusions (e.g., face reality as it is, not as one wishes it was).
         (d) Courage: Act with sustained initiative (e.g., change before it is required).
      (2) Leadership concepts (Koestenbaum, 2002)
         (a) Be effective. Emphasize results, both through management by objectives and by process.

(b) Understand that leadership is a mindset and a pattern of behaviors.

(c) Lead by teaching leadership, by empowering, by fostering autonomy, providing direction, and lending support. A teacher is an experienced and relentless learner.

(d) Have faith that leadership can be learned and that it can be taught.

(e) Know that the leader's mind can hold opposing ideas and contradictory feelings at the same time. It can achieve comfort with the tensions of ambiguity, polarity, and uncertainty.

(f) Be a leader in all six arenas of life: Work, family, self, ecologic responsibility, social responsibility, and financial strength.

(g) Use both reasons or models (living from the "outside in") and instincts or intuition (living from the "inside out").

c) Resources for nurse leaders

(1) The American Nurses Association (2009) has developed a resource for nurse administrators that is useful for the nurse manager.

(2) Anderson, Manno, O'Connor, and Gallagher (2010) used the American Nurses Association's National Database of Nursing Quality Indicators® to review nursing leadership.

(3) Clark (2009) provided a comprehensive discussion of nursing leadership and management.

(4) Meredith, Cohen, and Raia (2010) provided a description of the Magnet concept of transformational leadership and application to practice.

10. Future workforce issues

a) Advances in information technology: Consumer access to Internet, which can enable staff to communicate via secure Web sites with patients and other healthcare providers and can enable the consumer to access medical information, protocol availability, and recommended clinical guidelines

b) Focus on quality care

(1) Pay-for-performance initiatives are an incentive for nurses to improve care and control costs.

(2) Patient Protection and Affordable Care Act of 2010—Provisions in the legislation provide funding for nursing education and programs that focus on safety and quality.

(3) Patient satisfaction

(4) Staff satisfaction—National Database of Nursing Quality Indicators RN Survey

(5) Stakeholder interest

c) Globalization has brought new challenges (Tomey, 2009). Electronic communication facilitates instantaneous contact and worldwide collegial collaboration. The Internet allows the public to be aware of the latest diagnostic and treatment modalities and the "centers of excellence" at which those modalities are available.

References

Abruzzese, R.S. (1996). *Nursing staff development: Strategies for success* (2nd ed.). St. Louis, MO: Mosby.

American Academy of Ambulatory Care Nursing. (2006). *Core curriculum for ambulatory care nursing* (2nd ed.). Pitman, NJ: Author.

American Nurses Association. (2009). *Nursing administration: Scope and standards of practice*. Washington, DC: Author.

American Nurses Credentialing Center. (2010). ANCC Magnet® Recognition Program. Retrieved from http://www.nursecredentialing.org/Magnet.aspx

Americans with Disabilities Act. (1990). Public law 101-336. Retrieved from http://www.ada.gov/pubs/ada.htm

Anderson, B.J., Manno, M., O'Connor, P., & Gallagher, E. (2010). Listening to nursing leaders: Using National Database of Nursing Quality Indicators data to study excellence in nursing leadership. *Journal of Nursing Administration, 40*, 182–187. doi:10.1097/NNA.0b013e3181d40f65

Brant, J.M., & Wickham, R.S. (Eds.). (2004). *Statement on the scope and standards of oncology nursing practice*. Pittsburgh, PA: Oncology Nursing Society.

Carper, E., & Haas, M. (2006). Advanced practice nursing in radiation oncology. *Seminars in Oncology Nursing, 22*, 203–211. doi:10.1016/j.soncn.2006.07.003

Catlin-Huth, C., Haas, M., & Pollock, V. (Eds.). (2002). *Radiation therapy patient care record: A tool for documenting nursing care*. Pittsburgh, PA: Oncology Nursing Society.

Clark, C.C. (2009). *Creative nursing leadership and management*. Sudbury, MA: Jones and Bartlett.

Cotter, G.W., & Parsai, E.I. (Eds.). (2009). *American College of Radiation Oncology Red Book®: Guidelines for the ACRO practice accreditation program*. Bethesda, MD: American College of Radiation Oncology.

D'Amour, D., Ferrada-Videla, M., Rodriguez, L.S.M., & Beaulieu, M.D. (2005). The conceptual basis for interprofessional collaboration: Core concepts and theoretical frameworks. *Journal of Interprofessional Care, 19*(Suppl. 1), 116–131. doi:10.1080/13561820500082529

Eaton, L., & Tipton, J.M. (2009a). Evidence-based practice: Its role in quality improvement. In L.H. Eaton & J.M. Tipton (Eds.), *Putting evidence into practice: Improving oncology patient outcomes* (pp. 299–308). Pittsburgh, PA: Oncology Nursing Society.

Eaton, L.H., & Tipton, J.M. (Eds.). (2009b). *Putting evidence into practice: Improving oncology patient outcomes*. Pittsburgh, PA: Oncology Nursing Society.

Eaton, L.H., Tipton, J.M., & Irwin, M. (Eds.). (2011). *Putting evidence into practice: Improving oncology patient outcomes, volume 2*. Pittsburgh, PA: Oncology Nursing Society.

Gobel, B.H., & Tipton, J.M. (2009). PEP up your practice: An introduction to the Oncology Nursing Society putting evidence into practice resources. In L.H. Eaton & J.M. Tipton (Eds.), *Putting evidence into practice: Improving oncology patient outcomes* (pp. 1–8). Pittsburgh, PA: Oncology Nursing Society.

Gosselin-Acomb, T.K. (2006). Role of the radiation oncology nurse. *Seminars in Oncology Nursing, 22,* 198–202. doi:10.1016/j.soncn.2006.07.001

Hesselbein, F., Goldsmith, M., & Somerville, I. (Eds.). (2002). *Leading for innovation and organizing for results* (Drucker Foundation Wisdom to Action Series). San Francisco, CA: Jossey-Bass.

Institute of Medicine Committee on Quality of Health Care in America. (2001). *Crossing the quality chasm: A new health system for the 21st century* (Institute of Medicine report). Washington, DC: National Academies Press.

Knowles, M.S., Holton, E.F., III, & Swanson, R.A. (2005). *The adult learner: The definitive classic in adult education and human resource development* (6th ed.). Boston, MA: Elsevier.

Koestenbaum, P. (2002). *Leadership: The inner side of greatness: A philosophy for leaders* (2nd ed.). San Francisco, CA: Jossey-Bass.

Marquis, B.L., & Huston, C.J. (2009). *Leadership roles and management functions in nursing: Theory and application* (6th ed.). Philadelphia, PA: Lippincott Williams & Wilkins.

Meredith, E.K., Cohen, E., & Raia, L.V. (2010). Transformational leadership: Application of magnet's new empiric outcomes. *Nursing Clinics of North America, 45,* 49–64. doi:10.1016/j.cnur.2009.10.007

Moore-Higgs, G.J., Watkins-Bruner, D., Balmer, L., Johnson-Doneski, J., Komarny, P., Mautner, B., & Velji, K. (2003a). The role of licensed nursing personnel in radiation oncology part A: Results of a descriptive study. *Oncology Nursing Forum, 30,* 51–58. doi:10.1188/03.ONF.51-58

Moore-Higgs, G.J., Watkins-Bruner, D., Balmer, L., Johnson-Doneski, J., Komarny, P., Mautner, B., & Velji, K. (2003b). The role of licensed nursing personnel in radiation oncology part B: Integrating the ambulatory care nursing conceptual framework. *Oncology Nursing Forum, 30,* 59–64. doI:10.1188/03.ONF.59-64

Oncology Nursing Society. (2007). *Oncology nurse practitioner competencies.* Pittsburgh, PA: Author.

Oncology Nursing Society. (2008). *Oncology clinical nurse specialist competencies.* Pittsburgh, PA: Author.

Perez, C.A., & Halperin, E.C. (2004). Technology assessment, cost benefit, outcome analysis research and evidence-based radiation oncology. In E.C. Halperin, C.A. Perez, & L.W. Brady (Eds.), *Perez and Brady's principles and practice of radiation oncology* (4th ed., pp. 2022–2026). Philadelphia, PA: Lippincott Williams & Wilkins.

Smith, B.E., Arslanian-Carlin, L., & Cartwright-Alcarese, F. (2011). Radiation oncology guide for the nurse manager. In M.M. Gullatte (Ed.), *Nursing management: Principles and practice* (2nd ed., pp. 501–534). Pittsburgh, PA: Oncology Nursing Society.

Studer, Q. (2003). *Hardwiring excellence: Purpose, worthwhile work, making a difference.* Gulf Breeze, FL: Fire Starter Publishing.

Sullivan, E.J., & Decker, P.J. (2008). *Effective leadership and management in nursing* (7th ed.). Upper Saddle River, NJ: Pearson Prentice Hall.

Tomey, A.M. (2009). *Guide to nursing management and leadership* (8th ed.). St. Louis, MO: Elsevier Mosby.

Wakefield, M., & O'Grady, E. (2000). *Charting nursing's future.* Princeton, NJ: Robert Wood Johnson Foundation.

XII. Accreditation and quality improvement

A. The Joint Commission (TJC)
1. Mission: To continuously improve health care for the public, in collaboration with other stakeholders, by evaluating healthcare organizations and inspiring them to excel in providing safe and effective care of the highest quality and value (TJC, 2010a)
2. Independent, nongovernmental, nonprofit organization (TJC, 2010a)
3. Value of accreditation (TJC, 2010a)
   a) Provides a competitive advantage
   b) Strengthens community confidence
   c) Fulfills licensure requirements in more than 30 states. In many states, TJC accreditation fulfills some or all state licensure or regulatory requirements.
   d) Assists in recognition from insurers, associations, and other third parties. Accreditation is increasingly becoming a prerequisite for insurance reimbursement eligibility, association memberships, and participation in managed care plans and bidding on contracts.
4. Develops and updates state-of-the-art professionally based standards and evaluates compliance of healthcare organizations against these benchmarks
5. Types of accreditation/standards applicable to RT centers
   a) Hospital
      (1) Standards apply to hospital-based facilities.
      (2) Accreditation standards and requirements are delineated in the *2010 Portable Comprehensive Accreditation Manual for Hospitals*.
   b) Ambulatory care: Standards apply to free-standing facilities. Accreditation standards and requirements are delineated in the *2010 Portable Comprehensive Accreditation Manual for Ambulatory Care*.
   c) Additional standards/manuals exist for accreditation of other types of healthcare organizations: Long-term care, laboratory services, behavioral health care, home care, office-based surgery, and international accreditation.
6. Manual organization (TJC, 2010a, 2011b)
   a) TJC standards are organized by functions and processes that address patient-focused requirements, not by disciplines or departments.
   b) Standards included in the hospital and ambulatory manuals are similar except for additional standards in the hospital manual (see Table 21).
   c) Content in each is adapted to the appropriate healthcare setting.
7. Survey process (TJC, 2010a)
   a) Purpose of TJC accreditation survey
      (1) Assesses extent of an organization's compliance with applicable TJC standards, National Patient Safety Goals, and accreditation participation requirements
      (2) Provides on-site education as surveyors offer suggestions for approaches and strategies that may help the organization to meet standards and improve performance
      (3) Process emphasizes the importance of high-quality patient care.
      (4) During the on-site survey, surveyors evaluate the organization's performance of functions and processes by

Table 21. Comparison of Standards Included in Hospital and Ambulatory Care Accreditation Manuals

Standard	Hospital	Ambulatory Care
Environment of care	X	X
Emergency management	X	X
Human resources	X	X
Infection prevention and control	X	X
Information management	X	X
Leadership	X	X
Life safety	X	X
Medication management	X	X
Medical staff	X	
National patient safety goals	X	X
Nursing	X	
Provision of care, treatment, and services	X	X
Performance improvement	X	X
Record of care, treatment, and services	X	X
Rights and responsibilities of the individual	X	X
Transplant safety	X	X
Waived testing	X	X

Note. Based on information from Joint Commission, 2010a, 2011b.

assessing patient-centered and organizational functions that support safety and quality of patient care.

(5) The assessment is accomplished through

(a) Tracing the care delivered to patients: Surveyors "trace" the patient's experience, looking at services provided by various care providers and departments within the organization, including transition of the patients' care between departments.

(b) Verbal and written information provided to TJC

(c) On-site observations and interviews by TJC surveyors

(d) Documents provided by the organization (e.g., policy and procedure manuals, staff training documentation, machine-commissioning documentation, equipment maintenance logs).

b) Accreditation process does not end with the completion of the on-site survey.

(1) During the approximately three years between on-site surveys, TJC requires ongoing self-assessment and corrective actions (less focus on "ramp up" for survey).

(2) Organizations should continually improve systems and operations contributing to maintenance of safe, high-quality patient care environments and improved organizational performance.

(3) A random 5% sample of initially accredited organizations submitting Evidence of Standards Compliance will undergo an unannounced survey (TJC, 2010a).

c) Unannounced surveys

(1) Organizations that have completed their initial survey are re-surveyed on an unannounced basis.

(2) These surveys have been implemented to

(a) Enhance credibility of the accreditation process to ensure that surveyors observe organizational performance under normal circumstances

(b) Reduce unnecessary costs that organizations incur to prepare for survey

(c) Address public concerns that TJC receive an accurate reflection of the quality and safety of care

(d) Help healthcare organizations focus on providing safe, high-quality care at all times.

d) See Table 22 for accreditation decisions terminology.

8. National Patient Safety Goals (TJC, 2010b, 2010c): Purpose is to standardize evidence-based risk-reduction strategies that hospitals

Table 22. Joint Commission Accreditation Decisions

Decision	Definition
Accredited	Organization is in compliance with all applicable standards at the time of the on-site survey or has addressed all survey requirements for improvement in its Evidence of Standards Compliance within 45 or 60 days of posting the Accreditation Survey Findings Report.
Preliminary accreditation	Organization is in satisfactory compliance with a subset of the standards assessed during the first of two on-site survey events conducted under the Early Survey Policy. The preliminary accreditation decision remains in effect until the organization completes the second on-site survey event. (Early Survey Policy is for organizations not actively caring for patients but needing to provide evidence to payers or state/federal regulators of intent to obtain full accreditation.)
Provisional accreditation	This decision results when an organization fails to address all requirements for improvement in its Evidence of Standards Compliance within 45 or 60 days of posting of the Accreditation Survey Findings Report.
Conditional accreditation	This decision indicates that substantial compliance deficiencies exist in an organization. Correction of these deficiencies, which serve as the basis for further consideration of full accreditation, must be demonstrated through preparation and submission of Evidence of Standards Compliance and a follow-up survey.
Preliminary denial of accreditation	An organization receives this decision when there is either (1) an immediate threat to health or safety, (2) failure to resolve requirements from conditional accreditation, or (3) significant noncompliance with TJC standards. The decision is subject to review and appeal and may result in a final decision other than denial of accreditation.
Denial of accreditation	The organization has been denied accreditation. All review and appeal opportunities have been exhausted.

Note. Based on information from Joint Commission, 2010a.

use to reduce patient injury and enable evaluation of their effectiveness (Kirkpatrick, 2003).

a) Hospitals and ambulatory care facilities must comply with patient safety goals that are updated on a yearly basis.

b) Patient safety goals for 2011 (TJC, 2010b, 2010c)

  (1) Improve accuracy of patient identification

  (2) Improve the effectiveness of communication among caregivers (hospital only, not ambulatory care)

  (3) Improve the safety of using medications

  (4) Reduce the risk of healthcare-associated infections

  (5) Accurately and completely reconcile medications across the continuum of care

  (6) The hospital identifies safety risks inherent in its patient population (hospital only)

  (7) *Conduct a preprocedure verification process*

9. Universal protocol for preventing wrong site, wrong procedure, and wrong person surgery (TJC, 2010b, 2010c)

  a) Applies to hospital, critical care hospital, ambulatory care, and office-based surgery programs (applicable to ensure provision of safe RT treatments)

  b) Applies to all invasive procedures, surgical and nonsurgical

  c) Requires active involvement by all staff and the use of effective methods to improve communication among all members of the procedure team. Consistent implementation of a standardized protocol is most effective in achieving safety.

  d) Components of universal protocol

  (1) Conduct preprocedure verification process: Verify correct procedure, for the correct patient, at the correct site.

  (2) Mark the procedure site: Mark site before the procedure is performed per standard protocol and involve the patient when possible.

  (3) Time-out (i.e., the procedure is not started until all questions or concerns are resolved) is performed before the procedure and has the following characteristics.

   (a) Standardized as defined by the organization

   (b) Initiated by a designated member of the team

   (c) Involves the immediate members of the procedure team, including the individual performing the procedure

10. Performance measurement activities (TJC, 2008)

  a) Eight principles with regard to core performance measurement activities intended to guide TJC in the identification, implementation, and use of tools for measuring and improving patient care

  (1) Principles of core performance measurement activities

   (a) TJC performance measurement activities complement ongoing healthcare organization efforts to improve patient care. The goal of measurement is to improve both the quality of patient care and the cost of services.

   (b) Performance measures are identified and organized to address the highest priority measurement needs of specific users and stakeholders. Measures should be built around the Institute of Medicine's six specific aims of improvement of health care to be safe, effective, patient centered, timely, efficient, and equitable.

   (c) Performance measurement activities that are in agreement with TJC mission are useful for quality oversight purposes and facilitate internal quality improvement while meeting the needs of multiple stakeholders, including consumers and payers. Intention includes providing comparative information to assist consumers and purchasers, both public and private, to select among healthcare organizations based on the quality of their services.

(d) Each performance measure used for accreditation complies with TJC evaluation criteria: Targets improvement in populations; is precisely defined and specified; reliable; valid; interpretable; risk adjusted or stratified; data collection effort is assessed; useful in the accreditation process; under provider control; and publicly available. Where possible, measures meet criteria established by the National Quality Forum and are harmonized across settings.

(e) Performance measurement data have to be disseminated in such a way that they reach the intended audience(s), through public and private reporting, and in a format and time frame that meet the target audience's needs. To be useful, data must be disseminated to the intended audience in a timely fashion and be based on rigorous statistical techniques, permitting aggregation at different levels.

(f) The identification of performance measures and the establishment of performance measure requirements are designed to avoid duplication and reduce burden on healthcare organizations. Where possible, data-sharing elements, data element definitions, or the same measures are to be used that satisfy other entity requirements such as those of the Centers for Medicare and Medicaid Services (CMS), the National Quality Forum, the Hospital Quality Alliance, the American Medical Association, and the National Committee for Quality Assurance.

(g) TJC performance measurement requirements do not place undue burden of data collection on accredited organizations. Performance measures should be cost-effective and flexible enough to be relevant for the organization while still balancing the need to achieve comparability of data across organizations. Automation for data collection should be used wherever possible.

(h) TJC, performance measurement systems, and healthcare organizations collaborate to ensure performance measurement data are consistently accurate and complete. The usefulness of data for all parties depends on the quality of the data.

11. TJC-mandated performance improvement requirements (TJC, 2010d)

   a) Commitment to performance improvement is part of TJC's mission.

   b) TJC has adopted an inclusive approach to work with a variety of measure developers and adapt or adopt measures that allow it to participate in national initiatives, such as the Hospital Quality Alliance, and align with initiatives of the National Quality Forum and others.

   c) ORYX® (launched February 1997) (TJC, 2011b)

     (1) Goal: ORYX is an initiative that integrates outcomes and other performance measurement data into the accreditation process to support accredited organizations in their quality improvement efforts.

     (2) In 2002, accredited hospitals started collecting data on standardized or "core" performance measures.

     (3) Since 2004, TJC and CMS have been working together to align measures common to both organizations, called Hospital Quality Measures, which focus on actual care results.

     (4) Measurement alignment benefits hospitals because institutions can collect the same data to satisfy CMS and TJC, thus conserving resources.

   d) National hospital quality measures and other core measure data help to focus the on-site survey process (TJC, 2011a). These data are made publicly available on TJC Quality Check® Web site (www.qualitycheck.org/consumer/searchQCR.aspx).

   e) TJC supports the evolution of information technology infrastructure (i.e., electronic health records), so that performance improvement becomes a natural derivative of the care delivery process (TJC, 2010e).

   f) Related Web sites

     (1) TJC official Web site: www.jointcommission.org

     (2) Joint Commission Resources, for *Perspectives* and other newsletters: www.jcrinc.com

12. Principles of improving organization performance

a) Definition of *quality*: "The degree to which health service for individuals and populations increase the likelihood of desired health outcomes and are consistent with current professional knowledge" (Lohr, 1990, p. 21).

b) Quality management terminology: Although managers ensure the quality of daily operations, they must work toward changing the system to make it better (Juran, 1964).

   (1) Quality assurance: Any systematic process of checking to see whether a product or service being developed is meeting specified requirements (e.g., patient satisfaction surveys, routine equipment checks). "A quality assurance system is said to increase customer confidence and a company's credibility, to improve work processes and efficiency, and to enable a company to better compete with others" (Alexander, 2007, para. 1).

     (a) Productivity requirements

     (b) Labor standards

     (c) National Patient Safety Goals

     (d) CMS includes the requirement for quality care within its mission statement: "To ensure effective, up-to-date health care coverage and to promote quality care for beneficiaries" (CMS, 2010, "CMS' Mission").

   (2) Quality management: "How managers understand, explain, and continuously improve their organizations to allow them to deliver quality and safe patient care, promote quality patient and organizational outcomes, and improve health in their communities" (Kelly, 2007, p. 11).

   (3) Total quality: "A philosophy or an approach to management that can be characterized by its principles, practices, and techniques. The three principles are customer focus, continuous improvement, and teamwork" (Kelly, 2007, p. 10). The customer is anyone who has an expectation about the outcome of a service.

     (a) External: Parties outside the organization, patients, family members

     (b) Internal: Parties within the organization (e.g., pharmacy, radiology, registration)

     (4) Stakeholders: All groups that might be affected by an organization's service, such as insurance companies, employees, and accreditation agencies.

13. Quality improvement: The process of understanding the how and why with the goal to improve a work process or outcome. Also known as *continuous quality improvement* (Kelly, 2007).

  a) Shewhart cycle (also referred to as the Deming Cycle or Plan-Do-Check-Act cycle): A process that is used to help organizations to identify a process that needs to be improved, plan the intervention that will improve the process, implement the intervention, check to see what the outcomes of the intervention were on quality, and then act on the data (Deming, 1982). An example is provided using the NCCN distress screening tool (see Figure 33).

   (1) Plan: Requires an understanding of the process, the proposing of an improvement, and how data will be collected and tested

   (2) Do: Involves performing the test by implementing the action on a small scale

   (3) Check: Involves analyzing the effect of the action being tested

   (4) Act: Means to fully implement the action or reassess the improvement action and perhaps choose another action

  b) Improvement tools fall into four general categories.

   (1) Identifying customers' and stakeholders' expectations: Asking and observing the parties involved (informal/qualitative data)

   (2) Documenting a process (or processes)

     (a) Workflow diagram or simple flowchart: Shows details of a process, including tasks and procedures, alternative paths, decision points, and rework loops (see Figure 34)

     (b) Process flowchart: A simple tool for mapping out the process (see Figure 35)

     (c) Lead-time analysis: The user of this tool physically walks through the process that a document, a specimen, or a piece of equipment or patient would follow (Kelly, 2007, p. 50).

   (3) Diagnosing a problem

     (a) Fishbone diagram (cause and effect): Used to brainstorm pos-

Figure 33. Example of a Process Improvement Using the Shewhart Cycle

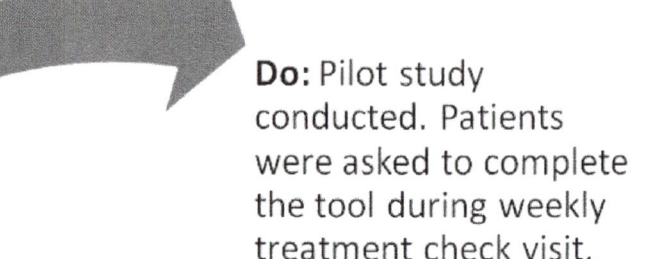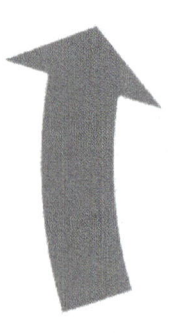

Plan: Implementing the use of the NCCN Distress Screening Tool into practice in an outpatient radiation clinic.

Do: Pilot study conducted. Patients were asked to complete the tool during weekly treatment check visit.

Act: NCCN Distress is given to each patient to complete during the first week of treatment. Nurses were able to identify problems early, leading to patient satisfaction with care.

Check: Nursing staff evaluated effectiveness of weekly assessment and decided that tool was most effective during the first week of treatment.

NCCN—National Comprehensive Cancer Network

Note. Created by Mary Ann Plambeck, RN, MSN, OCN®, Duke University Hospital, Durham, NC. Used with permission.

sible causes of a problem. The problem is written on the far right of the diagram. Categories of causes are represented by the diagonal lines (bones) connected to the horizontal line (spine), which leads to the problem (head) (Kelly, 2007) (see Figure 36).

(b) Check sheet: A simple data collection tool on which one makes hash marks to indicate how often something occurs (Kelly, 2007)

(c) Pareto chart: Used to look for the biggest pieces of a problem or contributors to a cause. A graph displays data in descending order using a bar graph and displays cumulative totals using a line graph when reading from left to right (Kelly, 2007).

(4) Monitoring progress: A run chart graphs data over time. Displaying data enables managers to more readily detect patterns or unusual occurrences in data (Kelly, 2007) (see Figure 37).

14. Six Sigma methodologies focus on the improvement of customer satisfaction, work

Figure 34. Flowchart Legend

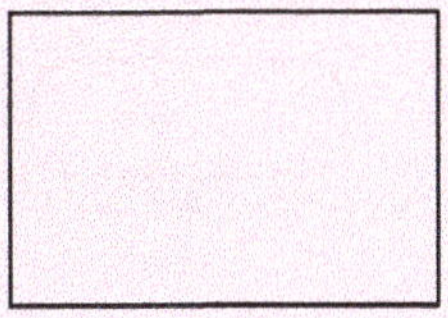

The **Process Symbol** represents any process, function, or action and is the most frequently used symbol in flowcharting.

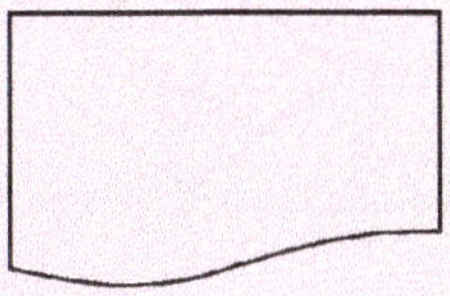

The **Document Symbol** is used to represent any type of hard copy input or output (i.e., reports).

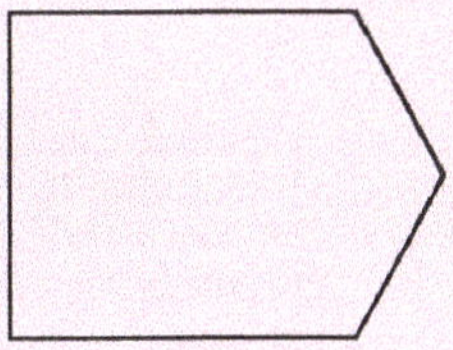

Offpage Connector Symbols are used to indicate the flowchart continues on another page. Often, the page number is placed in the shape for easy reference.

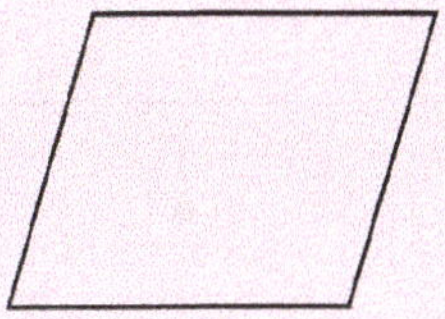

The **Input/Output Symbol** represents data that are available for input or resulting from processing (i.e., customer database records).

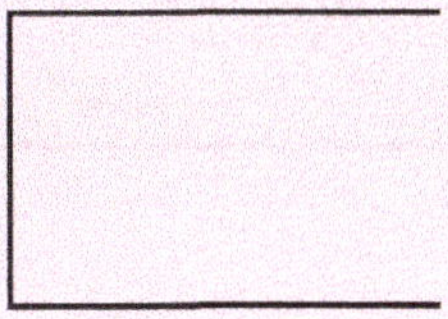

Comment Symbols are used when additional explanation or comment is required. This symbol is usually connected to the symbol it is explaining by a dashed line.

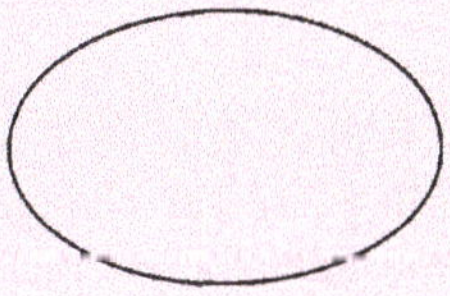

The **Decision Symbol** is a junction where a decision must be made. A single entry may have any number of alternative solutions, but only one can be chosen.

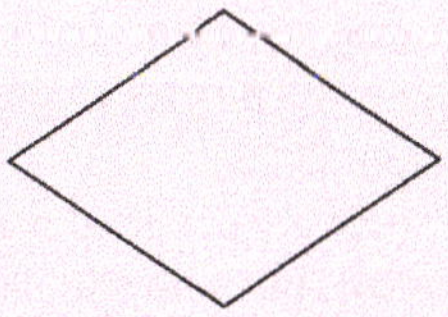

The **Process** start and stop point.

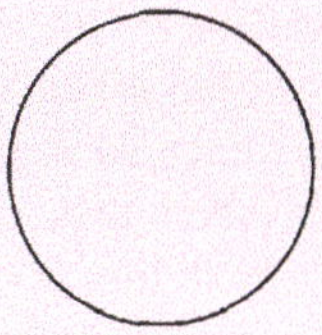

The **Connector Symbol** represents the exit to, or entry from, another part of the same flowchart. It is usually used to break a flow line that will be continued elsewhere. It is a good idea to reference page numbers for easy location of connectors.

Note. Figure courtesy of Steve Power, MBA, CQSE, CQA, Strategic Service Associate, Duke University Hospital, Durham, NC. Used with permission.

Figure 35. Process Flowchart

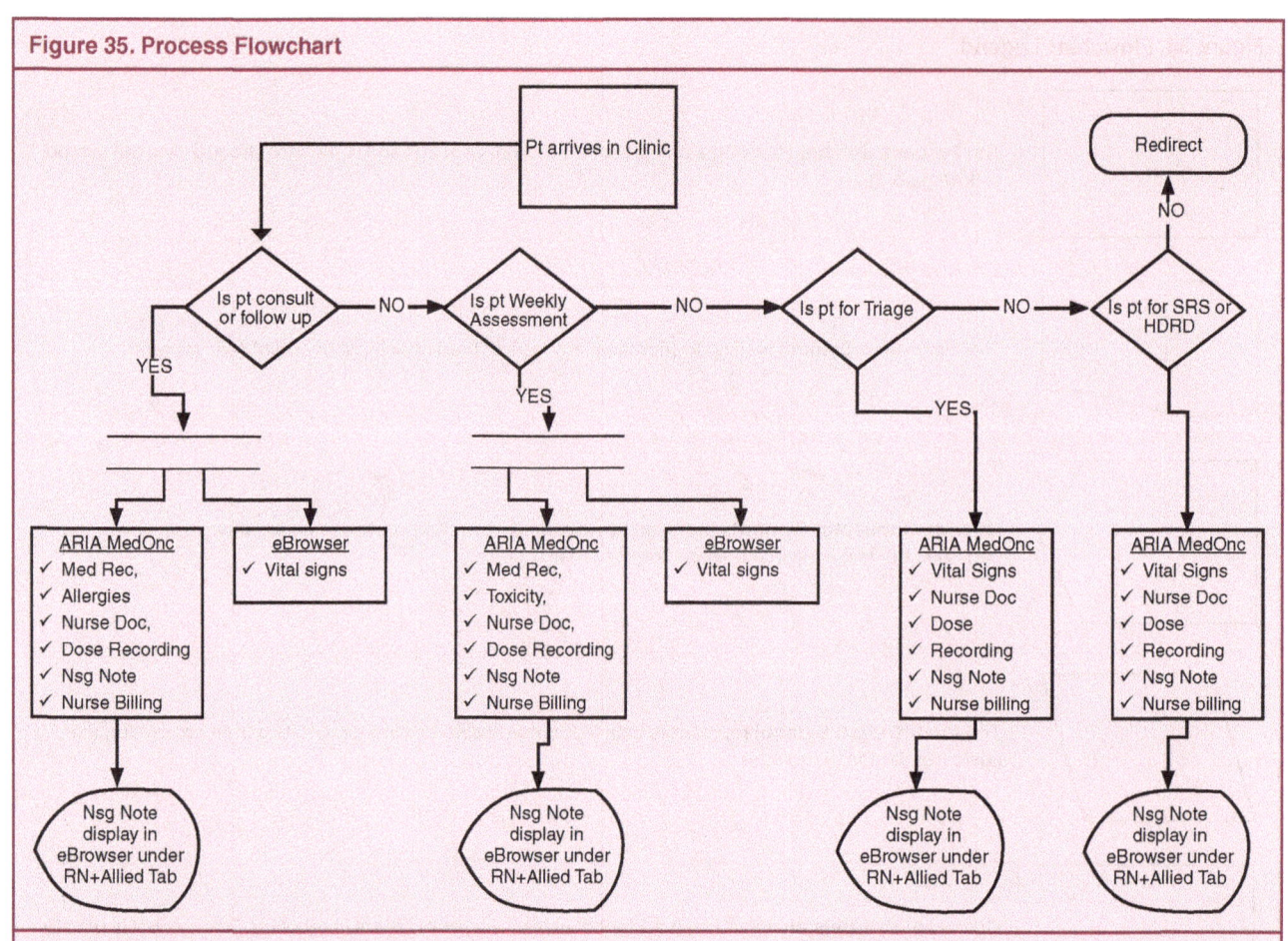

ARIA® MedOnc (Varian Medical Systems, Inc.) is a computer information system; eBrowser is a Web-based tool for patient reports and other clinical information.

HDRD—high-dose radiation; pt—patient; SRS—stereotactic radiosurgery

Note. Figure created by Katherine Becker, RN, MSN, Duke University Hospital, Durham, NC. Used with permission.

processes, profitability, speed, and efficiencies of all kinds (Pande & Holpp, 2002).

a) Six Sigma problem-solving model/ DMAIC model

(1) Define: Define the problem.

(2) Measure: Collect data about the problem.

(3) Analyze: Find the cause of the problem.

(4) Improve: Make changes to eliminate the problem.

(5) Control: Maintain effectiveness of change.

b) Six Sigma management team

(1) Executive leadership: Includes the chief executive officer or other top management responsible for Six Sigma implementation

(2) Champions: Senior leadership with ultimate accountability of the project

(3) Master black belts: Appointed by the champions. They are experts on Six Sigma methodology and often oversee multiple projects.

(4) Black belts: People dedicated full time to tackling critical changes. Primarily responsible for getting the team started, building confidence, observing, managing team dynamics, and keeping the project moving (Pande & Holpp, 2002).

(5) Green belts: These are people trained in Six Sigma skills but who still have a "real" job and serve as either a team member or a part-time Six Sigma leader. The role of the green belt is to bring the new concepts and tools to the day-to-day activities of the business (Pande & Holpp, 2002).

15. Root cause analysis is asking why the problem occurred and then continuing to ask why that happened until identification of the fundamental process element that failed (Kelly, 2007). Root cause analysis helps to reduce repeating the mistakes and frustration, maintain customer satisfaction, and reduce costs significantly. A *root cause*

Figure 36. Fishbone Diagram for Bloodstream Infection Reduction

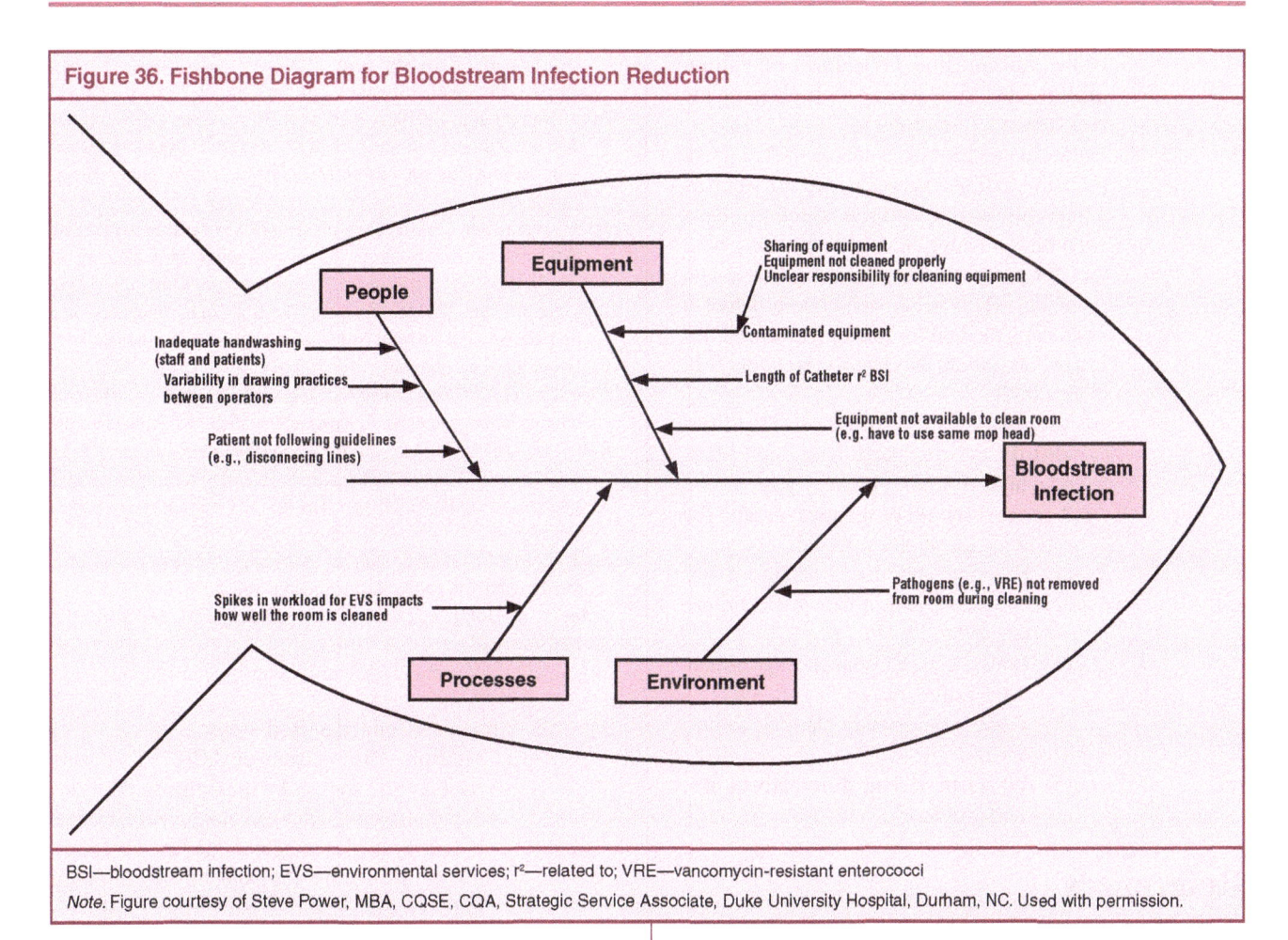

BSI—bloodstream infection; EVS—environmental services; r²—related to; VRE—vancomycin-resistant enterococci

Note. Figure courtesy of Steve Power, MBA, CQSE, CQA, Strategic Service Associate, Duke University Hospital, Durham, NC. Used with permission.

Figure 37. Example of Run Chart Tracking Falls

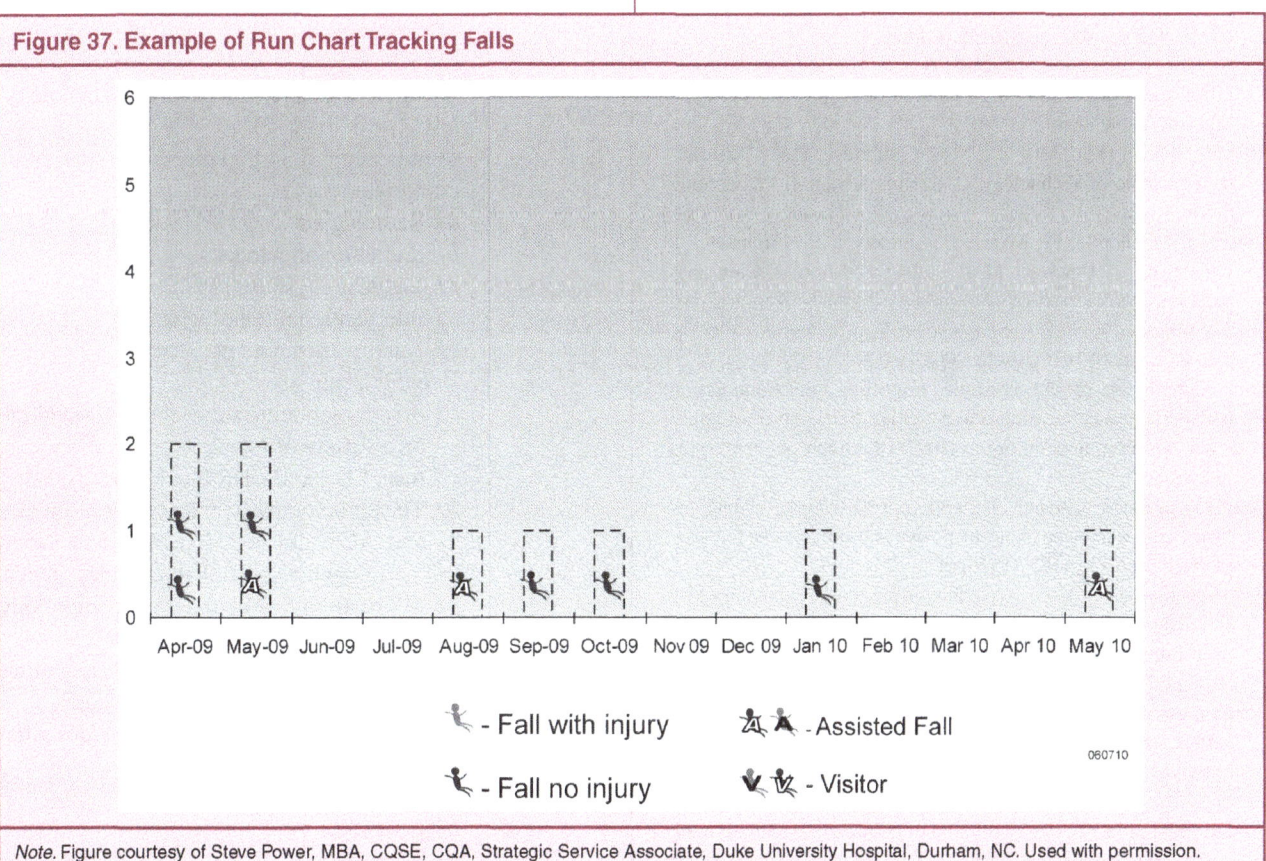

Note. Figure courtesy of Steve Power, MBA, CQSE, CQA, Strategic Service Associate, Duke University Hospital, Durham, NC. Used with permission.

is the fundamental breakdown or failure of a process that, when resolved, prevents recurrence of the problem.

16. Failure modes and effects analysis (FMEA) is a proactive look at what can go wrong, whereas a root cause analysis is a retrospective look at what did go wrong. FMEA is a widely used tool for prospectively evaluating safety and reliability. The FMEA technique provides a systematic method for finding vulnerabilities in a process before they result in an error (Ford et al., 2009).

   a) TJC requires that healthcare facilities identify and conduct at least one FMEA on a high-risk process every year.

   b) A process should be mapped out and the following questions assessed.

      (1) How frequently does the failure occur?

      (2) How easy is it to detect if a failure occurs?

      (3) What are the consequences or effects if the failure occurs?

      (4) What is the backup plan if a failure occurs?

      (5) What can be done differently to prevent a failure?

References

Alexander, J. (2007, February). Definition: Quality assurance (QA). Retrieved from http://searchsoftwarequality.techtarget.com/sDefinition/0,,sid92_gci816126,00.html

Centers for Medicare and Medicaid Services. (2010, June). Mission, vision and goals: Overview. Retrieved from http://www.cms.gov/MissionVisionGoals

Deming, W.E. (1982). *Out of the crisis.* Cambridge, MA: Massachusetts Institute of Technology, Center for Advanced Engineering Study.

Ford, E.C., Gaudette, R., Myers, L., Vanderver, B., Engineer, L., Zellars, R., ... Deweese, T.L. (2009). Evaluation of safety in a radiation oncology setting using failure mode and effects analysis. *International Journal of Radiation Oncology, Biology, Physics, 74,* 852–858. doi:10.1016/j.ijrobp.2008.10.038

Joint Commission. (2008). Principles respecting Joint Commission core performance measurement activities. Retrieved from http://www.jointcommission.org/assets/1/18/Attach_A_Principles_Review.pdf

Joint Commission. (2010a). *Accreditation handbook for ambulatory care.* Retrieved from http://www.jointcommission.org/assets/1/18/2011_AHC_Hdbk.pdf

Joint Commission. (2010b). Accreditation program: Ambulatory care national patient safety goals. Effective January 1, 2011. Retrieved from http://www.jointcommission.org/assets/1/6/2011_NPSGs_AHC.pdf

Joint Commission. (2010c). Accreditation program: Hospital national patient safety goals. Effective January 1, 2011. Retrieved from http://www.jointcommission.org/assets/1/6/2011_NPSGs_HAP.pdf

Joint Commission. (2010d). Evolution of performance measurement at the Joint Commission 1986–2010: A visioning document (At-tachment B). Retrieved from http://www.jointcommission.org/assets/1/18/SIWG_Prologue_web_version.pdf

Joint Commission. (2010e). 2005 to 2010 measure expansion and data use: Future goals and objectives. Retrieved from http://www.jointcommission.org/assets/1/18/SIWG_Vision_paper_future_goals.pdf

Joint Commission. (2011a). Facts about ORYX performance measurement systems. Retrieved from http://www.jointcommission.org/assets/1/18/ORYX_performance_measurement_systems_1_6_11.pdf

Joint Commission. (2011b). Hospitals: Facts about hospital accreditation. Retrieved from http://www.jointcommission.org/assets/1/18/Hospital_Accreditation_1_31_11.pdf

Juran, J.M. (1964). *Managerial breakthrough: The classic book on improving management performance.* New York, NY: McGraw-Hill.

Kelly, D.L. (2007). *Applying quality management in healthcare: A systems approach* (2nd ed.). Chicago, IL: Health Administration Press.

Kirkpatrick, C. (2003). Safety first: The JCAHO introduces new patient safety goals. *NurseWeek California, 16*(7), 20–22.

Lohr, K.N. (Ed.). (1990). *Medicare: A strategy for quality assurance.* Washington, DC: National Academies Press.

Pande, P., & Holpp, L. (2002). *What is Six Sigma?* New York, NY: McGraw-Hill.

B. American College of Radiology

   1. Mission: The mission of ACR "is to serve patients and society by maximizing the value of radiology, radiation oncology, interventional radiology, nuclear medicine, and medical physics by advancing the science of radiology, improving the quality of patient care, positively influencing the socioeconomics of the practice of radiology, providing continuing education for radiology and allied health professions, and conducting research for the future of radiology" (ACR, n.d., para. 2).

   2. Membership of 34,000 members (ACR, n.d.) comprising

      a) Radiologists

      b) Radiation oncologists

      c) Medical physicists

      d) Interventional radiologists

      e) Nuclear medicine physicians.

   3. Benefits to nurses

      a) Practice guidelines and technical standards on a variety of topics (e.g., use of IV contrast, LDR and HDR brachytherapy, SRS).

      b) The Radiological Society of North America and ACR developed a Web site (www.radiologyinfo.org) that provides patient information about diagnostic radiology, interventional radiology, and RT.

      c) Site provides a list of ACR-accredited facilities by modality and ZIP code.

   4. ACR's Web site (www.acr.org) provides information in the following areas.

      a) Accreditation

      b) Education

      c) ACR news

d) Healthcare headlines
e) Economics and health policy
f) Quality and safety resources
g) Government relations
h) Legal/business practices
i) Clinical research
j) Publications and products
k) Patient information

l) Meetings
m) Radiation oncology practice

Reference

American College of Radiology. (n.d.). About us. Retrieved from http://www.acr.org/MainMenuCategories/about_us.aspx

XIII. Radiation oncology resources

A. Oncology Nursing Society
  1. Radiation SIG
    a) Background: ONS is a national organization of more than 35,000 RNs and other healthcare professionals dedicated to excellence in patient care, teaching, research, and education in the field of oncology. To support oncology nurses in all subspecialties, ONS introduced a formal structure of SIGs to facilitate networking of members in an identified subspecialty or interest area. The Radiation SIG was established in 1989 and currently has more than 2,000 members.
    b) Mission: The mission of the Radiation SIG is to promote excellence in oncology nursing by improving the quality of nursing care delivered to patients receiving radiation treatment through research, education, leadership, and collaboration.
    c) Leadership team
      (1) Coordinator: This is an elected position and a four-year commitment. A team member is coordinator-elect for one year, coordinator for two years, and ex-officio for one year. The coordinator is responsible for preparing for an annual meeting at ONS Congress every year and supports the activities and projects of the SIG. The coordinator also attends the ONS leadership meeting held annually in July.
      (2) Editor(s) for newsletter: This is a volunteer position and does not have a time frame for commitment. The editor is responsible for producing a high-quality educational newsletter and updating information about SIG activities. The newsletter is produced three times per year and includes updates from the coordinator, educational articles, and other items of interest to the SIG. The newsletter is titled *The Boost*.
      (3) Webmaster(s) for Virtual Community and the SIG's page on Facebook: This is a volunteer position and does not have a time frame for commitment. The webmaster is responsible for updating and supervising the activity of the Radiation SIG Virtual Community and the group's page on Facebook.
      (4) Educational liaison: This is a volunteer position and does not have a time frame for commitment. The educational liaison is responsible for encouraging participation and presentation of radiation oncology nursing topics at local and national meetings. The liaison encourages publications in books, journals, and newsletters on current topics of interest in radiation oncology.
      (5) Historian: This is a volunteer position and does not have a time frame for commitment. The historian is responsible for maintaining records of national recognition of members, presentations at ONS meetings, and presenting and maintaining an informative poster for the annual ONS Congress.
      (6) ASTRO liaison: This is a volunteer position and does not have a time frame for commitment. The liaison is a member of the Radiation SIG and the ASTRO Nursing Committee. The liaison is responsible for encouraging joint sessions between the organizations to promote radiation oncology excellence.
    d) Goals: The goals of the Radiation SIG support the advocacy, knowledge, and partnership goals supported by ONS. Goals are updated and approved by ONS yearly.
      (1) Advocacy—Educate radiation oncology nurses about evidence-based principles and practice to enhance their nursing role when delivering care to patients receiving RT.
      (2) Knowledge—Update and develop educational resources for nurses working in a radiation oncology setting or working with patients receiving RT.
      (3) Partnership—Encourage nursing activities with other nursing organizations and encourage networking through the Virtual Community and the SIG's page on Facebook.
    e) Membership benefits to nurses: The SIG meets once per year during the ONS Con-

gress. The purpose of the meeting is to update members on SIG activities, present an educational topic, and encourage networking.

    (1) Newsletter (*The Boost*)—Published three times per year. Features a message from a SIG leader, relevant clinical practice articles, and reports of SIG activities.

    (2) Virtual Community and page on Facebook—Always available as means to communicate with other SIG members and stay updated with SIG activities.

    (3) ONS Excellence in Radiation Therapy Award—Presented once a year to a radiation nurse who demonstrates outstanding nursing excellence in the practice of radiation oncology nursing. This is a nominated award. The winner receives $1,000 and a plaque from ONS. The award is presented at the annual SIG meeting.

    (4) Authorship is encouraged through contributions to the SIG newsletter.

    (5) Participation in radiation oncology nursing mentorship programs is encouraged.

2. Web site resources

  a) ONS Radiation Therapy Clinical Resource Area: www.ons.org/ClinicalResources/Treatment/Radiation

    (1) The ONS Web site (www.ons.org) is the official site of ONS, a professional oncology association with membership of more than 35,000 RNs and other healthcare providers.

    (2) The ONS Clinical Resource Area is a gateway to information on radiation oncology.

  b) Excellence in Radiation Therapy Nursing Award: www.ons.org/Awards/ONSAwards/RadiationTherapy

    (1) The purpose of the award is to recognize and support excellence in RT nursing. One award winner each year (as long as funding availability continues) receives $1,000 and a plaque.

    (2) Additional information along with application information can be found at this site.

  c) ONS journals with peer-reviewed articles on RT

    (1) *Clinical Journal of Oncology Nursing*: www.ons.org/Publications/CJON

    (2) *Oncology Nursing Forum*: www.ons.org/Publications/ONF

  d) ONS Radiation SIG (see XIII.A.1): www.radiation.vc.ons.org

B. Additional online radiation resources

1. Web sites

  a) ACR (professionals)

    (1) www.acr.org

    (2) ACR's mission is to serve patients and society by maximizing the value of radiology, radiation oncology, interventional radiology, nuclear medicine, and medical physics by advancing the science of radiology, improving the quality of patient care, positively influencing the socioeconomics of the practice of radiology, providing continuing education for radiology and allied health professions, and conducting research for the future of radiology.

    (3) Radiation oncology practice guidelines and technical standards available at www.acr.org/SecondaryMainMenu Categories/quality_safety/guidelines/ro.aspx

  b) ACS (patients)

    (1) www.cancer.org/Treatment/Treatments and Side Effects/Treatment Types/Radiation/index

    (2) ACS is the nationwide, community-based, voluntary health organization dedicated to eliminating cancer as a major health problem by preventing cancer, saving lives, and diminishing suffering from cancer, through research, education, advocacy, and service. ACS provides patient and family guides on RT.

  c) American Brachytherapy Society (professionals)

    (1) www.americanbrachytherapy.org

    (2) The American Brachytherapy Society is a nonprofit organization that seeks to provide insight and research into the use of brachytherapy in malignant and benign conditions.

  d) American College of Radiation Oncology (professionals)

    (1) www.acro.org

    (2) The American College of Radiation Oncology strives to ensure the highest quality care for patients receiving RT and promote success in the practice of radiation oncology through education, responsible socioeconomic advocacy, and integration of science and technology into clinical practice.

  e) American Society of Radiologic Technologists (professionals)

    (1) www.asrt.org

(2) The American Society of Radiologic Technologists aims to advance the medical imaging and RT profession and enhance the quality of patient care through education, advocacy, and research.

f) ASTRO (professionals)

  (1) www.astro.org

  (2) ASTRO's mission is to advance the practice of radiation oncology by promoting excellence in patient care, providing opportunities for educational and professional development, promoting research, and disseminating research results.

g) Cancer.Net (patients)

  (1) www.cancer.net

  (2) Cancer.Net, the patient education site from ASCO, provides information to help patients and families make informed healthcare decisions. Site provides radiation resources.

h) European Society for Therapeutic Radiology and Oncology (ESTRO) (professionals and patients)

  (1) www.estro-ric.org/GeneralInformation/Pages/default.aspx

  (2) The ESTRO Radiotherapy Information Centre provides easily accessible, up-to-date information about radiation oncology and the benefits of treatment.

i) MedlinePlus: Radiation Therapy (patients)

  (1) www.nlm.nih.gov/medlineplus/radiationtherapy.html

  (2) MedlinePlus brings together authoritative information from the National Library of Medicine, the National Institutes of Health, and other government agencies and health related organizations.

j) NCI (professionals and patients)

  (1) www.cancer.gov/cancertopics/treatment/types-of-treatment

  (2) RT resources from NCI, including fact sheets in English and Spanish, a booklet for providers, and audio CDs for patients

k) Radiological Society of North America (professionals)

  (1) www.rsna.org

  (2) The mission of the Radiological Society of North America is to promote and develop the highest standards of radiology and related sciences through education and research. The organization seeks to provide radiologists and allied health scientists with educational programs and materials and to constantly improve the content and value of these educational activities. It seeks to promote research in all aspects of radiology and related sciences, including basic clinical research in the promotion of quality health care.

l) RadiologyInfo.org (patients)

  (1) www.radiologyinfo.org

  (2) RadiologyInfo is the public information Web site developed and funded by ACR and the Radiological Society of North America. It was established to inform and educate the public about radiologic procedures and the role of radiologists in health care.

m) RT Answers (patients)

  (1) www.rtanswers.org

  (2) ASTRO created this Web site to explain to patients, their families, and the public how RT is used to treat cancer.

n) RTOG (professionals)

  (1) www.rtog.org

  (2) RTOG is a key clinical research component of ACR and serves as a multi-institutional, international clinical cooperative group funded primarily by NCI.

o) Society for Radiation Oncology Administrators (professionals)

  (1) www.sroa.org

  (2) The Society for Radiation Oncology Administrators is committed to providing education, advocacy, and information to radiation oncology administrators.

2. Mobile applications

a) PEPID Medical Information Resources: Oncology Nursing Suite

  (1) www.pepid.com

  (2) PEPID provides continuously updated independent clinical content and mobile medical tools through its PDA applications. The Oncology Nursing Suite was developed in collaboration with ONS.

  (3) Available for iPhone, iPod Touch, iPad, BlackBerry, Web OS, Android, Mobile Wireless, Internet, Palm OS, and Windows Mobile

b) MedPage Today Mobile

  (1) www.medpagetoday.com

  (2) MedPage Today Mobile was codeveloped by MedPage Today and the University of Pennsylvania School of Medicine, Office of Continuing Medical Education. Each article alerts cli-

nicians to breaking medical news with summaries and actionable information enabling them to better understand the implications. News can be set to hematology/oncology. Meeting coverage from oncology meetings, including ASTRO, is available.

    (3) Available for iPhone, Android, and BlackBerry

  c) ACR Appropriateness Criteria®

    (1) www.acr.org/SecondaryMainMenu Categories/ACRStore/Featured Categories/QualityandSafety/ac_pda .aspx

    (2) The ACR Appropriateness Criteria Anytime, Anywhere™ application provides clinicians with instant point-of-care access to evidence-based clinical guidance for imaging decisions. This application features imaging decision support from ACR for more than 160 clinical topics, including radiation oncology.

    (3) Available for iPhone, iPod Touch, iPad, BlackBerry, and Palm

  d) Epocrates®

    (1) www.epocrates.com

    (2) Epocrates develops clinical information and decision support tools that enable healthcare professionals to find answers quickly and confidently at the point of care, especially related to medications.

    (3) Available for iPhone, iPod Touch, BlackBerry, Android, Palm, and Windows Mobile

C. American Society for Radiation Oncology

  1. History and purpose

    a) ASTRO (www.astro.org) was founded in November 1958 as the American Club of Therapeutic Radiologists by 58 radiation oncologists who were looking for their own specialty representation. In 1966, the membership changed the name to the American Society for Therapeutic Radiology and Oncology and created additional membership categories of corresponding and associate members. Another name change took place in 2009 to the American Society for Radiation Oncology (though the organization still uses the "ASTRO" acronym).

  b) ASTRO is the largest radiation oncology society in the world with more than 10,000 members who specialize in treating patients with radiation therapies representing the United States, Canada, and many countries worldwide.

    (1) Consists of radiation oncologists and affiliated staff and organizations within the field of radiation oncology such as nurses, medical physicists, dosimetrists, radiation therapists, biologists, and administrators. Five percent of members are RN, BSN, and/or OCN® certified (see www.astro.org/ Membership/MembershipInfo/ MembershipOverview).

    (2) Dedicated to improving patient care through education, clinical practice, advancement of science, and advocacy

      (a) Committed to continued excellence in patient care through a team-based treatment approach

      (b) Committed to helping the individual members of the treatment team grow within their profession

    (3) ASTRO focuses on fostering collaboration between radiation oncologists and the larger medical community and working together with medical oncologists, surgeons, urologists, gynecologists, internists, family practitioners, and other healthcare professionals to ensure that patients are offered the most up-to-date treatments available.

    (4) ASTRO works with the media to promote accurate articles on scientific breakthroughs involving RT.

    (5) ASTRO works with patient advocacy organizations to publish educational materials that keep patients and the public informed about RT as a safe and effective treatment option.

  2. Mission (www.astro.org/AboutUs/index.aspx)

    a) Advance the practice of radiation oncology by promoting excellence in patient care

    b) Provide opportunities for educational and professional development

    c) Promote research and disseminate research results

d) Represent radiation oncology in a rapidly evolving healthcare environment

3. ASTRO membership benefits

  a) Educational and professional development opportunities such as hands-on educational courses and annual meeting and other regional conferences

  b) Sponsorship of the premier radiation oncology research journal, *International Journal of Radiation Oncology, Biology, Physics*, also referred to as the Red Journal, and *Practical Radiation Oncology*, a journal that offers practical advice on treatments for radiation oncologists

4. Web site: www.astro.org

  (1) Provides specific information on all educational opportunities, including the annual meeting and other regional conferences

  (2) Provides information on radiation oncology equipment through the RO Marketplace

  (3) Access to ASTRO online membership

  (4) Wide variety of information including

    (a) Standards of care/consensus statements

    (b) Government relations, including current legislation and key bills in Congress

    (c) Health policy

    (d) Research

    (e) Publications

    (f) Coding and reimbursement

    (g) Patient advocacy groups and other professional organizations

    (h) Employment opportunities

    (i) ASTRO School of Radiation Oncology provides self-assessment modules, journal continuing medical education, virtual webinars, and more to continue education.

    (j) Association of Residents in Radiation Oncology provides students, residents, and other members with useful resources, information, and links.

  (5) ASTRO resources

    (a) Patient educational brochures created by ASTRO and RT Answers Web site

    (b) Patient- and family-focused educational Web site developed by ASTRO

    (c) *ASTROnews* and *ASTROgram* quarterly ASTRO professional publications

    (d) Links to other organizations such as ONS and Patient Advocate Foundation

    (e) Online updates and notification of educational opportunities related to radiation oncology

    (f) Discounts on registration at the annual meeting and other ASTRO-sponsored conferences

    (g) Discount on a subscription to the *International Journal of Radiation Oncology, Biology, Physics* and *Practical Radiation Oncology*

    (h) Online ASTRO membership directory

5. Nursing Committee: ASTRO Radiation Oncology Nurses (ARON)

  a) History

    (1) Formed in 1998

    (2) Consists of a group of radiation oncology nurses who are associate members of ASTRO

    (3) Led by the chair of the Nursing Committee

  b) Mission

    (1) Promote excellence in patient care

    (2) Advance the practice of radiation oncology nursing

  c) Strategic plan and goals of the ARON Committee

    (1) Focus on the needs of the nurse membership through education and support

    (2) Continue to increase nurse membership

    (3) Continue the development of ASTRO's patient education brochures

    (4) Marketing of ARON

    (5) Provide educational opportunities by presenting at ASTRO's annual meeting through educational sessions, panels, and scientific sessions

    (6) Maintain liaison/relationship with ONS and other professional organizations

    (7) Advocate for radiation oncology nurses through a Web site, networking, and supporting the role of radiation oncology nurse through education and resources

  d) Structure of Nursing Committee

    (1) Under the Education Council of the ASTRO Board of Directors

    (2) Nursing Committee membership

      (a) Eight radiation oncology nurses (RNs, APRNs)

      (b) One ASTRO board liaison and one ASTRO staff liaison

      (c) Committee members are employed at different facilities from all regions of the country and hold a wide variety of job titles and responsibilities.

      (d) Committee is directed by a chair who serves for two years. For the second year of the chair's term, a current committee member who has served at least two years is selected to become the vice chair. The vice chair supports the chair and learns the responsibilities of the role. After one year of service, the vice chair becomes the chair.

(3) Criteria for ARON Nursing Committee membership

      (a) Minimum of three years of experience in radiation oncology

      (b) Bachelor's degree in nursing or health-related field preferred

      (c) Leadership experience within work role or professional organization

      (d) Application: Submit curriculum vitae including leadership experience to ASTRO nursing liaison.

(4) Terms of committee membership: The term of board members is one year and is renewable up to five times. Responsibilities of nursing committee members include

      (a) Participate in monthly conference calls

      (b) Attend the annual meeting

      (c) Participate in one additional ASTRO-designated committee, activity, or project such as workforce, publications, educational council, or ONS liaison

      (d) Participate in planning the nursing-related educational sessions.

(5) ARON membership benefits

      (a) Opportunity to network with nurses and other radiation oncology professionals

      (b) ASTRO Web site (www.astro.org) can be linked to "The Nurses Corner," which provides information on the following.

        i. Educational opportunities

        ii. ASTRO nursing awards

        iii. ASTRO membership information

      (c) ASTRO resources as above

      (d) ASTRO Nurse Excellence Award

        i. Developed in 2008

        ii. Nominee must be currently licensed and employed as an RN.

        iii. The nominee must be an ASTRO member.

        iv. The Nursing Excellence Award is awarded to an RN who goes above and beyond the normal standards of nursing practice.

        v. This individual consistently portrays a positive image in the field of nursing within ASTRO, the individual's institution, and the community.

        vi. The award winner will demonstrate excellence in direct patient care delivered in a hospital or clinic setting.

      (e) Nurses Annual Meeting Abstract Award: Awarded to nurses who have conducted clinical research or presented at the annual meeting. Designed to recognize nurses for their achievements and outstanding service. Recipients must be the first author or coauthor and endorsed by their department chair. Up to two are awarded annually. Application can be submitted through abstract submission site.

6. Survivor Circle

    a) Created in 2003 to honor cancer survivors

    b) Features two local patient support organizations from the locale of the annual meeting

    c) Raises funds for the two organizations featured

7. ASTRO's Target Safely Plan (www.astro.org/targetsafely)

    a) Plan established in 2010 to enhance patient safety

    b) Six points

      (1) Work to create a national database for the reporting of medical errors

      (2) Advocate for new and expanded federal initiatives to help protect patients from radiation errors, and support the immediate passage of the Consistency, Accuracy, Responsibility, and Excellence in Medical Imaging and Radiation Therapy ("CARE") Act, which among other things requires national standards for RT treatment team members

      (3) Work with cancer support organizations to help patients with cancer and their families know what to ask their doctors when radiation is a possible treatment option

(4) Enhance the radiation oncology practice accreditation program and develop additional accreditation classes specifically addressing new technologies

(5) Expand educational training programs to include an intensive focus on quality assurance and safety

(6) Accelerate ongoing effort that seeks to ensure that device manufacturers can transfer treatment information from one machine to another seamlessly to reduce the chance of a medical error

8. Patient education site (www.rtanswers.org)
   a) Information booklets to explain how RT works to cure cancer are available.
   b) Radiation resources for patients in different parts of the United States are also available.
   c) Web site has a link for patients to find a radiation oncologist locally.

D. National Comprehensive Cancer Network
   1. NCCN (www.nccn.org) is a nonprofit alliance of 21 leading cancer centers worldwide dedicated to improving the quality and effectiveness of the cancer treatment trajectory for patients and families. This includes identifying appropriate diagnostic mechanisms, treatment guidelines, research protocols, and helping individuals adjust to life with a cancer diagnosis.
   2. NCCN publications, guidelines, and clinical resources
      a) NCCN Clinical Practice Guidelines in Oncology
      b) NCCN Drugs and Biologics Compendium
      c) NCCN Chemotherapy Ordering Templates
   3. NCCN educational events/programs and webinars
      a) Annual conference and clinical practice guidelines
      b) NCCN conferences related to disease-specific cancer guidelines
   4. NCCN research and business resources
      a) NCCN Oncology Research Program
      b) Reimbursement resources
      c) NCCN Best Practices—Practice standards by which all clinical care should be based
   5. Patient resources
      a) Treatment summaries
      b) Treatment decisions
      c) Living with cancer
      d) Paying for treatment
      e) Survivorship
   6. NCCN radiation oncology specific
      a) Clinical practice guidelines are multimodality focused.
      b) Guidelines include surgical, medical, and radiation treatment.
      c) Clinical practice oncology guidelines include site specific and symptom specific.
      d) Outcomes database
         (1) Measures adherence to NCCN Guidelines®
         (2) Clinical outcomes
      e) Resources
         (1) Institutional protocols
         (2) Treatment guidelines

E. National Cancer Institute
   1. NCI, established under the National Cancer Act of 1971, is a division of the National Institutes of Health, which is one of 11 agencies that compose the U.S. Department of Health and Human Services. NCI, a federal government agency, conducts cancer research and training (see www.cancer.gov).
   2. As the coordinator of the National Cancer Program, NCI conducts and supports extensive research, training, and the dissemination of a broad base of information related to cancer prevention, diagnosis, treatment, and rehabilitation.
      a) NCI cancer information for patients and healthcare professionals
         (1) Types of cancer: PDQ® (Physician Data Query, see www.cancer.gov/cancertopics/pdq) is NCI's comprehensive cancer database for patients and professionals. Focus is site-specific cancer information and multimodality treatment regimens.
         (2) Clinical trials (see http://clinicaltrials.gov)
            (a) Find a trial
            (b) View results
            (c) Review educational materials
            (d) Major NCI-supported trials
            (e) Conducting clinical trials
         (3) Specific topics
            (a) Treatment
            (b) Prevention
            (c) Genetics
            (d) Screening
      b) Cancer statistics
         (1) Interpreting statistical findings of site specific cancer diagnoses
         (2) Annual national report
         (3) Statistical tools and data/population-based statistics
         (4) Surveillance, Epidemiology, and End Results, or SEER, Data Cancer Statistics Review including incidence, mor-

tality, survival, prevalence, and lifetime risk (see http://seer.cancer.gov)

(5) Funding for biostatistics

c) Cancer research funding: Research priorities/resources/partnering with NCI

(1) Translational Research Working Group
(2) Center for Strategic Science Initiatives
(3) Office of Advocacy Relations
(4) NCI Small Business Initiative

d) Radiation-specific clinical information

(1) Extensive publications for professionals and patients
(2) Specific publication topics include general overview of EBRT as a cancer treatment modality, site-specific treatment and side effect profiles, brachytherapy, proton therapy, and audio files focusing on the trajectory of radiation treatment.
(3) NCI highlights focus on recent development of RT protocols.
(4) Multimodality clinical trials focus on the use of RT as an integral part of cancer treatment delivery.
(5) NCI supports research of RT-based protocols and offers an extensive array of clinical trials and treatment guidelines focusing on RT as primary treatment modality.

Index

The letter f *after a page number indicates that relevant content appears in a figure; the letter* t, *in a table.*